D0142231

The Female Pelvic Floor:

Disorders of Function and Support

The Female Pelvic Floor:

Disorders of Function and Support

Edited by

Linda T. Brubaker, M.D.

Associate Professor of Obstetrics and Gynecology
Rush Medical College
Head, Section of Urogynecology
Rush-Presbyterian-St. Luke's Medical Center
Chicago, Illinois

Theodore J. Saclarides, M.D.

Associate Professor of Surgery
Head, Section of Colon and Rectal Surgery
Rush Medical College
Rush-Presbyterian-St. Luke's Medical Center
Chicago, Illinois

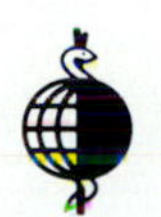

F. A. DAVIS COMPANY • Philadelphia

F. A. Davis Company
1915 Arch Street
Philadelphia, PA 19103

Printed in the United States of America

Last digit indicates print number: 10 9 8 7 6 5 4 3 2 1

Medical Editor: Robert W. Reinhardt
Medical Developmental Editor: Bernice M. Wissler
Production Editor: Glenn L. Fechner
Cover Designer: Louis J. Forgione

As new scientific information becomes available through basic and clinical research, recommended treatments and drug therapies undergo changes. The authors and publisher have done everything possible to make this book accurate, up to date, and in accord with accepted standards at the time of publication. The authors, editors, and publisher are not responsible for errors or omissions or for consequences from application of the book, and make no warranty, expressed or implied, in regard to the contents of the book. Any practice described in this book should be applied by the reader in accordance with professional standards of care used in regard to the unique circumstances that may apply in each situation. The reader is advised always to check product information (package inserts) for changes and new information regarding dose and contraindications before administering any drug. Caution is especially urged when using new or infrequently ordered drugs.

Library of Congress Cataloging-in-Publication Data

The female pelvic floor : disorders of function and support / edited by Linda T. Brubaker, Theodore J. Saclarides.
p. cm.
ISBN (invalid) 0-8036-0075-5
1. Pelvic floor—Pathophysiology. 2. Urogynecology.
I. Brubaker, Linda T., 1955– . II. Saclarides, Theodore J., 1956– .
[DNLM: 1. Pelvic Floor—physiopathology. 2. Urinary Incontinence. 3. Fecal Incontinence. 4. Prolapse. WP 155-F329 1996]
RG482.F447 1996
618.1—dc20
DNLM/DLC
for Library of Congress

96-2454
CIP

This work is dedicated to my family—wonderful parents, supportive and loving spouse, and marvelous children.

Linda T. Brubaker

I thank my teachers, for sharing their knowledge with me over the last two decades; Elena and the kids, for their understanding and patience; and Steven G. Economou, for his tutelage. Lastly, I am forever indebted to my parents, Deno and Evelyn; it is on their shoulders I stand.

Theodore J Saclarides

Foreword

Progress in medicine can take a number of routes: a brilliant flash of insight in the solution of a seemingly insoluble problem; an incremental growth and application of known and tested principles; a sudden, almost exponential coalescing and understanding of a number of separate pieces of knowledge—both old or just recently acquired—along with the availability of innovative technology into the solution of some long vexing questions. Such is the case of two young, gifted surgeons—one a urogynecologist and the other a specialist in diseases of the colon and rectum—who find themselves in the sorely needed position of leadership in an important field of medicine by editing their insightful and all-inclusive book, *The Female Pelvic Floor: Disorders of Function and Support.*

Abnormalities of the pelvis in women, especially those of advancing age, have been afflicting millions over the years, yet attention was not focused on them until the turn of the century. There it languished until about a generation ago, when serious attempts at seeking both cause and cure were made. Unfortunately, in keeping with a time of emerging surgical specialties, the problems seen in these women (as was also true in other areas of medicine) were addressed in a fractionated fashion: most were treated by gynecologists, whose clinical mainstay was obstetrics and some traditional surgery; some were treated by urologists, where it was natural and easy to pay the most attention to the complaint of urinary dribbling and how to correct it mechanically; still others were treated by general surgeons, whose therapeutic attention most often concentrated on perineal procedures. The pessary, of course, was used by everyone and by some practitioners as the only therapy. It is not surprising, then, that the multifaceted problem of pelvic disorders in women was treated by physicians who often were highly talented but who were disparate in their training, views, and practices. This led to results that have been so variable that they have baffled the surgeon and dismayed the patient.

For all of the above reasons, plus the sad fact that most pelvic disorders, however variable their presentation, have as a component the involuntary loss of urine, a problem that produces a deep concern in most patients and a self-imposed stigma in others, this is the last major "closet" disease. Important winners in all this have been the manufacturers of absorbent underwear, whose mellifluous pitchwomen have developed a significant lexicon of synonyms for diapers.

It is gratifying to realize, finally, that insight into the cause and necessary treatment of disorders of the pelvis in women appears to be in a modern-day renaissance. Drs. Linda Brubaker and Theodore Saclarides have presented us with a book whose seminal characteristics are self-evident. First, they recognized the need to assemble varied, broad, but relevant, information. They also realized that, despite their own considerable talents, a successful exposition would be more certain if they mined the rich storehouse of information from their colleagues throughout the nation. And they proceeded to do just that; they easily marshaled a remarkable group of interested and extremely resourceful physicians, whose ready acceptance of the invitation to participate speaks of their recognition of the urgent need for such a book.

The readers are fortunate indeed to have this array of stellar clinicians present their views, which the editors have woven into such a meaningful whole. *The Female Pelvic Floor: Disorders of Function and Support* will and should be read and referred to by those who have a direct interest in or an indirect exposure to this important and burgeoning area of medicine.

Steven G. Economou, M.D.

Preface

Disorders of the female pelvic floor can be complex and challenging to clinicians caring for patients afflicted with these disorders. Many of our colleagues have expressed a desire to have available expertise that complements, documents, and expands their fund of knowledge and opportunities for effective clinical care. These discussions prompted the creation of this text.

At Rush, we have been fortunate to have an interdisciplinary, collegial environment which allows us to provide efficient care for women with pelvic floor disorders. We strongly believe that such an environment is not only mandatory but also has the potential to advance patient care and enhance our scientific insights into the etiology of these disorders. Advances are being made in the fields of urogynecology, colorectal surgery, and reconstructive pelvic surgery, as well as other related fields. The rapidity of these developments is such that it is difficult to capture them in a timely manner for publication of a book of this magnitude. However, we hope that this collection of chapters will serve as an excellent source for pelvic floor clinicians.

It is our desire that our readers gain an appreciation of the extensive overlap between closely related disciplines. Increased awareness of associated clinical disorders and their evaluation and treatment should lead to focused and more informed consultation. It is our ultimate desire that the women who suffer with pelvic floor disorders will receive care from a growing cadre of clinicians whose knowledge is no longer limited by specialty.

LINDA T. BRUBAKER
THEODORE J. SACLARIDES
Rush-Presbyterian-St. Luke's Medical Center
Chicago, Illinois

Acknowledgment

We would like to acknowledge the outstanding secretarial support of Eileen Pehanich, whose attention to detail far surpassed our expectations.

Contributors

W. Allen Addison, M.D.
Professor of Obstetrics and Gynecology
Duke University Medical Center
Durham, North Carolina

William Altringer, M.D.
Mid-Dakota Clinic
Bismarck, North Dakota

Tamara G. Bavendam, M.D.
Assistant Professor of Urology
Director of Female Urology
University of Washington School of Medicine
Seattle, Washington

J. Thomas Benson, M.D.
Visiting Professor of Obstetrics and Gynecology
Rush Medical College
Chicago, Illinois
Clinical Professor of Obstetrics and Gynecology
Indiana University School of Medicine
Associate Director of Obstetrics and Gynecology Education
Methodist Hospital of Indiana
Indianapolis, Indiana

Alfred E. Bent, M.D.
Clinical Associate Professor of Obstetrics and Gynecology
Director, Section of Urogynecology
The Greater Baltimore Medical Center
Baltimore, Maryland

Elisa H. Birnbaum, M.D.
Associate Professor of Surgery
Washington University School of Medicine
Division of Colon and Rectal Surgery
Jewish Hospital of St. Louis
St. Louis, Missouri

Linda T. Brubaker, M.D.
Associate Professor of Obstetrics and Gynecology
Rush Medical College
Head, Section of Urogynecology
Rush-Presbyterian-St. Luke's Medical Center
Chicago, Illinois

Richard C. Bump, M.D.
Associate Professor and Chief
Division of Gynecologic Specialties
Duke University Medical Center
Durham, North Carolina

Geoffrey Cundiff, M.D.
Assistant Professor of Obstetrics and Gynecology
Division of Gynecologic Specialties
Duke University Medical Center
Durham, North Carolina

Daniel J. Deziel, M.D.
Associate Professor of Surgery
Rush Medical College
Rush-Presbyterian-St. Luke's Medical Center
Chicago, Illinois

José M. Dominguez, M.D.
Ferrell-Duncan Clinic
Springfield, Missouri

S. Renee Edwards, M.D.
Assistant Professor of Obstetrics and Gynecology
Rush Medical College
Rush-Presbyterian-St. Luke's Medical Center
Chicago, Illinois

Eugene Eisman, Ph.D.
Center for Bladder and Bowel Dysfunction
University of Illinois Hospital and Clinics
Chicago, Illinois
Clinic for Neurophysiological Learning
Milwaukee, Wisconsin

Dee E. Fenner, M.D.
Assistant Professor of Obstetrics and Gynecology
Rush Medical College
Director, Section of Benign Gynecology
Director, Integrated Residency Program
Department of Obstetrics and Gynecology
Rush-Presbyterian-St. Luke's Medical Center
Chicago, Illinois

James W. Fleshman, M.D.
Assistant Professor of Surgery
Section of Colon and Rectal Surgery
Washington University School of Medicine
St. Louis, Missouri

Michael Heit, M.D.
Instructor of Obstetrics and Gynecology
Director, Section of Urogynecology and Reconstructive Pelvic Surgery
University of Louisville
Louisville, Kentucky

Nicolette S. Horbach, M.D.
Associate Professor of Obstetrics and Gynecology
Director, Division of Gynecology and Urogynecology
George Washington University Medical Center
Washington, DC

Tracy L. Hull, M.D.
Staff Surgeon
Department of Colorectal Surgery
The Cleveland Clinic Foundation
Cleveland, Ohio

W. Glenn Hurt, M.D.
Professor of Obstetrics and Gynecology
Medical College of Virginia
Virginia Commonwealth University
Richmond, Virginia

Rhonda Kotarinos, M.S., P.T.
Women's Therapeutic Services, Ltd.
Rush-Presbyterian-St. Luke's Medical Center
Chicago, Illinois

Sang-Jeon Lee, M.D.
Department of Surgery
Chungbuk National University Hospital
Chungbuk, Korea

Ruth C. McMyn, R.N., M.S., C.E.T.N.
Coordinator, Enterostomal Therapy Nurse Consultation Service
Rush-Presbyterian-St. Luke's Medical Center
Clinical Instructor
Rush University College of Nursing
Chicago, Illinois

Alan P. Meagher, M.D.
St. Vincent's Clinic
Sydney, New South Wales
Australia

Amanda M. Metcalf, M.D.
Associate Professor of Surgery
University of Iowa Hospitals and Clinics
Iowa City, Iowa

Jeffrey W. Milsom, M.D.
Head, Section of Colon and Rectal Surgical Research
Department of Colon and Rectal Surgery
The Cleveland Clinic
Cleveland, Ohio

Peggy A. Norton, M.D.
Associate Professor
Departments of Obstetrics/Gynecology and Urology
University of Utah School of Medicine
Salt Lake City, Utah

John H. Pemberton, M.D.
Associate Professor of Surgery
Mayo Graduate School of Medicine
Rochester, Minnesota

Anita Pillai-Allen, M.D.
Clinical Assistant Professor
University of Hawaii
Obstetrics and Gynecology Residency Program
Straub Clinic and Hospital
Urogynecology and Pelvic Reconstructive Surgery
Honolulu, Hawaii

Sandra Retzky, D.O.
Director of Uro-gynecology
Mercy Hospital
Chicago, Illinois

A. Cullen Richardson, M.D.
Associate Clinical Professor
Emory University
Atlanta, Georgia
Assistant Professor of Surgery
Rush Medical College
Chicago, Illinois

Robert M. Rogers, M.D.
Attending Physician
The Reading Hospital and Medical Center
Reading, Pennsylvania
Assistant Clinical Professor
Department of Obstetrics and Gynecology
The University of Pennsylvania School of Medicine
Philadelphia, Pennsylvania

Theodore J. Saclarides, M.D.
Head, Section of Colon and Rectal Surgery
Associate Professor of Surgery
Rush Medical College
Rush-Presbyterian-St. Luke's Medical Center
Chicago, Illinois

Stephanie L. Schmitt, M.D.
Fellow, Department of Colorectal Surgery
The Cleveland Clinic—Florida
Fort Lauderdale, Florida

Anthony Senagore, M.D.
Associate Professor of Surgery
Michigan State University
East Lansing, Michigan
Director of Surgical Research
Ferguson-Blodgett Digestive Disease Institute
Grand Rapids, Michigan

B.L. Shull, M.D.
Professor and Chief of Gynecology
Department of Obstetrics and Gynecology
Scott and White Memorial Hospital and Clinic
Texas A & M Health Science Center
Temple, Texas

Sheldon Sloan, M.D.
Assistant Professor of Medicine
Rush Medical College
Chicago, Illinois

Claire S. Smith, M.D.
Professor of Radiology
Rush Medical College
Section Director, Gastrointestinal Radiology
Department of Diagnostic Radiology and Nuclear Medicine
Rush-Presbyterian-St. Luke's Medical Center
Chicago, Illinois

Lee E. Smith, M.D.
Professor of Surgery
Director, Division of Colon and Rectal Surgery
George Washington University Medical Center
Washington, DC

Steven J. Stryker, M.D.
Associate Professor of Clinical Surgery
Northwestern University Medical School
Chicago, Illinois

M. Chrystie Timmons, M.D.
Assistant Professor of Obstetrics and Gynecology
Duke University Medical Center
Durham, North Carolina

Jeannette Tries, M.S., O.T.R.
Sacred Heart Rehabilitation Hospital
Milwaukee, Wisconsin
Center for Bladder and Bowel Dysfunction
University of Illinois Hospitals and Clinics
Chicago, Illinois

José M. Velasco, M.D.
Professor of Surgery
Rush Medical College
Chicago, Illinois
Chairman, Department of Surgery
Rush North Shore Medical Center
Skokie, Illinois

Anne L. Viselli, M.D.
Department of Obstetrics and Gynecology
University of Vermont
Burlington, Vermont

Steven D. Wexner, M.D.
Chairman and Residency Program Director
Department of Colorectal Surgery
Vice Chairman, Division of Surgery
The Cleveland Clinic—Florida
Fort Lauderdale, Florida

Contents

SECTION THREE. DIAGNOSTIC ADJUNCTS 59

SECTION FOUR. DISORDERS OF PAIN 125

SECTION ONE

STRUCTURE AND FUNCTION

CHAPTER 1

Anatomy of Female Pelvic Support

Sandra S. Retzky • Robert M. Rogers, Jr.
A. Cullen Richardson

The pelvis encloses organs of storage and evacuation, functions that can be sustained only if normal anatomic relationships are maintained within this cavity. In the normal, nulliparous standing woman, the bladder, the proximal two thirds of the vagina, and the rectum are almost horizontal. The pelvic floor, especially the levator plate, parallels these organs and provides a hammock or dynamic backstop for them. The cervix is found at the level of the ischial spines.[1] In contrast to these horizontal structures, the urethra, the distal one third of the vagina, and the anal canal are almost vertical. These lower structures are supported by the levator hiatus, perineal body, and urogenital and anal triangles. Disruption of these normal anatomic relationships may cause incontinence and prolapse. The soundness of these critical relationships relies on the integrity of the elements that comprise the pelvis: bones and ligaments, muscles, and endopelvic fascia.

BONES AND LIGAMENTS

The pelvic bones are much more than a housing for the pelvic contents. The bony pelvis is the superstructure which surrounds, protects, and supports the soft tissues and pelvic viscera. These fused and articulated bones assist in weight bearing, locomotion, and transmitting pressure from the upper body to the lower extremities.

ILIUM

The ilium has a broad, flat surface called the alar, or wing, portion (Fig. 1–1). On its medial aspect course the muscles that produce hip flexion, primarily the iliacus, iliopsoas, and psoas muscles. The crest of the ilium is its most superior portion and serves as an attachment for the abdominal wall mus-

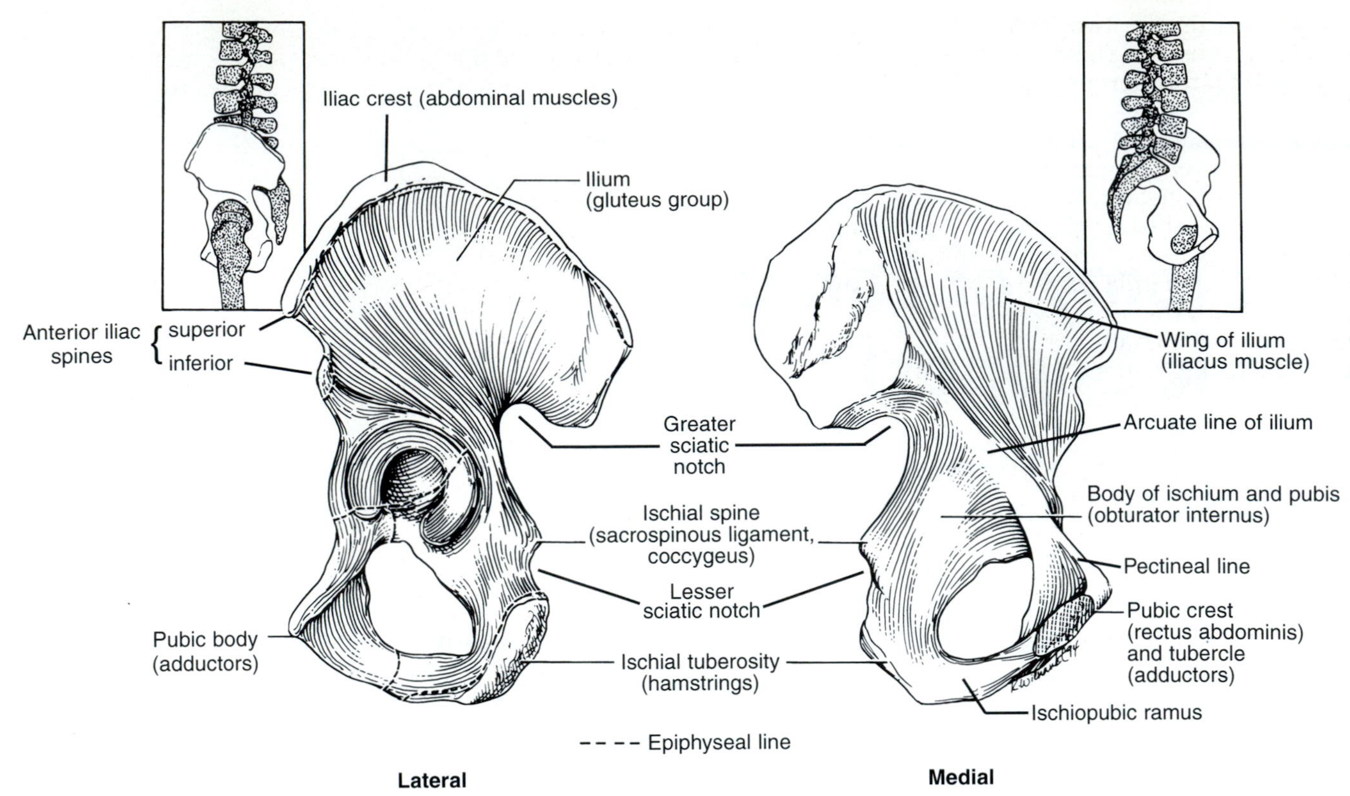

FIGURE 1–1. Medial and lateral views of the hip bones.

cles. Other clinically important bony prominences of the ilium include the anterior superior and inferior iliac spines. The bony ridge at the inferior border of the iliac fossa is called the **arcuate line** or **linea terminalis**, which demarcates the pelvic inlet. On the posterior side of the ilium, the greater sciatic notch forms the superior border of the greater sciatic foramen, through which important structures travel from inside the pelvis to the gluteal region. These include the tendons of the piriformis and gemelli muscles, the sciatic nerve, the posterior femoral cutaneous nerve, and the inferior gluteal and pudendal neurovascular bundles.

PUBIC BONE

The inferior pubic ramus fuses with the ischium to form the ischiopubic ramus. Spanning the gap between the ischiopubic rami is a structure unique to humans, the urogenital diaphragm. The superior pubic ramus has a bony ridge called the pectineal line, which is an important landmark for pelvic surgeons. The pectineal or Cooper's ligament is located on this line. This ridge flows from the **pubic tubercle** into the linea terminalis. Coursing over Cooper's ligament are the accessory obturator vessels, laceration of which may cause significant blood loss, because they connect directly with the inferior epigastric vessels. These obturator vessels traverse the obturator foramen; during retropubic surgery, this landmark should be identified in order to avoid inadvertent laceration.

A number of muscles have their origin on the pubic bone: the rectus abdominis from the crest of the pubis; the adductor muscles of the thigh from the superior and inferior rami of the pubic bone; and part of the levator ani muscle from the inner surface of the pubic bone.

Several important ligaments travel between the ilium and the pubic bone. The inguinal ligament is derived from the external oblique aponeurosis and courses between the anterior superior iliac spine and the pubic tubercle. Underneath the inguinal ligament are two large spaces, the lacuna musculorum and the lacuna vasculorum. They are separated by the iliopubic ligament, which drops from the inguinal ligament to the iliopubic eminence. The lacuna musculorum contains the lateral femoral cutaneous nerve, which innervates the lateral aspect of the thigh; the iliopsoas muscle; and the femoral nerve, which innervates the anterior thigh and leg. The lacuna vasculorum contains the femoral artery, the femoral vein, and, most medial, the deep inguinal lymph nodes; these latter structures are contained within the femoral sheath.

ISCHIUM

The third portion of the hip bone is the V-shaped ischium. In the sitting position, the weight of the body rests on the two ischial tuberosities. The hip extensor muscles (hamstrings and gluteus group) and the sacrotuberous ligament originate from the ischium.

The ischial spine points posteromedially and lies below the greater sciatic notch (Fig. 1–2). Obstetrician-gynecologists have long recognized the clinical usefulness of this structure, which can function as a landmark to assess progression during labor and as a guide for pudendal anesthesia. It is easily palpable through both the vagina and rectum and can also be felt transabdominally through the retropubic space. In the standing patient, the ischial spine is 2 to 3 centimeters above the top of the pubic crest (Fig. 1–1). Thus the posterior aspect of the pubic bone and the ischial spine are on an almost horizontal plane. This relationship is critical for understanding the lateral vaginal supports, which is discussed later in this chapter.

The sacrospinous ligament attaches the sacrum to the ischial spine, separating the sciatic notches into the greater and lesser sciatic foramina. This ligament shares the same origin and insertion as the coccygeus muscle. During a sacrospinous ligament suspension of the vagina, both the ligament and its overlying coccygeus muscle are visible at the time of dissection. Additionally, the medial half of the sacrospinous ligament intermingles with the sacrotuberous ligament as they both insert onto the sacrum.

Below the ischial spine and sacrospinous ligament is the lesser sciatic notch and foramen (Fig. 1–1). The obturator internus tendon exits the pelvis via the lesser sciatic foramen. Additionally, the pudendal neurovascular bundle and the nerve to the obturator internus muscle pass through this foramen as they enter the ischioanal fossa.

The ischial spine is an important site of attachment for muscles and fascia, both parietal and endopelvic, which are critical to pelvic support. The muscles of the pelvic floor ultimately attach to the ischial spine. The coccygeus muscle attaches directly, whereas the levator ani muscles attach through the arcus tendineus levator ani (muscle white line). In addition, endopelvic fascial elements attach to the spine. These include the pubocervical fascia and the rectovaginal septum.

SACRUM AND COCCYX

The sacrum serves as the central anchor for the sacrotuberous and sacrospinous ligaments. Its pelvic surface is marked by four transverse ridges representing fusion points of the original sacral vertebrae. At the ends of the ridges are the sacral foramina, which accommodate the ventral rami of the sacral nerves and the lateral sacral arteries. The sacrum is the line of insertion of the piriformis muscle and the superior portion of the coccygeus. Due to the concavity of the sacrum, these muscles are juxtaposed at approximately 45 degrees. This angulation be-

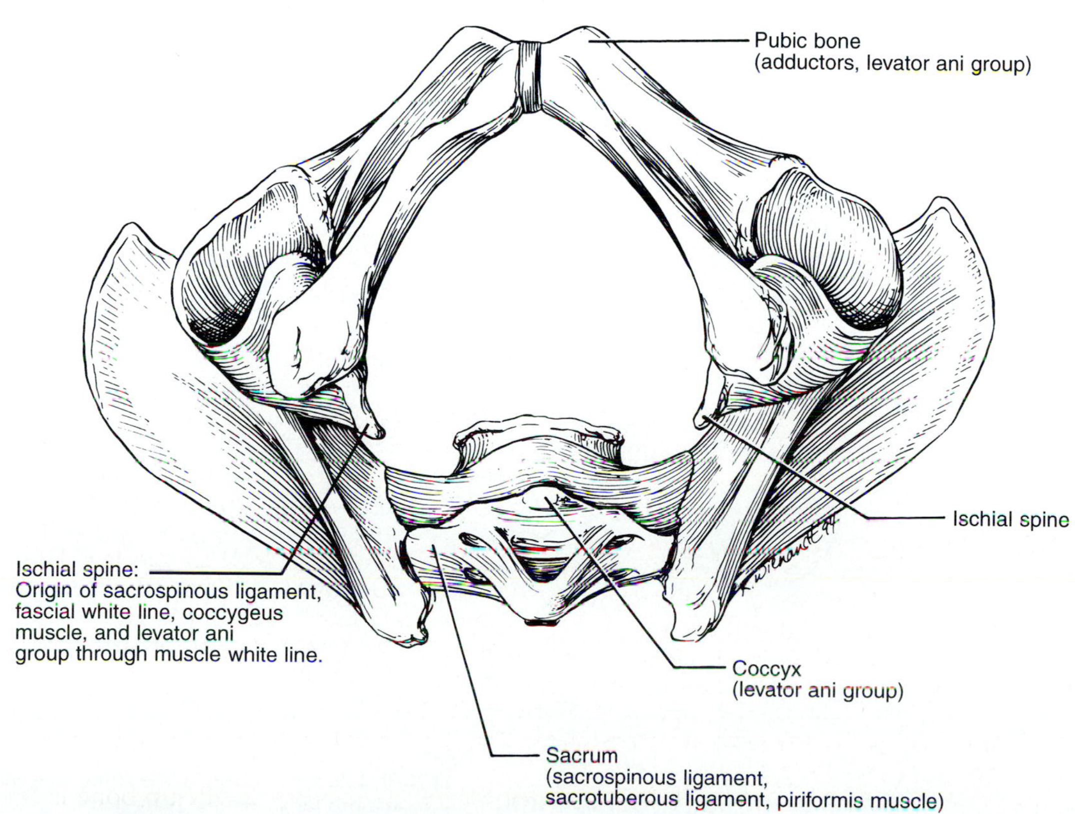

FIGURE 1–2. Important bony landmarks of the pelvic floor in dorsal lithotomy position.

tween the coccygeus and piriformis muscles provides a three-dimensional "bowl-shaped" configuration to the pelvic basin.

The coccyx is usually a single bone fused from four coccygeal elements. All muscles of the pelvic floor (pubococcygeus, iliococcygeus, and coccygeus) insert into the coccyx. In addition, the anococcygeal raphe extends from the coccyx to the external anal sphincter and is the point of midline fusion for the pubococcygeus and iliococcygeus muscles behind the rectum.

Thus, the bony pelvis is composed of the three portions of the hip bone (ilium, pubic bone, and ischium) and portions of the sacrum and coccyx.

ORIENTATION OF THE BONY PELVIS

A discussion of the proper orientation of the pelvis is necessary to understand its many functions. In the standing woman, the pelvis is held with the linea terminalis or pelvic inlet in an almost vertical plane, such that the ischiopubic rami and the first three sacral vertebrae are almost horizontal with the floor (Fig. 1–3). In this position, the pelvic and abdominal cavities are almost at right angles to each other, allowing proper transmission of weight from the upper body to the lower extremities. This perpendicular relationship directs pressure increases formed in the abdominal cavity away from the pelvic floor. Normally, pelvic contents rest against the pubic symphysis. This is in keeping with the physiologic role of bone in support and weight bearing. In contrast, muscles and endopelvic fascia are structurally adapted to bear *intermittent* pressure increases.

Consider an architectural paradigm wherein the pelvis can be thought of as an arch that transfers weight through an arched segment to columns (Fig. 1–4). In this analogy, the sacrum and coccyx form the keystone (center of arch), the linea terminalis and the pubic bone are the arched segments, and the femoral heads are the columns. The vector forces of pressure are carried through the lumbosacral spine and travel across the near-vertical linea terminalis to the femoral heads (Fig. 1–5). A stabilizing force traverses the pubic symphysis, steadying the sacroiliac and symphyseal articulations (Fig. 1–6).

Figure 1–7 shows the consequences that would result if the bony pelvis were oriented in a horizontal plane in a standing woman, as erroneously illustrated in many textbooks.[2] In such illustrations, increases in intra-abdominal pressure would actually disrupt the pubic symphysis. The ischial tuberosity would also no longer be posterior to the shaft of the femur and hip extension could not take place (Fig. 1–8). Thus, without the proper orientation of the pelvis, ambulation would be impossible and pressure transmission would be inappropriately directed toward the pelvic floor.

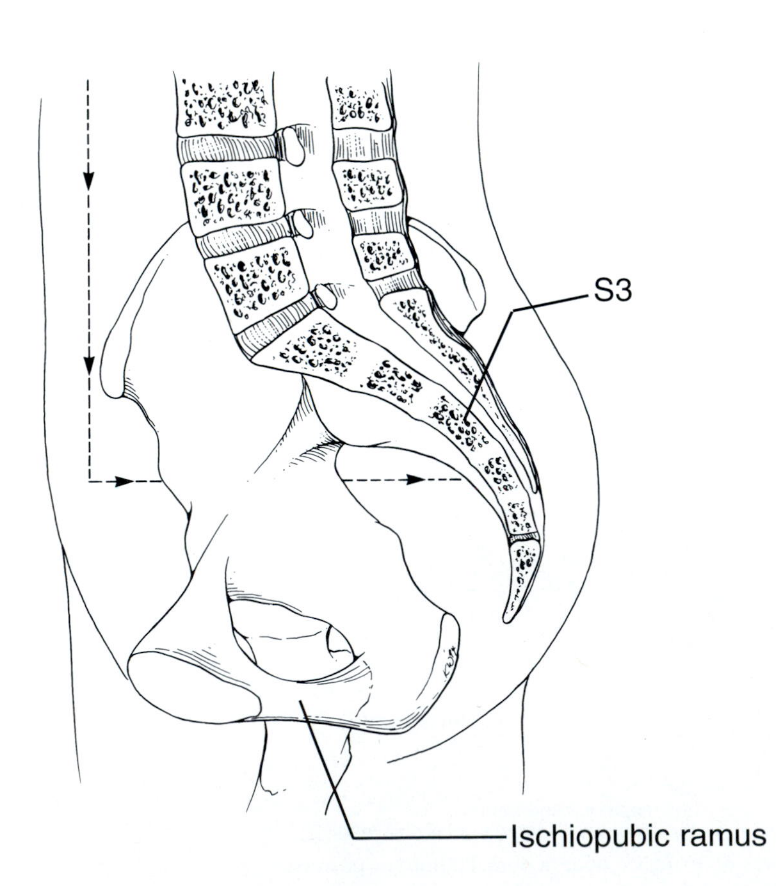

FIGURE 1–3. Relationship of the abdominal and pelvic cavities in a properly oriented bony pelvis.

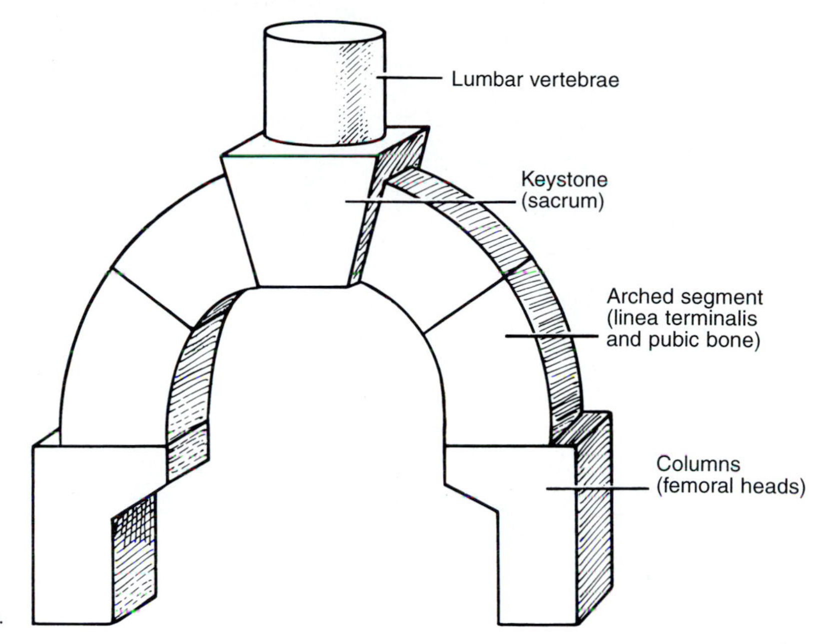

FIGURE 1–4. The bony pelvis resembles an arch.

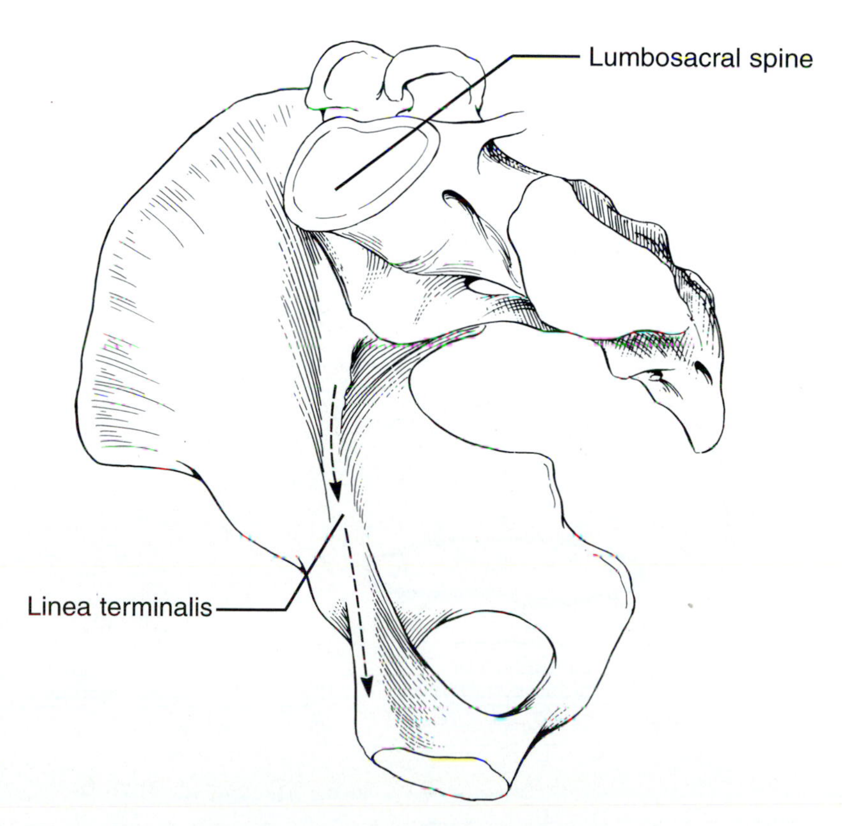

FIGURE 1–5. Medial view of the right half of the pelvis, showing the course of vector forces along the linea terminalis that occur when bearing weight.

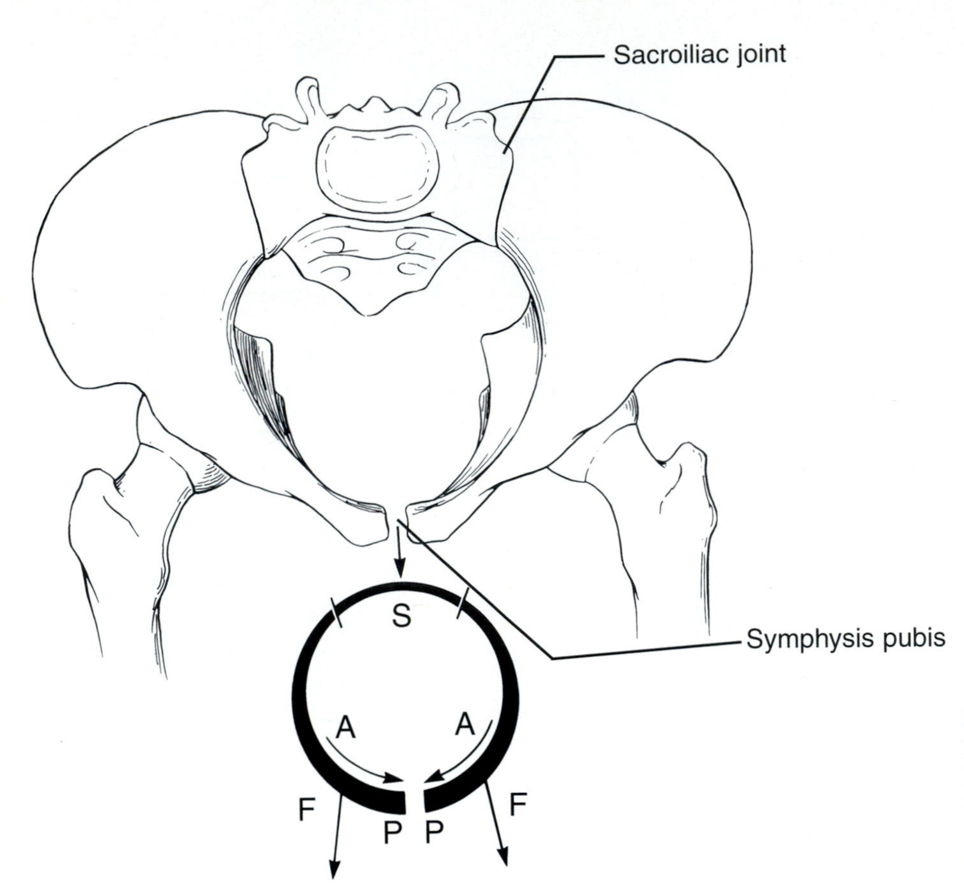

FIGURE 1–6. The standing pelvis shown with the inlet in a vertical position. Force is carried around the linea terminalis and is disseminated into the femoral heads. This position stabilizes the pubic symphysis. A = acetabulum; F = force; P = pubic bone; S = sacrum.

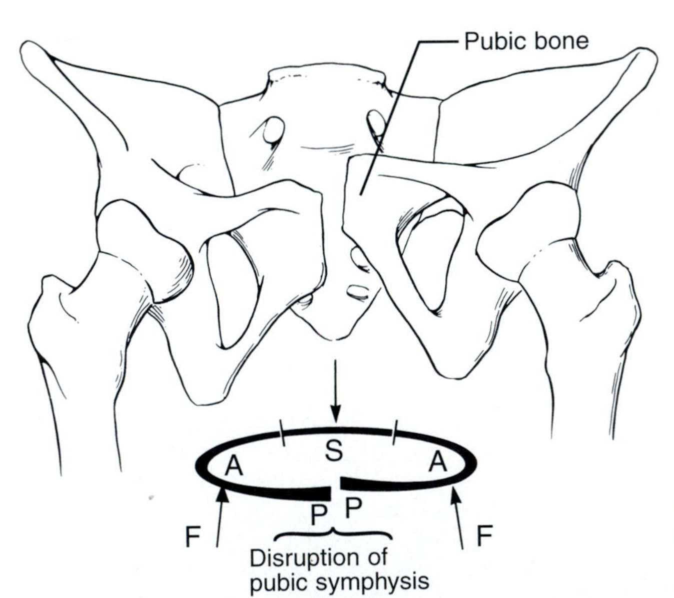

FIGURE 1–7. The consequences of a standing pelvis held with the linea terminalis in a horizontal position, with subsequent disruption of the pubic symphysis. A = acetabulum; F = force; P = pubic bone; S = sacrum.

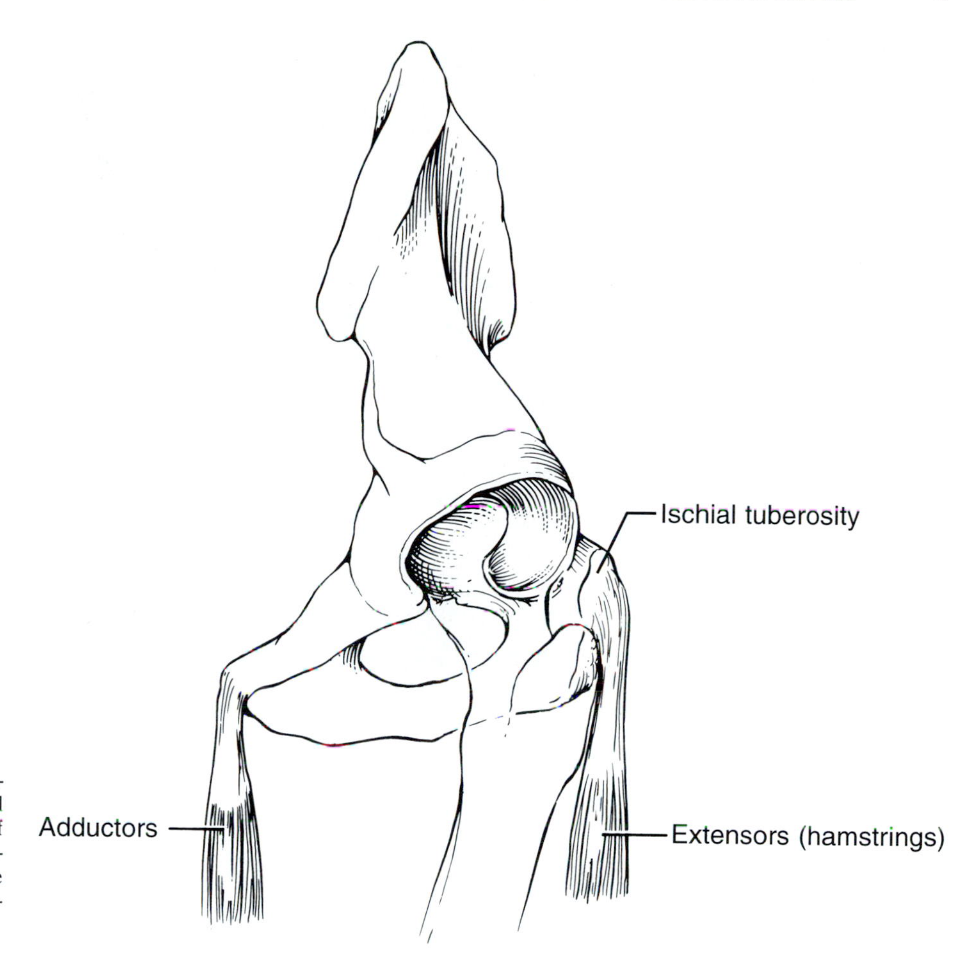

FIGURE 1–8. With the pelvis in the anatomically correct position, the ischial tuberosity is posterior to the head of the femur and above the pubis. This allows for flexion and extension of the lower limb, so that ambulation can occur.

MUSCLES AND PARIETAL FASCIA

The muscles of the pelvis are covered by parietal fascia, which is continuous with the transversalis fascia of the abdominal wall. Histologically, parietal fascia is distinct from the endopelvic facial structures, such as the pubocervical fascia and the rectovaginal septum. There are four groups of muscles particularly relevant to pelvic floor disorders in women. For the sake of simplicity, these muscles will be classified into those of the pelvic sidewalls, the pelvic floor, the perineum, and the accessory muscles.

MUSCLES OF THE PELVIC WALLS

The obturator internus and piriformis are the major muscles of the pelvic side walls. The obturator internus is a large fan-shaped muscle which arises from the bony margin of the obturator foramen, the pelvic surface of the obturator membrane, and the rami of the ischium and pubis (Fig. 1–9). This muscle forms the lateral wall of the pelvis and can be palpated transvaginally. The arcus tendineus levator ani or muscle white line is a linear thickening of the obturator fascia and is the semitendinous origin of the pubococcygeus and iliococcygeus muscles. The tendon of the obturator internus muscle passes through the lesser sciatic foramen, turning 120 degrees to insert onto the greater trochanter. The obturator internus is innervated by L5, S1-2 and produces external rotation of the hip. The parietal fascia of the obturator internus forms the lateral wall of the ischioanal fossa inferior to the muscle white line (Fig. 1–10).

The piriformis muscles form the posterior wall of the pelvis. These muscles originate from the anterior and lateral aspect of the sacrum in its middle to upper portion, coursing through the greater sciatic foramen and inserting on the greater trochanter. Like the obturator internus, the piriformis muscle externally rotates the hip. On top of this muscle is found the sacral plexus of nerves, which innervates the pelvic musculature and gives rise to the sciatic nerve. Posteriorly, in the subgluteal region, this muscle is an important landmark because the gluteal vessels and nerves pass from the pelvis to the gluteal region, either superior or inferior to it. The piriformis muscle is innervated by direct sacral efferents (motor) from the fifth lumbar and first and second sacral nerves.

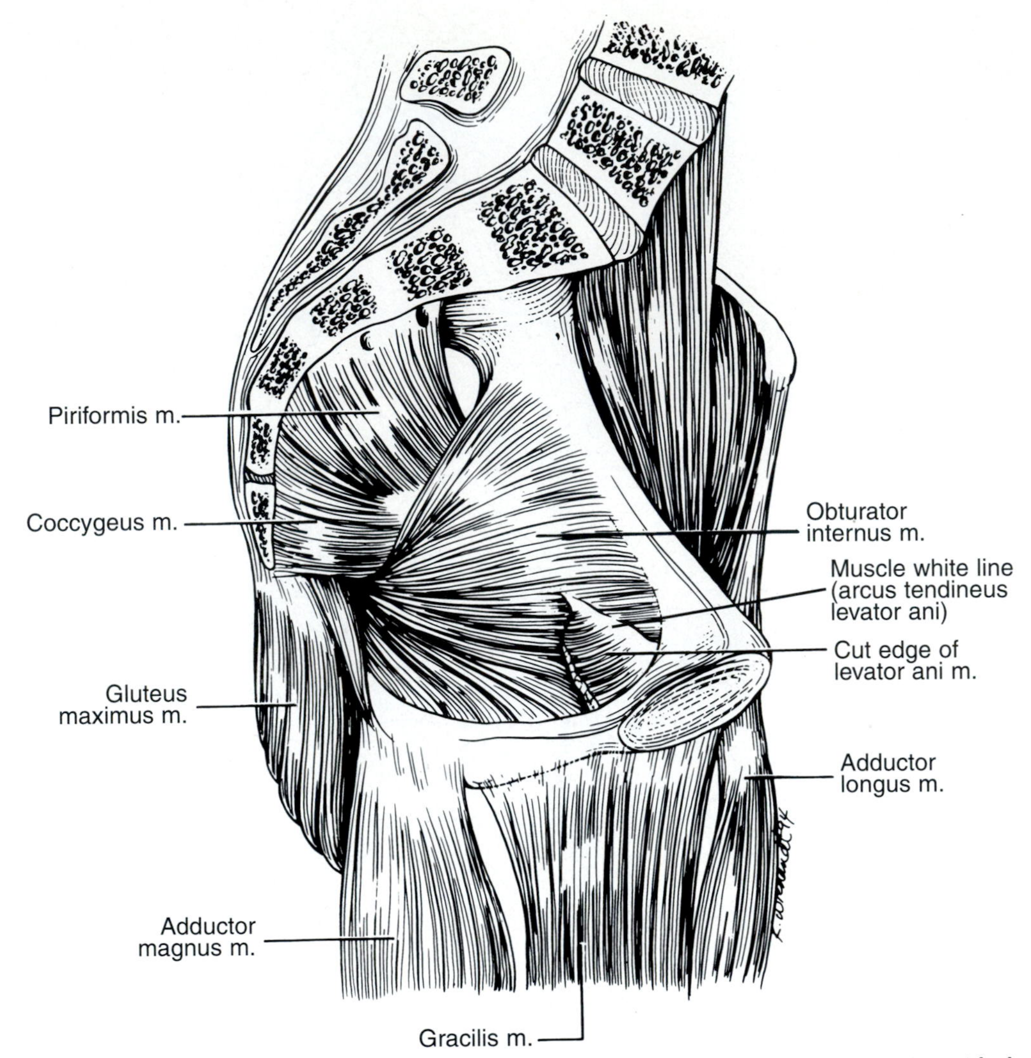

FIGURE 1–9. Midsagittal view of the pelvis with muscles. Accessory muscles, which function in conjunction with the levator ani, are shown.

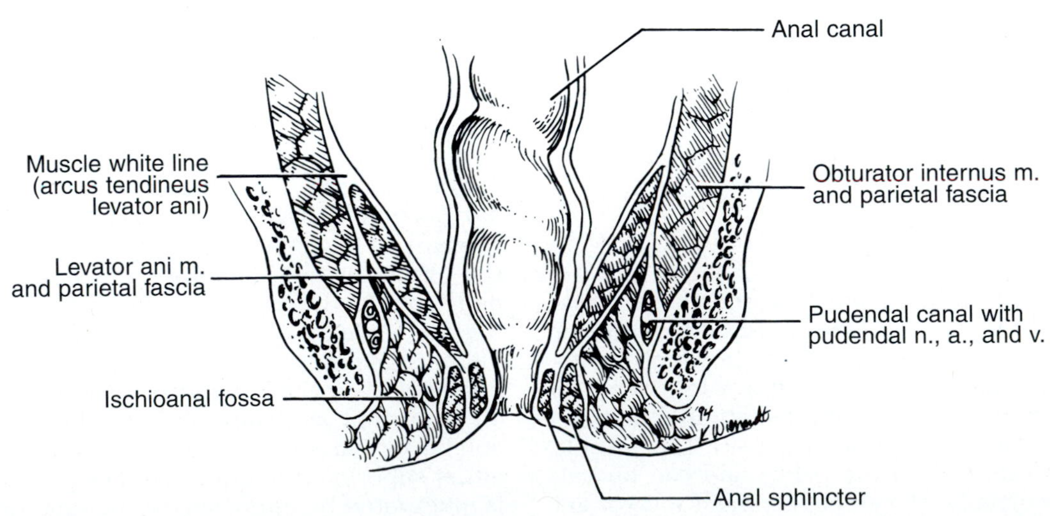

FIGURE 1–10. A coronal section of the pelvic floor showing the ischioanal fossa and the pudendal canal.

MUSCLES OF THE PELVIC FLOOR

An understanding of the muscles of the pelvic floor is critical for understanding many of the disorders discussed in this book. Physiologically, these muscles differ from most other skeletal muscles in that they exhibit constant activity (as shown by electromyography [EMG]) except during voiding and defecation. The near-constant activity of these muscles is necessary, as the pelvic viscera are suspended over these muscles by a network of endopelvic fascia.

The pelvic floor consists of the coccygeus muscles and levator ani muscles, together with their fascial coverings. As previously discussed, the coccygeus muscle originates from the ischial spine and the sacrospinous ligament and coccyx. This triangular muscle inserts on the lateral aspects of the lower sacrum and the upper coccyx. Innervation is supplied by branches S4 and S5.

The levator ani muscle consists of the pubococcygeus and iliococcygeus portions. The pubococcygeus arises from the superior ramus of the pubic bone and from the arcus tendineus levator ani. Its fibers blend with midline structures such as the vagina and perineal body. The puborectalis arises from the lower part of the pubic body, and its fibers pass posteriorly, forming a sling around the anorectal junction. The pubococcygeus inserts into the anococcygeal raphe and into the anterior and lateral sides of the coccyx.

The more posterior portion of the levator ani muscle, the iliococcygeus, is only 3 to 4 millimeters thick. It originates from the ischial spine and the arcus tendineus levator ani and slopes inferiorly toward the midline, sending off fibers that blend with the longitudinal muscle of the rectum. It fuses with its sister muscle from the opposite side in front of the anococcygeal raphe and forms the levator plate (Fig. 1–11).

Both muscles of the levator ani group receive dual innervation. The pelvic surface is innervated by direct branches from the second, third, and fourth sacral nerves, whereas the perineal surface receives innervation through the pudendal nerve (Fig. 1–12). This is an important concept, because pudendal nerve injury does not necessarily cause levator ani dysfunction (Fig. 1–13).

The muscular structures of the pelvic floor stretch from the pubis posteriorly to the coccyx and laterally to the arcus tendineus levator ani (Fig. 1–11). In the midline, the pelvic floor separates in front of the rectum to allow the passage of the urethra and vagina. This separation is called the levator or urogenital hiatus.

MUSCLES OF THE PERINEUM

The perineum is diamond-shaped; its lateral borders are the ischiopubic rami, ischial tuberosities, and sacrotuberous ligaments (Fig. 1–14). Anteriorly,

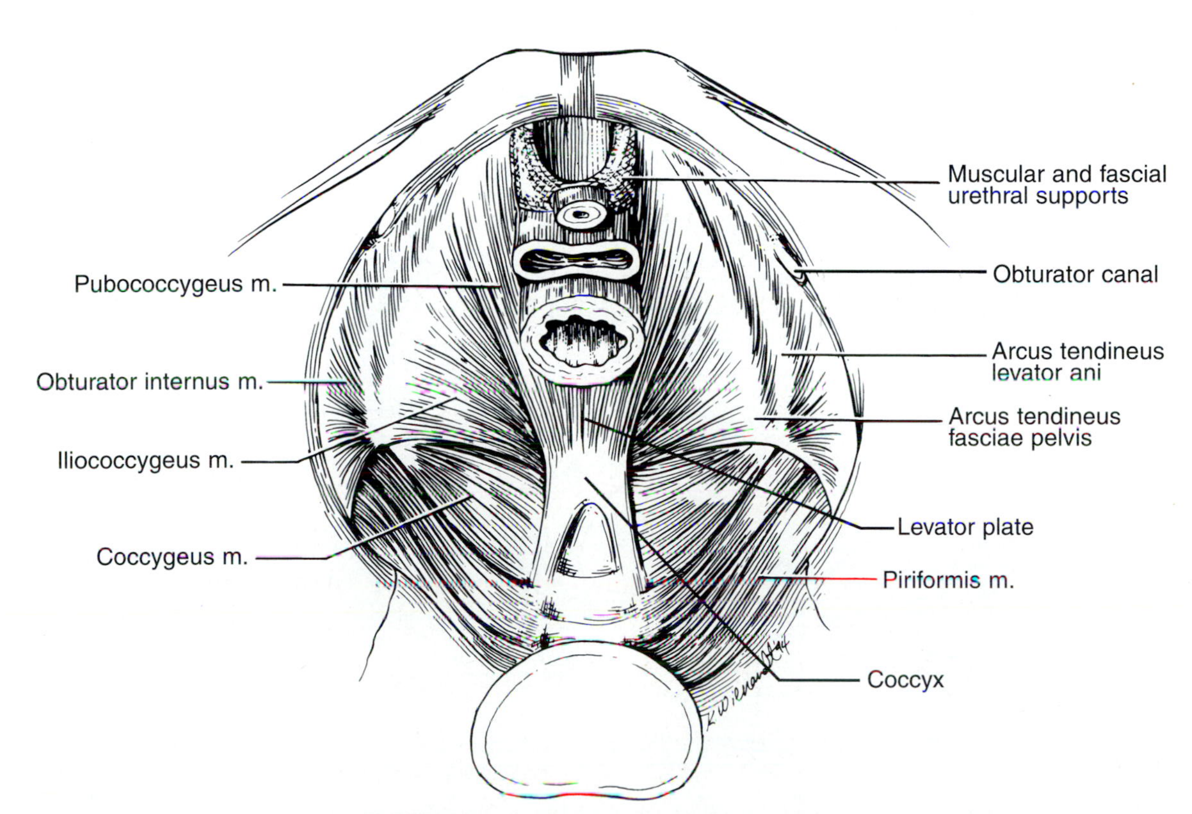

FIGURE 1–11. A superior view of the pelvic floor.

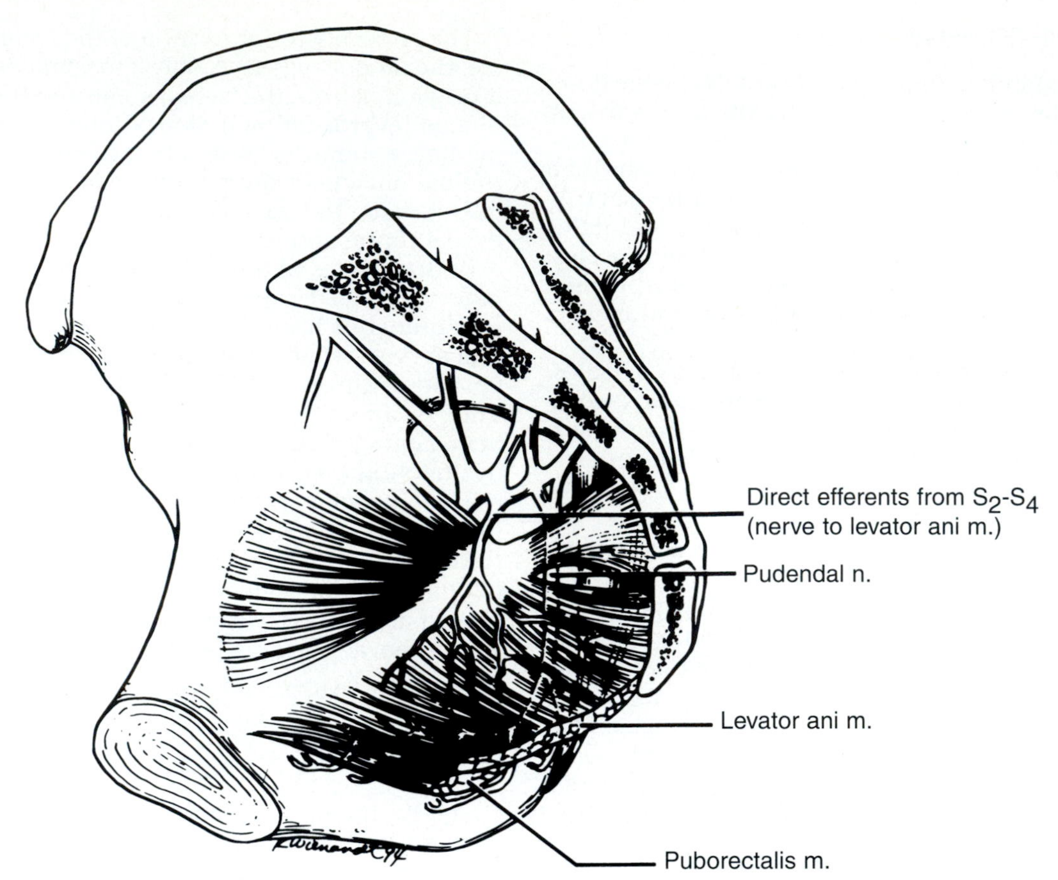

FIGURE 1–12. The dual innervation of the levator ani muscles.

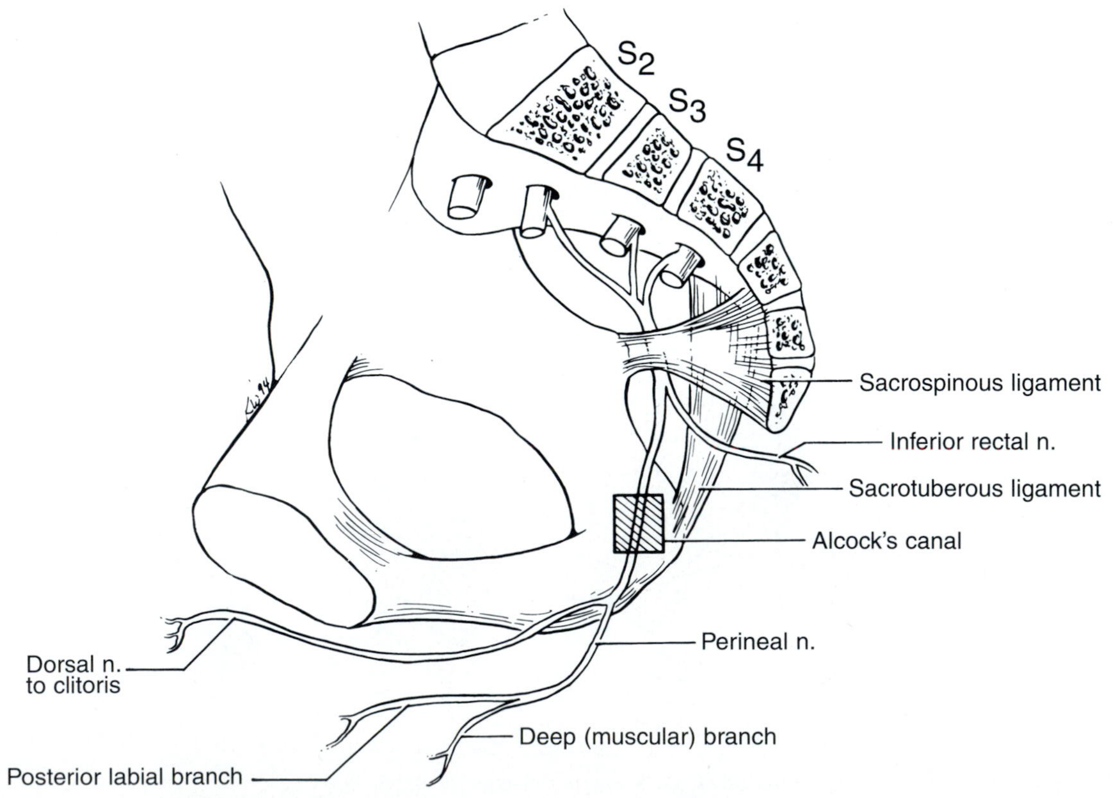

FIGURE 1–13. The course of the pudendal nerve with its terminal branches.

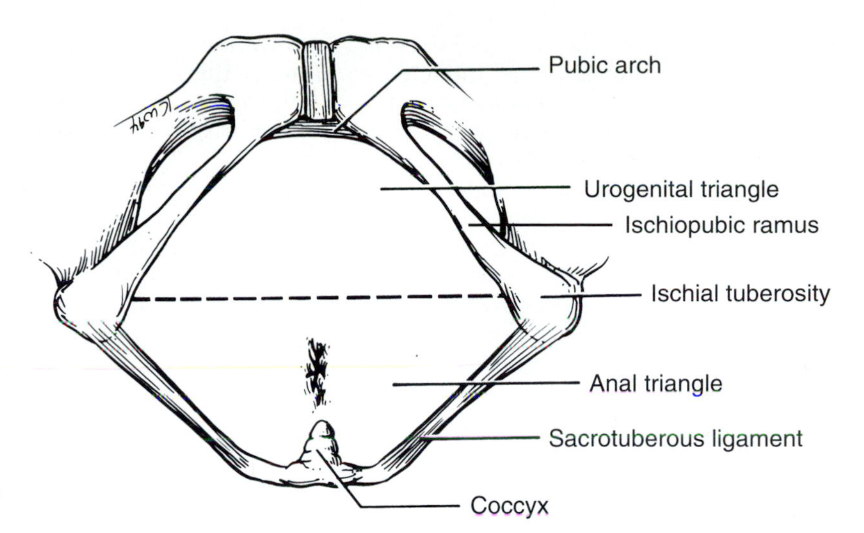

FIGURE 1–14. The boundaries of the perineum and its subdivisions, shown schematically.

the perineum is bounded by the pubic arch and posteriorly by the coccyx. The perineum can be divided into two triangular parts by drawing a line transversely between the ischial tuberosities. The posterior division is the anal triangle; the anterior portion is the urogenital triangle. The urogenital triangle is further divided into two compartments, the superficial and deep perineal compartments, which are separated by the perineal membrane. The perineal membrane spans the ischiopubic rami and is parallel to the floor in the standing patient.

The superficial perineal compartment contains the superficial transverse perinei, the bulbocavernosus and the ischiocavernosus muscles (Fig. 1–15). These muscles act to stabilize or compress the vaginal opening and erectile tissue within the superficial compartment. The bulbocavernosus inserts into the perineal body, interdigitating with fibers of the su-

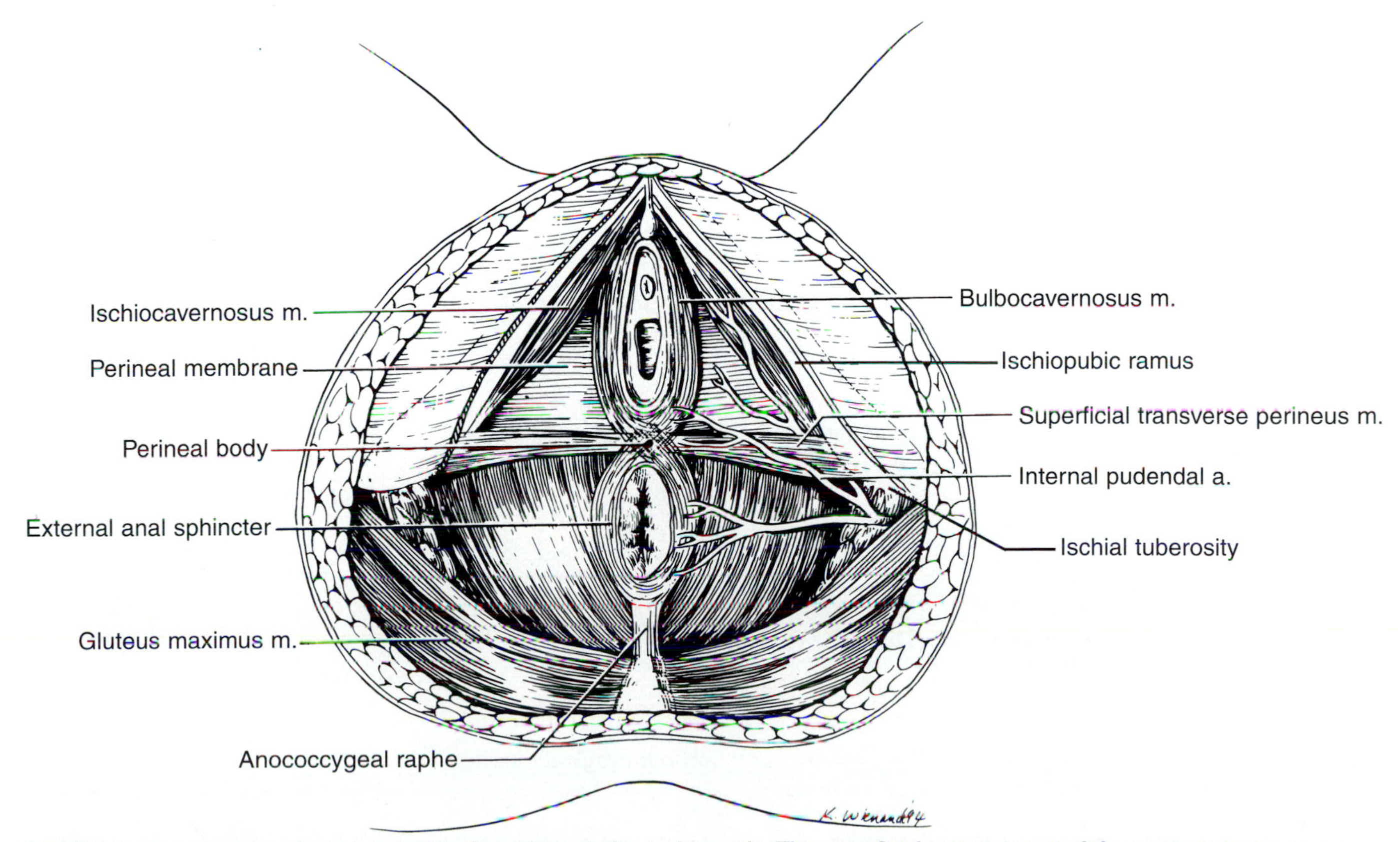

FIGURE 1–15. An inferior view of the pelvic floor through the anal triangle. The superficial compartment of the urogenital triangle surrounds the vagina and urethra.

perficial transverse perinei and external anal sphincter. The ischiocavernosus muscles compress the crura, thus impeding venous return and helping to maintain erection of the clitoris. These muscles originate from the medial side of the ischial tuberosities and from the ischiopubic rami. As their fibers course anteriorly, they encompass the crura and insert into the pubic angle. The superficial transverse perinei arise from the anterior and medial surfaces of the ischial tuberosities and course medially to insert into the perineal body. All the muscles of the superficial compartment are innervated by branches of the pudendal nerve (Fig. 1–13).

The deep perineal compartment is located on top of the perineal membrane. The neurovascular contents of the deep compartment include the deep dorsal vein and the dorsal nerves, arteries, and veins to the clitoris. The muscular contents of the deep compartment include the transversus vaginae muscles, the compressor urethrae, and the urethrovaginal muscles (Fig. 1–16).[3] The transversus vaginae muscle originates at the ischiopubic rami and courses medially, sending some fibers to blend with the vagina. The transversus vaginae meets its sister muscle in the midline at the perineal body. The compressor urethrae and urethrovaginal muscles form the distal portion of the external urethral sphincter. This is in contrast to the more proximal portion of the external urethral sphincter, called the **sphincter urethrae**, which is not part of the deep perineal compartment of the urogenital triangle.[3] The urethrovaginal muscle wraps around the distal portion of the urethra and vagina and inserts into the perineal body. The compressor urethrae muscles originate from the medial surfaces of the ischiopubic rami and course over the top of the urethra, where they fuse. The muscles of the deep perineal compartment act as sphincters of the urethra and vagina. It is thought that these delicate muscles provide a "backup" mechanism of urinary continence, allowing micturition to be put off for a short time.[4] Anterior reflections of the pubocervical fascia around the urethra to the pubic arch were formerly interpreted as "pubourethral" ligaments for suspension of the urethrovesical junction. They are now thought to help orient the urethra vertically and centrally, but not to suspend it. The neurovascular supply to these muscles is taken from the internal pudendal artery and vein and from the pudendal nerve.

The perineal body is the area of the perineum located between the vaginal outlet and the anus (Fig. 1–15). In the standing woman, the base of this three-dimensional pyramidal structure is parallel to the floor, with its apex at the junction of the lower third and middle third of the vagina. There are multiple important connections to the perineal body, including the bulbocavernosus muscles, the superficial transverse perinei, the transversus vaginae, the perineal membrane, the external anal sphincter, the rectovaginal septum, and the parietal fascia from the pubococcygeus muscles. The perineal body is critical for closure of the urethra, support of the lower third of the vagina, and proper function of the anal canal.

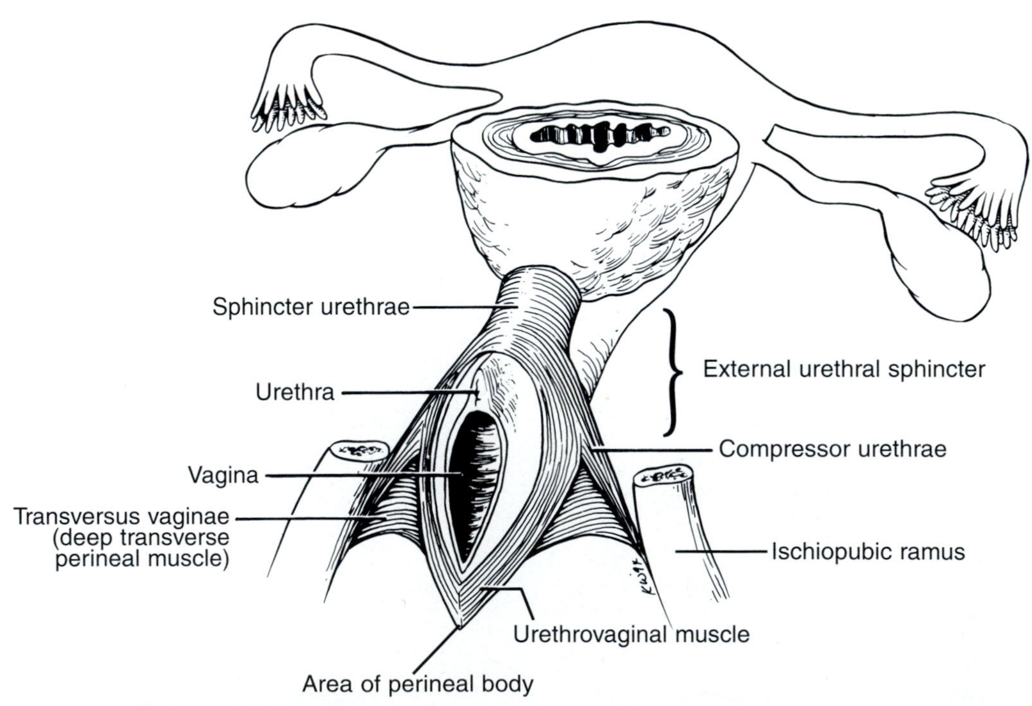

FIGURE 1–16. The muscles of the external urethral sphincter.

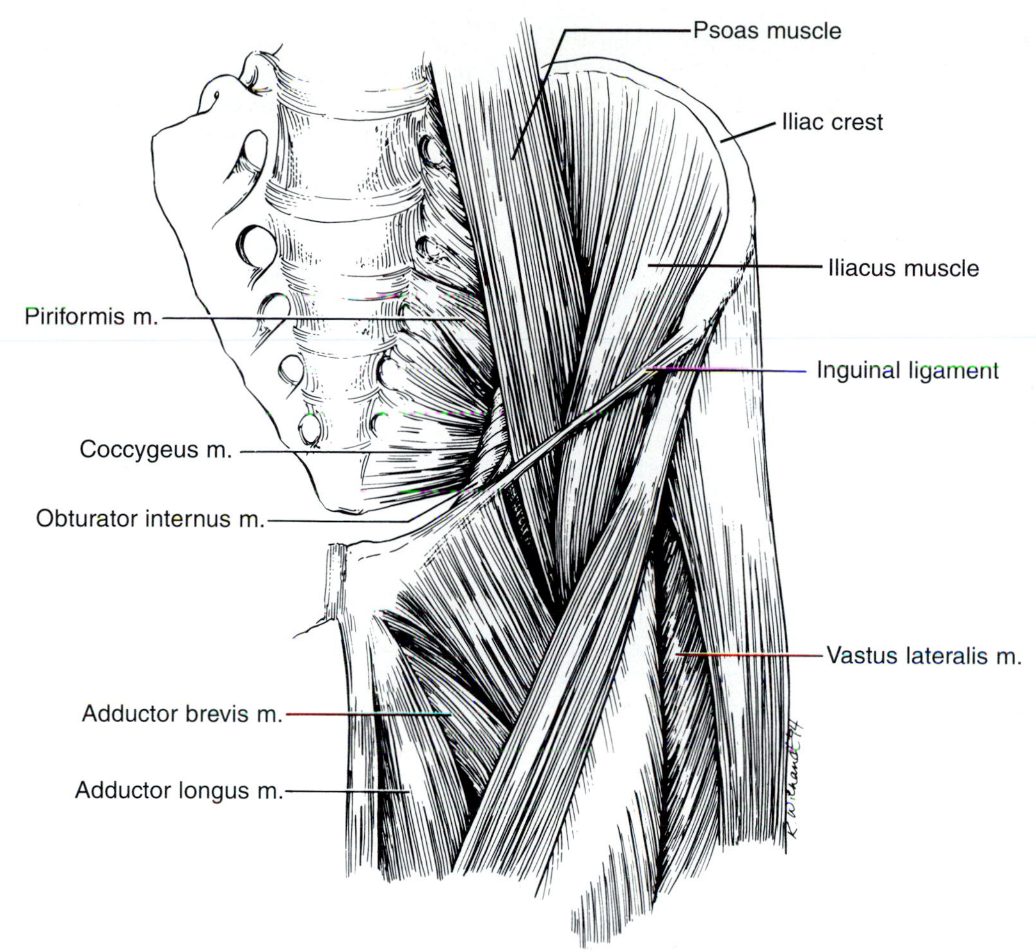

FIGURE 1–17. An anterior view of the muscular basin of the left side of the pelvis. Accessory muscles that flex the hip and adduct the thigh are shown.

ACCESSORY MUSCLES

The basic elements of pelvic visceral support include the bony foundation, pelvic floor musculature, and endopelvic fascia. In addition to these "main ingredients," however, the muscles of the perineum and hip girdle region provide added support at times of increased stress. EMG studies have shown that the hip girdle muscles act in conjunction with the levator ani muscles to contract the pelvic floor.[5] This is in keeping with principles of kinesiology, which state that no muscle works in isolation; rather, muscles work in groups.

The hip girdle muscles fall into three broad categories: those that externally rotate, those that extend, and those that adduct the thigh. The external rotators (obturator internus and piriformis) have already been discussed. The important hip extensors are the gluteus maximus and the hamstring muscles (Fig. 1–1). The gluteus maximus is a large muscle that originates from the sacrum, coccyx, ilium, and sacrotuberous ligaments. Besides being a powerful extensor of the thigh, the gluteus maximus may serve as a backup to the levator ani group. It is innervated by the inferior gluteal nerve. The other hip extensor is the hamstring group, which has its origin at the ischial tuberosity and inserts into the lateral and medial aspects of the tibia. The hamstrings are innervated by branches of the sciatic nerve.

The adductors of the thigh are also accessory pelvic floor muscles (Fig. 1–17). Collectively, this group of muscles originates from the ischium and pubic bone and inserts into the medial surface of the femur. The adductors are innervated by branches of the obturator nerve. These accessory muscles may be useful when rehabilitative techniques are employed to treat pelvic floor dysfunction, as discussed in Chapter 14.

ENDOPELVIC FASCIA

FUNCTION

Endopelvic fascia has two important functions. The first is to suspend the viscera over the levator plate of the pelvic floor. In a standing woman, the bladder, the upper two thirds of the vagina, and the rectum lie in an axis that parallels the floor. This horizontal orientation is critical to the maintenance of organ position. When intra-abdominal pressure increases, a perpendicular force is placed on the longitudinal axis of the pelvic viscera, pinning these organs against the simultaneously contracting pelvic floor. This prevents any oblique force from pushing the organs through the urogenital hiatus. The second function is to provide flexible conduits and physical supports for the vasculature, visceral nerves, and lymphatic tissue of the viscera.

Microscopically, endopelvic fascia is a meshwork of collagen, elastin, and smooth muscle, which surrounds and supports the viscera in the pelvis. Anatomists and surgeons have described this network in a piecemeal fashion, assigning names to isolated segments. On a gross level, it is actually a latticework of sheaths, continuous and interdependent, extending from the pelvic floor to the respiratory diaphragm. The endopelvic fascia is located in subperitoneal areas of the pelvis, between the parietal peritoneum and the parietal fascia of the muscular walls and floor.

TYPES

Portions of the endopelvic fascia envelop the bladder and urethra, the cervix and vagina, and the anal canal and rectum. These visceral capsules are intimately attached to the surrounding smooth muscle coat of each viscus. These capsules contain the vasculature, the visceral nerves, and the lymph nodes and channels, as well as adipose tissue. They also provide support during storage, distention, and evacuation. They connect the pelvic organs to parietal fascia and bone, anchoring them to the pelvic walls through sheaths and septa.[6] These endopelvic fascial sheaths and septa vary in their strength, thickness, and composition, depending on the support requirements for a particular area.

SUPPORT AXES

Conceptually, it is helpful to think of three distinct axes for fascial support—the upper vertical axis, the horizontal axis, and, distally, the lower vertical axis.[7] The upper vertical axis follows a vertical line from the sacroiliac joint along the anterior border of the greater sciatic foramen to the ischial spine, following

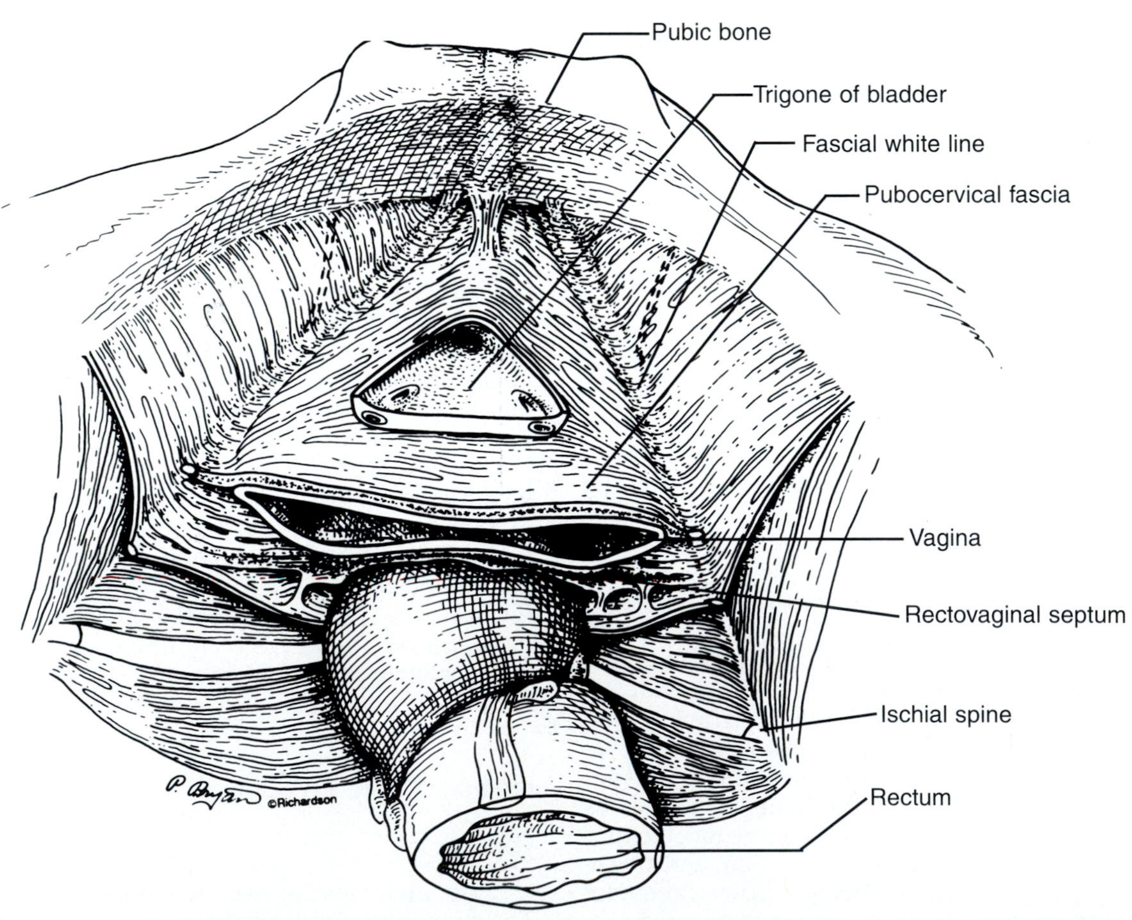

FIGURE 1–18. The pubocervical fascia supports the bladder and urethra (only the trigone is shown) and is attached laterally to the fascial white lines. The rectovaginal septum is a thin layer of fascia between the vagina and rectum. (Courtesy of Dr. Cullen Richardson).

the course and direction of the internal iliac vessels. The endopelvic fascia forms sheets which fuse around these blood vessels to form a sheath. The cardinal ligament portion of this fascial sheath is a broad, fan-shaped collection of fibers that continues along the uterine artery, eventually blending with the visceral fascial capsule of the cervix, upper vagina, and lower uterine segment. Posteriorly and laterally, the cardinal ligament merges with the parietal fascia of the piriformis and obturator internus muscles and the parietal fascia adherent to the anterior border of the greater sciatic foramen.

The uterosacral-ligament portion of this complex is a dense gathering of endopelvic fascia located in the medial and inferior areas of the cardinal ligament. These fibers fuse with the visceral fascial capsule of the cervix and upper vagina, suspending them to the presacral fascia over S2-4. The upper vertical axis contains suspensory fibers that serve to pull the top of the vagina, the cervix, and the lower uterine segment posteriorly toward the sacrum so that they are positioned over the levator plate. Detachment of these structures can cause uterovaginal prolapse.[8]

The second axis is a horizontal one that courses from the ischial spine to the posterior aspect of the pubic bone. The lateral or "paravaginal" supports to the bladder, the upper two thirds of the vagina, and the rectum are derived from this axis. This support is continuous with the fascial sheaths of the cardinal ligament–uterosacral ligament complexes, which take an abrupt right-angle turn at the level of the ischial spines and merge at the cervix into these horizontal or "paravaginal" supports. Unlike the long, spindle-like fibers of the cardinal ligament–uterosacral ligament complex, the fibers of these horizontal septa form short, firm bands.

The two structures of the horizontal axis of vaginal support are the pubocervical fascia anteriorly and the rectovaginal septum posteriorly. The pubocervical fascia is a thickening of the endopelvic fascial coat of the vagina anteriorly (Fig. 1–18). On each side, it attaches directly to the fascial white line through a short transverse vaginal septum. These attachments are responsible for the anterolateral sulci of the vagina. Posteriorly the pubocervical fascia attaches to the cervix, whereas anteriorly it attaches to the perineal membrane and helps support the urethra. The near-horizontal relationship between the posterior aspect of the pubic bone and the ischial spine provides the appropriate bony foundation for these horizontal supports. The arcus tendineus fasciae pelvis or "fascial white line" is a linear thicken-

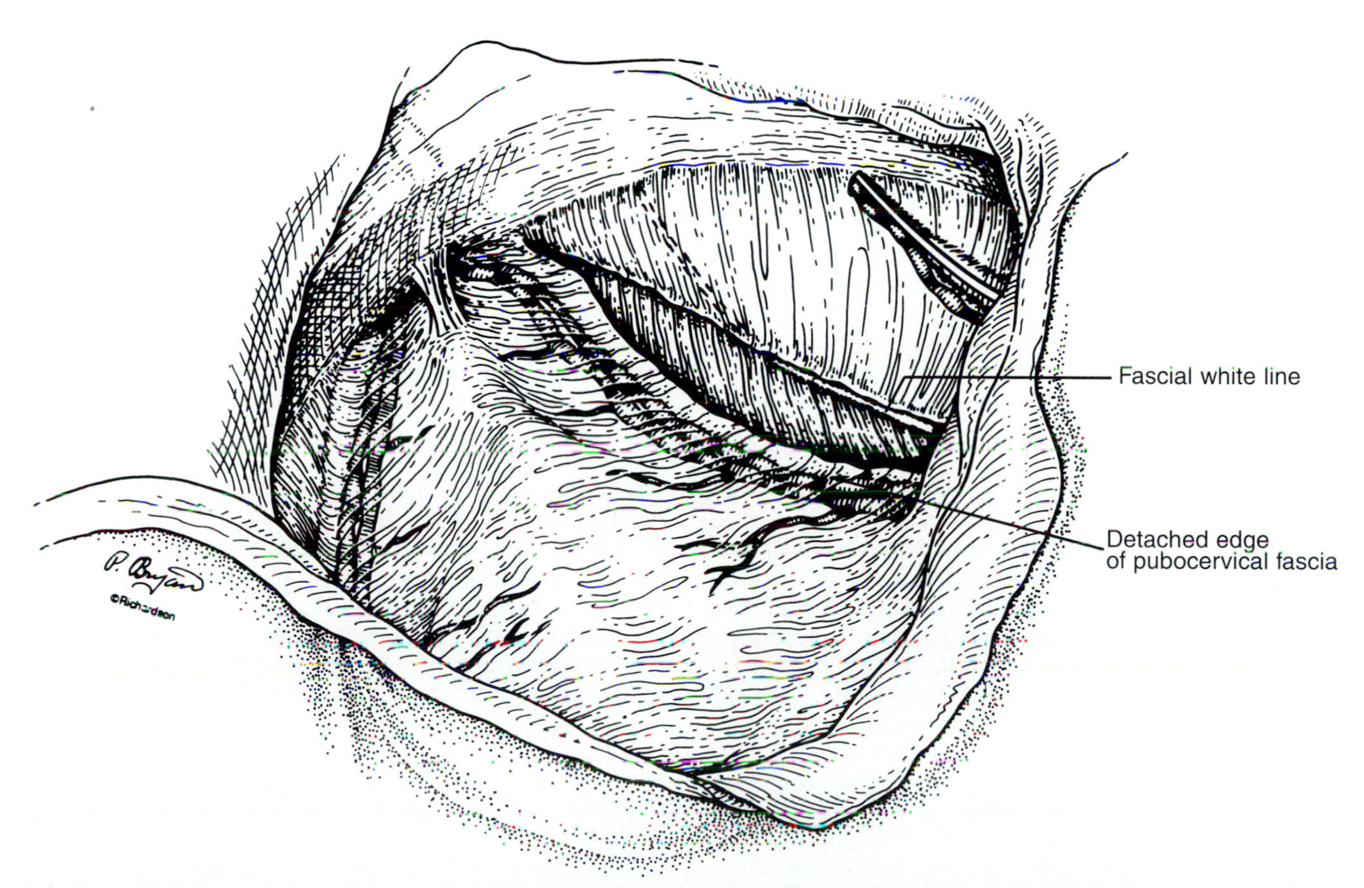

FIGURE 1–19. A complete detachment of the pubocervical fascia from the right fascial white line. This paravaginal defect is clinically manifested as a cystocele and urethrocele with loss of the right anterolateral vaginal sulcus. (Courtesy of Dr. Cullen Richardson).

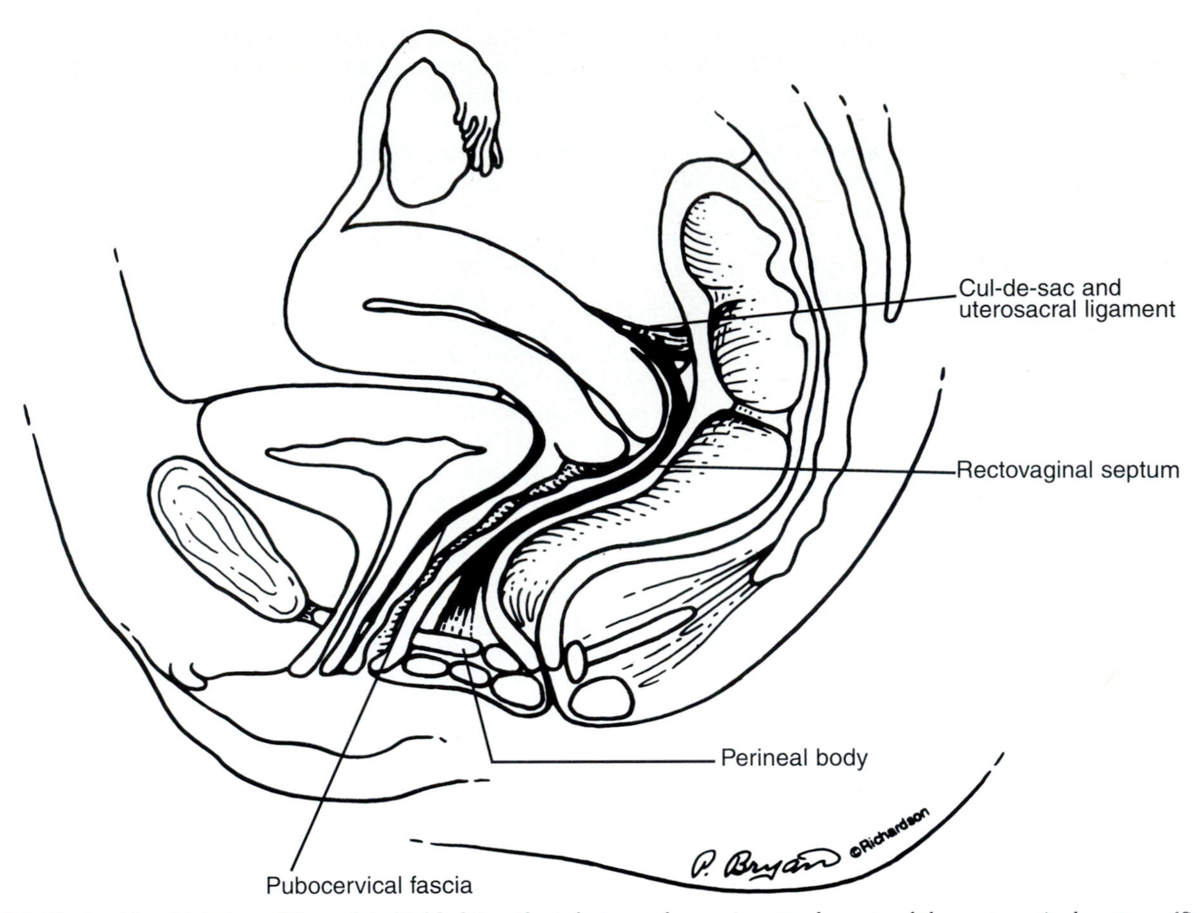

FIGURE 1–20. A midsagittal view of the pelvis highlighting the inferior and superior attachments of the rectovaginal septum. (Courtesy of Dr. Cullen Richardson).

ing of the levator ani fascia from the ischial spine to a point on the posterior aspect of the pubic bone, one centimeter lateral and one centimeter anterior to the pubic arch.[9] The arcus tendineus levator ani and the arcus tendineus fasciae pelvis fuse together posteriorly near the ischial spine, but anteriorly are separated on the posterior aspect of the pubic bone. Clinically, detachments of the pubocervical fascia from the fascial white line may cause cystoceles (Fig. 1–19).[10]

The rectovaginal septum, however, is not a thickening of the posterior vaginal coat, but is a separate endopelvic fascial layer between the vagina and rectum. The rectovaginal septum divides the anterior compartment of the pelvis, containing the bladder, urethra, and vagina, from the posterior compartment, containing the rectum (Fig. 1–20). Inferiorly, the rectovaginal septum is attached to the perineal body. Superiorly, it blends with the undersurface of the cul-de-sac and uterosacral ligaments.[11] This septum is an adherence of the anterior and posterior walls of the cul-de-sac peritoneum which, during fetal life, extends to the perineal body.[11] As the embryo develops, these layers fuse together and are modified histologically. The rectovaginal septum is attached to the lateral pelvic wall and ischial spine at the arcus tendineus fasciae pelvis (Fig. 1–21). Thus, the perineal body is essentially attached to the sacrum through its continuity with the rectovaginal septum and uterosacral ligaments. Clinically, rectoceles may be breaks in the attachments of the rectovaginal septum, as discussed in Chapter 31 (Fig. 1–22).

The third support axis is perpendicular to the planes of the urogenital and anal triangles and defines the vertical orientation of the lower one third of the vagina, the urethra, and the anal canal. In the standing woman, these organs connect directly to the horizontal urogenital triangle and perineal body. The lower portion of the vagina is supported by direct attachments of the pubococcygeus parietal fascia to the endopelvic capsule of the vagina with the fibers of Luschka. The distal urethra is embedded in the perineal membrane, whereas the proximal urethra is supported by a "hammock" of pubocervical fascia, which attaches laterally to the fascial white line (Fig. 1–23). Also related to the proximal urethra is the pubovesical muscle, which is composed of endopelvic fascia and a significant component of smooth muscle. Formerly thought to be the "posterior pubourethral ligament," this muscle is now believed to facilitate opening of the urethra at the time of voiding.

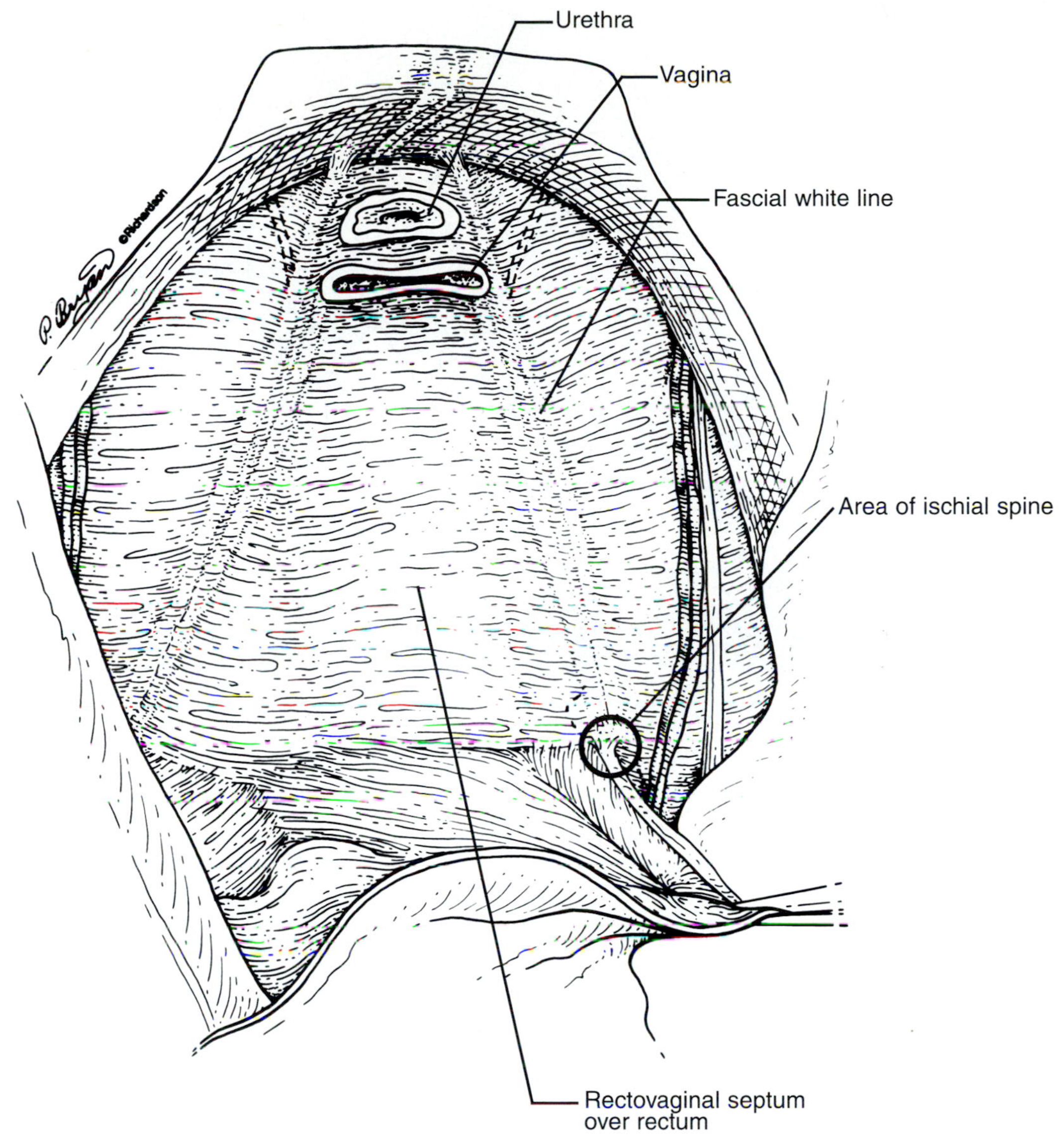

FIGURE 1–21. The bladder and upper two-thirds of the vagina have been removed. Shown is the rectovaginal septum with lateral attachments to the fascial white lines and posterior attachments to the cul-de-sac peritoneum and both uterosacral ligaments. (Courtesy of Dr. Cullen Richardson).

The anal canal is supported by direct fascial attachments to the pubococcygeus parietal fascia, the perineal body, and the external anal sphincter. These direct connections provide a compressive force to the openings of the pelvic viscera.

SUPPORTS OF THE FASCIAL NETWORK

Continuity of the endopelvic fascial network in the pelvis is focused on two key structures: the cervix and the perineal body. The endopelvic fascia of the upper vertical supports, the cardinal ligament–uterosacral ligament complexes, fuse into the posterolateral aspects of the supravaginal part of the cervix. From the horizontal support axis, the pubocervical fascia inserts into the anterior aspect of the cervix. The rectovaginal septum is linked to the cervix through its connections with the uterosacral ligaments. Together, these attachments form a paracervical ring of endopelvic fascia that ensures continuity and interdependency between the upper vertical support axis and the horizontal support axis. This paracervical fascial ring must be recreated at the time of hysterectomy and reconstructive vaginal surgery in order to provide uninterrupted support for the vaginal apex.

The perineal body is essential to the supportive structures of the urogenital and anal triangles. It serves as a mooring for the fascial coverings and muscular components of the superficial and deep perineal compartments that contain the supporting structures for the distal urethra, vagina, and anal ca-

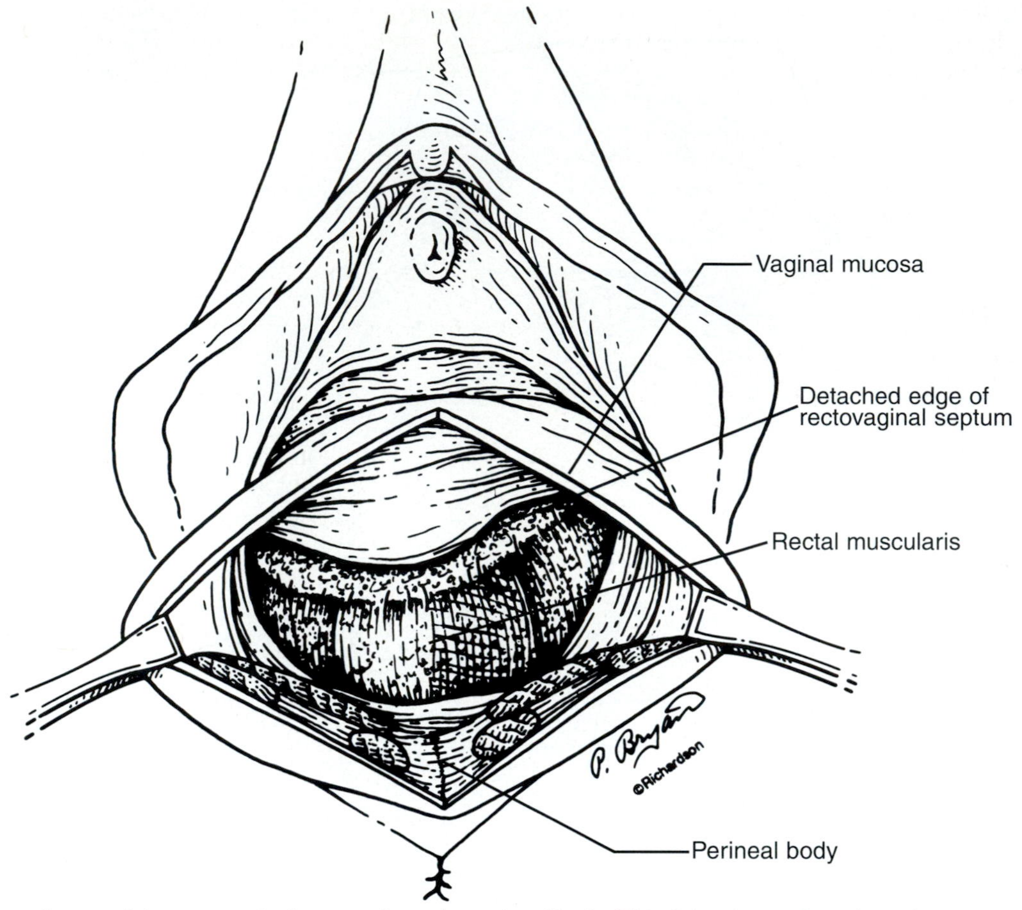

FIGURE 1–22. Detachment of the rectovaginal septum from the perineal body. This defect is manifested as a low rectocele. (Courtesy of Dr. Cullen Richardson).

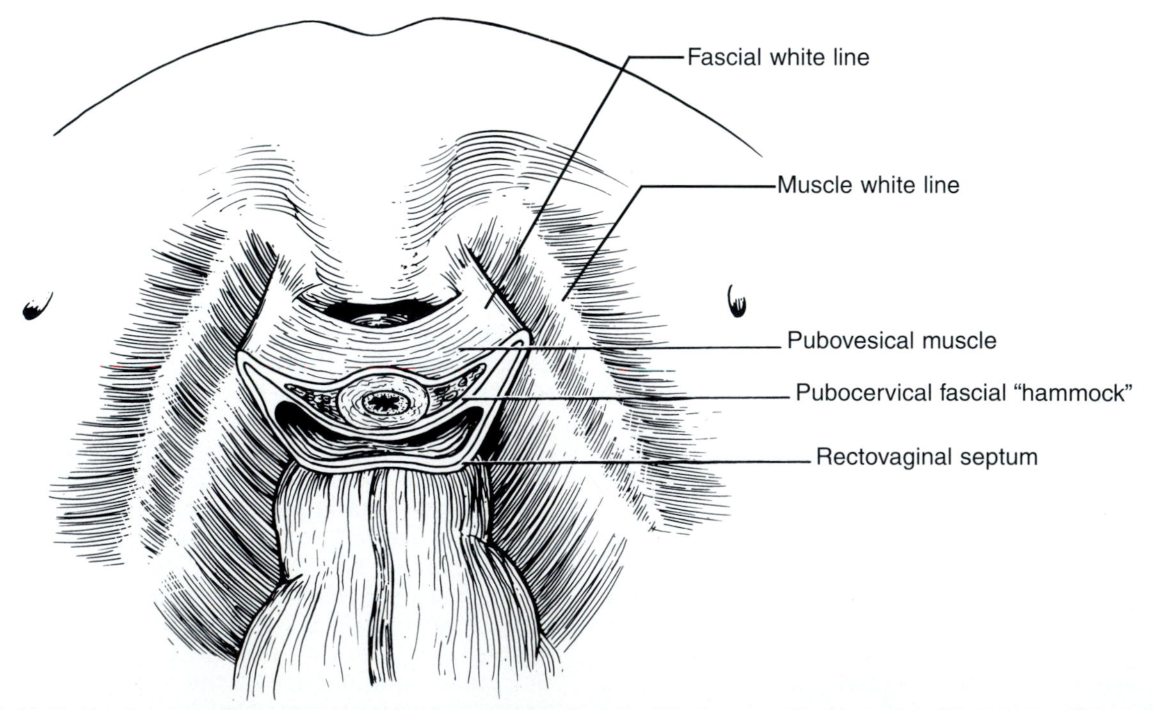

FIGURE1–23. Urethral support. The pubocervical fascia provides a "hammock" of support for the urethra. The function of the pubovesical muscle is not to provide support, however, but rather to allow opening of the urethra to facilitate micturition.

nal. This fibromuscular structure is a converging point for the horizontal supports and the lower vertical supports. The rectovaginal septum merges with it, whereas the pubocervical fascia connects to it through the perineal membrane of the urogenital triangle. Integrity of the perineal body helps to maintain competency of the visceral apertures. It is the keystone of support for the lower pelvic viscera.

SUMMARY

Multiple pelvic structures provide support and allow normal function of the pelvic organs. The human pelvis is a unique, multitiered system which provides support for organs with complex physiologic functions in the smallest possible space. The shape of the pelvic bones and their orientation to the vertebral column provides the first level of support. The "arch-like" arrangement of the pelvis enables abdominal pressure changes to be distributed to the femoral columns rather than to pelvic viscera and muscles. The near-vertical orientation of the pelvic inlet allows much of the weight of the pelvic contents to rest on a bony foundation rather than placing constant stress on muscles and ligaments.

Four muscle groups form the second tier of support for the pelvic organs. The muscles of the pelvic floor produce a dynamic backstop for the viscera. The hip-girdle and pelvic side wall muscles probably provide backup to the pelvic floor at times of increased stress. Additionally, compressive forces for organ closure are produced by the muscles of the perineum.

The last tier of support for the pelvic viscera comes from the endopelvic fascia. This intricate network of vertical and horizontal supports suspends and stabilizes the pelvic viscera in their central location over the levator plate of the pelvic floor.

The goal of reparative vaginal surgery is to reestablish the normal visceral relationships to the bones and soft tissues of the pelvis. The knowledgeable physician and surgeon understands, however, that proper surgical repair is only part of restoring normal physiologic function. An appreciation and understanding of the complexities of female pelvic anatomy and physiology is paramount in the treatment of disorders of function and support.

REFERENCES

1. DeLancey, JOL: Vaginographic examination of the pelvic floor. Int Urogynecol J 5:19, 1994.
2. Stromberg, MW and Williams, OJ: Misrepresentation of the human pelvis. J Biomed Commun 20:14, 1993.
3. Oelrich, TM: The striated urogenital sphincter muscle in the female. Anat Rec 205:223, 1983.
4. DeLancey, JOL: Structural aspects of the extrinsic continence mechanism. Obstet Gynecol 72:296, 1988.
5. Knott, M and Voss, D: Proprioceptive Neuromuscular Facilitation, ed 2. Harper & Row, New York, Chapter 4, 1968.
6. Uhlenhuth, E, Day, E, Smith, R, et al: The visceral endopelvic fascia and the hypogastric sheath. Surg Gynecol Obstet 86:9, 1948.
7. Peham, HV and Amreich, J: Operative Gynecology. JB Lippincott, Philadelphia, 1934.
8. DeLancey, JOL: Anatomic aspects of vaginal eversion after hysterectomy. Am J Obstet Gynecol 166:1717, 1992.
9. DeLancey, JOL: Structural support of the urethra as it relates to stress urinary incontinence: the hammock hypothesis. Am J Obstet Gynecol 170:1713, 1994.
10. Richardson, AC, Edmonds, PB and Williams, NL: Treatment of stress urinary incontinence due to paravaginal fascial defect. Obstet Gynecol 57:357, 1981.
11. Uhlenhuth, E, Wolfe, W, Smith, E, et al: The rectogenital septum. Surg Gynecol Obstet 86:148, 1948.

CHAPTER 2

Structure and Function of the Lower Gastrointestinal Tract

Sang-Jeon Lee • Alan P. Meagher
John H. Pemberton

STRUCTURE OF THE COLON

The large intestine is approximately 150 cm in length and consists of the cecum, ascending colon, hepatic flexure, transverse colon, splenic flexure, descending colon, sigmoid colon, rectum, and anal canal (Fig. 2–1). The internal diameter of the large intestine diminishes progressively from the cecum (7.5–8.5 cm) to the sigmoid (2.5 cm), increases again in the rectum (4.5 cm), and finally narrows in the anal canal.[1] Embryologically, bowel proximal to the mid-transverse colon is derived from the midgut, whereas the portion distal to this point is derived from the hindgut; consequently, their neurovascular anatomy is different, as discussed later in this chapter. The ascending and descending colon are retroperitoneal structures in most patients, in contrast with the sigmoid and transverse colon, which have mobile mesenteries.

Proximally, the colon begins at the ileocecal valve and ends at the rectosigmoid junction. This distal point is defined as the site wherein the taeniae coli merge to invest the bowel with a complete outer longitudinal muscle layer.[2] This occurs in the vicinity of the sacral promontory. Histologically, the colonic wall is composed of mucosa, muscularis mucosa, submucosa, circular muscle (mulcularis propria), longitudinal muscle (taenia coli), and serosa.

VASCULATURE

Arterial Supply

The arterial blood supply to the colon is shown in Figure 2–1. Proximal to the mid-transverse colon, the large bowel is supplied by branches of the superior

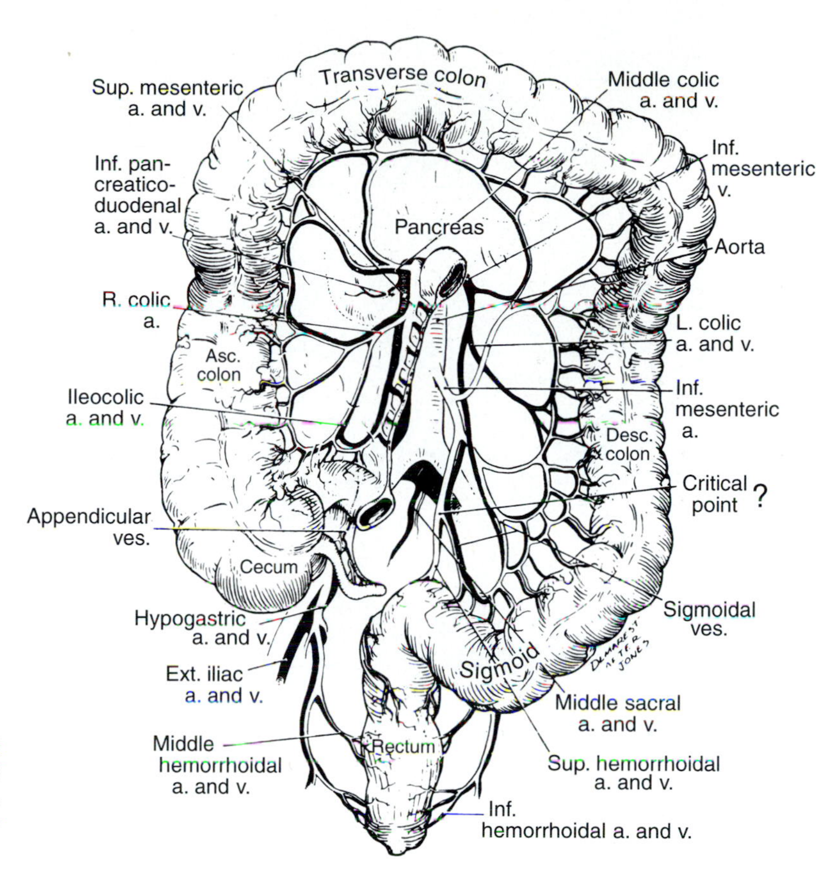

FIGURE 2–1. Anatomic divisions and blood supply of the colon. (From Zuidema, GD: Colon. In Condon, RE (ed.): Shakelfords Surgery of the Alimentary Tract, vol 4. WB Saunders, Philadelphia, 1991, p 10, with permission.)

mesenteric artery; distal to this point, it is supplied by branches of the inferior mesenteric artery. These two mesenteric arteries are connected by the marginal Drummond's artery, which provides collateral blood flow between them in the event one of the arteries is occluded.

Venous Drainage

Except for a slight difference in the course of the inferior mesenteric vein (Fig. 2–1), the veins of the colon accompany their corresponding arteries and drain into the portal circulation.

Lymphatic Drainage

Lymphatic drainage of the colon consists of an intramural network of lymphatic vessels and lymph follicles which lie along the muscularis mucosa; these vessels are interconnected and drain into an extramural network of lymphatic channels and lymph nodes which follow the regional arteries. These colonic lymph nodes have been classified:

1. Epicolic nodes, which lie on the colonic wall
2. Paracolic nodes, which lie along the marginal artery and on the vascular arcades within the mesentery
3. Intermediate nodes, which are near the main colonic arteries
4. Main (principal) nodes, which lie along the origin of the superior and inferior mesenteric arteries[3]

Lymphatics from the ascending and transverse colon reach the superior mesenteric group, whereas the lymphatics from the descending colon, sigmoid colon, and rectum drain into the inferior mesenteric group. The splenic flexure lymphatics may drain in either direction.[4] From the preaortic nodes, drainage is first into the cysterna chyli, then into the thoracic duct.

INNERVATION

The colon is innervated entirely by the autonomic nervous system. It is generally believed that parasympathetic (craniosacral) stimulation increases peristalsis and secretory activity and relaxes the ileocecal and anal sphincters. Sympathetic (thoracolumbar) stimulation has the opposite effect.

Sympathetic Innervation

Sympathetic preganglionic fibers for the proximal colon originate from the intermediolateral neurons of the lower five thoracic segments and the first three lumbar segments for the distal colon and rectum (Fig. 2–2).[4] These fibers pass to the paravertebral ganglia through white rami communicantes, without synapsing therein. Beyond the ganglia, these fibers are gathered into several bundles to form the splanchnic nerves (greater, lesser, least, and lumbar), which

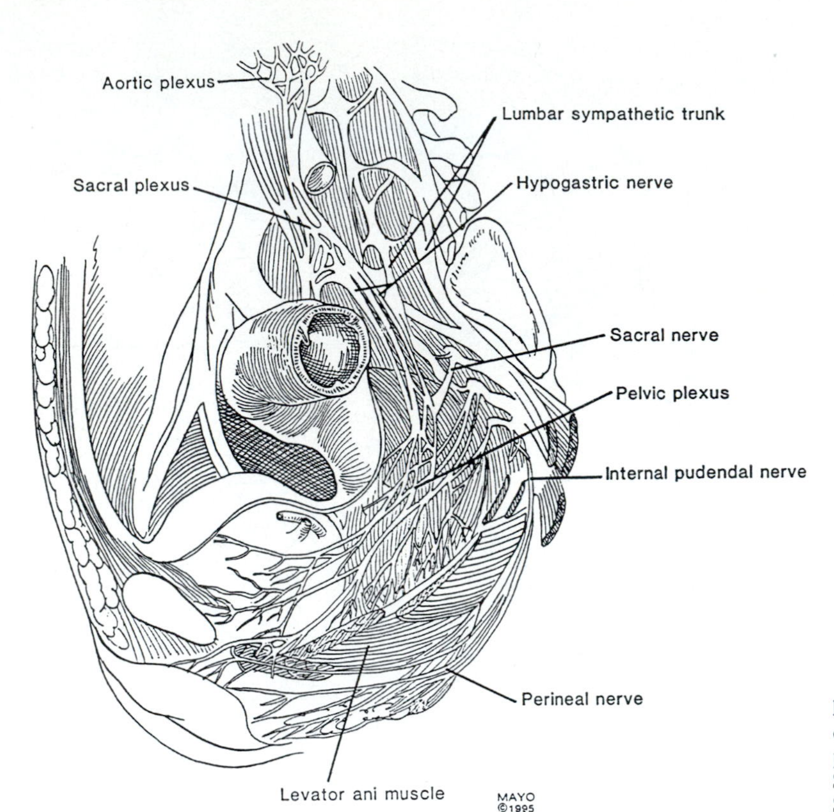

FIGURE 2–2. Innervation of the colon, rectum, and anal canal in women. (From Pemberton, JH: Anatomy and physiology of the anus and rectum. In Condon, RE (ed.): Shakelfords Surgery of the Alimentary Tract, vol 4. WB Saunders, Philadelphia, 1991, p 254, with permission.)

then pass to various plexi and their related ganglia (celiac, superior, and inferior mesenteric) at the roots of the correspondingly named arteries, where they synapse with postganglionic fibers. These postganglionic fibers form mesenteric nerves; their branches pass into the mesocolon and mesorectum. The sympathetic innervation of the proximal half of the colon comes from the celiac and superior mesenteric plexi, whereas the innervation of the distal half of the colon and upper rectum derives mainly from the inferior mesenteric plexus. The presacral (hypogastric) plexus, situated below the bifurcation of the aorta, arises from the preaortic plexus and the two lateral lumbar splanchnic nerves. The plexus thus formed generally diverges caudolaterally along each side of the pelvis (hypogastric nerves), where their nerves join the nervi erigentes to form the pelvic plexi.[5]

Parasympathetic Innervation

The parasympathetic innervation of the proximal colon is derived from the right vagus nerve.[5] Fibers pass to the preaortic and superior mesenteric plexi and accompany branches of the superior mesenteric artery. Parasympathetic innervation of the distal half of the colon and rectum is derived from the nervi erigentes (pelvic splanchnic nerves), which originate from S2-4.[5] Preganglionic fibers of these nerves exit from the ventral roots of the corresponding sacral somatic nerves, join the hypogastric nerves to form the pelvic plexi, and then supply the rectum and upper half of the anal canal (Fig. 2–2). Some fibers ascend through the presacral plexus to accompany the inferior mesenteric artery and supply the distal transverse, descending, and sigmoid colon. Preganglionic fibers entering the colon synapse in ganglia clustered in the myenteric and submucosal plexi within the colonic wall.

STRUCTURE OF THE RECTUM AND ANUS

RECTUM

Anatomists have defined the upper border of the rectum at the third sacral vertebra,[6] but surgeons usually locate it at either the sacral promontory[5] or the point at which the taenia have merged. The rectum has no appendices epiploicae, haustra, or obvious mesentery.[6] At the rectosigmoid junction, the transverse mucosal folds characteristic of the sigmoid colon give way to the smoother rectal mucosa.[7] The rectum follows the sacral curve down to the anorectal ring, which is formed by the puborectalis muscle and the external and internal anal sphincters. Below the anorectal ring, the anal canal turns abruptly downward and posteriorly to terminate at the anal verge.

The rectum has three lateral curves; on their inner aspect are folds known as Houston's valves. These infoldings incorporate all layers of the rectal wall except the outer longitudinal muscle layer. The middle valve is the most consistent and usually marks the location of the anterior peritoneal reflection.[8] Peritoneum covers the exterior surface of the upper third of the rectum completely, except posteriorly in the region of the mesorectum. In the middle third, only the anterior aspect of the rectum is covered by peritoneum; the lower third completely lacks a peritoneal covering. The level of the anterior peritoneal reflection is variable; in women it is located approximately 5 to 7.5 cm above the anal verge.[8] The peritoneum descends onto the rectum from the pelvic sidewalls and reflects anteriorly onto the vagina and uterus.

Fascial Relationships and Attachments

The rectum and mesorectum are enveloped by a thin layer of pelvic fascia, the **fascia propria**. Below the anterior peritoneal reflection, condensations of this fascia on each side of the rectum form the lateral ligaments, attaching the rectum to the pelvic side walls. Accessory branches of the middle rectal artery and autonomic nerves may traverse the lateral ligaments, just above the levator muscles. Posteriorly from the level of the fourth sacral vertebra, the rectosacral fascia (Waldeyer's fascia) courses downward and forward to reflect onto the fascia propria above the anorectal ring (Fig. 2–3*A*).[9] This is an avascular fascial layer of variable thickness, which must be divided during rectal mobilization in transabdominal prolapse repairs (Fig. 2–3*B*). Anteriorly, the extraperitoneal rectum is covered by Denonvilliers's fascia, which extends from the peritoneal reflection downward to the urogenital diaphragm, parallel to the rectum and dorsal to the urogenital structures.[10] In women, this fascia separates the rectum from the vagina. It is thought to represent the obliterated caudal end of the cul-de-sac.

ANAL CANAL

The anal canal extends from the hairy skin of the anal verge up to the anorectal ring. At rest, the lateral walls of the anal canal are opposed, creating an anterior-posterior slit,[11] which is surrounded by the internal and external anal sphincters.

Anal Canal Epithelium

The mucosa immediately above the dentate line is pleated into Morgagni's columns (Fig. 2–4), the lower ends of which are connected by small crescenteric mucosal folds, termed **anal valves** (Ball's anal valves[12]). Within each valve is a crypt to which is connected a variable number of ducts (4 to 10) that traverse the submucosa to terminate in glands located within the submucosa, internal anal sphincter, or the intersphincteric plane (Fig. 2–4). The mucosa extending from the anal valves to the tops of the columns is composed of cuboidal or transitional cells; this area, known as the **anal transition zone (ATZ)**,[13] connects the columnar epithelium of the rectum above to the modified squamous epithelium of the anal verge below.[14] Distal to the anal verge is the stratified squamous epithelium of the perianal skin, which possesses hair and sebaceous, sweat, and apocrine glands. These mucosal boundaries are variable and are not consistently located at the same level within the anal canal.

Musculature of the Anal Canal

The anal canal is enveloped by two muscular cylinders, one surrounding the other. The inner cylinder (internal sphincter) is composed of smooth muscle innervated by the autonomic nervous system; the outer cylinder (the external sphincter) is composed of skeletal muscle with somatic innervation.[15]

Smooth Muscle. The internal sphincter (Fig. 2–5) is the continuation of the circular muscle of the rectum; it terminates 1 to 1.5 cm below the dentate line, but above the end of the external sphincter.[6] The internal

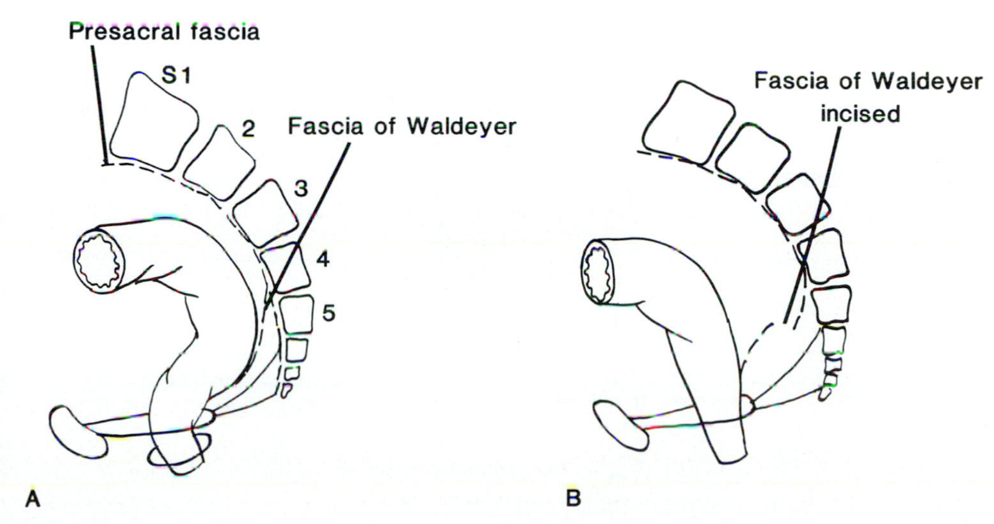

FIGURE 2–3. The presacral fascia and the fascia of Waldeyer. (*A*), Waldeyer's fascia reflects off of the presacral fascia above the anorectal ring. Sharply incising the fascia (*B*) frees the rectum posteriorly, thus facilitating complete mobilization. Blunt dissection of the fascia of Waldeyer at this level may tear the rectum. (From Pemberton, JH: Anatomy and physiology of the anus and rectum. In Condon, RE (ed.): Shakelfords Surgery of the Alimentary Tract, vol 4. WB Saunders, Philadelphia, 1991, p 246, with permission.)

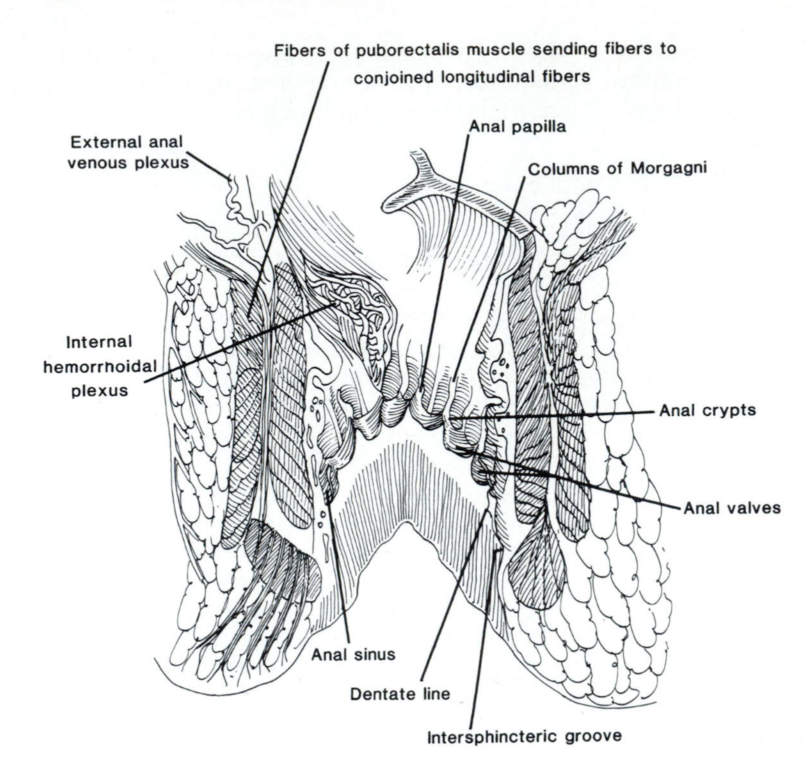

FIGURE 2–4. The anal canal. (From Pemberton, JH: Anatomy and physiology of the anus and rectum. In: Condon, RD (ed.): Shakelfords Surgery of the Alimentary Tract, vol 4. WB Saunders, Philadelphia, 1991, p 248, with permission.)

sphincter is 2.5 to 4 cm in length and 0.5 cm thick. The conjoined longitudinal muscle lies in the intersphincteric plane[16] and is a continuation of the longitudinal muscle of the rectal wall.[4] Inferiorly, these fibers may course through the internal and external anal sphincter to the perianal skin (corrugator cutis ani).

Striated Muscle. The external anal sphincter is continuous with the puborectalis muscle superiorly and consists of deep, superficial, and subcutaneous compartments. The clear separation of the muscle into three distinct parts has been questioned, however, and is rarely, if ever, observed during surgery or cadaveric dissections.[17,18] Posteriorly, the external

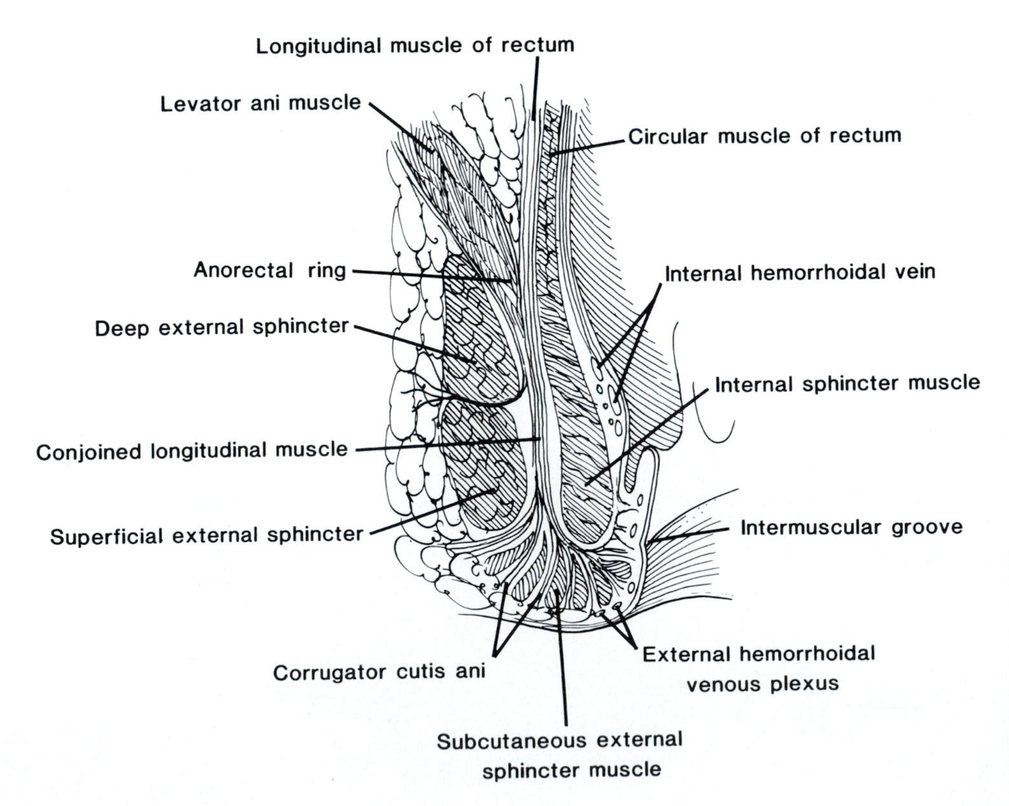

FIGURE 2–5. The voluntary and involuntary muscles of the anorectum and their relationships to the topography of the anal canal. (From Pemberton, JH: Anatomy and physiology of the anus and rectum. In Condon, RE (ed.): Shakelfords Surgery of the Alimentary Tract, vol 4. WB Saunders, Philadelphia, 1991, p 249, with permission.)

sphincter is attached to the skin superficially and to the anococcygeal raphe and coccyx more deeply. Anteriorly, the external anal sphincter is attached to the skin superficially, to the transverse perineus muscle more deeply, and proceeds with the puborectalis muscle toward the pubis at the level of the anorectal ring.

VASCULATURE OF THE RECTUM AND ANUS

Arterial Supply

The major arterial supply to the rectum and anal canal is from the superior and inferior rectal arteries; the middle rectal artery usually has a minor contribution. The superior rectal artery is the terminal branch of the inferior mesenteric artery (Fig. 2–6) and descends to the level of the third sacral vertebra, at which point it bifurcates into right and left branches.[19] The inferior and middle rectal arteries are branches of the internal pudendal artery, which is a branch of the internal iliac artery. The inferior rectal artery traverses the external anal sphincter to reach the submucosa of the anal canal and then ascends in this plane. A large middle rectal artery may be present if the superior rectal artery is small.[20] The middle rectal artery traverses the supralevator space on top of the levator ani musculature, deeper to the levator fascia. The three rectal arteries form an intramural arterial anastomotic network,[8,20] which explains why surgical division of both the superior and middle rectal arteries rarely causes necrosis of the rectum.

Venous Drainage

Venous drainage of the rectum and anal canal follows the arterial supply. The superior rectal vein drains into the portal system, whereas the middle and inferior rectal veins drain into the iliac veins and ultimately into systemic circulation.

Lymphatic Drainage

Lymphatic drainage also follows the route of vascular supply. Drainage from the upper two thirds of the rectum is exclusively to the inferior mesenteric lymph nodes. Lymphatic drainage from the lower third of the rectum and upper anal canal is to both the inferior mesenteric and internal iliac nodes. Drainage below the dentate line is usually to the inguinal lymph nodes but can also occur in a cephalad direction to the inferior mesenteric nodes. Retrograde lymphatic spread of cancer below the level of a rectal tumor occurs only if proximal lymphatic channels are obstructed by tumor.[21] Lymphatic drainage may also occur along the posterior vaginal wall, uterus, broad ligament, ovaries, and cul-de-sac.[22]

INNERVATION OF THE RECTUM AND ANUS

The rectum and anal canal are innervated by autonomic and somatic nerves. Sympathetic stimulation causes inhibition of the rectal smooth muscle and contraction of the internal sphincter, whereas parasympathetic stimulation causes contraction of

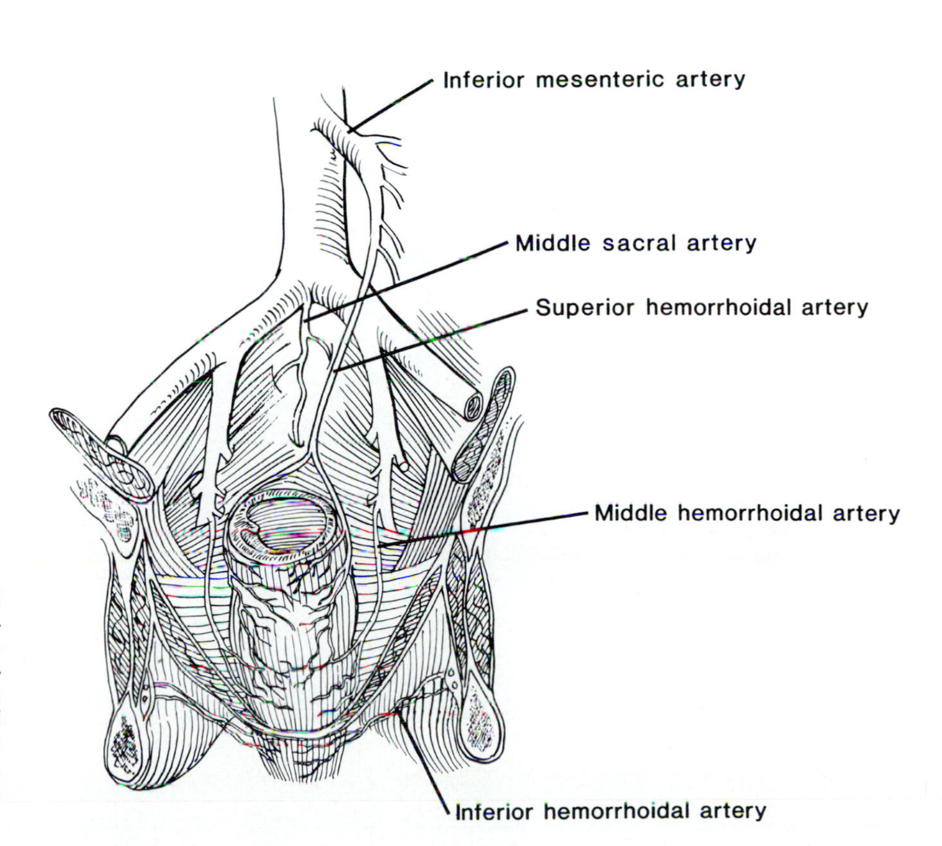

FIGURE 2–6. The vasculature of the rectal and anal canal. Note that the middle hemorrhoidal artery, if present, is small and lies immediately on top of the levator ani musculature, not in the lateral stalks. (From Pemberton, JH: Anatomy and physiology of the anus and rectum. In Condon, RE (ed.): Shakelfords Surgery of the Alimentary Tract, vol 4. WB Saunders, Philadelphia, 1991, p 252, with permission.)

the rectal wall and relaxation of the internal sphincter.

Internal Anal Sphincter

Motor nerves to the internal anal sphincter are derived from both sympathetic (L5 through the presacral plexus) and parasympathetic fibers (S2-4 through the pelvic splanchnic nerves).[7] Contraction of the internal anal sphincter is sympathetically mediated,[23] whereas relaxation in response to rectal distention occurs as part of an intramural (intrinsic) reflex called the **rectoanal inhibitory response**. This response is mediated by nonadrenergic, noncholinergic parasympathetic fibers.

External Anal Sphincter

The motor supply to the external sphincter is from the inferior rectal and perineal branch of the pudendal nerve. A crossover of fibers exists such that unilateral transection of a pudendal nerve does not abolish function of the external sphincter.[11]

Pelvic Floor

The puborectalis is innervated by direct pelvic branches of S3 and S4, by the inferior rectal branch of the pudendal nerve, or by a combination of the two. The pubococcygeus and iliococcygeus muscles are innervated on their superior portions by S4 and on their inferior aspects by perineal branches of the pudendal nerves.

Pudendal Nerve[24]

The pudendal nerve (Fig. 2–7) has both motor and sensory fibers. Its peculiar course may render it susceptible to injury, thus causing fecal and urinary incontinence. It is derived from the pelvic plexus, with fibers originating from S2-4. (The major contribution is from S2.) After the nerve roots traverse the sacral foramen, they divide into somatic and autonomic components. The autonomic branches form the pelvic plexus, which is the primary parasympathetic supply to the pelvic structures. The somatic branches combine to form one major trunk dorsal to the sacrospinous ligament on the coccygeal muscle.[25]

The pudendal nerve trunk then leaves the pelvis through the greater sciatic foramen between the piriformis and coccygeus and enters the gluteal region, crossing the sacrospinous ligament close to its attachment to the ischial spine, where the nerve lies medial to the internal pudendal vessels. The nerve re-enters the pelvis through the lesser sciatic foramen, passing into the pudendal canal (Alcock's canal) on the lateral wall of the ischiorectal fossa, accompanying the internal pudendal artery. In the posterior part of the canal, it first divides into the

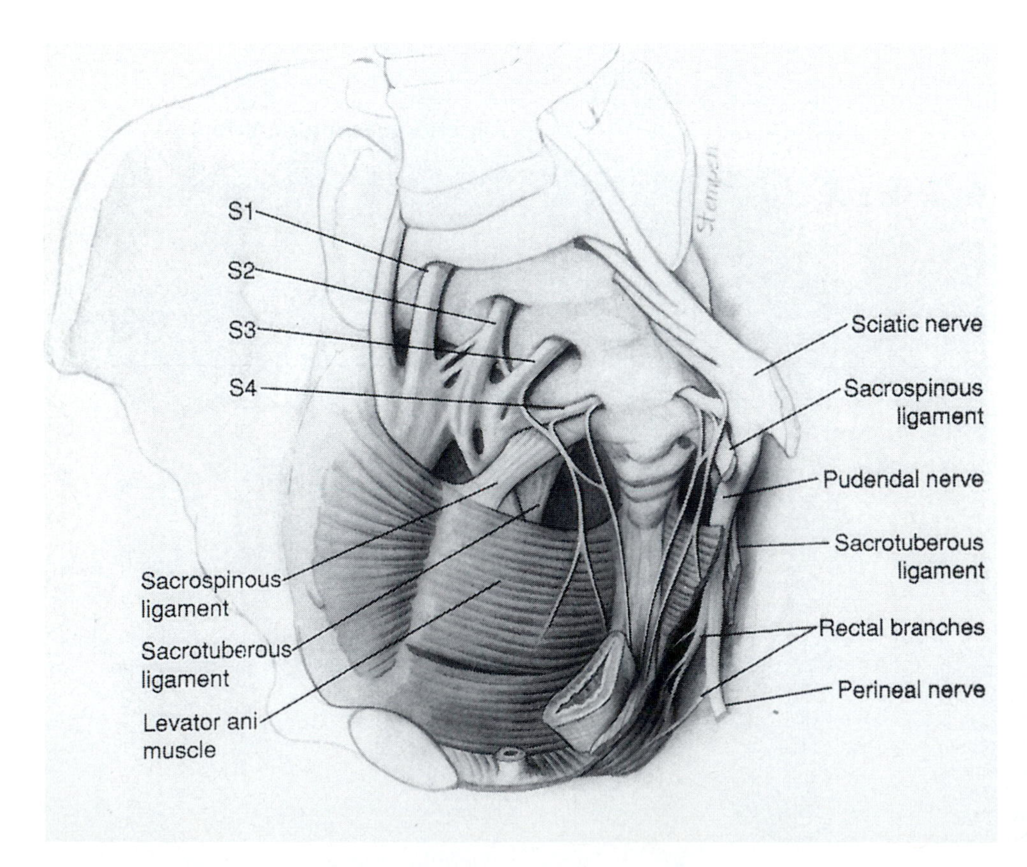

FIGURE 2–7. Origin and course of the pudendal nerve and the direct somatic nerves to the levator ani. To expose the topography of the sacrospinous and sacrotuberous ligament, the coccygeal muscles have not been rendered. Note the location of the pudendal nerve dorsal to the sacrospinous ligament but ventral to the sacrotuberous ligament. Note the two different peripheral nerve supplies of the levator ani and muscular anal canal. (From Matzel, KM, Schmidt, RA and Tanagho, EA: Neuroanatomy of the striated muscular continence mechanism. Dis Colon Rectum 33:668, 1990, with permission.)

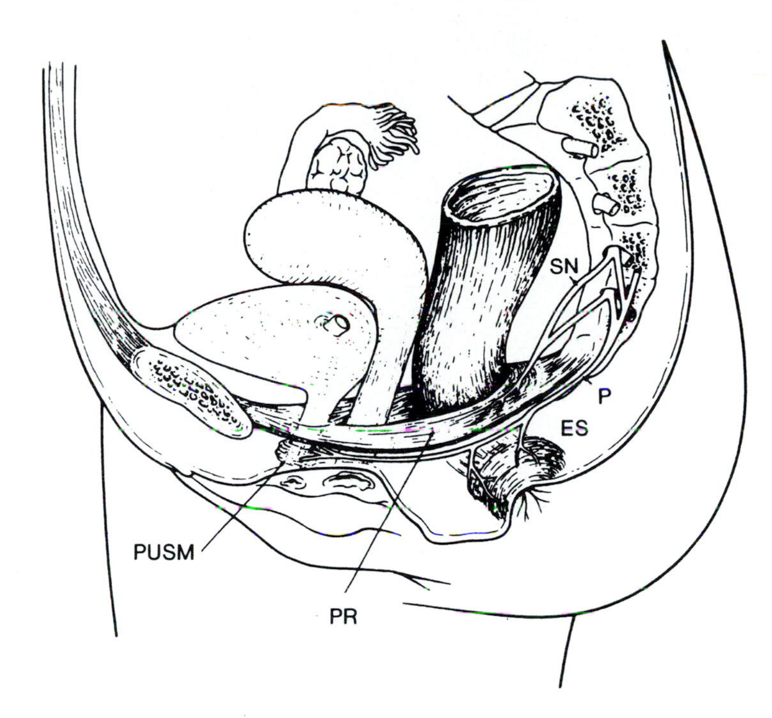

FIGURE 2–8. Sagittal diagram of female pelvis to show innervation of external anal sphincter muscle (ES) by inferior rectal branches; of periurethral striated sphincter muscle (PUSM) by perineal branches of the pudendal nerve (P); and of puborectalis muscle (PR) by direct somatic efferent motor branches from pelvic plexus (SN). (From Laurberg, S, Swash, M, Snooks, SJ, et al.: Neurologic cause of idiopathic incontinence. Arch Neurol 45:1252, 1988. Copyright 1988, American Medical Association, with permission.)

inferior rectal nerve, later into the perineal nerve and the dorsal nerve of the clitoris.[25]

The inferior rectal nerve pierces the medial wall of the pudendal canal, crosses the ischiorectal fossa with the inferior rectal vessels and supplies the external anal sphincter, the lining of the lower part of the anal canal, and the perianal skin (Fig. 2–8). Its branches connect with the labial nerves. Alternatively, the inferior rectal nerve may arise directly from the sacral plexus and may perforate the sacrospinous ligament and reconnect with the pudendal nerve.

The perineal nerve (the inferior and larger terminal branch of the pudendal nerve) passes forward below the internal pudendal artery, dividing into posterior labial and muscular nerve branches. These nerves pierce or pass over the inferior fossa of the urogenital diaphragm and run forward in the lateral part of the urethral triangle with the arteries of the same name, to the skin of the labia and the anterior part of the perineum. The muscular branches innervate the anterior portions of the external anal sphincter, levator ani, superficial transverse perinei muscle, bulbospongiosus, ischiocavernosus, deep transverse perinei muscle, and the urethral sphincter.

The dorsal nerve of the clitoris courses superior to the internal pudendal artery, along the ischial ramus and the margin of the inferior pubic ramus, deep to the inferior fascia of the urogenital diaphragm. Caudally, this small nerve divides into several motor and sensory fibers, supplying the corpus cavernosum of the clitoris. Clinical evidence suggests that the pudendal nerve supplies sensory branches to the lower part of the vagina, probably through fibers in the inferior rectal nerve and posterior labial branches of the perineal nerve.

Sensation

Rectum. Although many nonmyelinated nerve fibers exist, organized endings are generally absent in the rectal mucosa. Receptors for rectal distention likely lie outside the rectal wall itself.[26,27] Sensation from the rectum is carried by parasympathetic nerves S2-4.

Anal Canal. The epithelium of the anal transition zone contains free nerve endings, Meissner's corpuscles (touch), Krause's bulbs (cold), Golgi-Mazzoni bodies (pressure), and genital corpuscles (friction).[28,29] Sensation is carried in the inferior rectal branch of the pudendal nerve.[24]

PARA-ANAL AND PARARECTAL SPACES

Ischiorectal Space

The ischiorectal space (Fig. 2–9) is bounded inferiorly by the perineal skin, anteriorly by the transverse muscles of the perineum, posteriorly by the sacrotuberous ligament and gluteus maximus muscle, medially by the external anal sphincter and levator ani, and laterally by the obturator externus. Within the lateral wall of this space is Alcock's canal, through which course the internal pudendal vessels and the pudendal nerve. The contents of this space include fat, the inferior rectal vessels and nerves, the labial nerves and vessels, and the transverse perineal vessels.

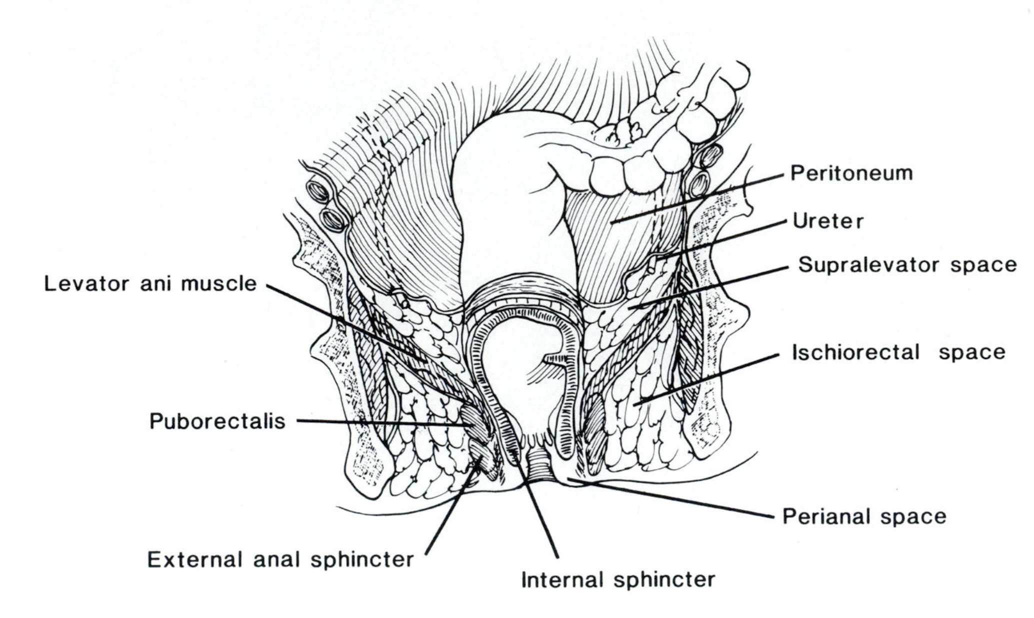

FIGURE 2–9. The para-anal and pararectal spaces. (Coronal view) (From Pemberton, JH: Anatomy and physiology of the anus and rectum. In Condon, RE (ed.): Shakelfords Surgery of the Alimentary Tract, vol 4. WB Saunders, Philadelphia, 1991, p 251, with permission.)

Perianal Space

This space surrounds the anal verge, is continuous with the fat of the buttocks laterally, and extends into the intersphincteric space (Fig. 2–9). It contains the most caudal part of the external anal sphincter, the external hemorrhoidal plexus, and the inferior rectal vessels.

Intersphincteric Space

This space is located between the internal and external sphincter muscles and is continuous with the perianal space.

Supralevator Space

The boundaries of this space (Fig. 2–9 and Fig. 2–10) are the peritoneum superiorly, the obturator fascia laterally, the rectum medially, and the levator plate inferiorly. This space may communicate in a horseshoe shape behind the rectum, deep to the anococcygeal raphe but superficial to the rectosacral fascia.

Superficial Postanal Space

The superficial postanal space (Fig. 2–10) lies under the skin and is superficial to the anococcygeal ligament. It is continuous with the superficial ischiorectal fossa posteriorly.

Deep Postanal Space

The deep postanal space (Fig. 2–10), also known as Courtney's retrosphincteric space, communicates with the deeper parts of the ischiorectal fossa posterior to the anal canal, deep to the anococcygeal ligament but superficial to the levator plate. Horseshoe abscesses generally occur through this space but may also occur in the supralevator and superficial postanal spaces.

Retrorectal Space

The retrorectal space (Fig. 2–10) is cephalad to the rectosacral ligament and continuous with the retroperitoneum above. Its boundaries are the fascia propria of the rectum anteriorly, the presacral fascia posteriorly, and the lateral rectal ligaments. Although this plane is usually avascular, it may occasionally contain a branch of the median sacral artery.

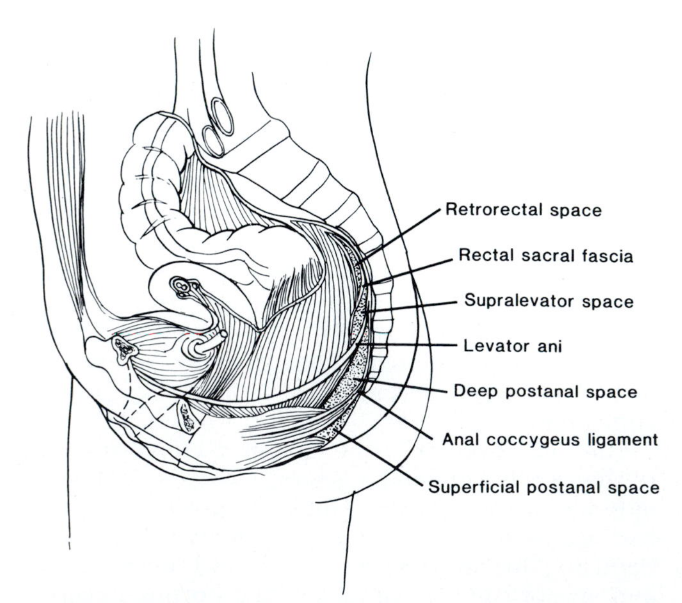

FIGURE 2–10. The posterior pararectal spaces seen in lateral projection. (From Pemberton, JH: Anatomy and physiology of the anus and rectum. In Condon, RE (ed.): Shakelfords Surgery of the Alimentary Tract, vol 4. WB Saunders, Philadelphia, 1991, p 251, with permission.)

FUNCTION OF THE COLON

The human large intestine has three functional regions:

1. Proximally, the cecum and the ascending and transverse colon serve as a site for temporary stasis, absorption, and bacterial fermentation.
2. The distal colon contributes to the formation, containment, and evacuation of solid stools.
3. The anorectal region provides temporary storage, programmed for convenient evacuation.

The major functions of the colon include:

1. Conversion of ileal liquid stool into semisolid feces
2. Conservation of water, sodium, chloride, short-chain fatty acids, and nitrogen substances
3. Secretion of potassium and bicarbonate
4. Propulsion of the luminal contents caudally
5. Storage of feces
6. Participation in defecation.

PRESERVATION OF SODIUM, CHLORIDE, AND WATER

Approximately 1500 mL of fluid enters the colon daily from the terminal ileum; 1350 mL of water, 200 mmol of sodium, 150 mmol of chloride, and 60 mmol of bicarbonate are subsequently absorbed. Most absorption of electrolytes and water occurs in the proximal colon;[29] the distal colon and rectum have considerably less absorptive capability. After passage through the colon, feces have low concentrations of sodium and chloride and higher concentrations of potassium and bicarbonate, relative to plasma.

In the proximal colon, sodium passively moves from the intestinal lumen across the mucosal cell membrane through sodium channels. This movement is driven by electrical and concentration gradients. Sodium is then actively transported from the cell in exchange for potassium across the basolateral membrane, against both electrical and concentration gradients. In the distal colon, sodium absorption is coupled with Na^+–H^+ and Cl^-–HCO_3^- exchanges.[30,31] Sodium is then actively transported through the basolateral membrane by a sodium pump. Chloride is actively absorbed in exchange for HCO_3^- across the apical membrane against a concentration gradient. Then, in contrast to sodium chloride follows its concentration and electrical gradients to exit through the basolateral membrane. The colon, unlike the kidney, has no independent mechanism for active absorption of water; water absorption from the colon is passive, following the osmotic pressure gradient created by sodium absorption.

POTASSIUM SECRETION

The concentration of potassium in stool is higher than in plasma, due to colonic water absorption and net potassium secretion. Active absorption of potassium from the lumen is achieved by a potassium pump linked with an enzyme, H^+-K^+ ATPase, on the luminal membrane of the colonic epithelial cell.[32] Active secretion of potassium depends on the entry of potassium into the cell through the basolateral membrane; this is mediated by either the sodium pump or by an exchange involving sodium and chloride ions. Potassium secretion is enhanced by mineralocorticoids.

ABSORPTION OF NUTRIENTS[30]

Other than salvaging calories from malabsorbed carbohydrate residues, the colon plays little role in digestion. Anaerobic bacteria ferment carbohydrate fragments, thus forming short-chain fatty acids such as acetate, butyrate, and propionate. These constitute the major fecal anions and are readily absorbed. These short-chain fatty acids also have several physiologic effects on the colon: (1) they promote the secretion of bicarbonate and the absorption of sodium, chloride, and water from the colonic lumen;[35] (2) they act as an energy substrate for the colonocytes;[36] and (3) butyrate may have an antineoplastic effect on colonic mucosa.[34]

Long-chain fatty acids are hydroxylated by colonic bacteria and can inhibit colonic absorption and promote secretion of water and electrolytes, thus functioning as laxatives. Some residues of protein digestion are also fermented by anaerobic bacteria into products such as indole, skatole, phenol, cresol, and hydrogen sulfide, which create the characteristic odor of feces. Colonic metabolism of urea produces ammonia, absorption of which occurs by passive coupled nonionic diffusion in which bicarbonate and ammonium ions form ammonia and carbon dioxide.

MOTILITY OF THE COLON

Motor activities of the colon include: (1) mixing of the contents to facilitate transmural exchange and transport of water and electrolytes; (2) propulsion of its contents distally; (3) maintenance of bacterial flora; (4) storage of feces; and (5) rapid emptying of at least part of the colon during defecation.[37] The rate of absorption in the colon is slow, because water absorption passively follows the absorption of sodium and potassium against concentration gradients. Moreover, the absorptive capacity itself is small, due to the absence of villi. Additionally, the process of bacterial fermentation is slow, so that a longer time is required for decomposition to fatty acids. Because of these limitations, colonic motility causes slow net distal propulsion, producing extensive mixing and uniform exposure of its contents to the mucosal surface.[36]

As the colon contracts, a net antegrade flow and mixing are produced. Due to the slowness of these processes and the difficulty in studying them, current clinical understanding is incomplete. Flow has been studied mainly by radiography; three contractile patterns have been observed:

1. Retrograde propulsion: Multiple colonic segments contract as a coordinated unit. This is observed predominantly in the ascending and transverse colon. Contraction originates in the midtransverse colon and may travel retrograde toward the cecum, retarding the aboral progression of feces.[37]
2. Segmental nonpropulsive movements: These are composed of retrograde or antegrade contractions in an isolated segment of the colon. They appear to mix the intraluminal contents and slow the colonic transit. They are observed mainly in the right colon, producing slower transit through the proximal colon when compared with the distal colon.[38]
3. Mass movements: These movements are characterized by propulsion of a large fecal bolus over long segments of the colon. They are infrequent (3 to 4 per day) and occur primarily in the transverse and descending colon, but they may also occur in the sigmoid colon during defecation.[39]

SUMMARY

Knowledge of the structure of the colon, rectum, and anus is of paramount importance for surgeons treating patients with the various disorders discussed in this text. This is especially true in those cases that have failed prior attempts at surgical correction because tissue planes and spatial relationships are frequently the most severely altered. Restoration of normal anatomy is the initial step in regaining normal function, however, it is not the only necessary ingredient. An understanding of normal physiology is important as well.

REFERENCES

1. Gordon, PH and Nivatvongs, S: Surgical anatomy. In Gordon, PH and Nivatvongs, S (eds.): Principles and Practice of Surgery for the Colon, Rectum and Anus. Quality Medical Publishing, St. Louis, 1992, p 3.
2. Fraser, ID, Condon, RE, Schulte, WJ, et al: Longitudinal muscle of muscularis external in human and nonhuman primate colon. Arch Surg 116:61, 1981.
3. Jameson, JK and Dobson, JF: The lymphatics of the colon. Proc R Soc Med (Surg Section) 2:149, 1909.
4. Siddharth, P and Ravo, B: Colorectal neurovasculature and anal sphincter. Surg Clinic North Am 68:1185, 1988.
5. Goligher, JC: Surgery of the anus, rectum and colon, ed 5, Baillière-Tindall, London, 1984, p 1.
6. Symington, J: The rectum and anus. J Anat 23:106, 1889.
7. Wood, BA and Kelly, AJ: Anatomy of the anal sphincters and pelvic floor. In Henry, MM and Swash, M (eds.): Coloproctology and the Pelvic Floor, ed 2. Butterworth-Heinemann, London, 1992, p 3.
8. Goldberg, SM, Gordon, PH and Nivatvongs, S: Essentials of Anorectal Surgery. JB Lippincott, Philadelphia, 1980.
9. Crapp, AR and Cuthbertson, AM: William Waldeyer and the rectosacral fascia. Surg Gynecol Obstet 138:252, 1974. Walsh, PC, Warwick, R, Dyson, M and Bannister, LH (eds.): Campbell's Urology, ed 6. WB Saunders, Philadelphia, 1992, p 3.
10. Phillips, SF and Edwards, DAW: Some aspects of anal continence and defaecation. Gut 6:396, 1965.
11. Williams, PL, et al (eds): Gray's Anatomy, ed 37. Churchill Livingstone, New York, 1989, p 1245.
12. Fenger, C: The anal transitional zone. APMIS 87:379, 1979.
13. Fenger, C: Histology of the anal canal. Am J Surg Pathol 12:41, 1988.
14. Park, AG: Hemorrhoidectomy. Adv Surg 5:1, 1971.
15. Lunniss, PJ and Phillips, RKS: Anatomy and functions of the anal longitudinal muscle. Br J Surg 79:882, 1992.
16. Goligher, JC, Leacock, AG and Brossy, JJ: The surgical anatomy of the anal canal. Br J Surg 43:51, 1955.
17. Oh, C and Kark, AE: Anatomy of the external anal sphincter. Br J Surg 59:717, 1972.
18. Foster, ME, Lancaster, JB and Leaper, DJ: Leakage of low rectal anastomosis: an anatomic explanation? Dis Colon Rectum 27:157, 1984.
19. Ayoub, SE: Arterial supply to the human rectum. Acta Anat (Basel), 100:317, 1978.
20. Quer, EA, Daklin, DC and Mayo, CW: Retrograde intramural spread of carcinoma of the rectum and rectosigmoid: a microscopic study. Surg Gynecol Obstet 96:24, 1953.
21. Block, IR and Enquist, IF: Studies pertaining to local spread of carcinoma of the rectum in females. Surg Gynecol Obstet 112:41, 1961.
22. Burleigh, DE and D'Mello, A: Neural and pharmacologic factors affecting motility of the internal anal sphincter. Gastroenterology 84:409, 1983.
23. Wunderlich, M and Swash, M: The overlapping innervation of the two sides of the external anal sphincter by the pudendal nerves. J Neurol Sci 59:97, 1983.
24. Juenemann, K, et al: Clinical significance of sacral and pudendal nerve anatomy. J Urol 139:74, 1988.
25. Scharli, AF and Kiesewetter, WB: Defecation and continence: some new concepts. Dis Colon Rectum 13:81, 1970.
26. Lane, RHS and Parks, AG: Function of the anal sphincters following colo-anal anastomosis. Br J Surg 64:596, 1977.
27. Duthie, HL and Gairns, FN: Sensory nerve-endings and sensation in the anal region of man. Br Surg 47:585, 1960.
28. Schuster, MM: Motor action of rectum and anal sphincters in continence and defecation. In Cade, CF and Heidel, W (eds.): Handbook of Physiology, vol 4, sect 6: Alimentary Canal. American Physiological Society, Washington, D.C., 1968, p 2121.
29. Pemberton, JH and Phillips, SF: Colonic absorption. Perspect Colon Rectal Surg 1:89, 1988.
30. Sapiro, HM (ed): Clinical gastroenterology, ed 4. McGraw-Hill, New York, 1993, p 503.
31. Binder, HJ, Foster, ES, Budinger, ME, et al: Mechanism of electroneutral sodium chloride absorption in distal colon of the rat. Gastroenterology 93:449, 1987.
32. Sweiry, JH and Binder, HJ: Active potassium absorption in rat distal colon. J Physiol 423:155, 1990.
33. Binder, HJ and Mehta, P: Short-chain fatty acids stimulate active sodium and chloride absorption in vitro in the rat distal colon. Gastroenterology 96:989, 1989.
34. Royall, D, Wolever, TM, Jeejeebhoy, KN, et al: The clinical significance of colonic fermentation. Am J Gastroenterol 85:1307, 1990.
35. Karaus, M and Wienbeck, M: Colonic motility in humans—a growing understanding. Clin Gastroenterol 5:453, 1991.
36. Sarna, SK: Physiology and pathophysiology of colonic motor activity. Dig Dis Sci 36:827, 1991.
37. Elliot, TR and Barclay-Smith, E: Antiperistalsis and other muscular activities of the colon. J Physiol (London) 31:272, 1904.
38. Ritchie, JA: Colonic motor activity and bowel function. Normal movements of contents. Gut 9:442, 1968.
39. Hertz, AF and Newton, A: The normal movements of the colon in man. J Physiol 47:57, 1913.

CHAPTER **3**

Clinically Relevant Neuroanatomy

Linda Brubaker • J. Thomas Benson

Many clinicians do not relish the thought of learning (or relearning) neuroanatomy; however, for proper care of women with pelvic floor disorders, some clinically relevant information must be mastered. A variety of sources present neuroanatomic concepts in detail.[1-3] This chapter broadly presents those concepts that are pertinent to clinicians.

GENERAL TERMINOLOGY

For non-neurologists, neurologic terminology can be intimidating. At a minimum, clinicians must understand several frequently used terms.

The **nervous system** can be divided into two main functional divisions: **motor** and **sensory**. The motor system is further divided into somatic and autonomic divisions. The **somatic** portion innervates the skeletal muscle and the body wall, whereas the **autonomic** portion innervates smooth muscle, glands, and viscera. In addition, nerve fibers receive a further designation regarding "which way" the neural message is being transmitted. Sensory fibers that carry a message to the central nervous system are called **afferent fibers**. The fibers carrying a message from the central nervous system are called **efferent fibers**. Generally, motor fibers are in the efferent system and sensory fibers are in the afferent system.

The sensory (afferent) supply to both visceral and somatic structures is by a similar system whereby the sensory fibers arise from cell bodies located in the dorsal root ganglion. These cells have a single process that divides into a peripheral and a central portion after leaving the cell body. The peripheral portion enters a peripheral nerve; the central portion passes from the dorsal root ganglion to the spinal cord.

The motor (efferent) system is more complicated and differs from the somatic and autonomic. Somatic fibers arise from nerve cell bodies located in the anterior part of the gray matter of the spinal cord, called **anterior horn cells**. A single long axon carries the efferent supply to the skeletal muscle that it innervates. The autonomic efferent fibers arise from nerve cell bodies in the intermediolateral cells column of the spinal cord and travel to their destination by at least a two-neuron chain. The autonomic portion is divided into two subsystems, sympathetic and parasympathetic. Anatomically the sympathetic (thoracolumbar system) fibers originate from the spinal cord and levels T1-L2, whereas the parasympathetic (craniosacral) fibers originate from S2-S4. There are additional cranial outflows which are not reviewed here.

The autonomic fibers that innervate viscera and organs are also called **visceral nerves**. These fibers are also designated according to which way the neural message is being transmitted. Sensory or afferent autonomic fibers carry messages **to** the central nervous system, and motor or efferent autonomic fibers carry messages **from** it.

Normal pelvic floor function depends on intact central and peripheral nervous systems, including both somatic and autonomic components. Although the brain and spinal cord are important in the regulation of pelvic floor function, the principal abnormalities dealt with in the clinical setting deal with the peripheral nerves of the pelvic floor. A peripheral nerve consists of an outside lining (epineurium) (Fig. 3–1) covering the entire nerve. Inside the epineurium are fascicles, which are lined by perineurium. At the core is the endoneurium and the individual nerve fibers. These nerve fibers vary greatly in size and myelination.

Large nerves typically provide somatic efferent, as well as sensory afferent, innervation for the muscles. Such nerves are usually myelinated and conduct neural impulses quickly. Touch and pressure receptors from the surface are also served by large, fast-conducting fibers. In contrast, autonomic nerves and nerves that provide pain and temperature sensation are the small, slow-conducting, lightly myelinated or unmyelinated nerves.

Myelinated nerves have a myelin sheath surrounding each nerve fiber. Larger fibers typically have more myelin. Small gaps between myelinated areas are called **Ranvier's nodes**. By contrast, unmyelinated nerve fibers share a single neurilemma (sheath) and are much smaller in diameter. Figure 3–2 shows both myelinated and unmyelinated fibers in a biopsy from a human female urethra.

The function of the nerve fiber is related to its size. Large myelinated fibers conduct very rapidly (velocities reaching 120 m/sec), whereas other myelinated nerves are smaller and conduct more slowly. The smallest myelinated and unmyelinated nerves conduct as slowly as 2 m/sec.

MECHANISMS OF INJURY

Many processes can damage nerves or the supporting structures of nerves. There can be damage to the myelin sheath, the nerve axon, or both. Common clinical examples of such processes include diabetes, alcoholism, nutritional deficiencies, inflammations, and toxic agents. In the pelvis, however, the most common form of nerve damage is mechanical, with direct damage to the nerve or supporting structures.

PUDENDAL NERVE

The pudendal nerve originates from sacral segments S2, S3, and S4 and is a *mixed* nerve, meaning that it contains both afferent and efferent fibers. The sacral roots join together to form this peripheral nerve, which then exits the pelvis through the

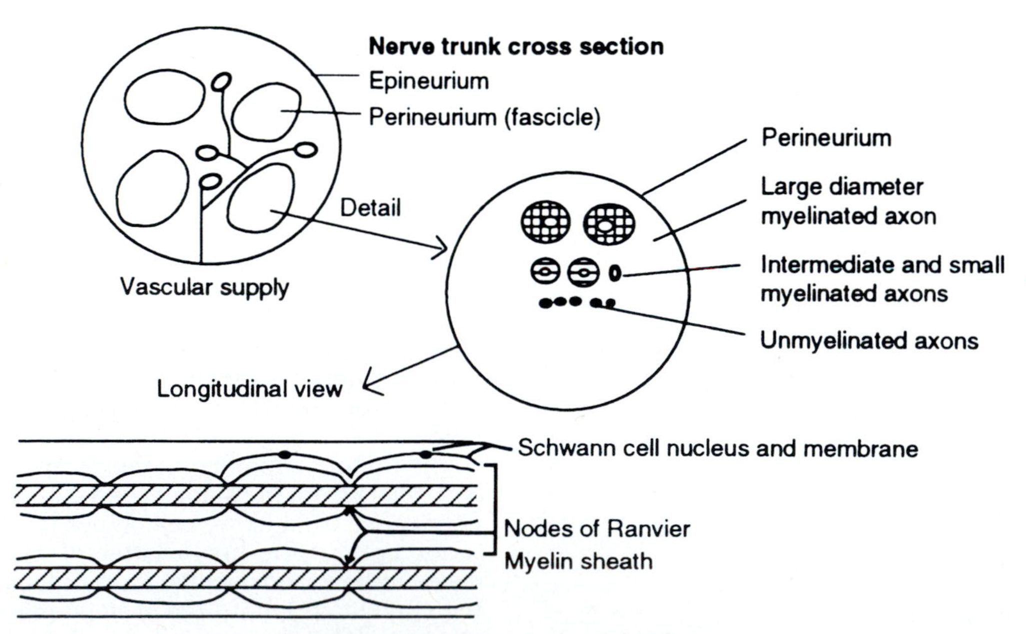

FIGURE 3–1. The anatomy of peripheral nerve.

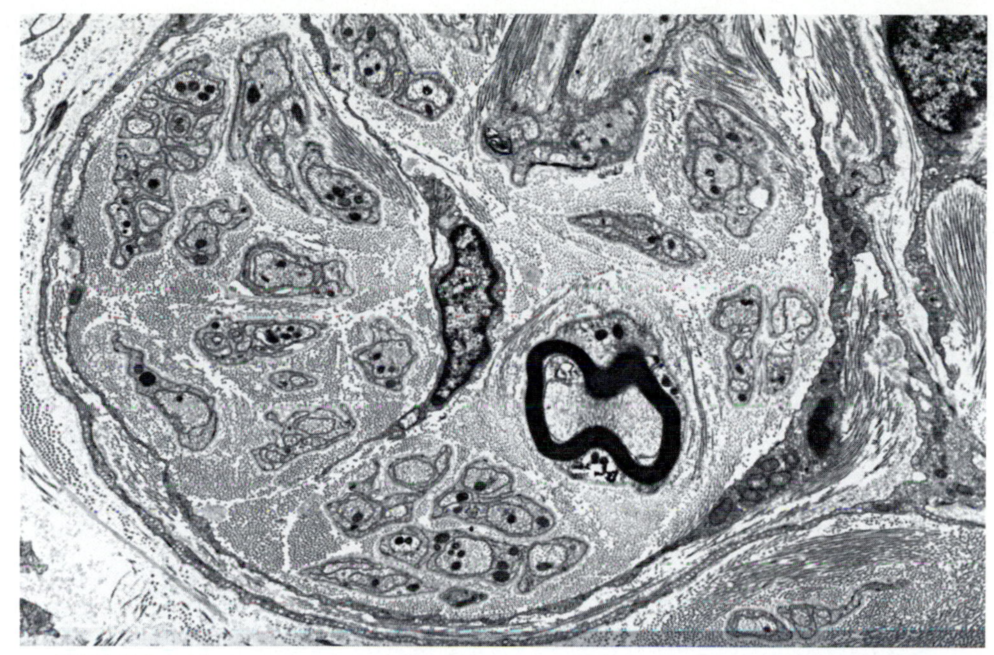

FIGURE 3–2. Myelinated and unmyelinated fibers in a biopsy from a human female urethra.

greater sciatic foramen. The nerve then loops around the ischial spine to re-enter the pelvis through the lesser sciatic foramen. The pudendal nerve then travels along the internal surface of the obturator internus muscle and traverses a split in the fascia known as **Alcock's canal.** This fascial tunnel is the putative site of injury during vaginal childbirth.[4-7] Confirmation of this hypothesis awaits scientific study. Following its exit from Alcock's canal, the pudendal nerve splits into three terminal portions: (1) the dorsal nerve of the clitoris; (2) the perineal branch, supplying the urethral sphincter, perineal muscles, and perineal sensation; and (3) the inferior hemorrhoidal nerve, supplying the external anal sphincter skeletal muscle and the sensation in the perianal area. This is further described in Chapters 1 and 2. Injuries to the pudendal nerve can be unilateral or bilateral.

PELVIC PLEXUS

The pelvic plexus is also an important neuroanatomic area for pelvic surgeons to understand. When the parasympathetic sacral nerves reach the pelvis, they are joined by visceral branches of the sympathetic nerves from the thoracic and first two lumbar spinal cord segments, thus forming the pelvic plexus. These nerves spread out anteriorly to the sacrum, surround the rectum, and go deep into the endopelvic fascia to supply the viscera. These delicate nerves travel in areas in surgical planes where they are difficult to visualize and prone to injury during pelvic surgical procedures (Fig. 3–3).

CAUDA EQUINA

During early development and growth, the vertebral column outgrows the bony spinal column (Fig. 3–4). In adulthood, the spinal column terminates at about the level of the L1 vertebra. Below the L1 level, ventral and dorsal nerve roots must travel all the way to the correct vertebral foramen. The peripheral nerve is then formed when the ventral and dorsal roots combine on exiting the foramen. Thus, the nerve roots of the lower lumbar and sacral nerves, which supply the pelvis, travel all the way from the

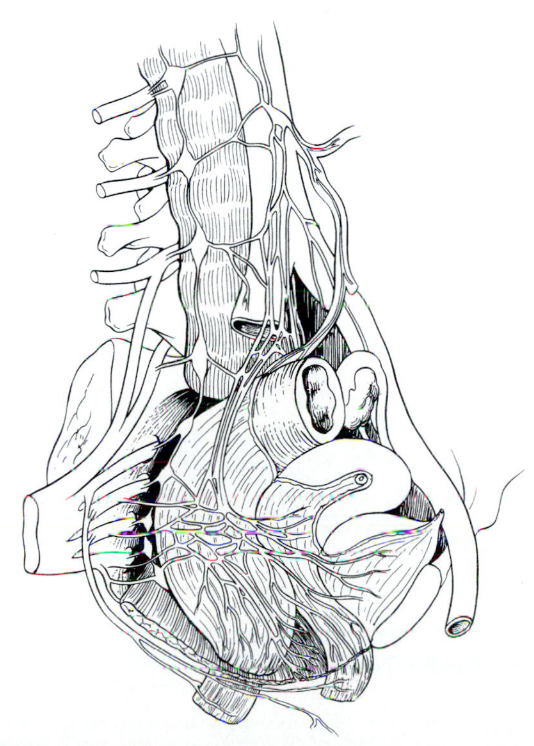

FIGURE 3–3. The pelvic plexus as it relates to pelvic viscera in the female.

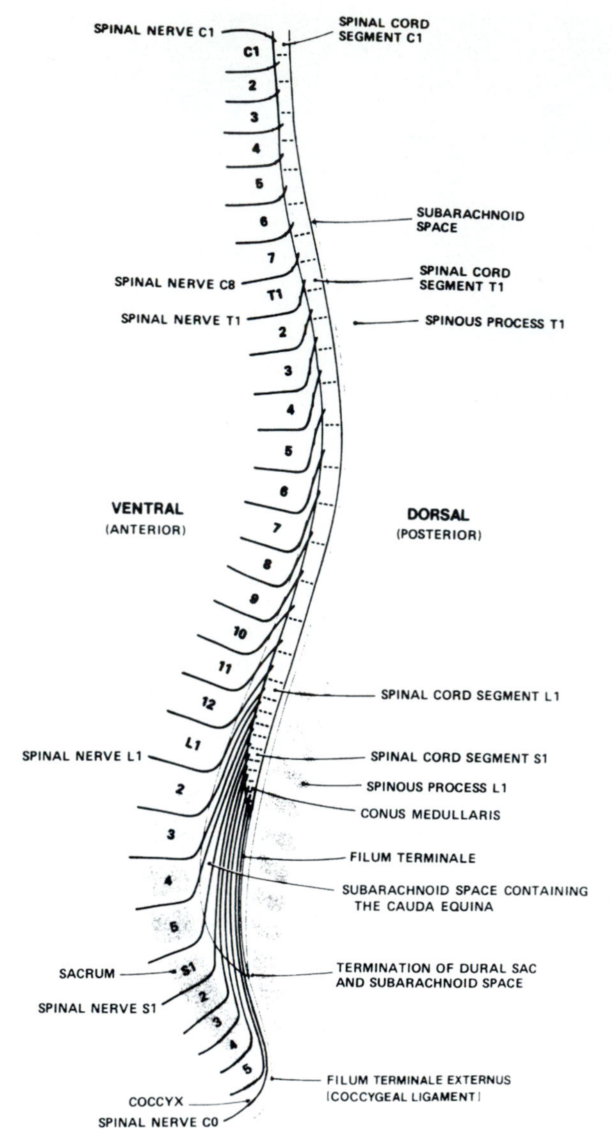

FIGURE 3–4. The bony vertebral column is longer than the spinal cord. Note the relationship of the conus medullaris and cauda equina. Source: Gilman S, Newman SW (eds): Manter and Gatz's Essentials of Clinical Neuroanatomy and Neurophysiology, Ed. 8. FA Davis, Philadelphia, 1992, p 11, with permission.

L1 vertebra to their specific exit foramen (e.g., S2, S3 and S4). This portion of the cord is called the **cauda equina**, the "horse's tail." In this area these nerve roots are particularly subject to damage from disk disease, inflammatory disease, and obstructive disease.

CLINICAL EFFECTS OF NEUROANATOMIC LESIONS

Muscle tone is a primary factor providing the pelvic floor with support; it is maintained by skeletal muscle reflex. Muscle spindles give rise to large, fast-conducting afferent fibers that carry a message through the peripheral nerve and enter the dorsal root. In the spinal cord a synaptic connection is made with an alpha motor neuron. The axon of this motor neuron goes through the ventral root and through the peripheral nerve to the extrafusal muscle fibers of the target muscle.

A lesion affecting the ventral root of the peripheral nerve will lead to motor loss of the skeletal muscle as well as significant atrophy and loss of contractility. A lesion affecting the dorsal root leads to loss of tone in the muscle while maintaining voluntary contractility. Thus, it is easy to see how nerve disease affecting the peripheral nerve or the nerve roots in the cauda equina can have significant impact on pelvic muscular support.

URINARY INCONTINENCE

The central nervous system has a significant relationship to urinary function. The **pons** (a brainstem structure) is the main connection between the brain and the spinal cord. The pons plays a critical role in coordinating lower urinary tract function. Lesions above the pons can affect two important centers in the cerebral cortex, the detrusor center and the pudendal center. Lesions affecting pathways from the specialized detrusor cortical center to the pons prevent the patient from being able to suppress a coordinated detrusor contraction voluntarily. Lesions in the pudendal cortical centers prevent relaxation of the external skeletal sphincter system and may also affect voluntary contraction of the sphincter.

Lesions below the pons and above the sacral cord may cause a loss of coordination of bladder and urethral sphincter. Clinically, detrusor hyperreflexia may be associated with discoordinate periurethral skeletal muscle contraction, the so-called **detrusor sphincter dyssynergia**. This diagnosis is pathognomonic for a spinal cord lesion.

Lesions in the sacral area can give rise to complex patterns of disturbance because the pudendal motor supply, the parasympathetic supply (which drives bladder contraction), and the afferent supply to the lower urinary tract are all centered in the sacral area. Lesions involving the cauda equina give effects similar to those produced by lesions involving the terminal portion of the spinal cord; the effects can be predominantly motor or sensory. The motor effects typically create a contracted, trabeculated bladder with decreased compliance, whereas the sensory effects give loss of sensation and increased compliance and capacity, frequently resulting in the overflow type of incontinence.

The etiology of genuine stress urinary incontinence has a major neurologic component. So-called **transference** of increased abdominal pressure to the urethra, such as with cough or stress, actually results from reflex skeletal muscle activity in the periurethral musculature. This reflex can be blocked with pudendal nerve blockade. Electrodiagnostic abnormalities in the perineal branch of the pudendal nerve are universally found in patients with genuine stress urinary incontinence[6,7] and in patients with severe neuropathic involvement, such as following repeated surgeries around the urethra.[8]

INABILITY TO VOID AND VOIDING DYSFUNCTION

Neuropathic changes in the peripheral innervation of the bladder may lead to detrusor areflexia. The most common cause is autonomic neuropathy due to diabetes. Other processes involving the cauda equina are also seen clinically.

Voiding dysfunction may also be seen following ganglionic damage within the wall of the bladder after marked overdistention, or after postoperative pelvic plexus disruption such as commonly occurs following rectal resection or radical hysterectomy. In the latter case, interference with the primarily parasympathetic detrusor activity exists.

Patients who present with the inability to void with no obvious neurologic stigmata are often found to have localized neuropathy involving the skeletal musculature of the periurethral area on electrodiagnostic study of this musculature. Over 90% of women with sustained retention without obvious neurologic or obstructive etiology are found to have evidence of neuromuscular involvement in this area.[9]

FECAL INCONTINENCE

Proper control of bowel activity requires storage in the rectum, sampling of bolus contents (gas, liquid, solid stool) in the anal canal, and elective skeletal muscle contraction to return fecal contents back to the rectal reservoir. This requires proper function of both the internal and the external anal sphincters. Sensory nerve function in the anal canal is provided by both pudendal and visceral afferent nerves. The internal anal sphincter (smooth muscle) constitutes approximately 70% of the closing pressure of the anal sphincter mechanism; it is kept in constant tone primarily by its sympathetic nervous system activity. The parasympathetic system causes relaxation, in contrast to the effects of the parasympathetic system on the rest of the enteric tract, where contraction (peristalsis) occurs.

Obstructed defecation is found in situations of failure of cooperative activity between pelvic floor relaxation and efforts at the Valsalva maneuver. Fecal incontinence can result from neuropathies involving either sensory, autonomic, or somatic neurogenic mechanisms.

SEXUAL DYSFUNCTION

Although the sexual response has been studied more extensively in the male, the neurologic basis for the female sexual response has many similarities. Both the sympathetic and parasympathetic systems affect blood vessels, erectile tissue, and smooth muscle in the vagina. During sexual stimulation, clitoral erection occurs because of blood pooling in the cavernosal tissue. Bulbocavernosus muscle tissues with fibers passing forward on each side of the vagina cover bulbs of the vestibule and attach anteriorly to the corpora cavernosa of the clitoris. Contraction of the anterior fibers and the small ischial cavernosus muscle contributes to erection by compression of the deep dorsal vein. The expansion of sinusoids with blood compresses veins against the tunica albuginea, partially occluding them and thus reducing venous outflow. Thus, a venous occlusion occurs passively.

Detumescence results from contraction of the smooth muscle of the arteries and reduction of blood flow to the lacunar spaces. Such contraction is largely a sympathetic effect. During orgasm, a rhythmic contraction of these muscles involving the somatic system is present. Thus, parasympathetic, sympathetic, and somatic systems are intimately involved in the sequence of events. Peripheral neuropathy can cause sexual dysfunction with difficulty with arousal or orgasm. Pelvic surgical procedures can damage the autonomic nerves in the pelvis and affect sexual function as well. In addition, a variety of drugs can reduce libido and affect the orgasmic response.

NEUROPATHIC PELVIC PAIN SYNDROMES

As with pain syndromes in other parts of the body, the patient with pelvic pain represents a distressing situation characterized by inaccurate diagnoses, multiple operative attempts at relief, and an excessive rate of failed therapy. The modern concept of neuropathic pain is divided into so-called "hot" and "cold" pain syndromes. Evaluation and diagnosis depends on taking a careful history and giving a complete physical examination, including determining the patient's response to both hot and cold stimuli, mechanical stimuli, and measurement of sweating, temperature, vasodilatation, and vasoconstriction.

The "hot" pain syndrome is explained by **ABC** or **a**ngry, **b**ackfiring, **c** nociceptors. These tiny unmyelinated nerves have antidromic stimulation, giving rise to burning pain. The condition parallels response to the local application of capsaicin. Typically, the area involved is red, warm, and has hyperesthesia to both mechanical and warm thermal stimuli. It is relieved by cold.

The "cold" pain syndrome is apparently due to denervation; subsequently the blood vessels become acutely sensitive to neurotransmitters and constrict. The denervation may be extensive enough that no dilatation of the pale, cold, vasoconstricted area occurs with nerve block. These patients have decreased cold sensation and hyperesthesia to mechanical and cold thermal stimuli. The pain is perceived as burning. Patients who get some relief with nerve block may be improved by vasodilation that occurs after sympathectomy.

SUMMARY

It is apparent that a variety of central and peripheral neuroanatomic lesions can give rise to clinically apparent pelvic floor disorders. Although neuroanatomy is a broad field which is undergoing a great deal of evolution, the clinician caring for a patient with pelvic floor disorders should understand the concepts that have been discussed in this chapter.

REFERENCES

1. Torrens, M and Morrison, JFB (eds.): The Physiology of the Lower Urinary Tract, Springer-Verlag, London, 1987.
2. Krane, RJ and Siroky, MB (eds.): Clinical Neuro-urology, ed 2. Little, Brown & Co, Boston, 1991.
3. Gilman, S and Newman, SW (eds.): Manter and Gatz's Essentials of Clinical Neuroanatomy and Neurophysiology, ed 8. FA Davis, Philadelphia, 1992.
4. Swash, M: The neurogenic hypothesis of stress incontinence. In: Neurobiology of Incontinence (Ciba Foundation Symposium 151). Wiley, Chichester, 1990, pp 156–175.
5. Swash, M, Snooks, SJ, Henry, MM et al. A unifying concept of pelvic floor disorders and incontinence. J R Soc Med 78:906–911, 1985.
6. Smith, ARB, Hosker, GL and Warrell, DW: The role of pudendal nerve damage in the etiology of genuine stress incontinence in women. Br J Obstet Gynecol 96:29–32, 1989.
7. Smith, ARB, Hosker, GL and Warrell, DW: The role of partial denervation of the pelvic floor in the etiology of genitourinary prolapse and stress incontinence of urine: a neurophysiological study. Br J Obstet Gynecol 96:24–28, 1989.
8. Benson, JT and McClellan, E: The effect of vaginal dissection on the pudendal nerve. Obstet Gynecol 82:387–389, 1993.
9. Fowler, CJ, Kirby, RS and Harrison, MJG: Decelerating bursts and complex repetitive discharges in the striated muscle of the urethral sphincter associated with urinary retention in women. J Neurol Neurosurg Psychiatry 48:1004–1009, 1985.

SECTION TWO

PRELIMINARY EVALUATION

CHAPTER 4

Initial Evaluation and Physical Examination

B. L. Shull

Initial evaluation of women who complain of disorders of the pelvic floor should include screening for risk factors related to cancer of the breasts, colon and rectum, and the female reproductive system. Patients with complaints suspicious for a malignant neoplasm should have those complaints thoroughly evaluated before a surgical management plan for the specific floor problem is instituted. In the absence of such complaints, the American Cancer Society has formulated a list of recommendations for the early detection of cancer in *asymptomatic* women. You should determine which screening tests are appropriate for your patient (Table 4–1).[1]

Initial evaluation and ultimate development of a management plan requires the physician to be a good listener, organized questioner, and accurate observer. Pelvic floor complaints are often complex because even though each of the pelvic organs has its own specific visceral or sexual function, they are in such close physical proximity that poor support or poor innervation for one organ is often associated with poor support or innervation for adjacent organs. Evaluation begins by listening and asking, looking and touching, and finally prioritizing a list of patient complaints and expectations of therapy as she herself perceives them. This priority list is useful to the clinician to decide which diagnostic tests are indicated and which therapeutic interventions are appropriate for a specific patient. A successful management plan for disorders of the pelvic floor requires this comprehensive approach, otherwise the opportunities for effective treatment are compromised.

HISTORY

Certain pelvic floor complaints result exclusively from poor support. The woman may feel well when she is lying down and have few complaints soon after arising, but the longer she stays erect, the more both-

TABLE 4–1. Summary of American Cancer Society Recommendations for the Early Detection of Cancer in Asymptomatic, Low-Risk People

Test or Procedure	Population: Age (y)	Population: Frequency
Sigmoidoscopy preferably flexible*	50 and over	Every 3 to 5 years
Fecal occult blood test	40 and over	Every year
Digital rectal examination	40 and over	Every year
Pap test	All women who are or have been sexually active, or have reached age 18, should have an annual Pap test and pelvic examination. After a woman has had three or more consecutive satisfactory normal annual examinations, the Pap test may be performed less frequently at the discretion of her physician.	
Pelvic examination	18–40 Over 40	Every 1–3 years with Pap test Every year
Endometrial tissue sample	At menopause, women with high risk†	At menopause
Breast self-examination	20 and over	Every month
Clinical breast examination	20–40 Over 40	Every 3 years Every year
Mammography‡	40–49 50 and over	Every 1–2 years Every year

*These are recommendations for asymptomatic *low-risk* people. Patients at high risk, such as those with ulcerative colitis or a strong family history of colorectal cancer or polyposis, should be screened with colonoscopy, even if asymptomatic.
†History of infertility, obesity, failure to ovulate, abnormal uterine bleeding, or estrogen therapy.
‡Screening mammography should begin by age 40 years.

ersome the complaints become. Typically she describes "a sense of things falling out," pelvic pressure or heaviness, a low backache, or the sense of sitting on something. It is helpful to document the duration of the complaints and whether they are stable, improving, or worsening. Document the extent to which these complaints alter her lifestyle; this may be the reason she chooses a conservative over a more aggressive management plan.

Symptoms of pelvic organ prolapse can also affect her sexual activity, because her sexual partner is concerned that foreplay or intravaginal intercourse is painful or dangerous. Specific information about the frequency of intravaginal intercourse as well as her desire to maintain or enhance the ability to have intravaginal intercourse is necessary in formulating a management plan.

UROGENITAL HISTORY

A recent set of clinical practice guidelines emphasizes the importance of the history in the basic evaluation of women with incontinence (see Table 4–2).[2] Open-ended questions such as "Do you have trouble with your bladder?" and "Do you have trouble holding your urine?" may be perceived by the patient as nonthreatening. Specific questions such as "Do you ever lose urine when you do not want to?" and "Do you ever wear a pad or other protective device to collect your urine?" may help you to learn the social impact of her complaints. You may find it helpful to ask your patients to record a urinary diary for several days prior to their visit (Table 4–3)[3] or to respond to a specific questionnaire (Table 4–4).[4] A number of transient causes of incontinence (Table 4–5) may respond to specific therapy. Alpha blockers, for example, reduce intraurethral pressure, leading to drug-induced stress incontinence.

PHYSICAL EXAMINATION

GENERAL EXAMINATION

The general examination addresses factors outside the pelvic floor that have a direct impact on pelvic floor function (Table 4–6). The patient's cognitive skills affect her social inhibitions as well as her ability to participate in the evaluation or execution of the management plan. Lack of normal mobility or manual dexterity adversely affects the patient's ability to care for her own personal hygiene, including bowel and bladder function. Even in the patient who is functionally independent, limitations in mobility or manual dexterity create significantly longer delays from the first urge to void or defecate until she can reasonably reach the toilet facility and undress herself. Dependent edema may be associated with nocturia or nocturnal enuresis. Abnormalities on a neurologic examination may suggest multiple sclerosis, stroke, or other neurologic diseases. Identification of any of these extrapelvic disorders will affect the development of a long-term management plan for pelvic organ prolapse and pelvic floor dysfunction.

PELVIC EXAMINATION

A detailed pelvic examination is critically important in developing a comprehensive management

TABLE 4–2. History: Basic Evaluation of Incontinence

Duration and characteristics of urinary incontinence (stress, urge, dribbling, other)
Frequency, timing, and amount of continent or incontinent voids
Precipitants and associated symptoms of incontinence (e.g., situational antecedents, cough, surgery, injury, trauma, new onset of diseases, and new medications)
Other lower urinary tract symptoms (e.g., nocturia, dysuria, hematuria)
Fluid intake pattern, including caffeinated or alcoholic beverages
Alterations in bowel habit or sexual function
Prior treatment and its effect on urinary incontinence
Use of pads, briefs, or other protective devices

TABLE 4–3. Bladder Record for Office Patients

Patient Name ______________________ Date __________

Instructions

Column 1–Please record the time you void–indicate when you get up and when you go to bed.
Column 2–Please record your fluid intake in ounces.
Column 3–Please record the volume you void in ounces. You can collect the urine in a measuring cup.
Column 4–Place a check next to the time an incontinent episode occurred and estimate the amount of leakage as follows:

+ means the leakage was just a few drops
++ means the leakage was enough to wet your underwear
+++ means the leakage was enough to run down your legs

Column 5–Note pad changes.
Column 6–Note any activity that may be associated with the incontinence, such as sneezing, coughing, lifting something heavy, "Couldn't make it to the bathroom," standing up after sitting a while, hand washing, or bed wetting.

Column 1	Column 2	Column 3	Column 4	Column 5	Column 6
Time Interval	Fluid Intake Ounces	Volume Voided Ounces	Had an Incontinent Episode	Changed a Wet Pad	Activity Associated with Incontinent Episode (Comments)
TOTALS					

plan for the patient with disorders of pelvic floor function and support. When the treatment strategy focuses exclusively on the support or function of one organ, long-term success for the function and support of the entire pelvic floor is unlikely. For instance, Dr. Burch reported in his first description of the colposuspension operation that although 100% of his patients were symptomatically relieved of their complaints of urinary incontinence, 8% had postoperative evidence of an enterocele.[5] Similarly, Wiskind, Creighton, and Stanton reported a series of 131 patients who had a Burch colposuspension for the treatment of urinary incontinence.[6] Although 82% of these patients were cured of stress incontinence, 27% required subsequent surgery to correct genital prolapse after the colposuspension.

Brubaker and Norton reviewed the English language literature for the period 1966 to 1990 to document the clinical classification or nomenclature for description of pelvic support defects. They concluded no universally accepted method exists for performing the pelvic examination or for reporting the physical findings.[7] The International Continence Society, the American Urogynecologic Society, and the Society of Gynecologic Surgeons are collaborating to develop recommendations to standardize terminology for pelvic organ prolapse. A standardized system for describing pelvic organ prolapse has recently been adopted by the International Continence Society (Appendix A).

Consensus is growing that the physical examination should be performed in such a way that support

TABLE 4–4. Questionnaire for Women with Incontinence

Do you lose urine by spurts during coughing, sneezing, or lifting? (*stress incontinence*)

Do you ever have an uncomfortably strong need to urinate and feel you will leak urine if you do not go to the bathroom immediately? (*sensory urgency*)

If "yes," do you ever leak before you reach the toilet? (*motor urge incontinence*)

How many times during the day do you urinate? (*frequency*)

How many times do you void during the night after going to bed? (*nocturia*)

Have you wet the bed in the past year? (*bed-wetting*)

When you are passing urine, can you usually stop the flow?

Do you ever leak during sexual intercourse?

Do you have pain or burning when you urinate? (*dysuria*)

Do you have blood in your urine? (*hematuria*)

Do you have difficulty intiating voiding or do you need to strain to empty your bladder?

After voiding, do you feel that your bladder is empty? (*postvoid fullness*)

TABLE 4–6. Physical Examination

General Examination: cognition, mobility, manual dexterity, edema, neurologic impairment

Abdominal Examination: masses, suprapubic tenderness

Pelvic Examination: perineal skin, genital atrophy, pelvic organ prolapse, muscle tone, vaginal capacity, bladder neck hypermobility

Rectal Examination: perineal sensation, sphincter tone (resting and active), bulbocavernosus reflex, fecal impaction, rectal mass

for individual sites in the vagins can be evaluated. The examination is generally performed with the patient recumbent on the examination table and straining as each site is evaluated. The single blade of a speculum is used to retract the posterior segment of the vagina, and as the patient strains, the anterior segment, comprising the urethra and bladder, can be evaluated. The speculum is then turned to retract the anterior segment while the cul-de-sac and rectum are evaluated. After determining which sites have poor support, the clinican ought to ask the patient to look with a hand held mirror to confirm that what she has previously seen or felt is the same as is presently seen. If not, the examination is repeated as she stands and strains. The standing position offers the advantage of assessing pelvic organ support with greater stress; practically, however, it is difficult to identify individual sites in the vagina with the patient erect. I prefer to examine the patient in the lithotomy position, with her bladder empty.

Objective classification of pelvic organ prolapse presupposes a knowledge of normal support. No objective data are available, at present, regarding normal support in women of different ages, childbearing histories, and surgical histories, nor do we have information directly correlating physical findings with subjective or objective measurements of pelvic organ function; therefore, clinicians are required to describe the physical findings as clearly as possible without assigning degrees of severity or presuming that certain symptoms are uniformly associated with specific physical findings. Every experienced clinician has examined patients who have poor support for one or more pelvic organs but who have no functional complaints and whose activities have not been restricted because of poor support. Other patients with little or no pelvic organ prolapse have significant complaints with bowel, bladder, or sexual function. Consequently the physical examination cannot be used to develop a treatment strategy in isolation.

Objective description of pelvic organ support can be done when the sites to be examined are specified and when the support for each site is described in relation to one or more fixed points within the pelvis. Two such fixed points are the ischial spines and the hymen. Using these two fixed points, it is possible to construct a horizontal plane called the midvaginal axis, extending from the hymen to the ischial spine. Pelvic organ support can then be described in relationship not only to the distance from the spines to the hymen but also in relationship to the midvaginal axis (Figs. 4–1 and 4–2). An organ prolapsing outside

TABLE 4–5. Common Causes of Transient Urinary Incontinence

D	Delirium
I	Infection
A	Atrophy
P	Pharmaceuticals
P	Psychologic
E	Excessive urine production
R	Restricted mobility
S	Stool impaction

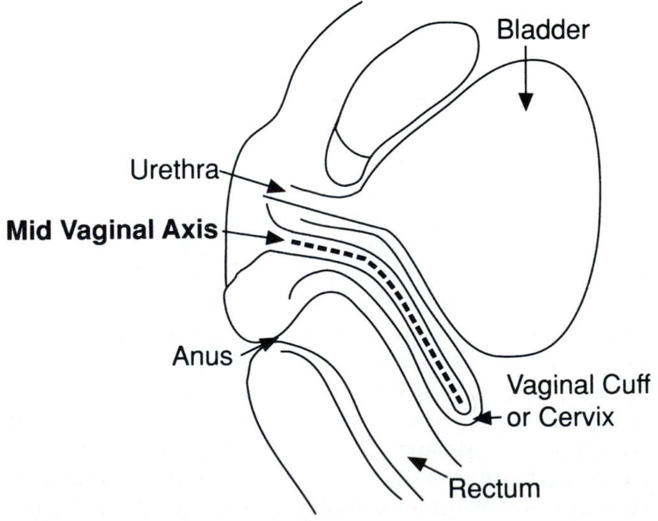

FIGURE 4–1. The mid vaginal axis.

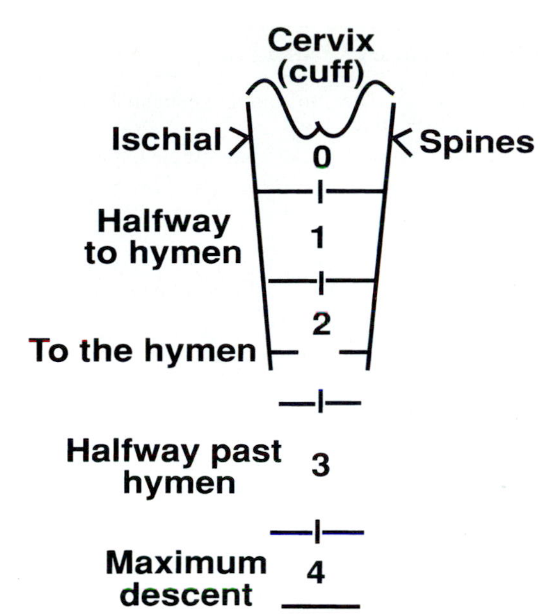

FIGURE 4–2. The ischial spines, hymen, and the half-way grading system.

the hymen can only be described in relation to the hymen. Using these ground rules for objective description, the urethra, bladder, cul-de-sac, and rectum can be said to have no support loss when they fail to cross the midvaginal axis as the patient strains. In addition, bilateral sulci adjacent to the urethra and the bladder mark the attachment of the pubocervical fascia and vaginal epithelium to the arcus tendineus (Fig. 4–3). The cervix or cuff has no support loss when it fails to descend past the ischial spines as the patient strains. A site with loss of support will cross the midvaginal axis or descend below the level of the ischial spines. Quantification of the support loss may be done by direct measurement in centimeters or may be graded as no descent (grade 0), descent halfway between the spines and hymen (grade 1), descent to the hymen (grade 2), descent halfway outside the hymen (grade 3), or descent fully outside the hymen (grade 4)[8] (Table 4–7). I have found this grading system to be useful clinically in the longitudinal evaluation of my gynecologic patients. It has been especially helpful in situations requiring long-term observations to determine if pelvic organ prolapse progresses with conservative management or to follow the long-term outcomes of pelvic reconstructive procedures.[9,10]

The physical examination should be performed in a reproducible, systematic, orderly fashion. With the patient in the dorsal lithotomy position, initially describe the urogenital hiatus: the distance from the urethral meatus to the 6-o'clock position of the hymen. Closure of the urogenital hiatus is a function of levator muscle tone. The wider the urogenital hiatus opens with straining, the less resistance there is for pelvic organs to prolapse. In most nulliparous women, the urogenital hiatus is closed when the patient is not straining and remains either closed or

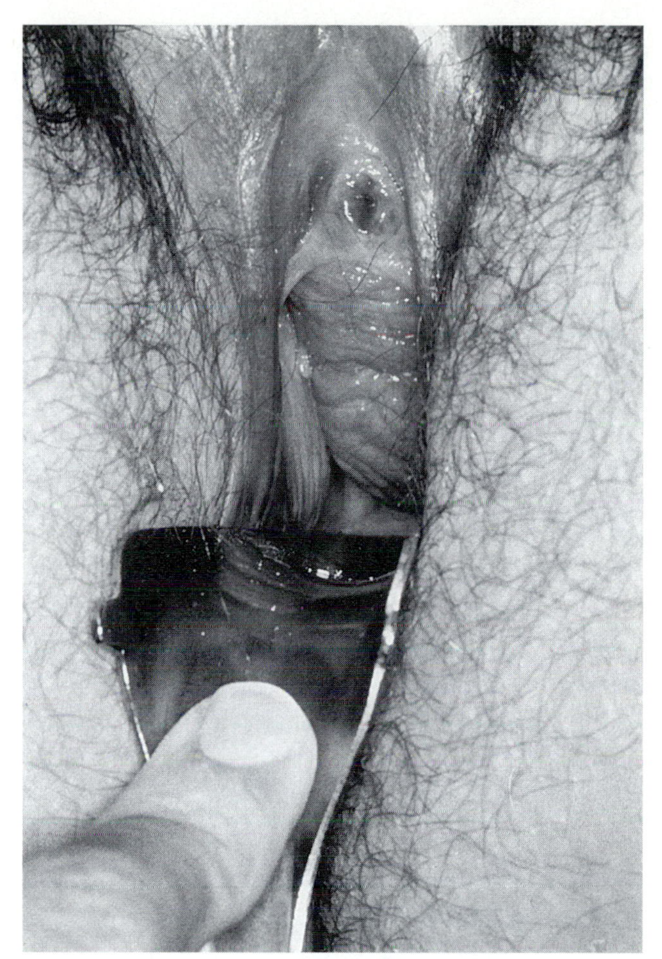

FIGURE 4–3. The anterior vaginal segment does not cross the midvaginal axis and the lateral vaginal sulci are intact.

opens less than two centimeters with straining (Fig. 4–4). A woman with pelvic organ prolapse frequently has an exaggerated increase in the size of the urogenital hiatus as she strains (Fig. 4–5). Traditionally clinicians have used such subjective, and sometimes pejorative, terms as **parous** or **gaping** to describe urogenital hiatus. A centimeter measurement from

TABLE 4–7. Objective Clinical Evaluation of Pelvic Organ Support

	Grade					
Site	**0**	**1**	**2**	**3**	**4**	**Comments**
Urethra						
Bladder						
Cervix/Cuff						
Cul-de-sac						
Rectum						

Grade Coding:
0 = No prolapse
1 = Prolapse half way to hymen
2 = Prolapse to hymen
3 = Prolapse half way outside hymen
4 = Maximum prolapse

Subpubic Arch:
< 2 finger breadths ______
= 2–3 finger breadths ______
= 3–4 finger breadths ______
> 4 finger breadths ______

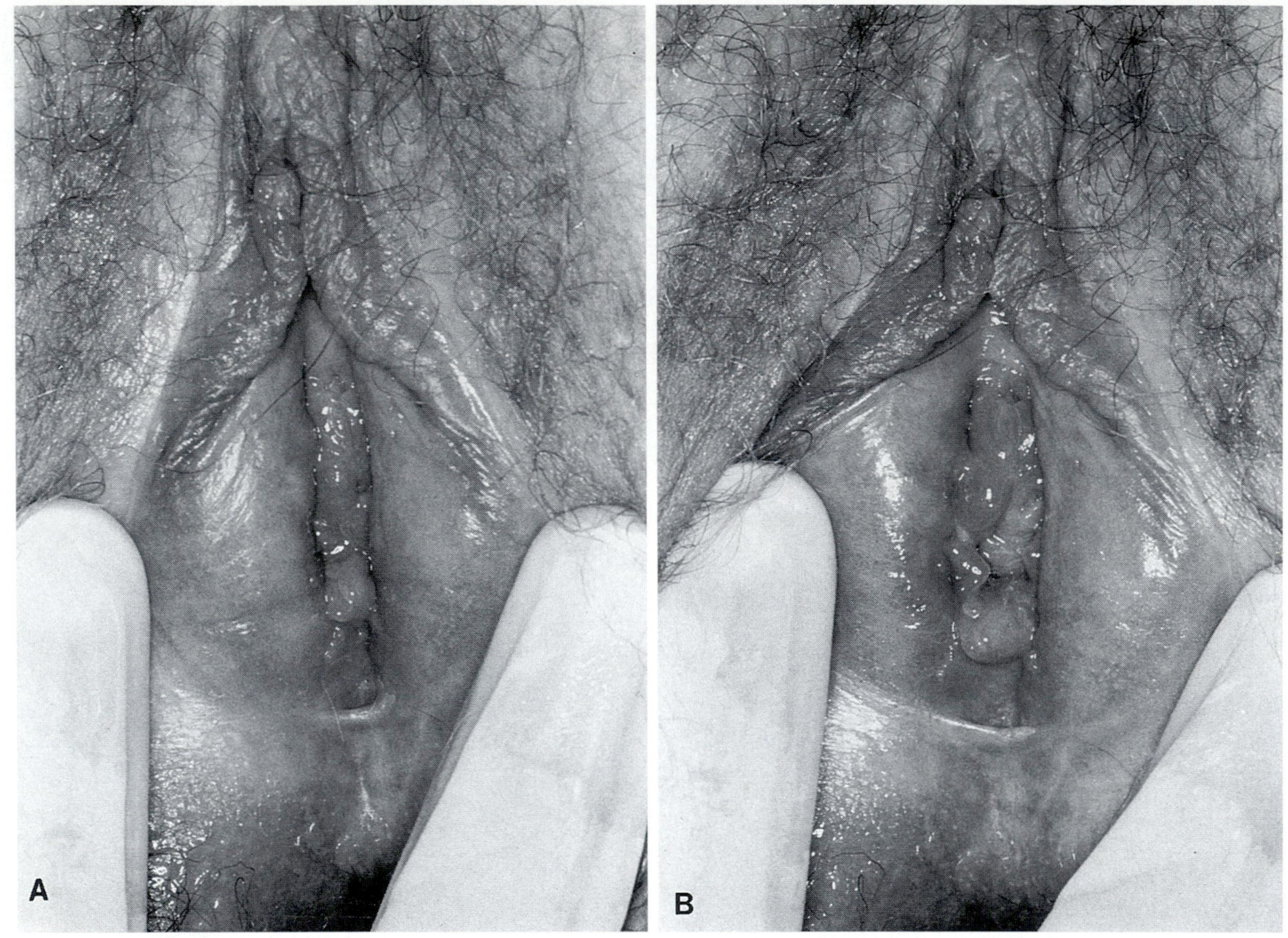

FIGURE 4–4 (A) The urogenital hiatus is closed in a nulliparous woman, and (B) barely opens when she strains maximally.

the urethral meatus to the 6-o'clock position of the hymeneal ring is more objective. This observation is important because an ultimate goal of management of pelvic organ prolapse, whether pelvic floor exercise or surgical reconstruction, is re-creation of a more normally functioning urogenital hiatus.

Anterior Segment

Site-specific analysis of pelvic organ support begins with evaluation of the *anterior segment*: the urethra, urethrovesical junction, and bladder. As the patient strains maximally, the physician must observe mobility and descent of the anterior vaginal wall. Clues to urethral mobility include not only descent of the distal anterior vaginal wall, but also movement of the external urethral meatus away from the back of the pubic bone. Mobility of the urethra and urethrovesical junction can be quantified by placing a cotton swab through the urethral meatus to the level of the urethrovesical junction.[11] The angle the cotton swab forms with a line horizontal to the floor is measured as the patient is not straining and measured again as she performs maximum straining. The greater the angle between the tip of the cotton swab and the horizontal plane, the greater the mobility of the urethra and urethrovesical junction; normal mobility is 30 degrees or less.

After the patient has performed maximum straining, she should be asked to contract the levator muscles as the physician observes her ability to bring the axis of the cotton swab closer to the horizontal. When the cotton swab returns to a more normal position with muscle contraction, a clinical clue is provided that the periurethral pubocervical fascia has significant attachment to the arcus tendineus fascia pelvis and that pubococcygeal muscle function is present. A pelvic floor exercise program may be beneficial. On the other hand, when the patient is unable to return the cotton swab applicator to a more horizontal plane, she may have poor fascial support, poor levator muscle function, or both. (See Chapter 5 for more on this test.)

The second site in the anterior segment is the base of the bladder. Physical examination must determine whether the bladder segment prolapses across the midvaginal axis halfway to the hymen, to the hymen, halfway outside the hymen, or fully outside the hymen. Analyzing localized support defects for the bladder is more complex than for any other site in

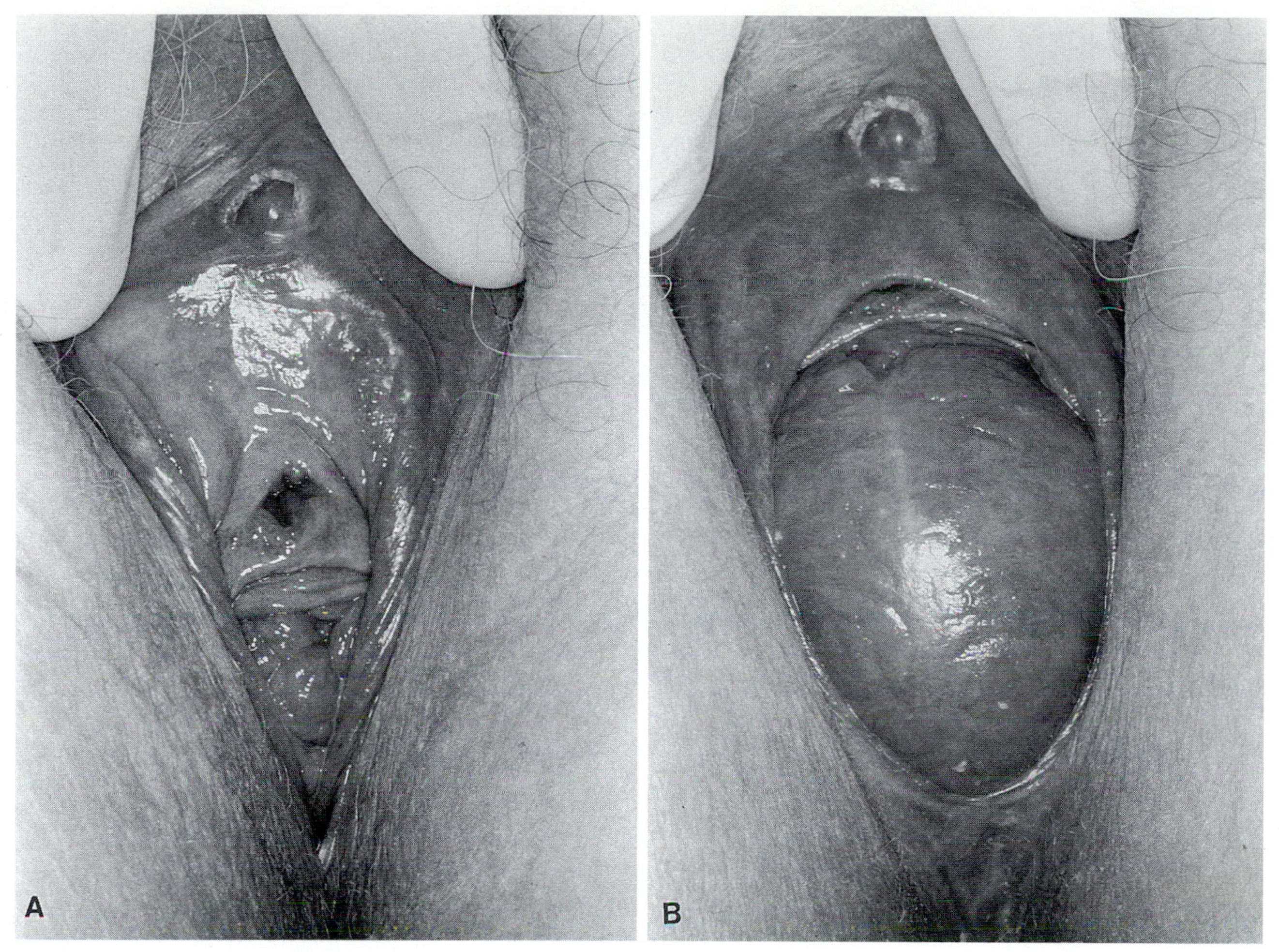

FIGURE 4–5 (A) A parous woman with pelvic organ prolapse has an open urogenital hiatus at rest. (B) As she strains, the hiatus opens to allow prolapse of the anterior vaginal segment.

the vagina. The urethra, urethrovesical junction, and bladder all rest on the trapezoidal pubocervical fascia. This fascial sheet fuses with the perineal membrane distally, is attached to the cardinal ligaments and cervix or cuff superiorly, and extends laterally to attach to the arcus tendineus fascia bilaterally. Support defects for the bladder classically have been thought to occur in the midline, but lateral or **paravaginal** support defects, **superior** defects, or any combination of these localized defects can occur. Patients with lateral or paravaginal defects have loss of the lateral vaginal sulci, suggesting detachment of the pubocervical fascia from the tendinous arch. The sulci can be recreated by using an open, ring sponge forceps to elevate the anterior vagina to its normal point of attachment along the lateral pelvic sidewalls. After the anterior vagina has been replaced laterally, the patient should strain to allow observation for central bulging through the open arms of the forceps. If she strains and has no evidence of anterior support defects, lateral or paravaginal loss of support is confirmed. If she strains and there is some improvement in anterior support, but there continues to be a midline bulge through the open arms of the forceps, she has both lateral and midline defects. The forceps should next be closed to support the base of the bladder centrally. The patient should strain again. If she has no midline descent and has evidence of normal sulci bilaterally, the **support defect** is **midline**. Superior loss of bladder support is characterized by the presence of thin, shiny anterior vaginal epithelium with loss of rugae extending from the vaginal cuff along the base of the bladder; the anterior vaginal wall itself is longer than the posterior vaginal wall. **Superior defects** are frequently associated with midline defects.

Cervix or Cuff

DeLancey's report[12] stressed the importance of the cardinal uterosacral ligament complex in maintaining normal support for the cervix or cuff. When the cardinal uterosacral ligament support is poor, the cervix descends from its normal position at or above the level of the ischial spines. This loss of support is also graded using the halfway system. In a postoperative patient who has a normally supported vaginal cuff, the cardinal uterosacral ligament attachments form dimples at the 3-o'clock and 9-o'clock positions. The linear scar at the vaginal cuff serves as a reference point to identify the location of the vaginal apex. Even with descent of the vaginal cuff from a normal position, it is possible to identify the dimples at the 3- and 9-o'clock positions. These dimples serve as an objective reference point, thus allowing discrimination between loss of support for the bladder anteriorly and loss of support for the cul-de-sac posteriorly.

Cul-De-Sac

The cul-de-sac is normally located at or above the level of the ischial spines and contains no small bowel. With loss of support, the epithelium overlying the cul-de-sac may become thin and shiny and the peritoneal lining may be distended by the intestines. Palpation of small bowel in the cul-de-sac or visualization of peristalsis in the cul-de-sac confirms the presence of an enterocele. Discrimination between an enterocele and a rectocele can be clinically difficult. The "double bubble," the discrete appearance of a hernia sac anterior to the surface of the rectum, is a helpful clinical sign of enterocele but is infrequently observed. Examination of the patient in the standing position may help discriminate between an enterocele and a rectocele. The standing patient should place one leg on a step or a riser. The clinician then places the index finger in the anterior rectal ampulla and thumb in the vaginal vault to palpate the rectovaginal septum for evidence of small bowel between the rectum and the vagina. It may be necessary to have the patient strain to force intestine into the elongated cul-de-sac.

RECTUM

The perirectal fascia joins the perineal body distally, extends laterally to attach to the levator fascia, and continues superiorly to the cul-de-sac. Defects in perirectal fascia support commonly occur in the midline but also may occur discretely in other sites. The examination is performed by using the speculum to retract the anterior vaginal segment. As the patient strains, the examiner observes whether the rectovaginal tissue crosses the midvaginal axis and prolapses to or through the hymen. Evaluation of localized defects in the rectovaginal septum is done in a manner similar to the evaluation of the anterior segment. The curved ring forceps are placed posteriorly and laterally to determine if the posterior support defect can be corrected by lateral replacement. When a bulge remains between the open arms of the forceps, it is possible to determine if the defect is midline by using the closed forceps to support the midline when the patient strains again. If the support loss is corrected, the defect is midline. Loss of support near the cul-de-sac is characterized by a bulge high in the rectovaginal septum but with normal support in the distal several centimeters in the rectovaginal septum. Loss of support in the distal rectovaginal septum near the perineal body is characterized by a bulge that originates in the distal 3 centimeters of the rectovaginal septum.

VAGINAL AXIS

Pelvic organ prolapse may be related to loss of the normal axis of the vagina. For a woman in the dorsal lithotomy position, the axis should be directed posteriorly into the hollow of the sacrum. When she stands, the vagina is horizontal to the floor, an orientation that protects her from prolapse of the upper vagina and cul-de-sac because intra-abdominal pressure forces the vagina into the hollow of the sacrum. All successful reconstructive procedures for pelvic organ prolapse are designed to enhance or recreate the posterior location of the vaginal apex and cul-de-sac.

GYNECOLOGIC PELVIMETRY

I find it helpful to evaluate the bony architecture of the pelvis. Clinical decisions regarding the choice of a surgical procedure may depend on the size of the subpubic arch or the bituberous diameter. A wide subpubic arch, three finger-breadths or greater, or a bituberous diameter greater than the width of a fist are clues that appropriate retractors can be used for good surgical exposure during vaginal reconstructive procedures. The distance from the ischial spines to the hymen provides information regarding the potential vaginal length following certain transvaginal reconstructive procedures. The final decision regarding a transvaginal or a transabdominal reconstructive procedure may depend on the bony architecture of the pelvis.

SUMMARY

Pelvic floor complaints may relate to poor function, poor support, or both. A clear understanding of the patient's complaints and an objective assessment of her pelvic organ support are requirements for the development of a therapeutic plan, for the longitudinal observation of the natural history of her pelvic floor disorders, and for the critical evaluation of surgical outcomes.

REFERENCES

1. Levin, B and Murphy, GP: Revision in American Cancer Society recommendations for the early detection of colorectal cancer. CA Cancer Clin 42:296, 1992.
2. Urinary Incontinence Guideline Panel: Urinary Incontinence in

Adults: Clinical Practice Guideline. AHCPR Pub. No. 92-0038. Agency for Health Care Policy and Research, Public Health Service, U.S. Department of Health and Human Services, Rockville, MD, 1992.
3. Norton, P: Nonsurgical management of stress urinary incontinence. Contemp OB/GYN 37:63, 1992.
4. Walters, MD and Fantl, JA: The problem of urinary incontinence. In Baden, WF and Walter T (eds.): Surgical Repair of Vaginal Defects. JB Lippincott, Philadelphia, 1991, p 63.
5. Burch, JC: Urethrovaginal fixation to Cooper's ligament for correction of stress incontinence, cystocele, and prolapse. Am J Obstet Gynecol 81:281, 1961.
6. Wiskind, AK, Creighton, SM and Stanton, SL: The incidence of genital prolapse after the Burch colposuspension. Am J Obstet Gynecol 167:399, 1992.
7. Brubaker, L, and Norton, P: Proceedings of International Continence Society 23rd Annual Meeting, Rome, Italy, September 1993, p. 200.
8. Baden, WF and Walker, TA: Physical diagnosis in the evaluation of vaginal relaxation. Clin Obstet Gynecol 15:1055, 1972.
9. Shull, BL, Capen, CV, Riggs, MW, et al: Preoperative and postoperative analysis of site-specific pelvic support defects in 81 women treated with sacrospinous ligament suspension and pelvic reconstruction. Am J Obstet Gynecol 166:1764, 1992.
10. Shull, BL, Capen, CV, Riggs, MW, et al: Bilateral attachment of the vagina cuff to iliococcygeus fascia: An effective method of cuff suspension. Am J Obstet Gynecol 168:1669, 1993.
11. Crystle, CD, Charme, LS and Copeland, WE: Q-Tip test in stress urinary incontinence. Obstet Gynecol 38:313, 1971.
12. DeLancey, JOL: Anatomic aspects of vaginal eversion after hysterectomy. Am J Obstet Gynecol 166:1717, 1992.

CHAPTER 5

First-Line Testing of Patients with Urinary Incontinence

Nicolette S. Horbach

Urinary incontinence, as defined by the International Continence Society (ICS), is the "involuntary loss of urine which is objectively demonstrable and a social or hygienic problem."[1] Although studies vary, urinary incontinence has been reported to affect up to 26% of women of reproductive age and 30% to 42% of women in the postmenopausal years.[2] A wide array of disorders can produce urinary incontinence, often with a myriad of overlapping and confusing symptoms. A thorough office evaluation can clarify the diagnosis in the majority of patients and identify the remainder of women who require more sophisticated urodynamic or radiographic testing.

Considerable controversy exists in the literature regarding the optimal clinical investigation of patients with urinary incontinence.[3–9] Most authors recommend at least taking a detailed history and giving a physical examination, measurement of residual urine with urinalysis and culture, a stress test, assessment of urethrovesical junction mobility, and a cystometrogram. The purpose of this section is to review these first-line diagnostic studies employed in the clinical evaluation of incontinent women.

URINALYSIS AND URINE CULTURE

A midstream or catheterized urine sample for routine urinalysis and culture should be obtained early in the evaluation of women with lower urinary tract symptoms. By obtaining the urine sample as a post-void residual determination, the possibility of an atonic bladder with overflow incontinence may be detected.

Up to 25% of women with acute cystitis may experience incontinence. Endotoxin produced by *Escherichia coli* has been shown to trigger abnormal detrusor activity resulting in detrusor instability, or to act as an alpha-adrenergic blocker.[10] The latter action may result in loss of urethral pressure and the subsequent development of stress incontinence. In one study, 4 of 12 women with stress incontinence and asymptomatic bacteriuria became continent following treatment with antibiotics.[11] Thus, consideration should be given to treating asymptomatic bacteriuria on culture in women with urinary incontinence. Treatment is especially important in women who require instrumentation of their lower urinary tract, such as cystoscopy or urodynamics.

An alternative to urine culture may be the microscopic evaluation of an unspun urine specimen. This sample should reveal one or more bacteria per high power field if there are more than 10^4 cfu/mL of bacteria in the urine. Pyuria is defined as more than 10 leukocytes/mL per high power field in unspun urine and is present in nearly all women with acute urinary tract infections. Microscopic hematuria may be seen in approximately 50% of women with cystitis.

At times urine dipstick tests have been used in place of urinary cultures or microscopic examination to identify patients with bacteriuria. The urinary nitrite test detects the conversion of urinary nitrate to nitrite by bacteria within the bladder. To optimize accuracy, the test should be performed on a concentrated first morning void. False negative results may be obtained with infections caused by enterococci, because they do not convert nitrate to nitrite. Additionally, the presence of urinary dyes such as bilirubin, phenazopyridine, or methylene blue may preclude accurate testing.

Urinary cytology should be considered in older patients with incontinence to rule out a neoplastic process, which can present as involuntary urinary leakage. A positive cytology or asymptomatic microscopic hematuria require further evaluation by radiographic or invasive studies.

DIRECT OBSERVATION OF URETHROVESICAL JUNCTION MOBILITY

Genuine stress incontinence is often associated with abnormal support of the proximal urethra and urethrovesical junction. Many surgical procedures are designed to correct genuine stress incontinence by repositioning these structures. In order to choose an appropriate surgical procedure, the anatomic support must be assessed. This determination is particularly important in women who have previously undergone unsuccessful surgery for incontinence. Anatomic support may be determined by direct observation during pelvic examination or the Q-tip test. Imaging studies include the bead chain cystogram, a straining cystogram, and ultrasound evaluation.[12–20]

The Q-tip test was initially introduced by Crystle and colleagues[12] to differentiate anatomic defects in Type I and Type II stress incontinence. Although Green's Type I and Type II classification is no longer recommended for the diagnosis and management of stress incontinence, the Q-tip test has continued to be used to determine the mobility of the urethrovesical junction.

With the patient adequately prepped and in lithotomy position, a wooden Q-tip lubricated with 2% xylocaine jelly is inserted through the urethra into the bladder. In most women resistance is encountered as the Q-tip is withdrawn into the urethrovesical junction, thus confirming correct placement. A resting angle is determined relative to the horizontal axis using an orthopedic goniometer. The patient is then asked to strain forcibly or to cough repetitively. Although no standard definition exists for a positive Q-tip test, a maximum straining angle of more than 30 degrees from the horizontal axis is usually defined to indicate positive increased mobility of the urethrovesical junction. Montz and Stanton[18] evaluated 100 women with urinary incontinence and found a straining Q-tip angle of more than 30 degrees to have a 61% sensitivity and 63% specificity in the diagnosis of genuine stress incontinence. The Q-tip test must be performed in a standardized fashion. Incorrect placement of the Q-tip in the bladder or in the mid- or distal urethra will alter the results and the reliability of the test, as reported by Karram and Bhatia.[13]

Several authors have shown that the Q-tip test is not a specific test for diagnosing genuine stress incontinence or for differentiating it from other disorders of the lower urinary tract.[13–18] It does, however, provide a noninvasive method for demonstrating excessive mobility of the urethrovesical junction in patients with suspected stress incontinence. Walter and Diaz compared[14] the maximum straining Q-tip angle from the horizontal in 48 incontinent women and 26 continent controls. A statistically significant difference was found between the asymptomatic women and those with genuine stress incontinence in both maximum straining angle and urethral hypermobility. No difference was found in the values between those women with genuine stress incontinence and the group with other urologic disorders, however.

A study by Caputo and Benson[15] has questioned the accuracy of the Q-tip test compared to sonographic visualization of urethrovesical junction anatomy. They examined 114 women with incontinence or prolapse. Using the ultrasound findings as the standard, the authors reported a false positive rate of 22% and a false negative rate of 75% for the Q-tip test. The positive and negative predictive values were 67% and 37%, respectively.

Because the purpose of many anti-incontinence procedures is to stabilize the urethrovesical junction in an intra-abdominal position, it is important to demonstrate a defect in support of the junction before surgical intervention is contemplated. The Q-tip test is an inexpensive screening test. In patients with a negative Q-tip test result, alternative surgical procedures that do not rely on repositioning of the urethrovesical should be chosen. More sophisticated radiographic or urodynamic studies are indicated in these women to confirm the diagnosis of genuine stress incontinence and to detect the presence of intrinsic sphincter dysfunction.[21] These tests are discussed in subsequent chapters.

STRESS TEST

Because objective evidence of urinary leakage with stress is necessary to establish the diagnosis of genuine stress incontinence, the stress test is an integral part of the evaluation of female urinary incontinence. A stress test can easily be performed during the routine pelvic examination by asking the patient to bear down. Loss of urine with a subjectively empty bladder in the lithotomy position implies significant impairment of the urethral continence mechanism. If the result of this initial stress test is negative, the test can be repeated after instilling at least 300 mL in her bladder. The patient is then asked to cough repetitively in the supine or standing position. Simultaneous loss of urine during coughing is highly suggestive of genuine stress incontinence. The stress test can easily be done at the beginning of an office examination if the patient is asked to arrive with a full bladder. After the stress test has been performed, the patient can be asked to void; postvoid residual volume can be measured. Alternatively, the stress test can be done at intervals during, or at completion of, a cystometrogram. Combining the stress test with a cystometrogram allows the clinician to determine the volume at which stress leakage occurs and to rule out the presence of uninhibited detrusor contractions as the cause for the urinary leakage.

Several modifications of the stress test have been devised in an attempt to predict the likelihood of surgical success in patients with stress incontinence. Bonney's test was designed to simulate the results of surgical elevation of the urethrovesical junction. To perform the test, the middle and index fingers are placed one centimeter laterally on each side of the urethra, and the junction is elevated to a retropubic position.[22] Marchetti's test, using Allis clamps and local anesthesia, or Read's test with rubber shod clamps, are performed similarly.[23,24] Patients who no longer lose urine when coughing during these examinations are considered to be excellent surgical candidates.

Although the reliability of these tests has been emphasized in the literature, more recent studies have questioned the validity of Bonney's test in selecting patients for surgical intervention.[25,26] Using urethral pressure profilometry in 12 patients with stress incontinence, Bhatia and Bergman[25] found no statistically significant difference in the urethral pressure recordings during Bonney's test as compared with results obtained with deliberate urethral occlusion. Thus, although Bonney's test was originally devised to predict the results of surgical intervention preoperatively, most investigators have abandoned its use as a prognostic test in the evaluation of female incontinence.

A variant of the stress test may be indicated in women with severe genitourinary prolapse, who may be paradoxically continent due to kinking, compression, or obstruction of the urethra.[27] The stress test can be performed as previously outlined after reduction of the prolapse with a loose-fitting pessary or using a Sims' retractor or the examiner's hand in the posterior fornix. If the patient demonstrates involuntary urinary loss with coughing following reduction of the prolapse, additional anatomic support of the proximal urethra and urethrovesical junction may be required at the time of surgical correction of genitourinary prolapse to prevent the development of postoperative stress incontinence.[28]

CYSTOMETRY

Cystometry is a pressure-volume relationship recorded during bladder filling. The purpose of a single channel cystometrogram (CMG) is to detect the presence of detrusor overactivity, which occurs in 8% to 63% of incontinent women.[20] Both the results and the conditions of cystometry must be reported, because many variables may affect interpretation, as listed in Table 5–1. During cystometry, the first sensation,

TABLE 5–1. Variables of Cystometric Testing Which Should Be Specified According to the International Continence Society

Variable	Option	Sub-option
Mode of access to the bladder		
	Transurethral	
	Percutaneous	
Equipment		
	Type of catheter	
		fluid-filled
		membrane
		microtip
	Recording device	
Filling method		
	Catheter	
		continuous
		incremental
	Diuresis	
Position of the patient		
	Supine	
	Sitting	
	Standing	
Filling medium		
	Carbon dioxide	
	Water	
	Saline	
Temperature of the fluid medium		
	Room	
	Body	
Rate of bladder filling		
	Slow (≤10 mL/minute)	
	Medium (11–100 mL/minute)	
	Fast (>100 mL/minute)	
Provocative maneuvers		
	Cough	
	Heel bounce	
	Hand washing	

maximum bladder capacity, and the presence of uninhibited detrusor contractions should be recorded. Most normal women report their first awareness of fluid within the bladder at 100 to 150 mL, an urge to urinate at 200 to 350 mL, and a strong need to void at 400 to 550 mL. At the beginning of bladder filling, there is a normal rise in intravesical pressure of 2 to 6 cm of water. Further increase in intravesical pressure as filling continues should not rise to more than 15 cm of water at normal cystometric capacity.

Detrusor overactivity is diagnosed when an increase in detrusor pressure occurs in the presence of urgency or urinary incontinence that reproduces the patient's presenting symptoms. Even small-amplitude detrusor contractions may be clinically significant, causing urinary incontinence in 10% and urgency in 85% of women who experience uninhibited contractions of less than 15 cm of water.[30] A gradual rise in intravesical pressure of over 15 cm water at normal bladder capacity indicates a low-compliance bladder. A high-compliance bladder is diagnosed when the maximum bladder capacity is significantly elevated without a rise in vesical pressure (no number is given by ICS). Because some women are able to train their bladders to increase bladder capacity over time, an increased capacity does not always indicate detrusor pathology. In a study by Weir and Jacques,[31] 30% of (n=109) patients with a maximum cystometric capacity over 800 mL were still able to generate a normal detrusor contraction for voiding.

Despite the widespread use of cystometry, no single technique has universal acceptance.[32,33] Most authors prefer fluid rather than gas as the distention medium. Although carbon dioxide cystometry may be easier and cleaner, it is less physiologic than water or saline as a distention medium. Carbon dioxide may irritate the bladder mucosa and mix with urine to form carbonic acid, leading to a 60% reduction in bladder capacity compared to fluid. As a gas, carbon dioxide is compressible, which may lead to less reproducible results. Urinary leakage is also difficult to visualize during cystometry if carbon dioxide is used and voiding studies cannot be performed.

Most studies are done using retrograde infusion of room-temperature saline or water using a transurethral catheter at a flow rate of 50 to 100 mL/minute. Flow rates are classified as either slow (physiologic) (<10 mL/minute), medium (10 to 100 mL/minute), or fast (>100 mL/minute).[1] Rapid filling of the bladder is discouraged. This rate does not allow sufficient time for normal bladder accommodation to take place and increases the likelihood of an erroneous diagnosis of uninhibited detrusor contractions.

Several convenient techniques have been developed to perform a simple cystometrogram in the office. A Foley catheter may be inserted into the patient's bladder and attached to a catheter-tip syringe with the piston removed, as shown in Figure 5–1. The patient is placed in the sitting or standing position and the top of the fluid column is held approximately 15 cm above the pubic symphysis. Using a medium fill rate, fluid is gradually poured into the syringe so that the level of the fluid column is constant. A rise in the fluid level associated with urgency or leakage is suggestive of detrusor overactivity.

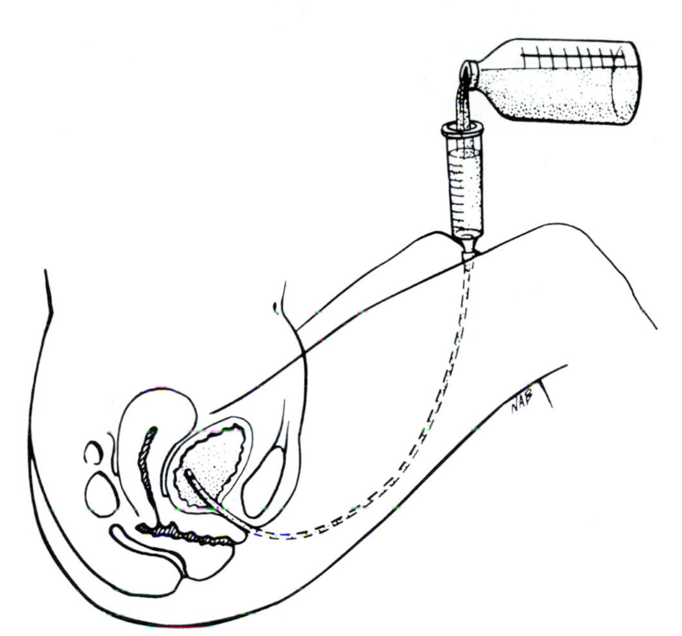

FIGURE 5–1. Simplified office cystometry to evaluate bladder sensation and to determine the presence of detrusor instability. The bladder is filled gradually with sterile fluid and the height of the fluid column indicates intravesical pressure. (Reprinted with permission from Walters, MD and Karram, MM, Clinical Urogynecology, CV Mosby, St. Louis, 1993, p 55.)

Alternatively, a spinal manometer may be used to determine intravesical pressure during bladder filling, as illustrated in Figure 5–2.[34] The bladder is filled incrementally at a medium fill rate and intravesical pressure is measured at 50 to 100 mL intervals by turning the stop-cock to the manometer port. Because only intravesical pressure is recorded during this type of cystometrogram, it may be difficult to differentiate an increased intravesical pressure caused by detrusor activity from an increase caused by an inadvertent Valsalva maneuver during bladder filling. One helpful technique is to ask the patient to inspire once a rise in intravesical pressure is observed. Women are rarely able to increase their intra-abdominal pressure while they inspire. Thus, a sustained increase in intravesical pressure during inspiration is usually due to a detrusor contraction. If the intravesical pressure returns to baseline when the patient inspires, the rise in pressure was due to effects of the Valsalva maneuver.

In an attempt to detect changes in intravesical and intra-abdominal pressures simultaneously during simple cystometry, some investigators have performed a continuous two-channel examination. Separate catheters are placed in the bladder and vagina or rectum to record both intravesical and intra-abdominal pressures. The vaginal or rectal catheters

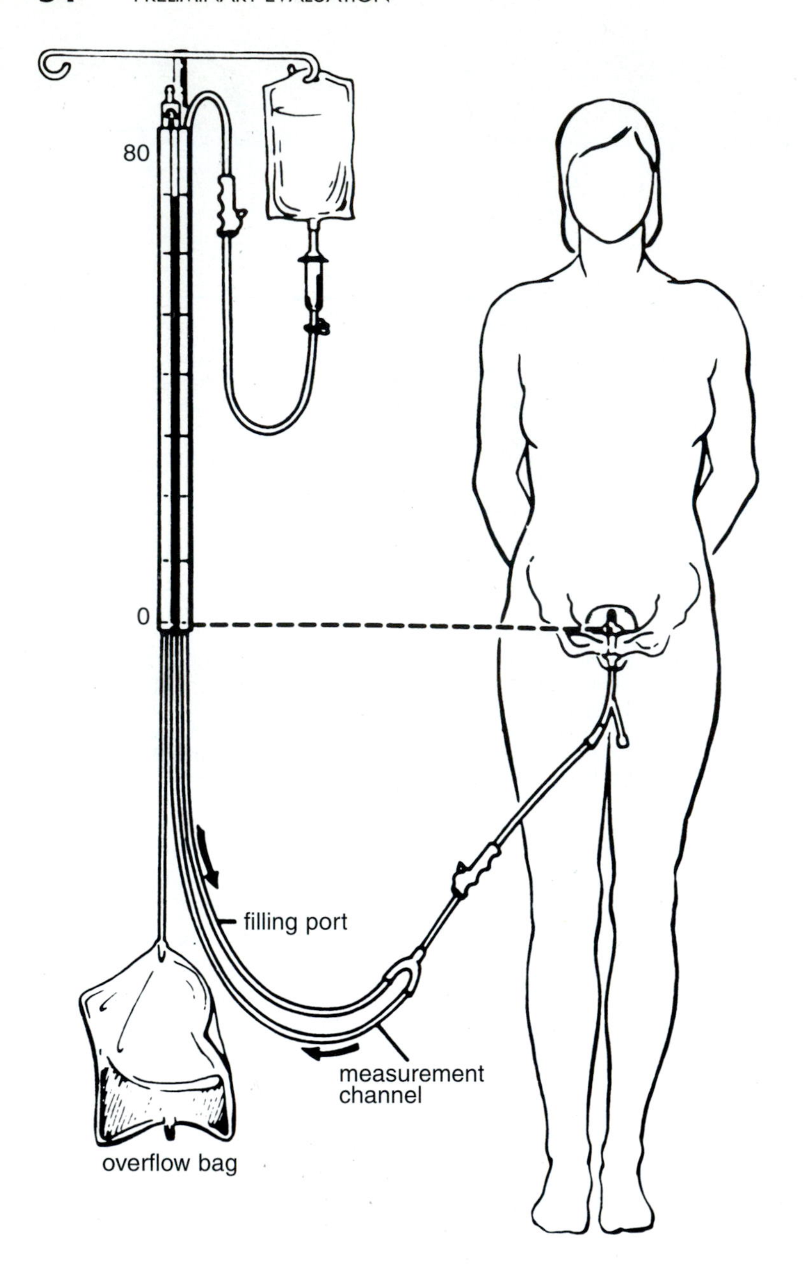

FIGURE 5–2. A manometer may be used to assess bladder function. Accuracy is improved by performing the test in the standing position. Intravesical pressure is determined for every 50 to 100 mL of bladder filling. (Reprinted with permission from Sand et al.,[34] Copyright 1991, The American College of Obstetricians and Gynecologists.)

should be inserted above the pelvic floor to approximate the measurement of intra-abdominal pressures. Vaginal catheters are preferred due to patient comfort, ease of cleaning the catheters, and lack of artifact that can be seen with rectal catheters due to rectal peristalsis. Vaginal catheters may be difficult to use in women with severe pelvic organ prolapse, however. In these women, an examination glove or condom may be tied around the catheter to facilitate the use of a rectal catheter. True detrusor pressure, the component of measured intravesical pressure that is due to the detrusor muscle itself, may be calculated by subtracting intra-abdominal pressure measurements from intravesical values, thus improving the accuracy of the evaluation.[35]

Specially designed electronic equipment is available to perform a single-channel cystometrogram. A catheter is inserted into the bladder and connected to an external pressure transducer to record intravesical pressure using either CO_2 or fluid as the distention medium at a medium fill rate. The patient should be standing and is asked to cough or heel bounce at every 50 to 100 mL during bladder filling, to attempt to provoke uninhibited bladder contractions. An intrauterine pressure catheter monitor used for obstetric patients may provide a cost-effective alternative to purchasing specific urologic equipment. An example of a normal CMG and the tracings of two women with detrusor overactivity are shown in Figure 5–3.

Supine single-channel cystometry will detect approximately 50% to 60% of women with detrusor overactivity.[33,36,37] The detection rate of this test may be improved an additional 20% to 40% by performing the cystometrics in the standing position and with the detrusor-provoking maneuvers of repetitive coughing, hand washing, or heel bounce. A report by Sand, Brubaker, and Novak[34] compared two standing

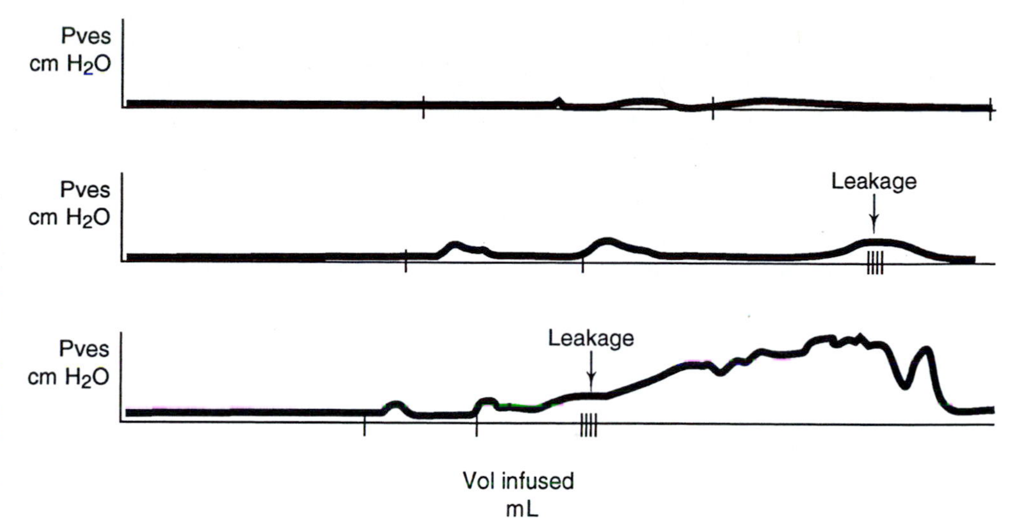

FIGURE 5–3. An example of single-channel cystometrogram tracings. (Top) Normal study; (Middle) Small-amplitude phasic uninhibited detrusor contractions produced urgency at first without urinary leakage. As bladder volume increased, the patient experienced incontinence. (Bottom) A series of large-amplitude uninhibited detrusor contractions were noted without relaxation between contractions associated with complete bladder emptying.

incremental single-channel CMGs performed on two different days with supine and standing multichannel urethrocystometry in 100 women. The ability of the first and second single-channel CMGs to detect detrusor instability was 84% and 90% respectively, in a patient population with a 64% prevalence rate of detrusor instability. Using the two single-channel CMGs together, uninhibited detrusor contractions were detected with a sensitivity of 92% and a negative predictive value of 87%.

Inadequate filling may also result in a falsely negative CMG. Arnold found that 6 of 11 women with a stable bladder at half bladder capacity developed detrusor overactivity when filled to maximum cystometric capacity.[33] Thus, care must be taken to ensure adequate filling, ideally to a maximum bladder capacity of 350 to 500 mL or until the patient's symptoms are reproduced. Because some patients may experience significant leakage, discomfort, or pain at more than 350 mL, however, filling may have to be terminated before reaching a normal cystometric capacity.

The reliability of single-channel cystometry compared with multichannel urodynamics has been debated extensively.[37,38] The reported advantage of multichannel cystometry is that artifactual increases in intravesical pressure due to a rise in intra-abdominal pressure (.e.g, activity caused by Valsalva maneuver) can be recognized and subtracted. This results in an accurate recording of true detrusor pressure. Thus, multichannel testing is thought to decrease the incidence of an erroneous diagnosis of detrusor overactivity. Sand, Hill, and Ostergard[36] reported that 40% of women with an unstable bladder on standing single-channel cystometry had no evidence of detrusor instability during urodynamic testing. Sutherst and Brown[38] compared single-channel and multichannel urodynamics in a blind cross-over study of 100 incontinent women. Seven women with uninhibited detrusor contractions on single-channel evaluation were noted to have stable bladders after urodynamic evaluation. In this study, single-channel cystometry was found to be 100% sensitive and 89% specific compared with multichannel urodynamics in detecting the presence of uninhibited detrusor contractions.

The use of multichannel urodynamics as the standard by which the accuracy of other tests is evaluated remains controversial. Women with a history highly suggestive of detrusor overactivity may not demonstrate uninhibited contractions even during multichannel testing. Patients with detrusor overactivity may experience days without urinary leakage. Bhatia and Ostergard have suggested that ambulatory multichannel urodynamics may be a more sensitive method of detecting detrusor abnormalities than standard urodynamic testing.[39] In their study, the patient's diagnosis, previously based on multichannel urodynamics, was significantly revised in 60% of patients after continuous monitoring was performed. See Chapter 6 for more information on multichannel urodynamic testing.

UROFLOWMETRY

Uroflowmetry assesses voiding function by measuring the volume of urine voided and the time interval required for doing so. The purpose of uroflowmetry is to detect anatomic or functional voiding abnormalities. **Anatomic** obstructive voiding is less common in women than in men and is characterized by a low flow rate and a prolonged voiding interval. This pattern may also be seen in women with a poor detrusor contraction during voiding. **Functional** obstructive voiding patterns may occur in women with recurrent urinary tract infections, urethral spasms, or detrusor sphincter dyssynergia.[40,41] Uroflowmetry may also be helpful preoperatively in detecting gross voiding abnormalities which may predispose a patient to prolonged voiding following anti-incontinence surgery. These include the inability to generate a detrusor contraction of ≤15 cm of water during

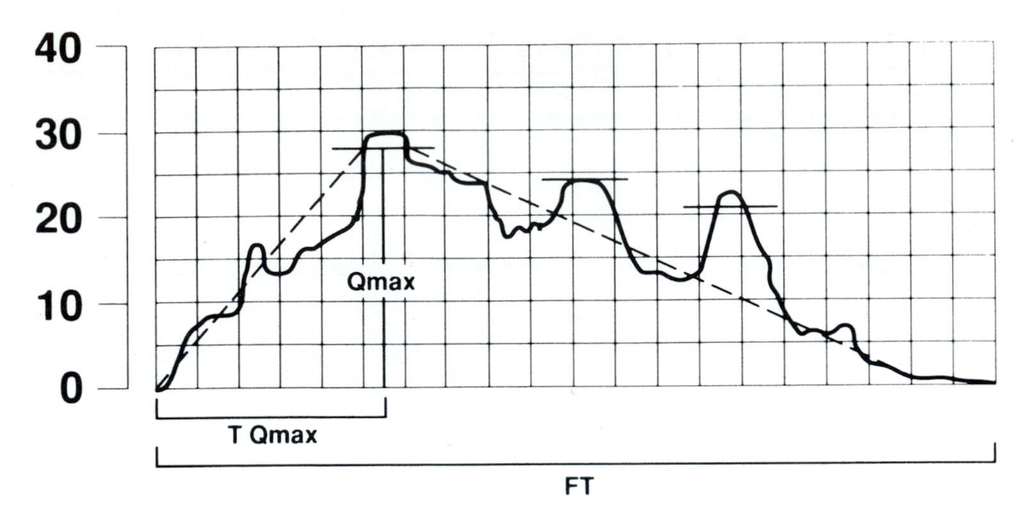

FIGURE 5–4. Graphic representation of a normal uroflow curve with measured parameters illustrated. Qmax is the maximum flow rate (mL/sec) during voiding; T Qmax is the time (sec) until maximum flow is achieved, and T is the total voiding time (sec). (Reprinted with permission from Walters, MD, and Karram, MM: Clinical Urogynecology, CV Mosby, St. Louis, 1993, p 80.)

TABLE 5–2. Normal Values for Uroflowmetry*

Total time for voiding	< 20 sec
Time to peak flow	2–8 sec
Peak flow rate	> 20 mL/sec
Average flow rate	> 10 mL/sec

*Assuming that patient voids at least 200 mL.

micturition, or voiding using the Valsalva maneuver alone.[42] Bhatia and Bergman[42] performed preoperative uroflowmetry in 43 women who underwent Burch's retropubic urethropexy. Of 13 patients (38%) with reduced flow rates, 5 required catheter drainage for 7 or more days postoperatively, compared with only 10% of women with normal preoperative flow patterns. More sophisticated evaluation with pressure-flow studies and electromyography is indicated in women with underlying neurologic disease who present with incontinence or voiding dysfunction, or preoperatively in women who demonstrate a significant voiding abnormality during uroflowmetry.

A simple screening uroflow can be performed using a stopwatch and a measuring container that fits over the commode. The patient is asked to come to the office with a full bladder and to void into the measuring container while recording the total time of voiding with the stopwatch. Alternatively, electronic recording equipment is available. Figure 5–4 illustrates the parameters that are measured. For the test to be accurate, a patient must void at least 200 mL. Normal values are listed on Table 5–2.

Voiding may be classified as normal, intermittent, intermittent interrupted, and obstructive, based on the uroflow pattern. An **intermittent** flow pattern is characterized by a drop in flow rate followed by a subsequent increase, producing a multiple-peak tracing. If the drop in flow rate is to 2 mL per second or less, the pattern is defined as intermittent interrupted, as seen in Figure 5–5. This type of tracing may be encountered in a patient who voids primarily by increases in intra-abdominal pressure.

PAD TEST

The perineal pad test is used clinically to document urinary loss in women who have not demon-

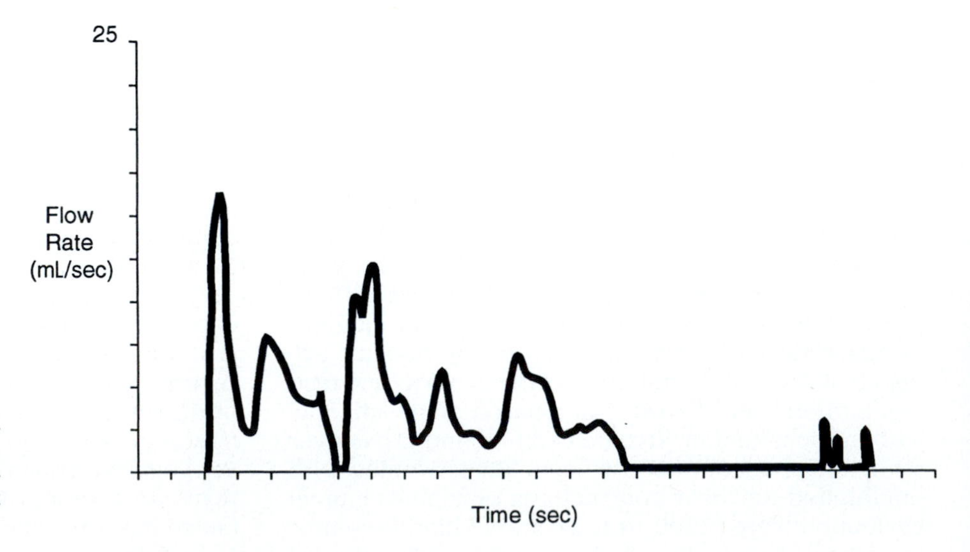

FIGURE 5–5. Intermittent interrupted uroflow tracing from a woman who voided using the Valsalva maneuver without detrusor activity. Note the multiple peak curve with normal values for voiding.

strated loss during previous testing. Because the pad test incorporates more extensive activity than that which can be performed during routine cystometric testing, it may more accurately reflect the "stresses" to which the bladder is subject during normal day-to-day activities. Although the pad test does not delineate the cause of incontinence, a positive test verifies its presence.[43–45] The test does not necessarily correlate with the severity of the incontinence. Given a positive test result, the clinician should pursue more sophisticated studies to determine the cause of the incontinence. If the pad test is negative with more than 250 mL in the bladder, the diagnosis of urinary incontinence should be questioned. Small increases in the pad weight may be due to "pseudoincontinence" from vaginal secretions or perspiration.

The pad test may be performed as a 1-hour office test, or a 12-hour or 24-hour home test. In the 1-hour test outlined by the ICS, a preweighed pad is applied to the patient's perineum after she has emptied her bladder.[1] She is then asked to drink 500 mL of fluid and to rest for 15 minutes. For the next 30 minutes the patient is instructed to walk and climb the equivalent of one flight of stairs. The pad is then checked for evidence of urinary leakage and can be weighed if damp. Following this, the test continues with a variety of maneuvers including position change, coughing, running in place, picking up objects from the floor, and placing hands under running water for 1 minute. The pad is reweighed at the end of the hour. A greater than 2 gram increase in pad weight indicates urinary loss.

The home pad test may at times be facilitated by giving a patient phenazopyridine to color the urine before the onset of testing.[45] This coloration test may also be helpful in detecting women with pseudoincontinence. Rarely, women may have urine enter the vagina during voiding. These patients report postvoid spills because this "vaginal" urine leaks out when they assume the upright position. Simple alterations in hygiene habits will eliminate urinary leakage in this group of patients.

SUMMARY

Approximately 10% of patients with urinary incontinence will require more extensive testing, such as multichannel urodynamics or radiographic studies, to elucidate their diagnosis. Historic information or findings during clinical testing that may indicate the need for urodynamic testing are shown in Table 5–3. Elderly patients may require urodynamic testing due to their diverse symptoms and the increased prevalence of detrusor instability and intrinsic sphincter dysfunction in the older population which may particularly affect the outcome of any contemplated surgical intervention. Radiographic studies are indicated when anatomic relationships cannot be clarified on clinical examination. Because of the expense of these more sophisticated tests, they should be used only when specific information is needed, such as when: (1) the diagnosis should be determined given the results of the previous testing; (2) the patient has failed conservative therapy that was based on a presumptive diagnosis from limited testing; or (3) surgical intervention for incontinence or prolapse is contemplated and the operative approach may be altered based on the radiographic or urodynamic data.

TABLE 5–3. Indications for Urodynamic Testing

History
Elderly (older than 60 years of age)
Failed incontinence surgery
Prior radical pelvic surgery or radiation therapy
Symptoms of continuous incontinence or leakage with minimal stress or urge
History of neurologic disease
Clinical Examination
Abnormal neurologic examination
High postvoid residual volume
Negative Q-tip test (well-supported or immobile urethra)
No demonstrable leakage on stress test
High or low maximum bladder capacity during simple cystometrics
Absent sensation during bladder filling
Symptoms of urgency, frequency, nocturia and urge incontinence and a negative screening cystometrogram
Gross voiding abnormalities

REFERENCES

1. Abrams, P, Blaivas, JG, Stanton, SL, et al: The standardization of terminology of lower urinary tract function produced by the International Continence Society Committee on Standardization of Terminology. Scand J Urol Nephrol 114(suppl):5, 1988.
2. Consensus Conference: Urinary incontinence in adults. JAMA 261:2685, 1989.
3. Green, TH: Urinary stress incontinence: differential diagnosis, pathophysiology, and management. Am J Obstet Gynecol 122:368, 1975.
4. Kaufman, JM: Urodynamics in stress urinary incontinence. J Urol 122:778, 1979.
5. Ouslander, J, Staskin, D, Raz, S, et al: Clinical versus urodynamic diagnosis in an incontinent geriatric female population. J Urol 137:68, 1987.
6. Fischer-Rasmussen, W, Hansen, RI and Stage, P: Predictive values of diagnostic tests in the evaluation of female urinary stress incontinence. Acta Obstet Gynecol Scand 65:291, 1986.
7. Cardozo, LD and Stanton, SL: Genuine stress incontinence and detrusor instability—a review of 200 patients. Br J Obstet Gynecol 87:184, 1980.
8. Diokno, AC, Wells, TW and Brink, CA: Urinary incontinence in elderly women: urodynamic evaluation. J Am Geriatr Soc 35:940, 1987.
9. Bryne, DJ, Stewart, PKA and Gray, B: The role of urodynamics in female urinary stress incontinence. Br J Obstet Gynecol 59:228, 1987.
10. Nergardh, A, Boreus, LO and Holme, T: The inhibitory effect of E. coli endotoxin on alpha-adrenergic receptor functions in the lower urinary tract. An in vitro study in cats. Scand J Urol Nephrol 11:219, 1977.
11. Bergman, A and Bhatia, NN: Urodynamics: the effect of urinary tract infection on urethral and bladder function. Obstet Gynecol 66:366, 1985.
12. Crystle, CD, Charme, LS and Copeland, WE: Q-tip test in stress urinary incontinence. Obstet Gynecol 38:313, 1971.
13. Karram, MM and Bhatia, NN: The Q-tip test: standardization of

the technique and its interpretation in women with urinary incontinence. Obstet Gynecol 71:807, 1988.
14. Walters, MD and Diaz, K: Q-tip test: a study of continent and incontinent women. Obstet Gynecol 70:208, 1987.
15. Caputo, RM and Benson JT: The Q-tip test and urethrovesical junction mobility. Obstet Gynecol 82:892, 1993.
16. Bergman, A, McCarthy, TA, Ballard, CA, et al: Role of the Q-tip test in evaluating stress urinary incontinence. J Reprod Med 32:273, 1987.
17. Fantl, JA, Hurt, WG, Bump, RC, et al: Urethral axis and sphincteric function. Am J Obstet Gynecol 155:554, 1986.
18. Montz, FJ and Stanton, SL: Q-tip test in female urinary incontinence. Obstet Gynecol 67:258, 1986.
19. Bergman, A, McKenzie, C, Ballard, CA, et al: The role of cystourethrography in the preoperative evaluation of stress urinary incontinence in women. J Reprod Med 33:372, 1988.
20. Gordon, D, Pearce, M and Norton, P: Comparison of ultrasound and lateral chain urethrocystography in the determination of bladder neck position and descent. Neurourol Urodyn 5:181, 1987.
21. Bergman, A, Koonings, PP and Ballad, CA: Negative Q-tip test as a risk factor for failed incontinence surgery. J Reprod Med 4:193, 1989.
22. Berkeley, C and Bonney, V: A Textbook of Gynecologic Surgery, ed 3. Cassell, London, 1935, pp 511–513.
23. Marshall, UF, Marchetti, DA and Krantz, KE: The correction of stress incontinence by simple vesicourethral suspension. Surg Gynecol Obstet 88:509, 1949.
24. Stamey, TA: Urinary incontinence in the female. Campbell's Urology, ed 4. WB Saunders, Philadelphia, 1979, pp 2292–2293.
25. Bhatia, NN and Bergman, A: Urodynamic appraisal of the Bonney test in women with stress urinary incontinence. Obstet Gynecol 62:696, 1983.
26. Migliorini, GD and Glenning, PP: Bonney's test—fact or fiction. Br J Obstet Gynecol 94:157, 1987.
27. Rosenzweig, BA, Pushkin, S, Blumenfeld, D, et al: Prevalence of abnormal urodynamic test results in continent women with severe genitourinary prolapse. Obstet Gynecol 79:539, 1992.
28. Berman, A, Koonings, PP and Ballard CA; Predicting postoperative urinary incontinence development in women undergoing operation for genitourinary prolapse. Am J Obstet Gynecol 158:1171, 1988.
29. Wall, LL: Diagnosis and management of urinary incontinence due to detrusor instability. Obstet Gynecol Surv 45(suppl):1S, 1990.
30. Coolsaet, BLRA, et al: Subthreshold detrusor instability. Neurourol Urodyn 4:309, 1985.
31. Weir, J and Jacques, PF: Large-capacity bladder: a urodynamic survey. Urology 4:544, 1974.
32. Gleason, DM, Bottaccini, MR and Reilly RJ: Comparison of cystometrograms and urethral profiles with gas and water media. Urol 9:155, 1977.
33. Arnold, EP: Postural effects in incontinent women. Urol Int 29:185, 1974.
34. Sand, PK, Brubaker, LT and Novak, T: Simple standing incremental cystometry as a screening method for detrusor instability. Obstet Gynecol 77:453, 1991.
35. Goncalves, SC, et al: Continuous two-channel water cystometry: description of an alternative test for evaluating incontinent women. Int Urogynecol J 2:212, 1991.
36. Sand, PK, Hill, RC and Ostergard, DR: Supine urethroscopic and standing cystometry as screening methods for the detection of detrusor instability. Obstet Gynecol 70:57, 1987.
37. Frigerio, L. Ferrari, A and Candiani, GB: The significance of the stop test in female urinary incontinence. Diag Gynecol Obstet 3:301, 1981.
38. Sutherst, JR and Brown, MD: Comparison of single and multichannel cystometry in diagnosing bladder instability. Br Med J 288:1720, 1984.
39. Bhatia, NN and Ostergard, DR: Urodynamics in women with stress urinary incontinence. Obstet Gynecol 60:552, 1982.
40. Karl, C, Gerlach, R, Hannappel, J, et al: Uroflow measurements: their information yield in a long-term investigation of pre- and postoperative measurements. Urol Int 41:270, 1986.
41. Stanton, SL, Ozsoy, C and Hilton, P: Voiding difficulty in the female: prevalence, clinical and urodynamic review. Obstet Gynecol 61:144, 1983.
42. Bhatia, NN and Bergman, A: Use of preoperative uroflowmetry and simultaneous urethrocystometry for predicting risk of prolonged postoperative bladder drainage. Urology 28:440, 1986.
43. Fantl, JA, Harkins, SW, Wyman, JF, et al: Fluid loss quantitation test in women with urinary incontinence: a test-retest analysis. Obstet Gynecol 70:739, 1987.
44. Jakobsen, H, Vedel, P and Andersen, JT: Which pad-weighing test to choose: ICS one hour test, the 48 hour home test or a 40 min test with known bladder volume. Neurourol Urodyn 4:23, 1987.
45. Wall, LL, Wang, K, Robson, I, et al: The pyridium pad test for diagnosing urinary incontinence. J Reprod Med 35:682, 1990.

SECTION THREE

DIAGNOSTIC ADJUNCTS

CHAPTER **6**

Multichannel Urodynamic Testing

Richard C. Bump

Clinical multichannel urodynamic testing uses electronic instruments to measure and display multiple physiologic parameters from the lower urinary tract simultaneously. The ability to transform mechanical parameters, such as pressure or flow, into electrical signals capable of being displayed and manipulated is a relatively recent development. The uroflowmeter, first described in 1948, was not commercially available until the 1960s.[1] Enhorning's landmark studies using electromanometry to measure vesical and urethral pressures were also reported during that same decade.[2] The intervening three decades have witnessed a plethora of reports using multichannel urodynamics to investigate various hydrodynamic and neurophysiologic aspects of urine storage and evacuation. The over 4000 articles related to urodynamics published since 1966 have, in their bulk, greatly enhanced our knowledge of the physiology of lower urinary tract function and dysfunction. This great mass of literature has also generated controversy, confusion, and competition among various authors' techniques with respect to their clinical value. It is my opinion that there is no single standard test. Rather, there are often several urodynamic techniques that allow us to answer different clinical questions and thereby facilitate effective management of an individual patient. Before considering specific tests in this chapter, I pose the questions clinicians should ask when performing a urodynamic evaluation on a woman with symptoms of filling phase dysfunction (e.g., incontinence, urgency and frequency syndromes) or of emptying phase dysfunction (e.g., retention, hesitancy, incomplete emptying). Various tests that, singly or in combination, can answer these questions are considered next. First, however, some technical and philosophic aspects of multichannel urodynamic testing are addressed briefly.

MULTICHANNEL URODYNAMIC EQUIPMENT

A complete review of the technical specifications for multichannel urodynamic equipment is beyond the scope of this chapter. Such specifications were considered in a comprehensive report from the International Continence Society (ICS) in 1987[3] and are included in a more accessible 1989 review[4] for interested readers. An appreciation of potential limitations imposed by the technical characteristics of any urodynamic measuring system is essential to ensure accurate interpretations and to avoid spurious interpretation of artifact. It is particularly important to decide which parameters are to be measured and what is required of a system to allow their measurement before investing thousands of dollars in equipment. For example, if relatively slow events such as bladder contractions or strains resulting from the Valsalva maneuver are to be measured, a system with a frequency response of 4 Hz is adequate. If more rapid pressure events such as a cough are to be captured, the system frequency response should be 15 Hz; to record an electromyographic (EMG) signal accurately, the frequency range must extend to 10 kHz.[3] Other technical specifications that are important in the selection of equipment, in addition to frequency response, include measurement range, sensitivity drift, linearity, and hysteresis, all of which factors relate to the accuracy of recorded measurements.

TRANSDUCER

Each of the three major components of a urodynamic measuring system (transducer, signal processor, and display) can affect the overall system's frequency response and accuracy. The transducer converts a mechanical parameter (e.g., pressure or flow) into a proportional electrical signal that can be processed and displayed. Pressure transducers can be either external to the urinary tract, with the pressure transmitted physically through a fluid-filled catheter, or catheter-mounted (internal), with the electrical signal being generated at the site of pressure measurement. Internal transducers have a much higher frequency response and are easier to use but are more fragile and expensive than external transducers. A uroflow transducer or flowmeter generates an electrical output proportional to the quantity of fluid passed per unit time. The two most commonly used flowmeter types, gravimetric and rotating disk, differ significantly in the way they produce and process the electrical signal but are comparable in their accuracy. Because the former calculates flow by measuring accumulated mass and is calibrated for water, however, it must be recalibrated if used with a radiopaque medium with a density, significantly greater than that of water.[3] For EMG; the parameter being measured originates as electrical activity from contracting skeletal muscle; thus, no transducer is necessary and an electrode conveys the bioelectrical signal to the measuring system. Monopolar needle electrodes and bipolar wire or surface electrodes can be used to measure the level of electrical activity of the striated urethral sphincter.

SIGNAL PROCESSOR

Signal processing of the electrical signal from a transducer or electrode can include amplification, filtration, differentiation, integration, subtraction, and digitalization. The amplifier magnifies the very small applied signal from the transducer or electrode. Filters limit the frequency range of the system, with the aim of eliminating artifactual *noise.* Other processors allow the mathematic derivation of new parameters from directly measured events, such as converting an increase in mass over time into a flow rate or subtracting one pressure from another to obtain a pressure difference. Digital conversion of continuous analog data allows computer disk storage, processing, and analysis of urodynamic parameters. Although signal processing is essential to transform electrical signals into usable forms, it should do so with minimal distortion; each step in processing can detract from the accuracy of the system. For example, a 4 Hz filter or an 8 Hz digitalizer eliminates the frequency response advantage of a 100 Hz transducer.

RECORDING DEVICES

Recording devices allow the graphic display of directly measured and derived data; they include paper chart recorders, plotters, and video display terminals. Most widely used devices allow the display of four to eight channels. Mechanical analog chart recorders must have a frequency response sufficient to ensure accurate graphic reproduction of the signal; measurements and calculations are made directly from the real-time tracing. As already noted, computer-based recording devices must digitalize at a sampling frequency that is adequate to accurately capture the event of interest. After this has been ensured, these devices eliminate much of the tedious labor of measurement and calculation.

PHILOSOPHY OF MULTICHANNEL URODYNAMICS

In an era when sophisticated medical technology is valued more highly than clinical judgment, danger exists that the vast amount of data generated by a multichannel urodynamic study will become more the focus of attention than the patient and her symptoms. Validity of a diagnosis based upon such data is inexorably linked to the patient's symptoms and to the reproduction of those symptoms during the study.[5,6] A normal study that does not reproduce the patient's presenting symptoms is inconclusive. Conversely, a diagnosis based on a study that produces symptoms that never bother the patient is likely to be erroneous. The two basic requirements for an accurate urodynamic diagnosis are: (1) reproduction of only the symptom(s) of concern, and (2) accurate measurement of appropriate parameters while the symptom is occurring. Implicit are requirements that the urodynamicist knows the details of the patient's symptoms, is aware of and has tried to minimize potential artifacts imposed by the laboratory environment and equipment, and has formulated the specific questions to be answered by the study.

QUESTIONS TO BE ANSWERED BY MULTICHANNEL URODYNAMICS

FILLING (STORAGE) PHASE DYSFUNCTION

The most common filling phase symptoms are incontinence and irritative symptoms (urgency, frequency, nocturia) without incontinence. The urodynamic evaluation of the incontinent patient should answer the following questions:

1. What physiologic condition is causing the incontinence? That is, does the patient have genuine stress incontinence (GSI), detrusor instability (DI), mixed incontinence (GSI and DI), a noncompliant bladder, unstable urethral pressure, reflex incontinence and detrusor hyperreflexia, overflow incontinence, or some combination of these conditions?
2. Does the patient have a physiologic subtype of incontinence that may increase her risk for therapeutic failure or complications? Examples include the woman with GSI due to intrinsic urethral deficiency (ISD) with or without urethral hypermobility, the woman with detrusor instability who also has impaired detrusor contractility, or the woman with significant unstable urethral pressure associated with detrusor instability or mixed incontinence.
3. Is there information not directly related to the physiologic type or subtype of incontinence that might impact on management? Is the patient able to sense bladder filling with enough forewarning to be able to avoid incontinence, can she effectively suppress a detrusor contraction, or can she increase her urethral pressure by contracting her pubococcygeus muscle?

The evaluation of the continent woman with irritative symptoms should determine if there is any abnormal motor component (urethral or detrusor instability or poor bladder compliance) as opposed to a purely abnormal sensory cause (i.e., urgency or pain at an unusally low bladder volume) for the symptoms. Multichannel urodynamic tests that examine the filling phase include urethrocystometry, urethral pressure profilometry, and leak point pressure determinations.

EMPTYING (VOIDING) PHASE DYSFUNCTION

Symptoms of emptying phase dysfunction include hesitancy; prolonged, interrupted or incomplete voiding; and retention. The multichannel urodynamic evaluation of a woman with such symptoms should measure pertinent parameters in the bladder and urethra during a voiding attempt and correlate these parameters with the measured flow rate. With such information, a specific diagnosis such as detrusor acontractility, detrusor underactivity, detrusor areflexia, detrusor and urethral dyssynergia (involving smooth or skeletal muscle), striated sphincter overactivity, and mechanical obstruction can be established. Multichannel urodynamic tests that examine the emptying phase include uroflowmetry, pressure flow studies, and external urethral sphincter EMG studies.

ANCILLARY TESTING

Urodynamics traditionally refers to the study of hydrodynamics and muscle activity to define the functional status of the lower urinary tract. These measurements are always correlated with the patient's symptoms. Other methods of lower urinary tract investigation, such as radiographic, ultrasonographic, and endoscopic visualization; neurologic examination; pelvic support defect analysis; or urethral axial mobility determination, are useful adjuncts to multichannel urodynamic testing. These adjunctive tests are not covered in any detail in this chapter, but some examples of how they facilitate patient assessment and management are noted here.

MULTICHANNEL URODYNAMIC ASSESSMENT OF THE FILLING PHASE

SIMULTANEOUS ELECTRONIC MULTICHANNEL URETHROCYSTOMETRY

Cystometry is the measurement of the pressure-volume relationships of the bladder. Multichannel electromanometry permits the continuous measurement, derivation, and display of pressures from multiple anatomic sites during bladder filling, allowing a more precise analysis of lower urinary tract function than is possible with single-channel or mechanical manometry. There are many important variations and subtle nuances of urethrocystometry and no standard technique has been mandated. The ICS has established variables of technique that should be specified by authors and clinicians performing these tests. (See Chapter 5, Table 5–1.) Urethrocystometry is most physiologic when performed with liquid medium, at as low a flow rate as is compatible with timely completion of the study, with catheters that are as small as possible, with the patient in a comfortable position, and with every effort being made to provide physical and emotional support. Attention to these factors minimizes, but does not eliminate, the physical and psychologic artifact inevitably imposed by the laboratory environment.

Pressure is measured directly from the following anatomic sites: the bladder (p_{ves} or vesical pressure), the urethra (p_{ura}), and either the vagina (p_{vag}) or the rectum (p_{rect}). Of these sites, only the bladder is a fluid-filled cavity to which the measurement of pressure applies in the strict physical sense. In the other sites, directional force applied to the catheter or transducer has been equated with pressure and is referred to as such by convention. This directionality of measurement can be an important source of artifact and is likely to compromise the reproducibility of some measurements.

The p_{vag} and p_{rect} measurements are indirect estimations of abdominal pressure (p_{abd}). Simultaneous measurement of p_{abd} with p_{ves} allows the urodynamicist to differentiate contraction of the detrusor from abdominal muscle contraction or strain from the Valsalva maneuver (Fig. 6–1*A*, and 6–1*B*). I prefer to use a vaginal catheter; its placement is generally more comfortable for the patient, and p_{rect} represents both abdominal pressure and bowel peristaltic activity, which may confuse or obscure an appreciation of detrusor activity (Fig. 6–1*D*).[6,7] Similar confusion may also result from shifting of the position of the vaginal catheter when the patient changes position (Fig. 6–1*C*). It is necessary to record p_{ves}, p_{ura}, and p_{abd}, as well as p_{det} and p_{uc}, to avoid misinterpretations due to these phenomena. The rectum must be used as the site of estimation of p_{abd} in women with severe pelvic-organ prolapse or significant vaginal shortening.

Two additional pressures are usually derived by the electronic subtraction of one directly measured pressure from a second. Detrusor pressure (p_{det}) is derived by subtracting p_{abd} from p_{ves}; it represents the portion of the vesical pressure that is created by active and passive forces in the bladder wall.[6] Urethral closure pressure (p_{uc}) is the pressure gradient between the urethra and the bladder and is derived by subtracting p_{ves} from p_{ura}.

During retrograde urethrocystometry, the directly measured and derived pressures are recorded during filling. The patient is asked to state when she experiences her first sensation to void (when she is first aware that her bladder is filling), her normal sensation to void (when she would want to urinate at the next convenient moment, but could tolerate delay if necessary), a strong desire to void (persistent desire to void without fear of leakage), and when she feels she can no longer delay micturition (maximum cystometric capacity [MCC]).[6] In practice, differentiating

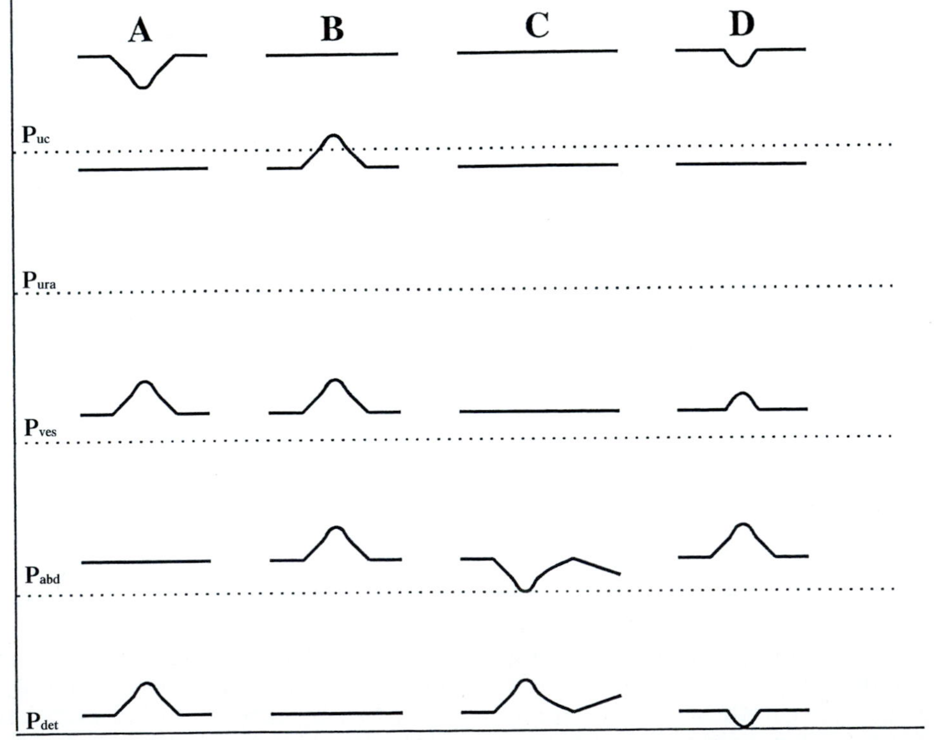

FIGURE 6–1. These urethrocystometry excerpts demonstrate the importance of recording pressures from multiple sites to allow accurate interpretation. (*A*) The increase in p_{ves} is due to a detrusor contraction and results in a decrease in p_{uc} (top). (*B*), The increase in p_{ves} is due to abdominal straining, seen as a simultaneous increase in p_{abd}. The increase in p_{abd} is transmitted to the urethra in this normal, stress-continent patient, so that there is no change in p_{uc}. (*C*), The apparent detrusor contraction recorded in p_{det} is the result of movement of the vaginal transducer used to record p_{abd}. Movement causes a change in the directional force applied to the transducer, resulting in an apparent decrease in pressure (see text for further discussion). (*D*), A small bladder contraction, seen in p_{ves}, results in a parallel decrease in p_{uc} in this stress-continent patient. Because of concurrent rectal peristaltic activity which hides the detrusor contraction, however, a decrease in p_{det} is recorded, rather than an increase. P_{uc} = urethral closure pressure; P_{ura} = urethra pressure; P_{ves} = vesical (bladder) pressure; P_{abd} = abdominal pressure; P_{det} = detrusor pressure.

among these four grades of sensation as defined by the ICS is subjective and thus not terribly useful. I generally ask the patient to tell me when she would normally first consider urinating if it were convenient (first sensation) and when she would find a way to empty her bladder even if it were inconvenient (strong desire or functional MCC). The former sensation usually occurs around 200 mL and the latter between 400 and 600 mL. I have termed the difference between these two measurements the **proprioceptive sensory threshold** and have observed that it tends to be shortened in some women, especially hypoestrogenic and elderly women.[8] An unusually short proprioceptive threshold, with first sensation delayed until at or near MCC, may be an important contributing factor for incontinence in some patients.

Bladder filling should not be stopped prematurely based solely on the patient's sensation of urgency if no bladder or urethral activity is documented. It is useful to compare the infused volume to the patient's normal functional capacity (estimated from her frequency-volume voiding diary or from her uroflow volume with a comfortably full bladder prior to cystometry) and to reassure her that her low-volume urgency is probably due to stress from the testing situation. Urethrocystometry can be performed with the patient in any position, from supine through sitting to standing. Although evidence suggests that standing cystometry may be more provocative than supine or sitting cystometry for detrusor contractions,[9] the most important criterion for an adequate test is reproduction of the patient's symptoms. Unavoidable patient movement associated with standing cystometry makes measurement of maximum p_{ura} unreliable and makes diagnosis of unstable urethral pressure suspect due to concurrent catheter or transducer movement within the urethra (Fig. 6–2).

Urethrocystometric testing is performed only in a woman who is known to be free of urinary tract infection (UTI), because UTI can cause spurious test results[10] and because prolonged catheterization, manipulation, and retrograde infusion may contribute to increased morbidity from UTI. I perform the test with the patient in the 45-degree upright position in a birthing chair, using an 8-Fr dual-sensor, microtip transducer infusion catheter with one transducer in the bladder and the other in the midurethra in the area of maximum p_{ura} (Fig. 6–2) and a second single-sensor catheter in the vagina or rectum. The transurethral catheter is attached to an external profilometer arm to maintain catheter stability, and the patient is asked to remain still during the retrograde infusion. Room-temperature sterile water is infused at 30 mL per minute until MCC is reached. If no bladder instability is recorded during this passive filling, progressive provocative maneuvers are performed in the following order:

1. Coughing in the 45-degree position
2. Sitting upright
3. Coughing while sitting upright
4. Standing
5. Coughing while standing
6. Heel bouncing
7. Listening to the sound of running water
8. Walking
9. Hand washing

If the patient had the presenting complaint of urge incontinence and that symptom has not been reproduced, further filling of the bladder in the standing position is performed.

The diagnosis of DI is made when the patient complains of involuntary loss of urine associated with a strong desire to void and the urethrocystogram demonstrates a detrusor contraction and leakage, spontaneously or on provocation, while the patient is attempting to inhibit micturition (Fig. 6–3).[8] Diagnosis of GSI can be made during urethrocystometry, meeting all criteria of the ICS definition, when urinary leakage is observed simultaneously with a physical stress, with p_{ves} exceeding p_{ura} in the absence of a detrusor contraction (Fig. 6–4*D*). GSI can also be diagnosed if these criteria are met during a dynamic urethral pressure profile, if leakage is observed si-

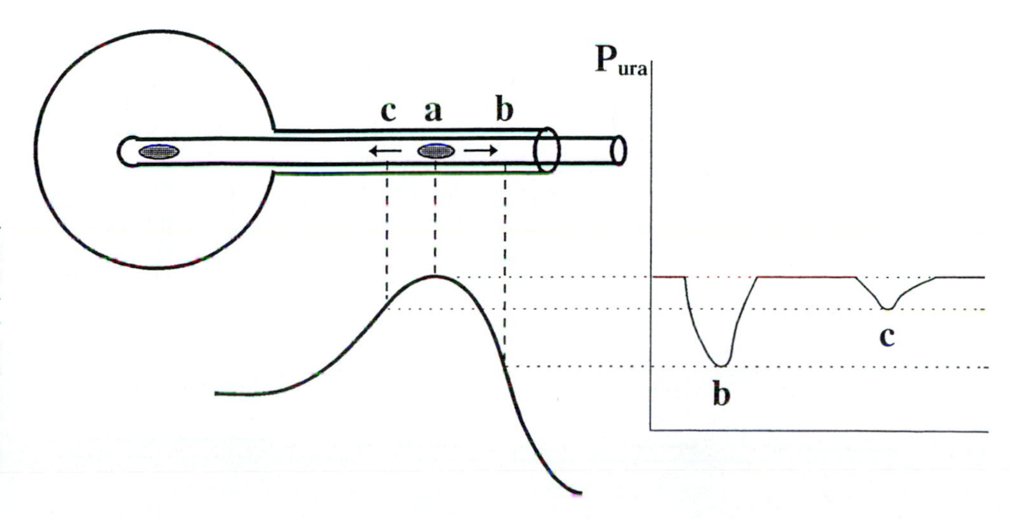

FIGURE 6–2. The apparent decreases in urethral pressure (p_{ura}) demonstrated in the tracing on the right are not due to unstable urethral pressure but rather to movement of the urethral pressure transducer from the high-pressure zone of the urethra (*point a*) to a more proximal (*point c*) or distal (*point b*) location. Such artifact is currently impossible to control in standing or ambulating patients.

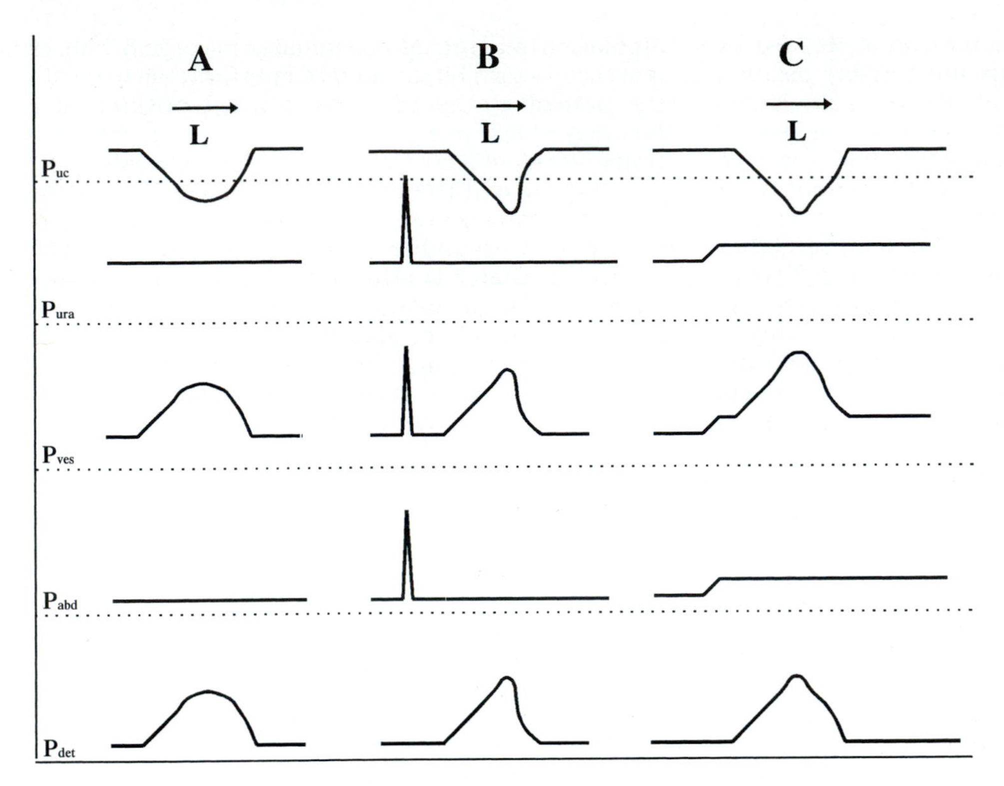

FIGURE 6–3. (*A*), Spontaneous detrusor instability with a detrusor contraction, equalization of p_{uc}, and observation of sustained urine leakage (*L*). (*B*), Detrusor instability following a cough (indicated by a sharp rise in p_{abd}, p_{ves}, and p_{ura}), an example of provoked instability. (*C*), Another example of provoked detrusor instability, which was noted shortly after the patient went from a supine to a standing position. The small sustained rise in p_{abd}, p_{ves}, and p_{ura} with standing results from an increase in abdominal pressure.

multaneously with a stress without concurrently demonstrable DI during cystometry (without measuring p_{ura}), if leakage is observed from the urethra at the instant of a stress immediately after the urethral catheter is removed, or if detrusor instability was totally absent during the preceding urethrocystometry. Diagnosis of mixed incontinence is made when the patient meets the diagnostic criteria for both DI and GSI.

Unstable urethral pressure (UUP—a term not defined by the ICS) is diagnosed if variations in urethral pressure greater than 15 cm water pressure (positive

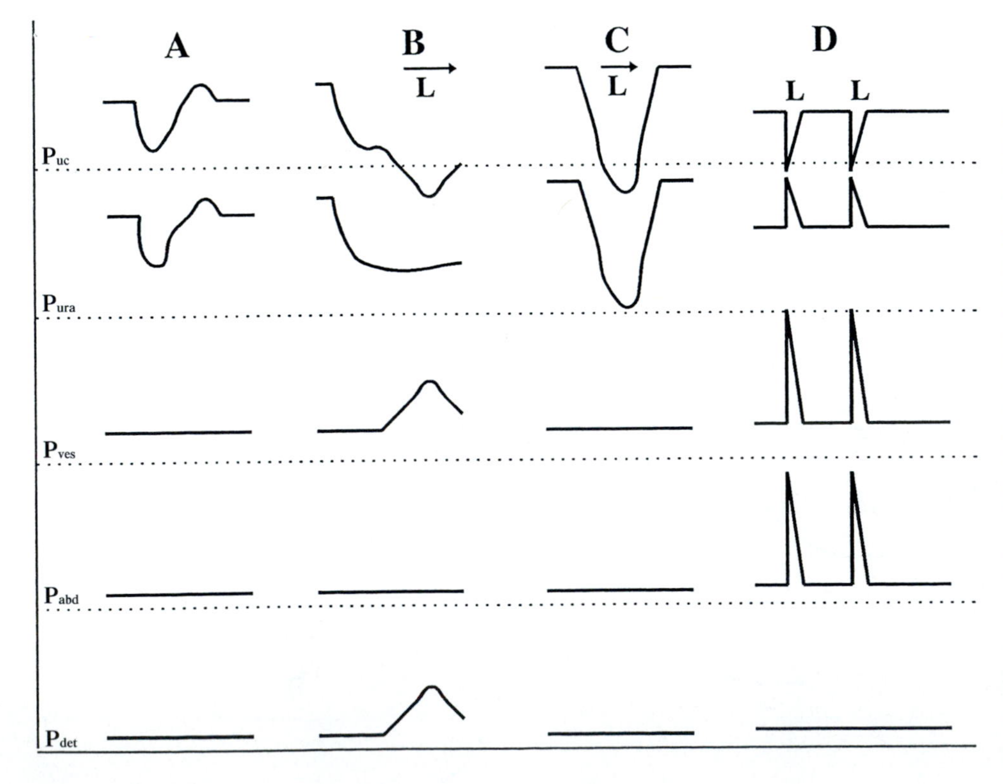

FIGURE 6–4. (*A*), Unstable urethral pressure (UUP) manifested by a fall in p_{ura} and p_{uc} not associated with a change in p_{abd} or p_{ves}; p_{uc} does not equalize and leakage does not occur. Patients often complain of abrupt urgency concurrent with such a drop in urethral pressure. (*B*), An incontinent episode initiated by a drop in p_{ura} followed by a detrusor contraction which results in the equalization of p_{uc} and leakage (*L*). (*C*), An incontinent episode resulting from pure UUP. Leakage occurs when urethral relaxation results in equalization of p_{uc}; no bladder or abdominal pressure changes are noted. (*D*), Leakage due to genuine stress incontinence contrasts with UUP in that the equalization of p_{uc} results from preferential transmission of rapid increases in p_{abd} to the bladder compared to the urethra. The difference in pressure transmission exceeds the resting pressure gradient between the urethra and the bladder, and leakage occurs.

or negative), not associated with an increase in abdominal pressure or with vascular pulsations, are demonstrated (Figs. 6–4*A*, *B*, *C*).[11] UUP has been associated with chronic urethral syndrome, sensory urgency, and "sensory" urge incontinence (i.e., urgency incontinence without the demonstration of detrusor contractions on cystometry).[12,13] It is also commonly seen preceding bladder contractions during urodynamic testing in patients with DI[14–16] (Fig. 6–4*B*) and in patients with mixed incontinence.[17] In such patients the finding of UUP may have important therapeutic implications; patients with UUP preceding their DI may respond poorly to anticholinergic therapy unless it is combined with an alpha adrenergic agonist[18]; those with UUP and mixed incontinence may be the subset of patients with mixed incontinence who respond well to continence surgery.[17] It should be emphasized that a wide overlap exists between urethral pressure variations in normal women and in those with various types of incontinence.[19,20] Variations in urethral pressure not temporally associated with significant urgency, not preceding detrusor instability, or not resulting in incontinence with equalization of p_{ves} and p_{ura} are likely physiologic and of no clinical significance.

Compliance is calculated by dividing the change in bladder volume by the change in p_{det} during retrograde filling ($C = \Delta V/\Delta p_{det}$) and is expressed as mL/cm H_2O. During normal bladder filling, little or no increase in p_{det} is observed; the ICS calls this normal compliance. There is no generally accepted definition of abnormal compliance. A steady rise in p_{det} that leads to urine leakage is unquestionably abnormal (Fig. 6–5). The p_{det} at which leakage starts from the urethra is referred to as the **detrusor leak point pressure** (DLPP). A DLPP in excess of 40 cm H_2O poses a high risk for vesicoureteral reflux, hydronephrosis, and upper tract deterioration.[21] Such extreme examples of abnormal compliance are limited to patients with myelodysplastic conditions and spinal cord injuries.

Detrusor hyperreflexia is detrusor overactivity caused by disturbances affecting neurologic control. **Reflex incontinence** is urine loss caused by detrusor hyperreflexia with or without involuntary urethral relaxation in the absence of the sensation of urgency in patients with neuropathic disorders.[6] **Overflow incontinence** is loss associated with over-distension of the bladder and is really a filling phase symptom that is due to emptying phase dysfunction.

AMBULATORY URODYNAMICS

Prolonged ambulatory monitoring techniques, originally developed for electrocardiographic and esophageal manometric studies, have been adapted to urodynamics.[22–24] Ambulatory urodynamics uses internal pressure transducers mounted on small-caliber catheters, with digitalization of the pressure signal allowing storage on magnetic tape or in microprocessor solid-state memory for later computer retrieval and analysis.[22] The technique eliminates the physical constraints and psychologic stress of the

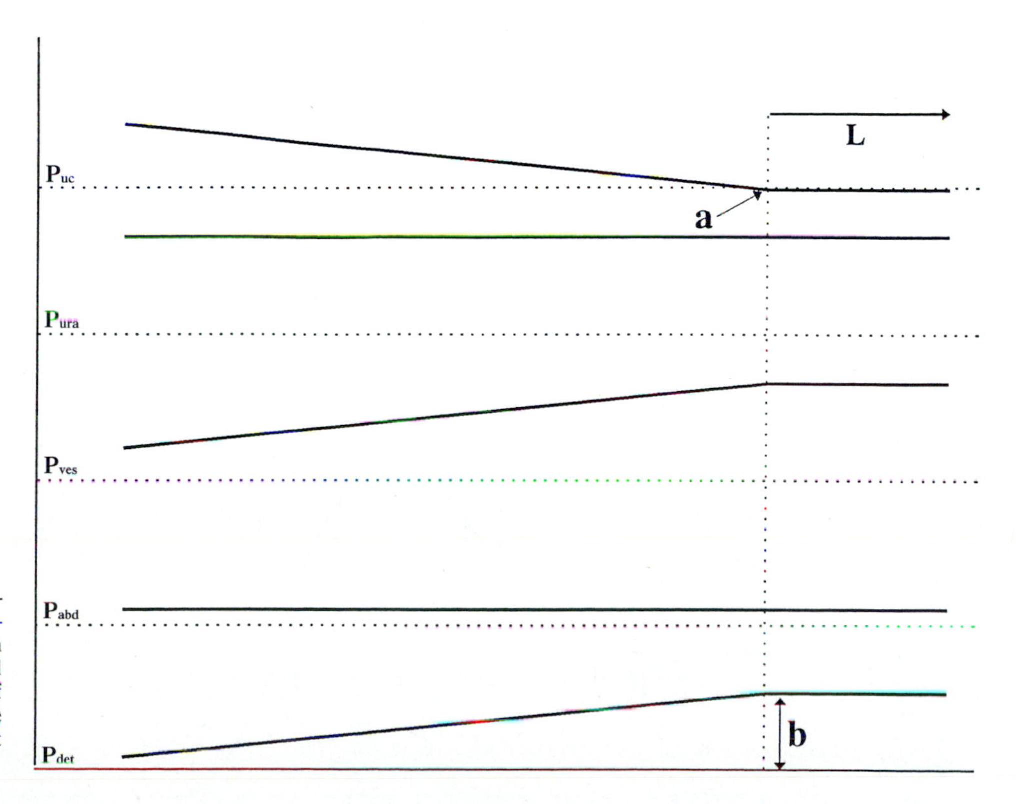

FIGURE 6–5. A noncompliant bladder with a steady increase in p_{det} resulting in a decrease in p_{uc} with eventual pressure equalization and urine leakage at *point a*. The level of detrusor pressure at which leakage starts (*B*) is the detrusor leak point pressure (DLPP).

laboratory setting and the artifact of retrograde filling. It allows extended observation (from several hours to 1 day) of lower urinary tract function during physiologic bladder filling under normal daily circumstances and conditions that normally cause symptoms for the patient. The technique has considerable potential for the study of women with urge incontinence in whom traditional urodynamic studies have been normal and in those with symptoms limited to certain activities or sleep.[23]

Because the procedure is time-consuming and high costs of equipment limit the number of studies that can be performed, its likely role is as a supplement to nondiagnostic studies rather than a replacement of conventional laboratory urodynamics. Current techniques are limited to the measurement of bladder and abdominal pressure, because inevitable catheter movement renders urethral pressure measurements unreliable.[24] It should also be noted that detrusor instability was observed in 69% of 36 healthy, asymptomatic female volunteers monitored for 5 hours with this technique.[24] Thus, it is important that events recorded during ambulatory monitoring be rigorously correlated with the simultaneous occurrence of symptoms.

URETHRAL PRESSURE PROFILE (UPP)

Urethrocystometry records urethral pressure at one location in the urethra during filling. The UPP measures pressure along the urethra by pulling a transducer from the internal to the external meatus at a constant speed using a mechanical pulling device (profilometer); the pressure curve is displayed on a chart recorder or video display system whose plotting speed is matched to the withdrawal speed of the transducer (Fig. 6–6). The functional urethral length (FUL; the distance through which p_{ura} exceeds p_{ves}) and the maximum p_{uc} (also commonly referred to as MUCP) are the most commonly reported measurements. The total profile area and mean p_{uc} (MnUCP; [profile area in mm $\times$ cm H_2O]/[FUL in mm]) can also be derived and may correlate better with other measures of sphincteric function than FUL or MUCP.

The role of the UPP in the evaluation of the incontinent woman is controversial. The major goal of urethral studies during urodynamics is to identify the stress-incontinent patient who has a severely compromised intrinsic urethral sphincteric mechanism (intrinsic sphincter deficiency [ISD]—previously called type III GSI) and to differentiate her from the patient with simple hypermobility GSI (type II), because this distinction has important therapeutic implications.[25] Urethral pressure profilometry can help to identify the patient with ISD. Other methods that can aid in the diagnosis include fluoroscopic video-urodynamic evaluations, urethral ultrasound studies, and leak point pressure determinations. None of these studies alone absolutely establishes the diagnosis of ISD; each should be correlated with the overall clinical picture and total urogynecologic evaluation.[25]

As with urethrocystometry, the specific testing circumstances during the UPP should be stated. In addition to those specified in Table 5–1, the bladder volume, internal transducer orientation (anterior, lateral, or posterior) and transducer withdrawal speed should be specified. The UPP is most often per-

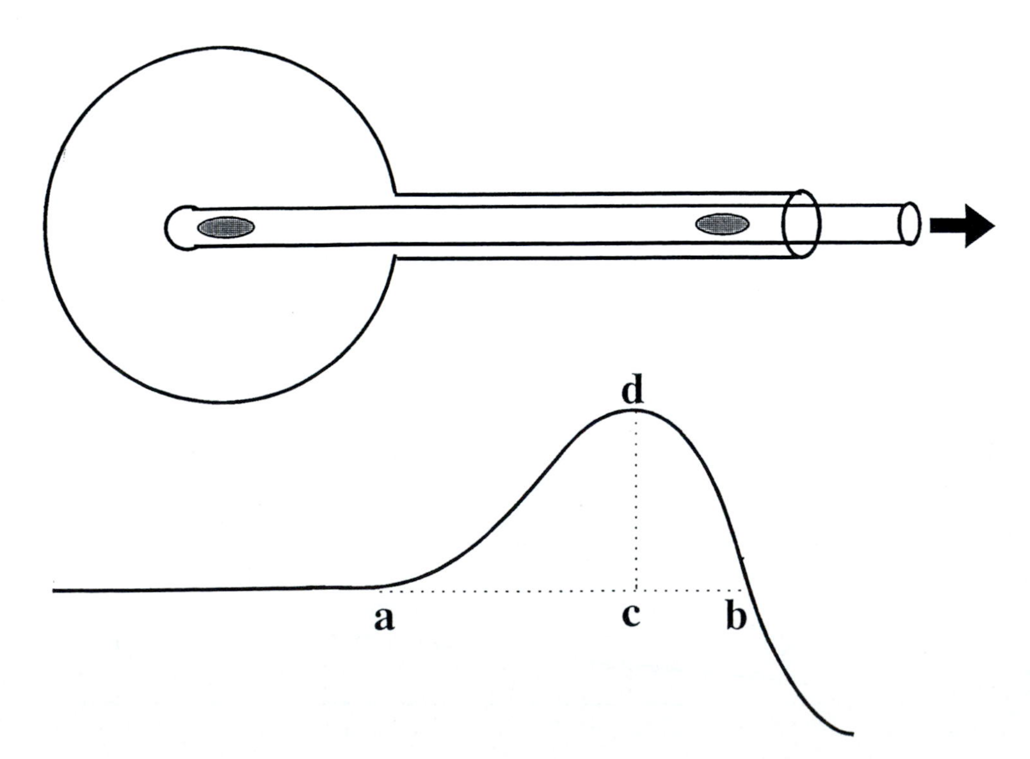

FIGURE 6–6. The urethral transducer on the dual internal transducer catheter is positioned 6 cm proximal to the distal vesical transducer, so that it can be withdrawn through the entire length of the female urethra while the distal transducer remains in the bladder. The urethral pressure profile (UPP) curve is traced by a recorder with a tracing speed equal to the catheter withdrawal speed. Line a–b represents the functional urethral length (*FUL*, starting at the point when the UPP curve rises above baseline p_{ves} and ending when the curve returns to that level) and line c–d represents maximum urethral closure pressure (MUCP). The area of a–b–d–a can also be calculated and a mean urethral closure pressure (MnUCP) obtained by dividing this area by the FUL.

formed with the patient at rest (passive UPP), as in Figure 6–6, and with the patient coughing repeatedly (dynamic UPP; Fig. 6–7). The undamaged urethra in a young woman has an MUCP of 80 to 120 cm H_2O, the product of the multifactorial urethral sphincteric mechanism derived from skeletal muscle, smooth muscle, vascular, epithelial, and connective-tissue sources.[26–28] The sphincteric mechanism deteriorates and MUCP is decreased by a variety of life's events, including childbirth, neurologic disease or injury, aging, hormonal deprivation, and surgery. Critical deterioration to the point at which the mechanism is no longer capable of maintaining coaptation of the urethral mucosal surfaces represents ISD. An MUCP below 15 to 20 cm H_2O suggests this diagnosis.[25,29]

Dynamic UPP can be used to establish the diagnosis of GSI (Fig. 6–7). It can also be used to calculate a pressure transmission ratio (PTR, Fig. 6–8). The PTR expresses in quantitative terms the relative magnitude of pressure rises in the urethra and bladder with stress.[30] A PTR of 100% signifies that the urethral and vesical pressure spikes are of equal magnitude; one below 100% means that the vesical pressure spike is greater than the urethral spike, and one above 100% means that the urethral spike is greater.

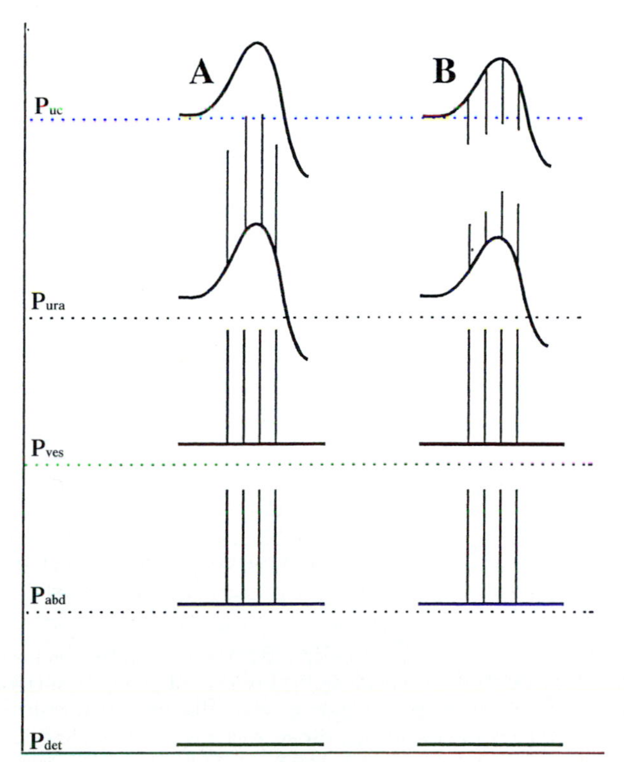

FIGURE 6–7. *(A)*, A dynamic urethral pressure profile (UPP) in a stress-continent patient with equal cough pressure spikes in the bladder and the urethra, resulting in unchanged p_{uc}. *(B)*, A dynamic UPP in a patient with genuine stress incontinence. The cough pressure spikes in the bladder are much higher than those in the urethra, the difference being sufficient to eliminate the positive urethral pressure gradient. Leakage is observed concurrent with equalization of p_{uc} in the absence of any detrusor activity.

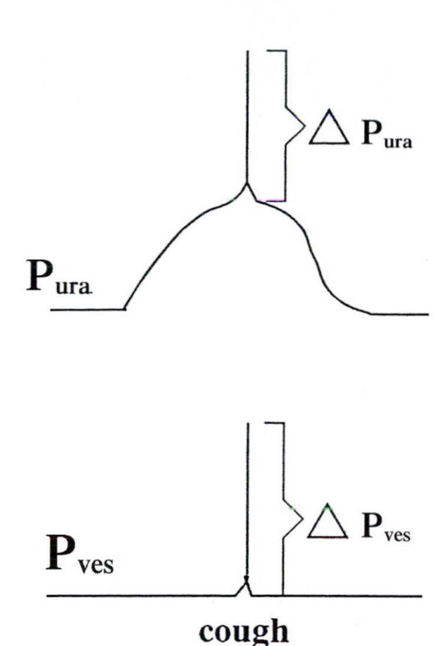

FIGURE 6–8. Calculation of the pressure transmission ratio (PTR). The cough-induced pressure rise in urethral pressure (Δp_{ura}) is divided by the simultaneous rise in vesical pressure (Δp_{ves}) and the quotient is multiplied by 100. PTRs can be calculated at several locations along the urethra, with the location noted as a percentage of the functional urethral length or as a particular quarter or third of the urethra.

Groups of patients with GSI have significantly lower PTRs than groups of normal women[31] and patients with other forms of lower urinary tract dysfunction.[30] Although virtually all women with GSI have PTRs below 100%, many women with PTRs below this level remain stress continent either because their resting urethral closure pressure is great enough or their daily stresses are small enough to allow them to maintain a positive, though diminished, pressure gradient with stress. Although normal pressure transmission appears to have both active neuromuscular and passive anatomic bases,[32] significant depression of PTR is usually associated with urethral hypermobility. Women with type II GSI typically have MUCP well above 15 to 20 cm H_2O, PTR much below 90%, and significant urethral hypermobility. GSI with MUCP below this level and with PTR above 90% suggests the diagnosis of ISD even when hypermobility is present; they are diagnostic of ISD in the presence of a normally positioned urethra. An increase in PTR toward or above 100% is the most consistent urodynamic finding associated with successful continence surgery designed to elevate and stabilize the urethrovesical junction.

Urethral pressure profiles can also be performed during Kegel's pelvic muscle contraction **(Kegel's UPP)** and during the Valsalva maneuver **(strain UPP)**. Kegel's UPP can be used to assess how effectively an individual patient can perform a pelvic muscle contraction and may assist in the training of the patient in the technique (Fig. 6–9).[33] The strain UPP observes the effect of straining during the Valsalva maneuver on the urethral pressure gradient; if leakage is observed during the profile, the bladder leak point pressure with the Valsalva maneuver can be determined.

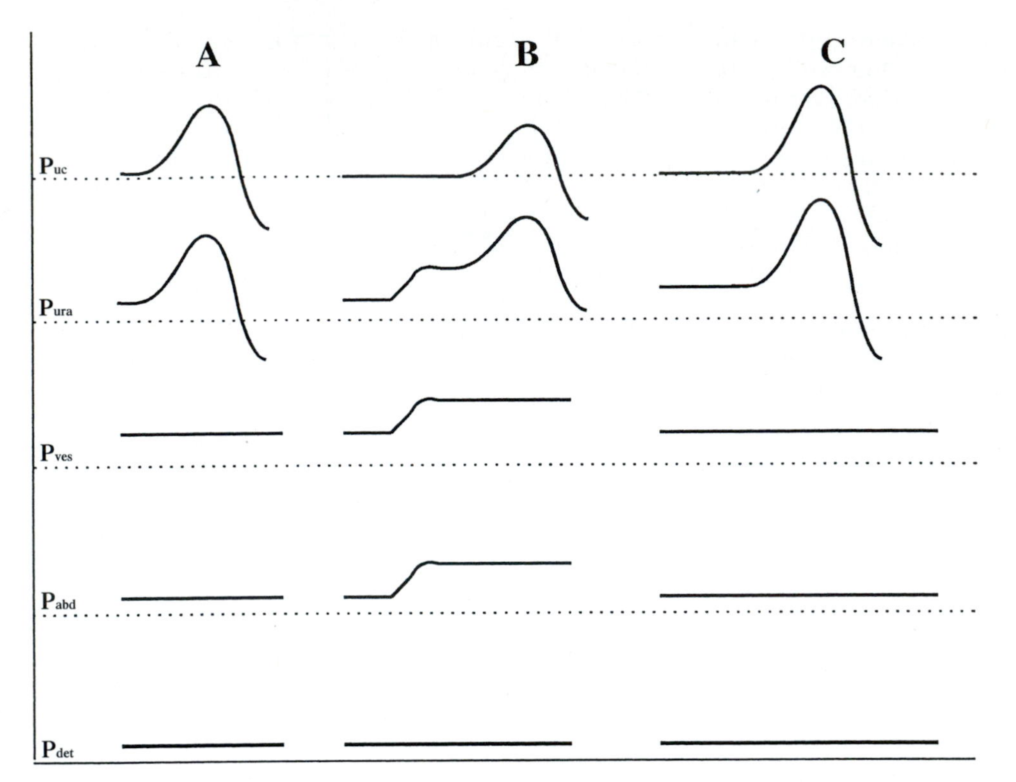

FIGURE 6–9. (*A*). Resting urethral closure pressure compared with (*B*) an ineffective and (*C*) an effective Kegel pelvic muscle contraction. In (*B*), the Kegel effort was accompanied by a significant Valsalva effort with an increase in abdominal and vesical pressure which was transmitted only partially to the urethra in this patient who had genuine stress incontinence. The net effect was a decrease in total profile area, maximum urethral closure pressure, and mean urethral closure pressure. In (*C*), the patient substantially increases the strength of urethral closure with no abdominal straining. Analysis of the Kegel urethral pressure profile can help in training patients to perform Kegel exercises correctly.

LEAK POINT PRESSURE (LPP)

The DLPP has already been considered in the discussion of the noncompliant bladder. The **abdominal** or **Valsalva LPP (VLPP)** is recorded by measuring the increase in p_{ves} at the precise instant that fluid leakage is observed at the external urethral meatus while the patient is performing a Valsalva maneuver (Fig. 6–10). The VLPP has been used in the evaluation of women with GSI and promoted as an accurate diagnostic test for ISD.[34–36] A VLPP less than 60 cm H_2O has been significantly correlated with the diagnosis of ISD on video-urodynamic studies.[35,36] The measurement is easy to perform with less sophisticated and expensive equipment than the UPP requires and is highly reproducible in the majority of women with GSI.[36,37] Its measurement can depend on several variables of technique, however, including bladder volume, patient position, and catheter size.[37,38] VLPP is poorly correlated with MUCP and only weakly correlated with MnUCP.[37]

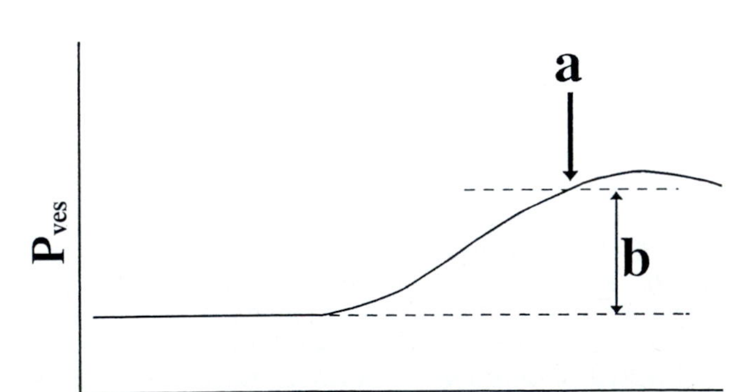

FIGURE 6–10. Measurement of Valsalva leak point pressure (VLPP). The periurethral area is swabbed dry, after which the patient is asked to bear down progressively while holding her breath. The precise instant that fluid is observed at the external urethral meatus is recorded on the vesical pressure record using a remote event marker, denoted by the arrow at point *a*. The rise in p_{ves} over baseline (*b*) is measured at the instant leakage begins and represents the VLPP.

VIDEO-URODYNAMICS USING FLUOROSCOPY OR ULTRASONOGRAPHY

Fluoroscopic video-urodynamics combines multichannel urethrocystometry using radiocontrast as the fluid medium, EMG, and fluoroscopy with simultaneous video monitor display of the urodynamic data and fluoroscopic image.[5] The technique can identify patients with a mobile urethrovesical junction, supporting a diagnosis of hypermobility as the cause of a patient's GSI, as well as those with an open bladder neck at rest, supporting a diagnosis of ISD. Video-urodynamics can also confirm a constant position of the urethral sensor during urethrocystometry and can visually confirm detrusor contractions, detrusor sphincter dyssynergia, outlet obstruction, and abnormal detrusor contractility, further validating diagnoses based on pressure tracings.[5,25] Many experts agree with Blaivas in his analysis that video-urodynamics "provides the most precise, artifact-free display of normal and abnormal physiology" of the lower urinary tract.[5] Disadvantages of the study include a substantial increase in costs for equipment and facilities, longer study duration, higher patient charges, and exposure to radiation for both patient and staff. In an effort to overcome some of these limitations, several authors have reported the use of real-time ultrasound instead of fluoroscopy for the continuous visualization of the bladder and urethra during urethrocystometry, especially to evaluate bladder neck mobility and funneling in patients with GSI.[39–42] The superiority of these simultaneous visualization techniques over lower-cost and "lower-tech" procedures (such as selected resting and straining lateral cystourethrography, urethrocystoscopy, Q-tip testing) has not been established.

MULTICHANNEL URODYNAMIC ASSESSMENT OF THE EMPTYING PHASE

PRESSURE-FLOW STUDIES

Uroflowmetry is the recording of instantaneous urine flow rate (in mL/sec^{-1}) versus time during voluntary micturition. Parameters measured or derived include the voided volume, the maximum flow rate (Q_{max}), the mean flow rate (Q_{mean}), the flow time, and the micturition time (Fig. 6–11).[6] A postvoid residual urine measurement is also considered a part of the study. Flow patterns are classified as normal/continuous (Fig. 6–11*A*), multiple-peaked/continuous, or interrupted (Fig. 6–11*B*).[1,43] Flow rates are proportional to the starting bladder volume and there is considerable intra- and interindividual variation. Normal studies display a $Q_{max} \geq 15$ mL/sec^{-1}, a $Q_{mean} \geq 10$ mL/sec^{-1}, continuous flow, and a postvoid residual ≤ 50 mL. A single abnormal study, particularly in the stressful confines of an often intimidating urodynamic laboratory, should be verified on several occasions; no study should be considered abnormal if the total bladder volume (voided volume plus residual) was less than 200 mL.[44] Noninstrumented uroflowmetry is a reasonable screening test for voiding dysfunction. Pressure-flow (P/Q) studies, especially when combined with external sphincter electromyography, allow definition of the patient's voiding mechanism and establish the basis of any voiding dysfunction. P/Q studies may also have some value for the identification of patients with GSI (patients with poor detrusor contractility and those who void during the Valsalva maneuver) who are more likely to develop prolonged retention after continence surgery.[45]

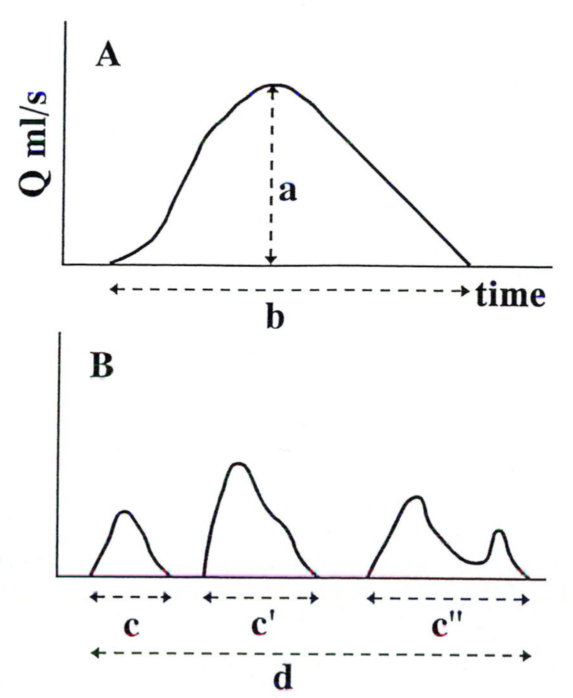

FIGURE 6–11. (*A*), A normal continuous uroflow curve, plotting instantaneous flow (Q) versus time. Line *a* represents maximum flow (Q_{max}) and line *b* represents flow time. Mean flow is calculated by dividing the voided volume by the flow time. (*B*), A multiple-peak, interrupted uroflow curve. The flow time = (c + c′ + c″) and the micturition time = *d*. Flow time is always used to calculate mean flow rates. For continuous uroflow patterns, flow time and micturition time are the same.

The PQ study is performed with a small-gauge (3-Fr), nonobstructing transurethral catheter to measure p_{ves} and a vaginal (or rectal) catheter to measure p_{abd}. Despite years of effort, urologists do not agree as to how P/Q studies should be interpreted and how the diagnosis of bladder outlet obstruction in benign prostatic hypertrophy should be established. Normal values and diagnostic criteria in women who rarely have natural obstruction have received little attention. Agreement exists that high flow at low pressure excludes obstruction (and may suggest sphincter weakness), and that low flow at high pressures defines obstruction. There is no accepted absolute normal cutoff level of either flow or pressure, however, and results of many studies fall in equivocal ranges. It should also be noted that rises in p_{ves} and p_{det} depend on both the increase in bladder tone and the urethral resistance. Patients with very low resistance may not show a sustained detrusor contraction because the detrusor contraction generates increased flow without a significant increase in pressure. Thus diagnosis of an acontractile or underactive detrusor may be difficult in these situations unless flow is stopped by artificially obstructing the outlet.[47] This pressure (termed **p_{det}iso**) is normally in the range of 50 to 100 cm H_2O in adult men and women and probably is the best general measure of the adequacy of detrusor contractility. A significant lowering of p_{det}iso and a prolongation in time required to achieve the maximum p_{det}iso are the major urodynamic characteristics of a condition termed **detrusor hyperactivity with impaired contractility (DHIC),** a cause of urgency incontinence and paradoxic ineffective emptying of the bladder commonly observed in incontinent elderly women.[48] Pharmacologic treatment of the detrusor hyperactivity in an effort to control incontinence places these women at risk for developing urinary retention.

Other important variables with respect to the evaluation of emptying phase dysfunction determined during PQ studies are the opening pressure, the bladder pressure at maximum flow (Fig. 6–12), and the source of the bladder pressure (i.e., detrusor contraction versus strain during the Valsalva maneuver). In a study of 19 healthy, asymptomatic female volunteers, the mean opening pressure (p_{ves}op) was

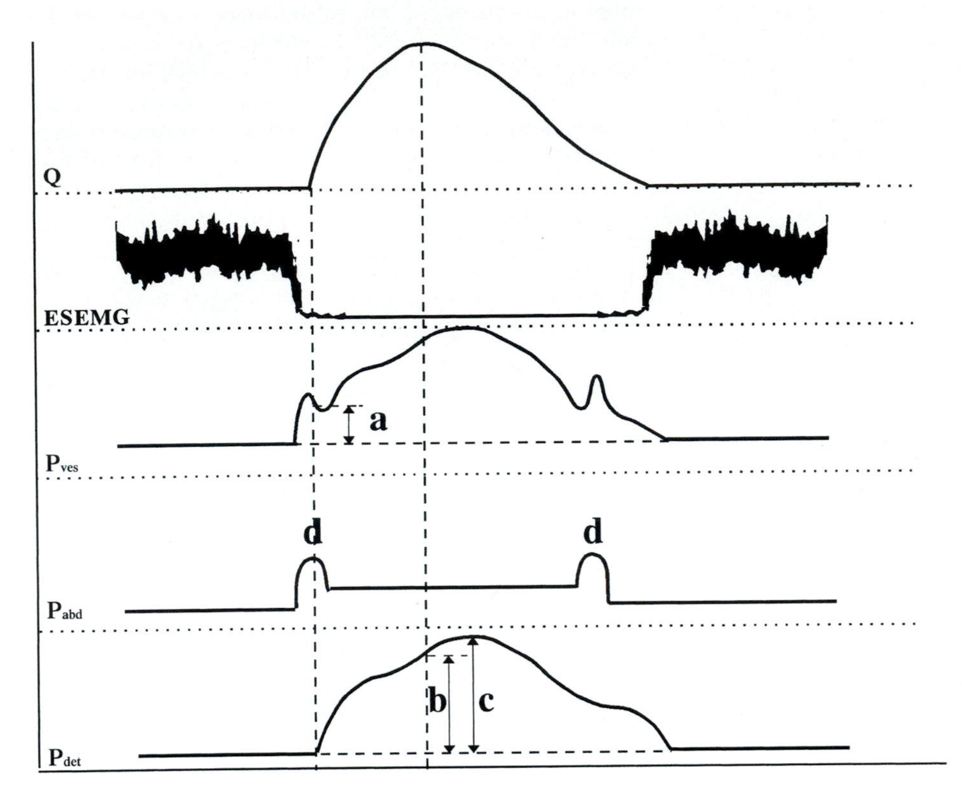

FIGURE 6–12. A pressure/flow/electromyographic (EMG) study: The external sphincter EMG is silent during the continuous void. Line *a* is the opening vesical pressure, *b* is the detrusor pressure at maximum flow, and *c* is the maximum detrusor pressure. Points *d* represent slight abdominal straining at the start and end of the voiding episode.

around 40 cm H_2O and the mean detrusor pressure at maximum flow ($p_{det}Q_{max}$) was around 30 cm H_2O.[47] When poor flow is seen despite a normally contracting detrusor, external sphincter EMG, in combination with an anatomic evaluation of the bladder outlet, is used to differentiate among mechanical obstruction, detrusor/external sphincter dyssynergia (DSD), and detrusor/urethral smooth muscle dyssynergia.

EXTERNAL SPHINCTER ELECTROMYOGRAPHY (ESEMG)

Bioelectrical activity generated when a skeletal muscle motor unit depolarizes represents the motor unit action potential that can be measured as the ESEMG using various inserted and surface electrode systems. Skeletal muscle is electrically silent at rest, a state that is observed in the external urethral sphincter only during micturition.[49] At other times, the multiple contracting motor units of the sphincter generate a complex record of potentials known as a **complete interference pattern.** Parameters of this interference pattern are qualitatively related to contraction strength of the sphincter. Analysis of the interference pattern is used to evaluate the micturition reflex and to see if the normal sequence of external sphincter relaxation preceding detrusor contraction is seen (Fig. 6–13). Failure of a good-quality ESEMG to silence during a micturition effort is diagnostic of DSD.[50] Poor flow in the face of a normal increase in p_{ves} due to a detrusor contraction and a silenced ESEMG in the absence of physical obstruction is diagnostic for detrusor/urethral smooth muscle dyssynergia.

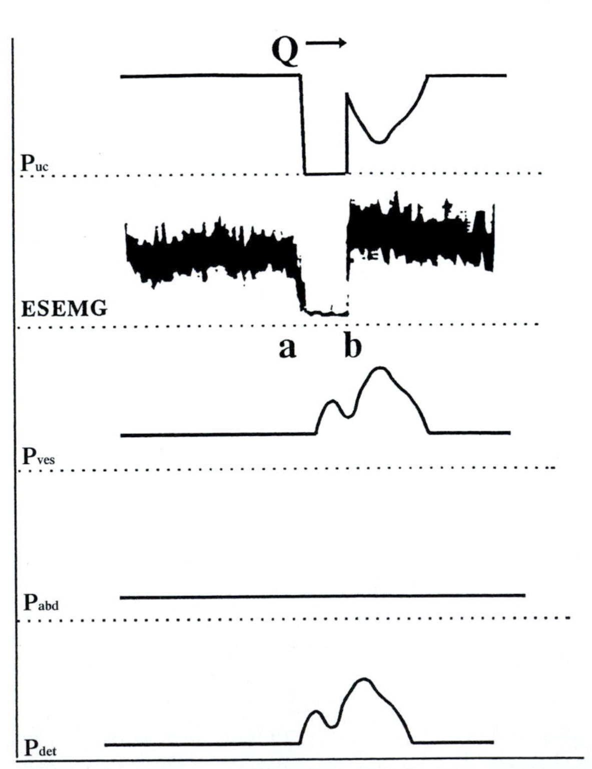

FIGURE 6–13. A normal void and stop-void study. The external sphincter electromyographic (ESEMG) silences at point *a* and p_{uc} decreases, just before the detrusor contraction begins. The process is reversed when the patient is asked to stop her stream (point *b*).

REFERENCES

1. Nielsen, IKT, Bruskewitz, RC and Madsen, PO: Urodynamics of the lower urinary tract. Urol Res 16:271, 1988.
2. Enhorning, G: Simultaneous recording of intravesical and intraurethral pressure. Acta Chir Scand 276 (Suppl):1, 1961.
3. Rowan, D, James, ED, Kramer, AE, et al: Urodynamic equipment: technical aspects. Produced by the International Continence Society Working Party on Urodynamic Equipment. J Med Eng Technol 1:57, 1987.
4. Bump, RC: The urodynamic laboratory. Obstet Gynecol Clin North Am 16:795, 1989.
5. Blaivas, J: Multichannel urodynamic studies. Urol 23:421, 1984.
6. The International Continence Society Committee on Standardization of Terminology; Abrams, P, et al: The standardization of terminology of lower urinary tract function. Scand J Urol Nephrol 114S:5, 1988.
7. Richardson, DA: Use of vaginal pressure measurements in urodynamic testing. Obstet Gynecol 66:581, 1985.
8. Fantl, JA, Wyman, JF, Anderson, RL, et al: Postmenopausal urinary incontinence: comparison between non-estrogen-supplemented and estrogen-supplemented women. Obstet Gynecol 71:823, 1988.
9. Sand, PK, Hill, RC and Ostergard, DR: Supine urethroscopic and standing cystometry as screening methods for the detection of detrusor instability. Obstet Gynecol 70:57, 1987.
10. Bergman, A and Bhatia, NN: Urodynamics: effect of urinary tract infection on urethral and bladder function. Obstet Gynecol 66:366, 1985.
11. Ulmsten, U, Henriksson, L and Iosif, S: The unstable female urethra. Am J Obstet Gynecol 144:93, 1982.
12. Weil, A, Miege, B, Rottenberg, R, et al: Clinical significance of urethral instability. Obstet Gynecol 106:106, 1986.
13. Kulseng-Hanssen, S: Prevalence and pattern of unstable urethral pressure in one hundred seventy-four gynecologic patients referred for urodynamic investigation. Am J Obstet Gynecol 146:895, 1983.
14. Hindmarsh, JR, Gosling, PT and Deane, AM: Bladder instability: is the primary defect in the urethra? Br J Urol 55:648, 1983.
15. Penders, L, de Leval, J and Petit, R: Enuresis and urethral instability. Eur Urol 10:317, 1984.
16. Papa, PE and Ulmsten, U: Bladder instability in women: a premature activation of the micturition reflex. Neurourol Urodyn 12:235, 1993.
17. Koonings, P, Bergman, A and Ballard, CA: Combined detrusor instability and stress urinary incontinence: where is the primary pathology? Gynecol Obstet Invest 26:250, 1988.
18. Bergman, A, Koonings, PP and Ballard, CA: Detrusor instability: is the bladder the cause or the effect? J Reprod Med 34:834, 1989.
19. Kulseng-Hanssen, S and Kristoffersen, M: Urethral pressure variations in females with and without neurological symptoms. Scand J Urol Nephrol 114S:48, 1988.
20. Sørensen, S: Urethral pressure variations in healthy and incontinent women. Neurourol Urodyn 11:549, 1992.
21. McGuire, EJ, Woodside, JR, Borden, TA, et al: Prognostic value of urodynamic testing in myelodysplastic patients. J Urol 126:205, 1981.
22. Griffiths, CJ, Assi, MS, Styles, RA, et al: Ambulatory monitoring of bladder and detrusor pressure during natural filling. J Urol 142:780, 1989.
23. McInerney, PD, Vanner, TF, Harris, SA, et al: Ambulatory urodynamics. Br J Urol 67:272, 1991.
24. van Waalwijk van Doorn, ESC, Remmers, A and Janknegt, RA: Conventional and extramural ambulatory urodynamic testing of the lower urinary tract in female volunteers. J Urol 147:1319, 1992.
25. Urinary Incontinence Guideline Panel: Urinary Incontinence in Adults: Clinical Practice Guideline. AHCPR Pub. No. 92-0038. Agency for Health Care Policy and Research, Public Health and Human Services, Rockville, MD, March 1992, pp 1–25; and 53–58.
26. Tanagho, EA, Meyers, FH and Smith, DR: Urethral resistance: its components and implications. I. smooth muscle component. Invest Urol 7:136, 1969.
27. Rud, T: Factors maintaining the intraurethral pressure in women. Invest Urol 17:343, 1980.
28. Bump, RC, Friedman, CI and Copeland, WE, Jr: Non-neuromuscular determinants of intraluminal urethral pressure in the female baboon: relative importance of vascular and nonvascular factors. J Urol 139:162, 1988.
29. Sand, PK, Bowen, LW, Panganibank, R, et al: The low pressure urethra as a factor in failed retropubic urethropexy. Obstet Gynecol 69:399, 1987.
30. Bump, RC, Copeland, WE, Jr, Hurt, WG, et al: Dynamic urethral pressure profilometry pressure transmission ratio determinations in stress-incontinent and stress-continent subjects. Am J Obstet Gynecol 159:749, 1988.
31. Hilton, P and Stanton, SL: Urethral pressure measurement by microtransducer: the results in symptom-free women and in those with genuine stress incontinence. Br J Obstet Gynaecol 90:919, 1983.
32. Bump, RC, Huang, KC, McClish, DK, et al: Effect of narcotic anesthesia and skeletal muscle paralysis on passive and dynamic urethral function of stress continent and incontinent women. Neurourol Urodyn 10:523, 1991.
33. Bump, RC, Hurt, WG, Fantl, JA, et al: Assessment of Kegel pelvic muscle exercise performance after brief verbal instruction. Am J Obstet Gynecol 165:322, 1991.
34. Appell, RA: Injectables for urethral incompetence. World J Urol 8:208, 1990.
35. Fitzpatrick, CC, McGuire, EJ, Wan, J, et al: Abdominal leak point pressure as an index of urethral sphincter function (abstr). American Urogynecologic Society Scientific Program. Int Urogynecol J 4:387, 1993.
36. Gormley, EA and McGuire, EJ: Reproducibility of abdominal leak point pressure in the diagnosis of stress urinary incontinence (abstr). American Urogynecologic Society Scientific Program. Int Urogynecol J 4:387, 1993.
37. Bump, RC, Elser, KM and McClish, DK: Valsalva leak point pressures in adult women with genuine stress incontinence: reproducibility, effect of catheter caliber, and correlations with passive urethral pressure profilometry (abstr). International Continence Society Scientific Program. Neurourol Urodyn 12:307, 1993.
38. Decter, RM and Harpster, L: Pitfalls in determination of leak point pressure. J Urol 148:588, 1992.
39. White, RD, McQuown, D, McCarthy, TA, et al: Real-time ultrasonography in the evaluation of urinary stress incontinence. Am J Obstet Gynecol 138:235, 1980.
40. Brown, MC, Sutherst, JR, Murray, A, et al: Potential use of ultrasound in place of X-ray fluoroscopy in urodynamics. Br J Urol 57:88, 1985.
41. Kohorn, EI, Scioscia, AL, Jeanty, P, et al: Ultrasound cystourethrography by perineal scanning for the assessment of female stress urinary incontinence. Obstet Gynecol 68:269, 1986.
42. Johnson, JD, Lamensdorf, H, Hollander, IN, et al: Use of transvaginal endosonography in the evaluation of women with stress urinary incontinence. J Urol 147:421, 1992.
43. Fantl, JA, Smith, PJ, Schneider, V, et al: Fluid weight uroflowmetry in women. Am J Obstet Gynecol 145:1017, 1983.
44. Abrams, P: Uroflowmetry. In Stanton SL (ed.) Clinical Gynecologic Urology. CV Mosby, St. Louis, 1984, p 127.
45. Bhatia, NN and Bergman, A: Urodynamic predictability of voiding following incontinence surgery. Obstet Gynecol 63:85, 1984.
46. Abrams, P, Feneley, R and Torrens, M: Urodynamics. Springer-Verlag, New York, 1983, p 73.
47. Sjöberg, B and Nyman, CR: Hydrodynamics of micturition in healthy females: pressure and flow at different micturition volumes. Urol Int 36:23, 1981.
48. Resnick, NM and Yalla, SV: Detrusor hyperactivity with impaired contractile function: an unrecognized but common cause of incontinence in elderly patients. JAMA 257:3076, 1987.
49. Wein, AJ and Raezer, DM: Physiology of micturition. In Krane, RJ and Siroky, MB (eds.): Clinical Neuro-Urology. Little, Brown & Co, Boston, 1979, p 1.
50. Dibenedetto, M and Yalla, SV: Electrodiagnosis of striated urethral sphincter dysfunction. J Urol 122:361, 1979.

CHAPTER 7

Anal Manometry

Lee E. Smith

Anal manometry provides an objective assessment of sphincter function and pressure. Due to the complexity of sphincter physiology, complete functional assessment requires the evaluation of multiple factors in addition to sphincter pressures, such as neuromuscular integrity, rectal reservoir compliance, and colonic motility. Manometry, electromyography (EMG), pudendal nerve testing, colon transit time, defecography, rectal compliance, and rectal capacity are physiologic tests that might be employed in such an assessment. Clearly, anal manometry by itself is seldom the only test needed to define a problem, yet only manometry measures the pressures generated by the anorectal sphincter mechanism. Objective data obtained from manometry are resting tone, voluntary squeeze, presence of the rectoanal inhibitory reflex, compliance, and qualitative sensation. These findings may verify, classify, and diagnose specific causes of fecal incontinence and constipation.

INDICATION

Whenever the integrity of the anal sphincter needs to be evaluated, manometry may be employed to quantify the pressures generated. For example, the degree of sphincter impairment caused by obstetrical, surgical, and traumatic injury may be evaluated and documented prior to initiating treatment. The faulty portion of the sphincter mechanism may be identified and subsequent treatment modified by the extent and location of the injury.

Constipation disorders may likewise be classified by physiologic testing; manometry is one of the primary tests used in this regard. Hirschsprung's disease, which results from the absence of intramural ganglion cells, may manifest as chronic constipation. The classic manometric finding in this disorder is the absence of the anorectal inhibitory reflex (ARIR), which is described later in this chapter.

MANOMETRIC SYSTEMS

There is no standardized method for anorectal manometry. Each of several systems has advantages and disadvantages. The basic equipment in each system includes a catheter which is inserted into the anus and rectum, a transducer system, an air or water perfusion system, and a recorder (Figs. 7–1 and 7–2). Primary differences lie in whether the catheters are open or closed and whether balloons are used within the anal canal.

OPEN WATER PERFUSION SYSTEM

The open system employs a hydraulic water perfusion pump, which directs water through a catheter (Fig. 7–2); the water exits through holes near the tip of the catheter, which has been placed within the anus (Fig. 7–3). The sphincter provides resistance over the holes, generating a retrograde pressure which is transmitted through the catheter back to the transducer. Pressures recorded are therefore an index of resistance to the flow of water through the end of the catheter. In the transducer, mechanical force is converted to an electric signal that can be amplified and recorded.

The holes in the catheter may be arranged circumferentially around the tip (usually eight holes), or longitudinally at 0.5 to 1.0 cm intervals; simultaneous recordings reflect the circumferential or longitudinal pressure profile of the anal sphincter. At the catheter tip, side holes are preferable to the end holes because the anus closes in a side-to-side fashion.[1–3] A small balloon is mounted on the tip of the catheter and rests in the rectal vault; when insufflated, the balloon simulates gas or feces and presses against the rectal wall, initiating relaxation of the internal sphincter. This is the anorectal inhibitory reflex (ARIR); it is normally present.

The open water perfusion sysem is used most frequently, but its major disadvantage is error introduced by leakage of water. Water infused into the rectum may leak out onto the skin; the patient reacts and squeezes, causing an artificial tracing.[4] This may be circumvented by using catheters with low flow rates (0.2 mL/min) to minimize the volume of water.

CLOSED, LARGE BALLOON SYSTEM

Closed systems employ small or large balloons which may be filled with either air or water. Popularized by Marvin Schuster, the large balloon method uses double-molded balloons that are tied onto a hollow metal cylinder.[5] Two balloons can be inflated independently; pressures from each balloon are therefore recorded separately. When both balloons are

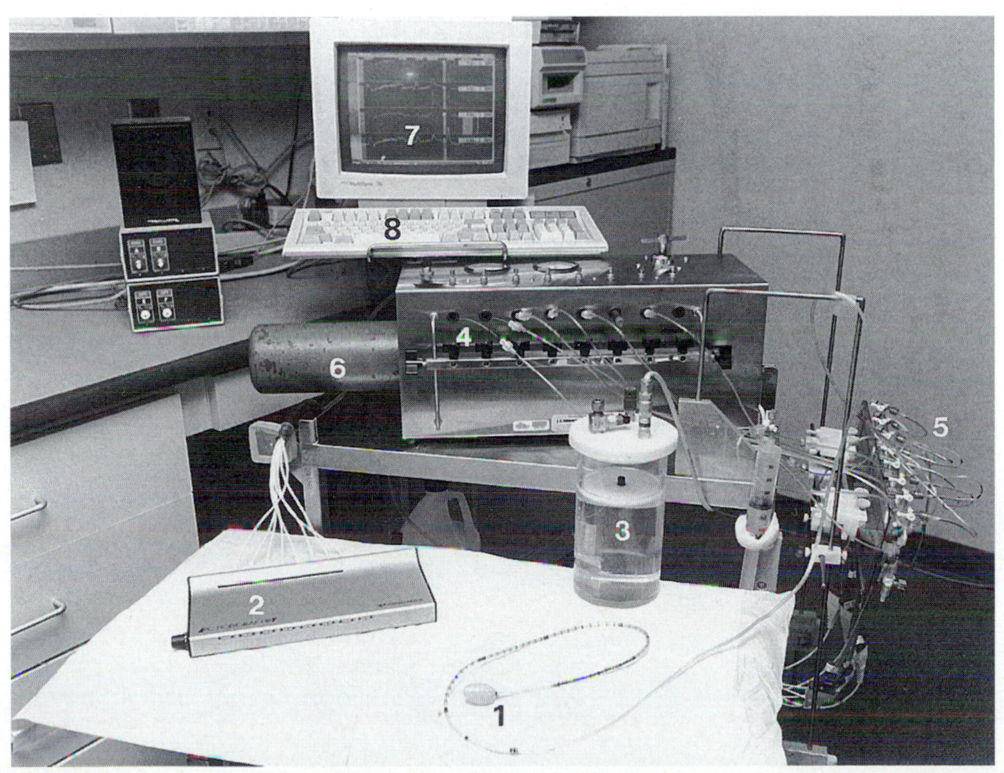

FIGURE 7–1. Water perfusion manometry unit. (1) Eight-channel catheter with rectal balloon. (2) Recorder. (3) Water reservoir. (4) Water perfusion pump. (5) Transducers. (6) Carbon dioxide tank. (7) Monitor. (8) Computer keyboard.

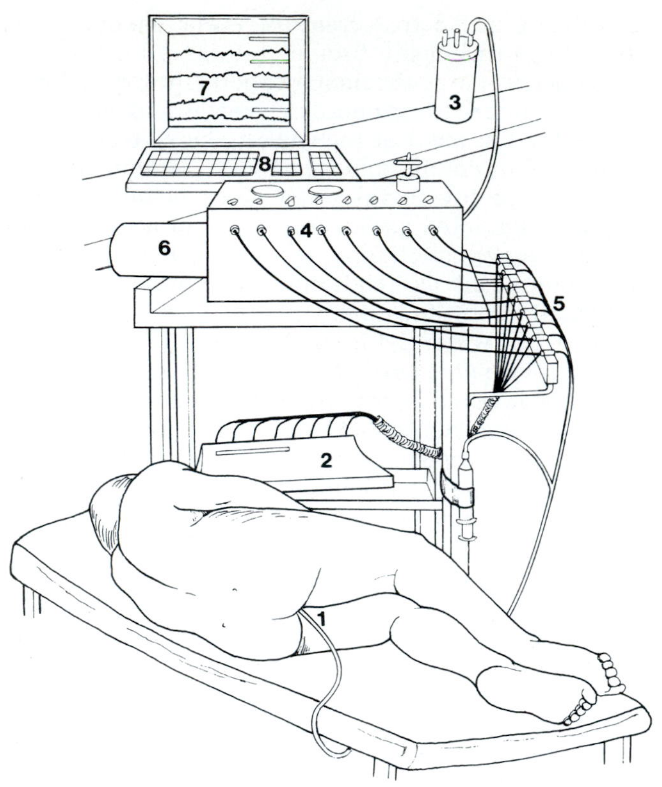

FIGURE 7–2. Diagram of water perfusion manometry unit. The numbering is the same as shown in Figure 7–1. The patient is in the left lateral decubitus position with the catheter inserted.

inflated, the proximal balloon impacts at the anorectal ring, preventing extrusion and fixing the distal balloon externally onto the sphincter mechanism. Fixation is an advantage of the closed system, but the large size of the cylinder introduces potential error; the pressures may be falsely increased if the probe stretches the sphincter.[1,6] The proximal balloon records internal sphincter pressures (resting pressure) and the distal balloon measures the external sphincter pressure (voluntary squeeze pressures). Another balloon is placed into the rectal vault and is used to elicit the anorectal inhibitory reflex and measure reservoir compliance and function. A disadvantage of this system is that balloons become more compliant over time, so that the baseline drifts and pressures at different points in the anal canal cannot be assessed.[7]

CLOSED, SMALL BALLOON SYSTEM

The small balloon system employs a catheter with two small balloons mounted on the tip. The two balloons are placed such that one rests in the upper half of the anus and the other in the lower half. An additional balloon is attached at the tip, up in the rectum, in order to elicit the anorectal inhibitory reflex. The balloons are filled with water. Smaller balloons create less stretch and less distortion than larger balloons.

MICROTRANSDUCERS

Microtransducer systems employ strain gauges mounted on the tip of the catheter.[8] A balloon must be introduced into the rectum in parallel with the microtip pressure transducer to elicit the rectal inhibitory reflex. The advantage of this system is the small size of the catheter and the lack of a water leak. The disadvantages are the limited number of microtransducers that can be mounted on the catheter, the cost of the system, the rigidity of the catheters, and the inability to record simultaneous circumferential or longitudinal measurements. In the future the microtransducers may become smaller and cheaper.

SLEEVE SENSORS

A sleeve-tipped catheter has water flowing into and out of the "hollow" tip. This sensing segment of the catheter spans the sphincter, recording resistance along its entire length. This system cannot distinguish the internal from the external sphincter, a potential disadvantage.

COMPUTERIZED MANOMETRY

Computer software programs have been employed to help analyze data,[9] which may be plotted and displayed in many useful ways. This method uses a mo-

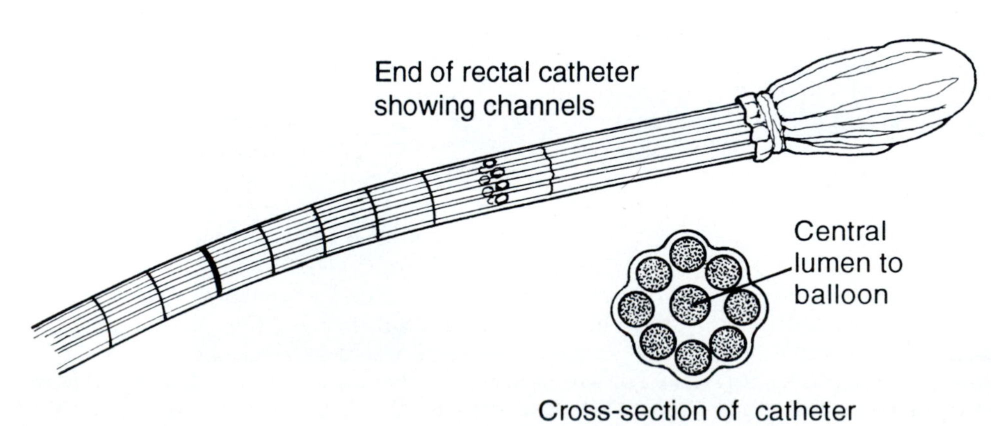

FIGURE 7–3. Diagram of the catheter, showing eight channel holes for recording circumferentially. The central hole connects to the balloon to elicit the rectoanal inhibitory reflex.

tor that pulls the catheter through the anal canal at a constant rate, thereby helping to produce reproducible data. Three-dimensional sphincter analysis can be determined by plotting both circumferential and longitudinal points.

TECHNIQUE OF THE EXAMINATION

Ideally, manometry should follow a clearly defined protocol, so that results are reproducible and differences between patients can be appreciated.

EQUIPMENT

Our system consists of a catheter, a perfusion pump, eight transducers, and an eight-channel recorder (Fig. 7–1). The long catheter has eight holes located circumferentially 10 centimeters from the tip (Fig. 7–3). At the end of the catheter is a balloon, which is connected to a syringe by a central channel through the catheter. The pump perfuses water at a rate of 0.1 mL per minute through the eight channels, each of which is connected to a separate transducer capable of measuring up to 15 pounds per square inch.

PREPARATION

The patient is instructed to take a small enema prior to the examination, but incontinent patients may not be able to do this. The patient must be counseled as to what to expect and how to aid in completing a meaningful examination.

POSITION

The patient is placed in the left lateral decubitus position with the buttocks at the edge of the examination table (Fig. 7–2). The knees and hips are flexed to allow access to the anal area. The anal skin is well-lubricated for introduction of the catheter.

TECHNICAL PROTOCOL

The perfusion openings near the catheter tip should be positioned in the rectum, above the anal canal. The catheter is withdrawn in increments; the resting pressure is measured. The length of the anal canal can be determined with reasonable accuracy; as the lumens are pulled into the anal canal, pressures rise, and the distance over which the pressures are high reflects the length of the anal canal. In our protocol the catheter is pulled out in 1 cm stations from 5 to 3 cm; from 3 cm, we measure in 0.5 cm increments.[10]

As an alternative to the "station pull-through" method, the catheter is pulled through by a motor at a specified rate. Continuous pull-through gives a better longitudinal profile and a better estimate of the functional length, but ultra slow waves are not detected. Movement artifact is also a problem with continuous pull-through.[11,12]

The second step of manometric testing measures squeeze pressures. Generally, squeeze pressure is recorded at the level of highest resting pressure observed, so the catheter should be positioned at this level. The patient is asked to squeeze as hard and long as possible; this maneuver is repeated two or three times. If the squeeze pressure observed is at or below 100 mmHg, the catheter is moved to the 1 cm level and the squeeze test is repeated.

Third, the anorectal inhibitory reflex is tested. At the level of highest resting pressure, the rectal balloon is inflated with increasing volumes to evoke the reflex. If the ARIR is intact, one should see relaxation of the internal sphincter as the rectal balloon is inflated[5,13] (Fig. 7–4*A*). The volume needed to evoke the reflex is normally sensed by the patient; if not, the sphincter will permit stool to descend without patient awareness. Measurement of intrarectal pressure with increases in balloon volume also gives useful information regarding rectal sensation and compliance.

INTERPRETATION

RESTING PRESSURES

Normal values for the resting tones and squeeze pressures are poorly defined, due to the lack of method standardization. The resting pressures reflect the resistance provided by the internal anal sphincter (IAS), which accounts for 80% of the resting tone. (The remainder is due to the external sphincter muscle bulk.) As the catheter is pulled out at 1 cm increments, the pressure progressively increases toward the distal end of the sphincter[13] (Fig. 7–4*A*). This gradient from lower pressure proximally to high pressure distally theoretically acts to maintain continence. The normal resting pressures may vary between 40 mmHg and 80 mmHg.

Values vary according to sex, age, and other factors such as prior history of childbearing and anorectal surgery. Pressures in men tend to be higher; women generally have lower resting tones, lower voluntary contractions, shorter anal canals, lower rectal compliance, and an anorectal inhibitory reflex that reacts to smaller volumes.[10,14] Aging results in a progressive lowering of resting and squeeze pressures.[15–17] Childbearing also contributes to lessened anal pressures.[18] Other factors that influence pressures are time of day (fluctuations have been noted), posture, and the presence of feces within the rectum.[19] Standing and sitting cause a fourfold increase in rectal pressure,[20] thereby maximizing the potential for normal continence during changes in body position. Increases in intra-abdominal pressures cause reflex external anal sphincter (EAS) contraction.[21–23]

Although slow waves are found in all patients, they are not continuous. Slow waves vary in amplitude

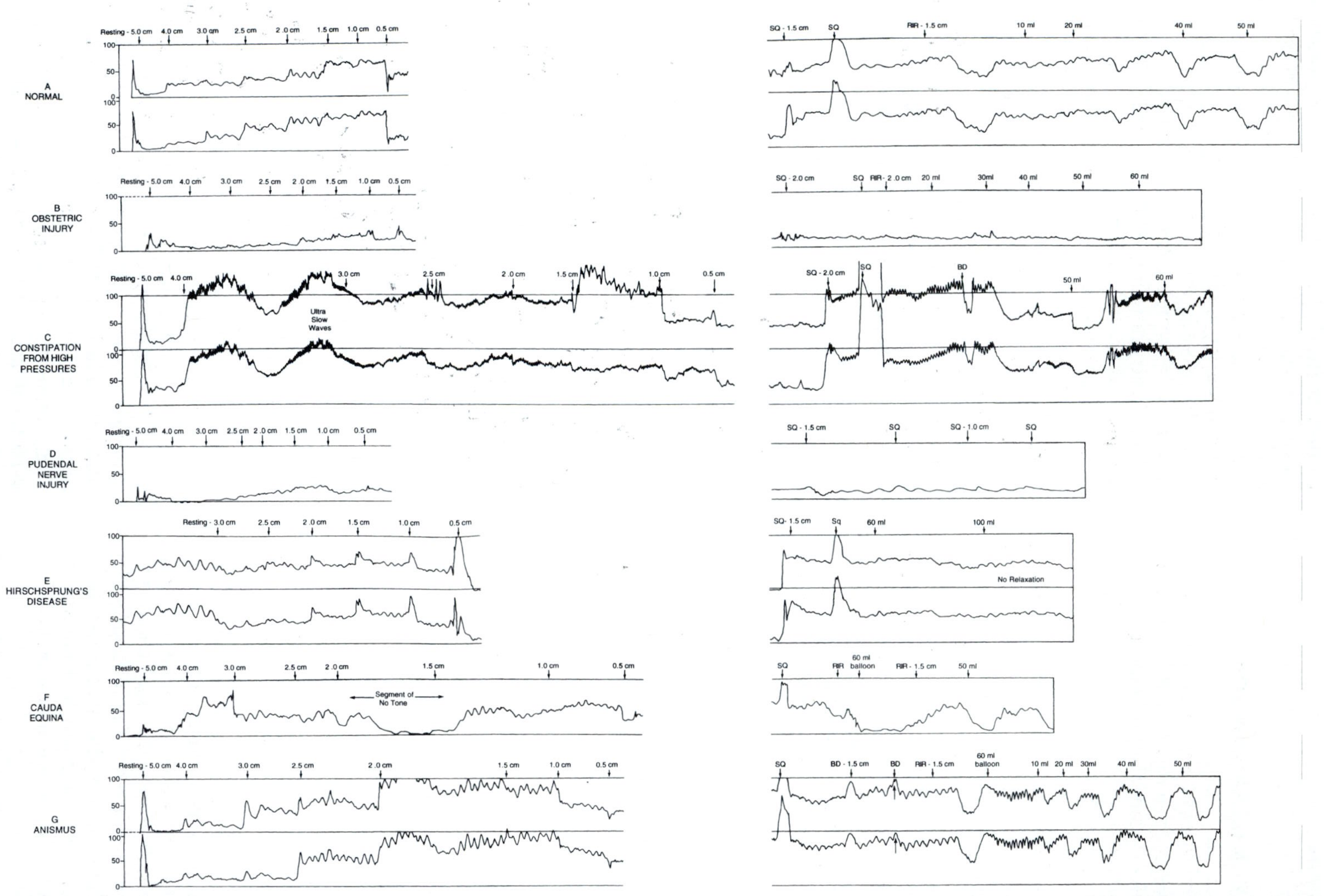

FIGURE 7–4. Manometry tracings (selected segments). (*A*), Normal. The steps in a station pull-through show a stair-step configuration. Squeeze (SQ) voluntarily doubles the pressure. The rectoanal inhibitory reflex (RIR) shows progressively larger relaxations with larger balloon insufflations. (*B*), An obstetric injury is manifested by low pressures throughout. (*C*), Constipation is shown by high pressures with ultraslow waves. When the patient bears down (BD), there is an expected relaxation. (*D*), In Hirschsprung's disease there is no relaxation even with 100 mL balloon insufflation. (*E*), Anismus shows a high pressure profile, but also shows a paradoxic increase in pressure when bearing down (BD) as if to have a bowel movement.

(5–25 cm of H_2O) and frequency (6–20/min). Ultra slow waves are present in patients with higher resting pressures (Fig. 7–4*C*). These waves also vary in amplitude (30–100 cm of H_2O) and frequency (less than 3/min).[24,25] These waves are probably generated by the IAS and are seen in 5% of normal subjects.[25]

SPATIAL RELATIONSHIPS

Pressure varies along the anal canal, both longitudinally and circumferentially.[7,16,18] At the proximal end of the functional anal canal, sphincter pressure is greater posteriorly, where the puborectalis muscle encircles the anorectum. In the middle of the anal canal, pressures are reasonably uniform circumferentially. Distally, the pressures are greater anteriorly.[18] Longitudinally, the pressure is greatest in the distal third of the anus. The functional anal canal measures from 2.5 cm to 5.0 cm.[17]

SQUEEZE PRESSURES

The voluntary squeeze pressure is a measure of EAS competence (Fig. 7–4*A*). The recorded measurement is actually a summation of both the resting tone and the voluntary squeeze. Generally, EAS squeeze pressure should be approximately twice the resting pressure. Voluntary squeeze is greater in men, but it diminishes in both sexes with aging.[26]

SENSATION

Sensation is a qualitative phenomenon. Most patients can sense a balloon that has been distended to a volume of 10 mL to 20 mL, yet a large rectum may not sense such a small volume. As the rectal balloon is gradually inflated, the patient may experience an urge to defecate; with larger volumes, this urge may become intolerable. The volumes and pressures needed to produce these sensations vary from patient to patient and reflect compliance of the rectum.

ABNORMAL MANOMETRY

TRAUMA

Anorectal tears may result from obstetric injury, fistulectomy,[27] or impalement, in which cases a portion of the sphincter may be torn. Injury will produce an overall lower resting tone and squeeze pressure (Fig. 7–4*B*). By using circumferential measurements, the injured quadrant may be identified, because it will have lower pressures than the other quadrants. After obstetric injury, defects may not become clinically significant until years after the last delivery[28]; therefore, one should never exclude trauma as a possible cause of incontinence, even if it was sustained many years earlier. Anal sonography in these instances demonstrates the defect.

HEMORRHOIDS

As mentioned previously, ultra slow waves (USW) may be seen in 5% of healthy people (Fig. 7–4*C*), yet 40% of patients with abnormally large hemorrhoids will have USW.[29] Large hemorrhoids may result in increased anal tone, especially in men.[30]

HIRSCHSPRUNG'S DISEASE

In this disease, the ganglion cells within the internal sphincter are absent; as a result, the anorectal inhibitory reflex is absent (Fig. 7–4*D*). Megarectum may occur, so that rectal sensation is low and compliance high.

FISSURE

Patients with fissures have a high resting tone.[31] In addition, USW are seen in 80% of these unusually hypertensive internal sphincters.[32] When sphincterotomy is employed to treat the fissure, sphincter pressure frequently drops 50%.[33]

IDIOPATHIC MEGARECTUM

Megarectum is seen in the elderly and in children and occurs as a result of faulty toilet habits. Patients complain of constipation and impaction by large, hard stools. Often the stool is not sensed until there is a large volume. Even though the sphincter is intact, leakage of feces may occur; the stool elicits the inhibitory reflex and the sphincter relaxes, producing soilage. This sequence of events occurs without the patient's being aware.

IRRITABLE BOWEL SYNDROME

Increased sensitivity of the rectum may lead to a frequent, urgent need to defecate,[34,35] but when the patient attempts elimination, only small amounts pass. This same hypersensitivity may be seen in patients with inflammatory bowel disease, prior radiation, or solitary rectal ulcer syndrome.[36,37] During manometry the balloon is sensed at low volume, compliance is low, and the pain threshold is abnormally low.

ANISMUS

Patients with anismus complain of constipation and prolonged straining at stool. If a 50-mL balloon is placed inside the rectum, frequently it cannot be evacuated. Furthermore, the resting tone and voluntary squeeze are increased (Fig. 7–4*E*). The puborectalis muscle appears to be contracting paradoxically during attempts to defecate;[38–40] this abnormality can be proven with defecography or concentric needle EMG.

SUMMARY

Manometry is one of several physiologic tests that aid in defining anorectal abnormalities. Both constipation and incontinence disorders may be better understood by analyzing the history, clinical examination, and physiologic tests.

REFERENCES

1. Gibbons, CP, Bannister, JJ, Trowbridge, EA, et al: An analysis of anal sphincter pressure and anal compliance in normal subjects. Int J Colorect Dis 1:231, 1986.
2. Duthie, HL, Kwong, NK and Brown, B: Adaptability of the anal canal to distention. Br J Surg 57:388, 1970.
3. Schouten, WR and van Vroonhoven, Th JMV: A simple method of anorectal manometry. Dis Colon Rectum 26:721, 1983.
4. Hancock, BD: Measurement of anal pressure and motility. Gut 17:645, 1976.
5. Schuster, MM, Hookman, P, Hendrix, TR, et al: Simultaneous manometric recording of internal and external anal sphincter reflexes. Bull Johns Hopkins Hosp 116:79, 1965.
6. Collins, CD, Brown, BH, Whittaker, GE, et al: New Method of measuring forces in the anal canal. Gut 10:160, 1969.
7. Jonas, U and Klotter, HJ: Study of three urethral pressure recording devices; Theoretical considerations. Urol Res 6:119, 1978.
8. Vela, AR and Rosenberg, AJ: Anorectal manometry: a new simplified technique. Am J Gastroenterol 77:486, 1982.
9. Coller, JA: Clinical application of anorectal manometry. Gastroenterol Clin North Am 16:17, 1987.
10. Sun, WM and Read, NW: Anorectal function in normal subjects: the effect of gender. Int J Colorect Dis 4:188, 1989.
11. McHugh, SM and Diamant, NE: Anal canal pressure profile: A reappraisal as determined by rapid pullthrough technique. Gut 28:1234, 1987.
12. Sun, WM and Read, NW: Reflex anal dilatation; the effects of parting the buttocks on anal function in normal subjects and patients with anorectal and spinal disease. Gut 32:670, 1990.
13. Bannister, JJ, Read, NW, Donnelly, TC, et al: External and internal anal sphincter responses to rectal distention in normal subjects and in patients with idiopathic fecal incontinence. Br J Surg 76:617, 1989.
14. Womack, NK, Morrison, JFB and Williams, NS: Impaired recruitment of the pelvic floor musculature by intraabdominal pressure in fecal incontinence. Gut 26:26, 1985.
15. Read, NW, Harford, WV, Schmulen, AC, et al: A clinical study of patients with fecal incontinence and diarrhea. Gastroenterology 76:747, 1979.
16. Taylor, BM, Beart, RW and Phillips, SF: Longitudinal and radial variations of pressure in the human anal sphincter. Gastroenterology 86:693, 1984.
17. Nivatvongs, S, Stern, HS and Fryd, DS: The length of the anal canal. Dis Colon Rectum 24:600, 1981.
18. Varma, JS and Smith, AN: Anorectal profilometry with the microtransducer. Br J Surg 71:867, 1984.
19. Kerremans, R: Morphological and physiological aspects of anal continence and defecation. Presses Académiques Européennes, Brussels, 1969.
20. Johnson, GP, Pemberton, JH, Ness, J, et al: Transducer manometry and the effect of body position on anal canal pressure. Dis Colon Rectum 33:469, 1990.
21. Haynes, WG and Read, NW: Anorectal activity in man during rectal infusion of saline: a dynamic assessment of the anal continence mechanism. J Physiol 330:45, 1982.
22. Floyd, WF and Walls, EW: Electromyography of the sphincter ani externum in man. J Physiol 122:599, 1953.
23. Parks, AG, Porter, NH and Melzak, J: Experimental study of the reflex mechanisms controlling the muscles of the pelvic floor. Dis Colon Rectum 5:407, 1962.
24. Karlin, PL, Zinsmeister, A and Phillips, S: Motor responses to food of the ileum, proximal colon and distal colon of healthy humans. Gastroenterology 84:762, 1983.
25. Hancock, BD and Smith, K: The internal sphincter and Lord's procedure for hemorrhoids. Br J Surg 62:833, 1975.
26. McHugh, SM and Diamant, NE: Effect of age, gender and parity on anal canal pressures. Contribution of impaired anal sphincter function to fecal continence. Dig Dis Sci 32:726, 1987.
27. Belliveau, P, Thomson, JP and Parks, AG: Fistula-in-ano: A manometric study. Dis Colon Rectum 26:152, 1983.
28. Lubowski, DZ, Nicholls, J, Swash, M, et al: Neural control of internal anal sphincter function. Br J Surg 74:668, 1987.
29. Sun, WM, Read, NW and Shorthouse, AG: Hypertensive anal cushions as a cause of high anal pressure in patients with hemorrhoids. Br J Surg 77:458, 1990.
30. Hancock, BD: Internal sphincter and the nature of hemorrhoids. Gut 18:651, 1977.
31. Hancock, BD: The internal sphincter and anal fissure. Br J Surg 64:92, 1977.
32. Gibbons, CP and Read, NW: Anal hypertonia in fissures: cause or effect. Br J Surg 73:443, 1986.
33. Bennett, RC and Duthie, HL: The functional importance of the internal sphincter. Br J Surg 51:355, 1965.
34. Prior, A, Maxton, DC and Whorwell, PJ: Anorectal manometry in irritable bowel syndrome: differences between diarrhea and constipation. Gut 31:458, 1990.
35. Whitehead, WE, Engel, BT and Schuster, MM: Irritable bowel syndrome. Dig Dis Sci 25:404, 1980.
36. Rao, SSC, Holdsworth, CO and Read, NW: Anorectal sensitivity and reactivity in patients with ulcerative colitis. Gastroenterology 83:1270, 1987.
37. Sun, WM, Read, NW, Donnelly, TC, et al: A common pathophysiology for full thickness rectal prolapse anterior mucous prolapse and solitary ulcer. Br J Surg 76:290, 1989.
38. Barnes, PR, Hawley, PR, Preston, DM, et al: Experience of posterior division of the puborectalis muscle in the management of chronic constipation. Br J Surg 72:475, 1985.
39. Preston, DM and Lennard-Jones, JE: Anismus in chronic constipation. Dig Dis Sci 30:413, 1985.
40. Bannister, JJ, et al: Urological abnormalities in young women with severe constipation. Gut 29:17, 1988.

CHAPTER 8

Fluoroscopic Evaluation of the Pelvic Floor

Claire Smith • Linda Brubaker
Theodore J. Saclarides

Diagnostic evaluation of patients with pelvic floor disorders has undergone a significant evolution over the past decade. Advances in the understanding and diagnosis of pelvic floor pathophysiology have opened the way for new treatment modalities, both surgical and nonsurgical.

Meticulous site-specific physical examination of patients with pelvic floor disorders is the mainstay of evaluation. Electrophysiologic and manometric testing of pelvic floor structures are new additions to the diagnostic armamentarium that were previously unavailable. Recently, radiologic studies have gained an important place in this diagnostic array.[1–7] These studies can be individually tailored to obtain valuable information. This chapter reviews our technique and experience with the fluoroscopic evaluation of patients with pelvic floor disorders.

DIAGNOSTIC METHODS OF EVALUATION

Evaluation by urodynamic and anorectal tests (as discussed in Chaps. 6 and 7) yields valuable information regarding the physiology of pelvic floor structures, but visualization of gross anatomic alterations is best obtained by radiologic methods. Fluoroscopic evaluation, ultrasonography, and magnetic resonance imaging (MRI) are the possible radiologic tools available for study of the pelvic floor. Due to limitations imposed by the supine position needed for MRI scanning and the limited "window" available for ultrasound scanning by the perineal approach, fluoroscopic evaluation has emerged as a vital component of patient evaluation. This approach allows events to be recorded more easily with the patient in the upright or sitting position, performing any and all of the normal or exaggerated physiologic maneuvers that contribute to her clinical complaints.

Because urinary incontinence, urogenital prolapse, fecal incontinence, rectal prolapse, and constipation rarely present as isolated entities, the pelvic floor must be totally evaluated before initiating treatment. Inadequate identification of all abnormalities may lead to an unsuccessful surgical repair. We have found that the fluoroscopic technique described later in this chapter provides an accurate assessment of the entire pelvic floor, rather than concentrating on a single anatomic region, as other diagnostic tests do.[2]

DYNAMIC FLUOROSCOPY

To evaluate pelvic floor disorders fluoroscopically, opacification of the pelvic viscera is needed. Barium sulfate suspension is ingested to opacify the small bowel, allowing visualization of any enteroceles present. Contrast material should also be placed in the urinary bladder, the vagina, and the rectum, so that cystoceles, vaginal vault prolapse, sigmoidoceles, and rectoceles can be identified and their spatial relationship to each other appreciated.

This prerequisite of complete visceral opacification contributes to the complexity of the examination. In truth, the study requires a high degree of motivation and cooperation on the part of the patient. In our experience, we have found that a key component to success is to maintain a sense of dignity during what is a "personally invasive" study for the patient. Both the physician and technologic staff must discuss the procedure with the patient at length and address any questions or concerns openly and sympathetically. Patient modesty is of utmost importance and must be maintained scrupulously throughout the study.

Equipment needed for the examination is shielded from the patient's view. Radiology personnel are situated close enough to the patient to provide help if needed, but far enough away to remain unobtrusive. No glaring lights are used; patient gowning is always discreet.

MATERIALS AND METHODS

Between 1 and 2 hours before the patient enters the fluoroscopic suite, 2 cups of low-density (60% W/V) barium sulfate suspension and one 8-ounce glass of cold water are ingested by the patient. In our experience, the vast majority of patients have adequate small bowel opacification within 1 hour.

Bladder catheterization with a small-caliber opaque-lined feeding tube is done in a sterile manner. The bladder is filled with 150 to 200 mL of water-soluble contrast material (Hypaque 25% W/V; Winthrop Pharmaceutical Division, Sterling Drugs, New York City, NY). The catheter is left in place for the initial radiographs, but may be removed for the voiding portions of the study. A paste of thickened barium powder and water is placed in the vagina using a lu-

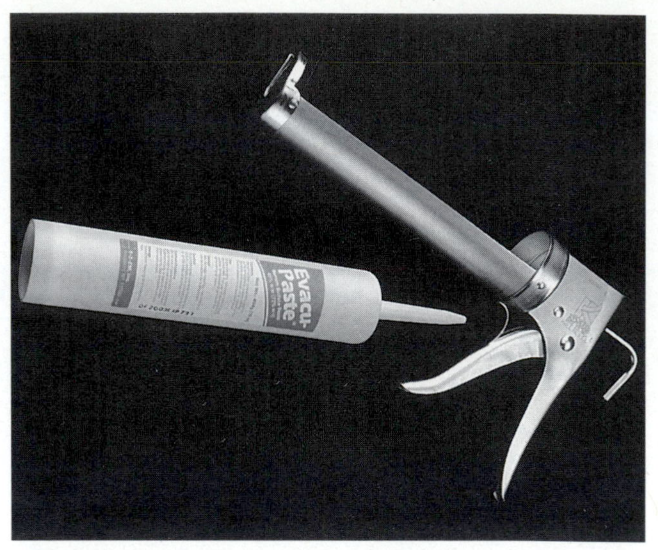

FIGURE 8–1. Rectal contrast agent with delivery device. A variety of commercial semisolid rectal contrast agents are available for use in proctographic studies. Administration is facilitated using a "caulking gun" device. (Photograph compliments of E-Z EM, Inc., Westbury, NY.)

bricated syringe. A tube of commercially available barium paste (Evacupaste, 100% W/V: E-Z-EM, Inc., Westbury, NY: Anatrast 100% W/V: Lafayette Pharmaceuticals, Lafayette, IN) is inserted into the rectum using a device similar to a caulking gun (Fig. 8–1). Finally, two radiopaque markers are placed on the surface of the perineum; one marker is placed as close to the anus as feasible, the other on the perineal body between the vagina and rectum. These markers allow adequate assessment of structures in relationship to the perineal body.

When all contrast agents have been administered, the patient sits on an upright commode especially designed for this procedure. We use a commercially available device (E-Z-EM, Inc., Westbury, NY) (Fig. 8–2), but many institutions use commodes designed by internal engineering teams. The commode is secured to the footboard of the fluoroscopy table. When the commode is brought to the upright position, both vertical and horizontal movement of the fluoroscopic tower and table are still possible.

We use digital fluoroscopy to reduce the patient's exposure to radiation, although conventional fluoroscopy also can be employed for this study. Fluoroscopic examination time varies depending on how quickly evacuation can be accomplished. Usual fluoroscopic times range from 20 to 40 seconds.

FILMING PROTOCOL

Views of the pelvis are obtained with the patient at rest, when the patient squeezes her pelvic muscles "as if trying to stop her urine flow," and when the patient is straining in attempted defecation. These maneuvers allow estimation of the function of the pelvic muscles by visualization of anorectal angle changes (Fig. 8–3).

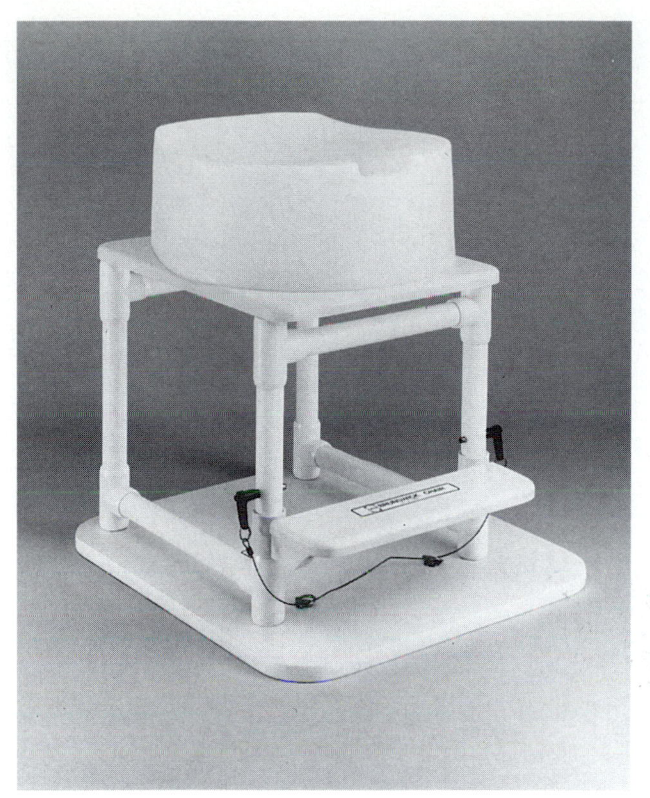

FIGURE 8–2. Commode for radiographic examination of the pelvis. This commode is commercially available, but any device that allows physiologic positioning with the ability to perform adequate spot radiographs through a radiolucent commode is appropriate. (Photograph compliments of E-Z EM, Inc., Westbury, NY.)

The dynamic portion of the examination is performed as the patient evacuates the contrast material from both the bladder and the rectum. This evacuation may be done simultaneously or consecutively. Dynamic images are recorded by video fluoroscopic tape-recording or by rapid filming sequences at 2 frames per second. Alterations in the structure and relationship of the pelvic organs to each other, which occur during the patient's normal urinary voiding and defecation, are recorded. The results are reviewed before the patient leaves the department so that additional views in different positions may be obtained if needed. We have found that delayed views should be routinely performed, because maximal straining maneuvers are frequently required to demonstrate defects that may not be seen even during the normal evacuation process.

FLUOROSCOPIC FINDINGS

ANTERIOR VAGINAL DEFECTS

Urethral Abnormalities

Support defects of the anterior vaginal wall include abnormalities at both the urethrovesical junction and the base of the urinary bladder. Normally, the bladder base should have a horizontal configuration (Fig. 8–4). The urethrovesical junction is supported in such a way that it remains slightly below the bladder base. Analysis of posterior urethrovesical angles was thought to be an important step in determining the causes and possible solutions for urinary incontinence. Subsequent investigations have shown that urinary continence is due to a complex interplay of muscular, fibromuscular, and neural components.[8] Even though measurement of anatomic angles does not readily explain all the mechanisms of urinary continence, visualization of the bladder base can provide important information that may not be available by other means.

The bladder base is fluoroscopically assessed at rest and during straining. The urethrovesical junction should be closed at rest; it normally opens with a funnel-shaped configuration when the patient voids. If the junction is funnel-shaped at rest, this is an abnormal finding consistent with an intrinsic sphincter deficiency[9] (Fig. 8–5). Because clinical examination provides only a gross estimate of the mobility of the urethrovesical junction, evaluation by ultrasonography or by contrast cystourethrography, as is done during fluoroscopy of the pelvic floor, can provide more specific information.

Cystoceles

Disruptions in the endopelvic fascial support of the urinary bladder produce cystoceles. In such instances, increases in intra-abdominal pressure cause abnormal descent of the urinary bladder, urethral rotation, and unequal pressure transmission to the urinary bladder base; they may produce genuine stress incontinence.[8]

If a cystocele is present, the urinary bladder prolapses below the pubic symphysis and causes extrinsic pressure on the anterior and superior aspect of the vagina. The spectrum of appearances is wide, ranging from minimal bulging of the bladder base to a classic "hour-glass" appearance (Fig. 8–6). Although there has been little objective correlation between the appearance of the urinary bladder and surgical outcome, appearance and degree of cystocele descent may provide some indication as to the specific surgical procedures that may succeed or fail in each individual patient.

APICAL DEFECTS

Enteroceles

Herniations of the small bowel through fascial defects in the inguinal, femoral, and umbilical regions have long been recognized and are usually treated surgically to avoid complications such as obstruction or strangulation. Although herniations of the small bowel through weak points in the pelvic floor are not easily recognizable, they are just as capable of causing distressing symptoms. Diagnostic testing for such defects was performed as early as 1962.[10]

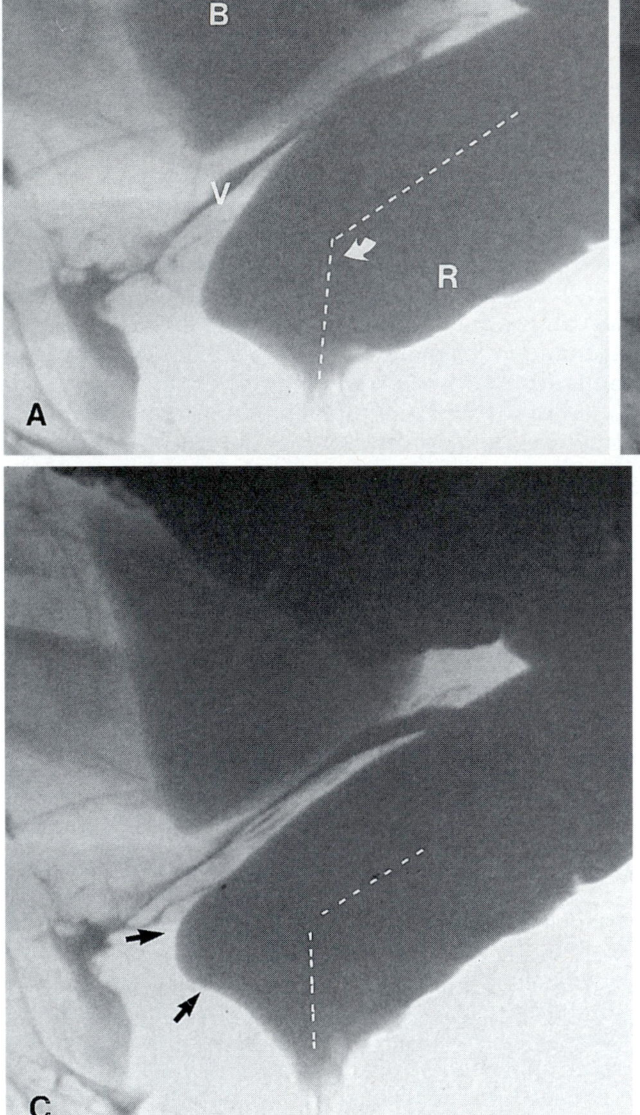

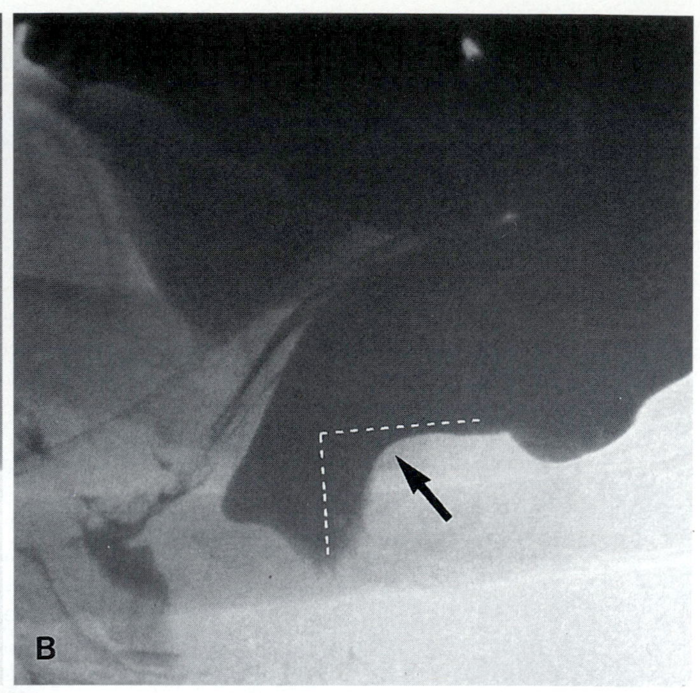

FIGURE 8–3. Lateral radiograph of the pelvis. (*A*), At rest, this patient has contrast material in the urinary bladder (B), in the small bowel (SB), in the vagina (V), and in the rectum (R). At rest, the angle (curved arrow) between the anal canal and the orientation of the rectum is 130 degrees. (*B*), With squeezing of the pelvis muscles (Kegel maneuver), note the prominent muscular indentation (arrow) at the distal anus due to contraction of the puborectalis muscle. The anorectal angle becomes more acute at 90 degrees. (*C*), With attempted defecation, the puborectalis muscles relax with subsequent widening of the anorectal angles, allowing defecation. The anterior rectal wall appears somewhat protuberant (arrows), raising the question of a small rectocele. The patient was not symptomatic.

Unfortunately, ways to determine normal depth of the cul-de-sac and perineal descent and consistent nomenclature for classifying enteroceles have been problems facing physicians for years.[9]

We have found that instead of assuming the presence of an enterocele using the standard finding of "widening of the rectovaginal septum,"[11] direct opacification of the small bowel and evaluation by dynamic fluoroscopy provide a more reliable study of small-bowel herniation. Distortion of the vaginal or rectal wall by small-bowel loops should be studied.

When enteroceles are large and prolapsing, visualization with fluoroscopic imaging is not difficult (Fig. 8–7). The clinical significance of many of these enteroceles is not understood, however, and symptoms do not always match the severity of the hernia. Severe symptoms may be experienced with only small to moderate-sized hernias. In contrast, some women with large enteroceles may be entirely asymptomatic.

In a study[11] using only physical examination, experienced urogynecologists failed to detect a significant number of radiographically demonstrable enteroceles. When small-bowel loops are located low in

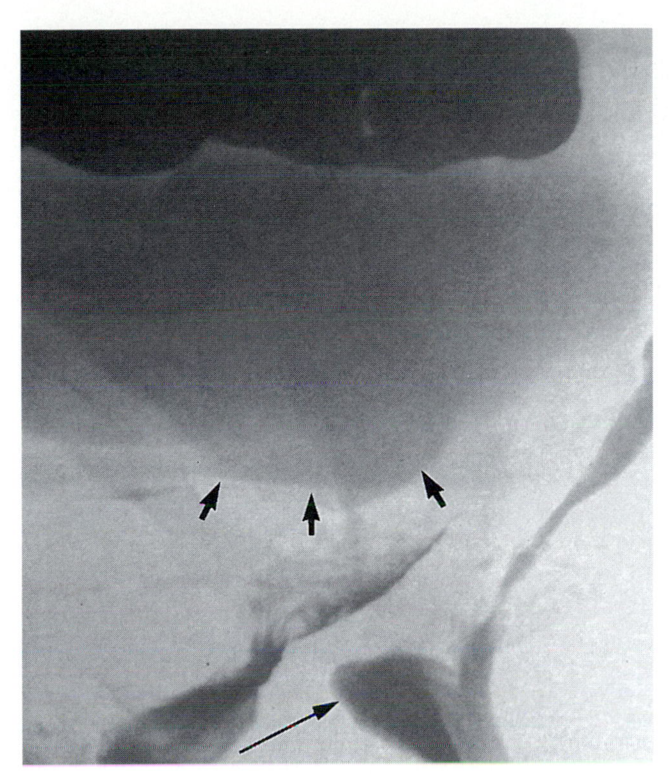

FIGURE 8–4. Normal bladder base. Postdefecation film before urinary voiding shows a normal rounded base to the urinary bladder (arrows). A small rectocele (long arrow) is present.

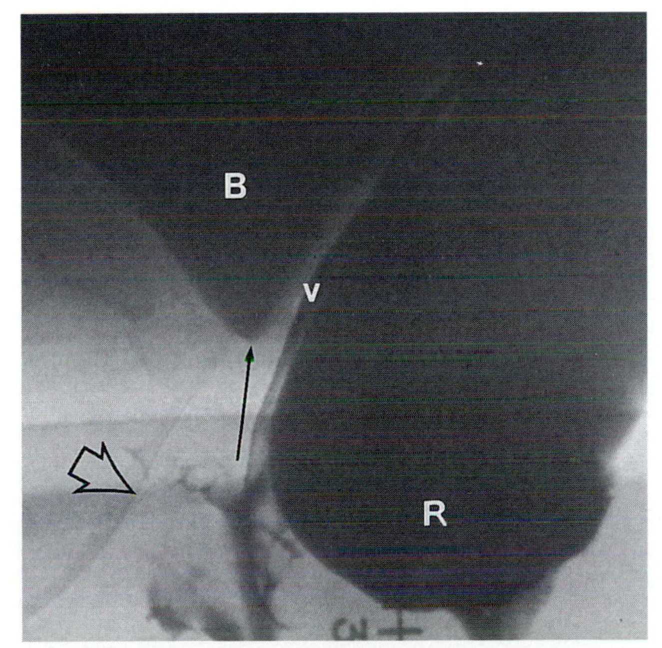

FIGURE 8–5. Abnormal funneling of the urinary bladder. Film of the pelvis obtained at rest shows an abnormal pointing of the base of the urinary bladder (B) (long arrow). There is a radiopaque catheter (open arrow) in the urethra. This appearance in the absence of urinary bladder contraction suggests that there may be an intrinsically damaged urethral sphincter (Type III stress incontinence). Rectal contrast is present in the rectum (R), and contrast material outlines the vagina (V).

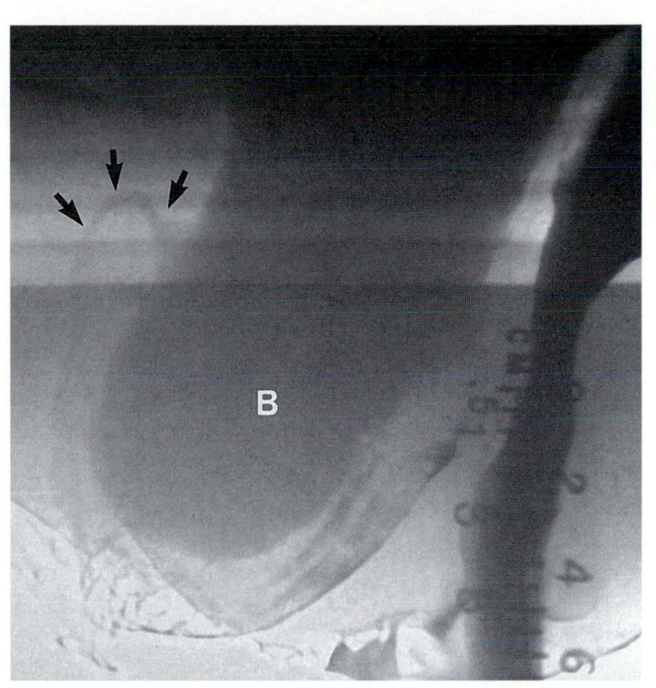

FIGURE 8–6. Cystocele. The urinary bladder (B) has prolapsed to half its length. Note the abnormal contour of the urethra (arrows), which would correspond to a clinically positive "Q-tip test."

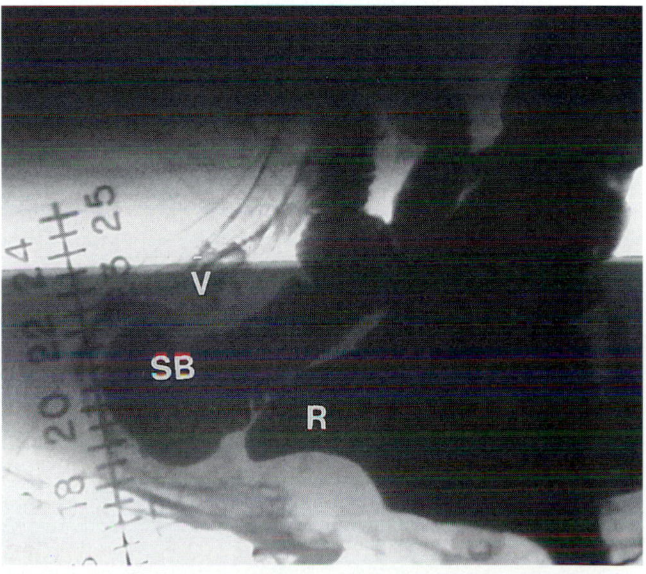

FIGURE 8–7. Enterocele. Multiple small bowel loops (SB) have herniated into the pelvis, causing deformity of the vagina (V). There is an associated posterior compartment defect (rectocele—R).

the pelvis but do not cause any deformity of the vagina or rectum, diagnosing an enterocele even radiologically is controversial. In such patients, if symptoms are severe enough and consistent with an enterocele, treatment for this condition may be justified.

Vaginal Vault Prolapse and Uterine Descensus

In the normal upright patient, the apex of the vagina is attached horizontally. If there are weakened support structures, the cervix can invaginate and migrate downward on a vertical axis into the vagina. Because contrast material is placed in the vagina during fluoroscopic evaluation, vaginal vault prolapse or uterine descensus can be visualized easily, confirming the clinical findings.

POSTERIOR VAGINAL DEFECTS

Rectoceles

Defects of the posterior vaginal wall or supporting attachments result in rectoceles that can produce a spectrum of symptoms. Some patients are completely asymptomatic, whereas others have distressing feelings of obstructed defecation and incomplete evacuation. The straining efforts that accompany these feelings may aggravate minor degrees of damage and can result in progressive injury. Rectoceles are easily seen during dynamic fluoroscopy of the pelvic floor and may have a heterogenous appearance. Most rectoceles are placed anteriorly and become evident in the early or middle stages of the examination, but they may not occur until the defecation process is almost complete. The contour of rectoceles varies, as does location with respect to the perineal body (Fig. 8–5).[8–10] Although nomenclature, classification, and clinical significance are still being investigated, rectoceles that retain contrast material after the rectum has been emptied are considered abnormal[12,13] (Figs. 8–8 to 8–10).

Sigmoidoceles

Patients with abnormally deep cul-de-sacs and redundancy of the sigmoid colon may prolapse this portion of the bowel into the pelvis. Radiographic diagnosis is not difficult, because the bowel causing extrinsic pressure on the contrast-filled vagina can clearly be distinguished as sigmoid colon rather than small bowel (Fig. 8–11). Clinically, sigmoidoceles mimic an enterocele or a rectocele.

RECTAL DEFECTS

Rectal Intussusception and Prolapse

Rectal intussusception may assume a funnel-shaped or ringlike configuration during straining (Fig. 8–12). Intussusception may remain above the rectal ampulla or may travel either into or through the anal canal, thus producing complete external rectal prolapse.[14] The significance of finding internal rectal prolapse during fluoroscopy is unclear. It can be seen in asymptomatic patients; the extent to which it is responsible for defecatory dysfunction in symptomatic patients is debatable.

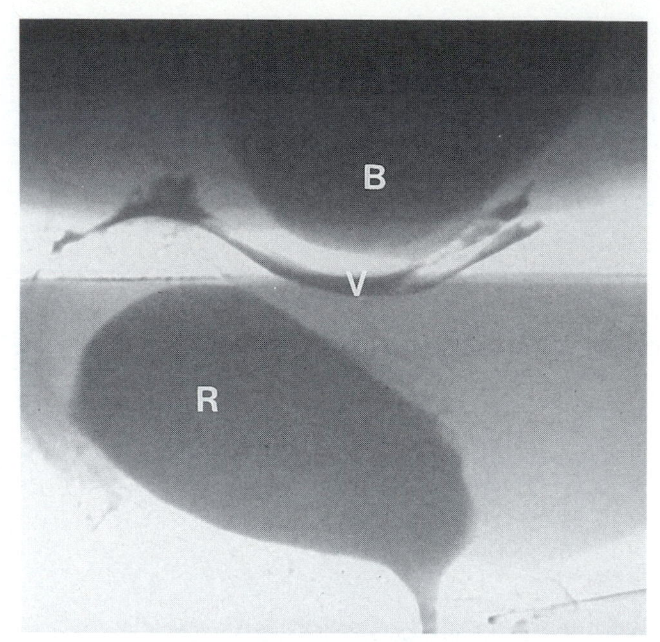

FIGURE 8–8. Rectocele. Post-evacuation film shows a large obliquely oriented rectocele (R). The patient could not evacuate this contrast material spontaneously and required digital evacuation. There is slight bulging of the urinary bladder base consistent with a small cystocele (C) that was detected clinically. Note distortion of the contrast-filled vagina (V) by both the cystocele and the rectocele.

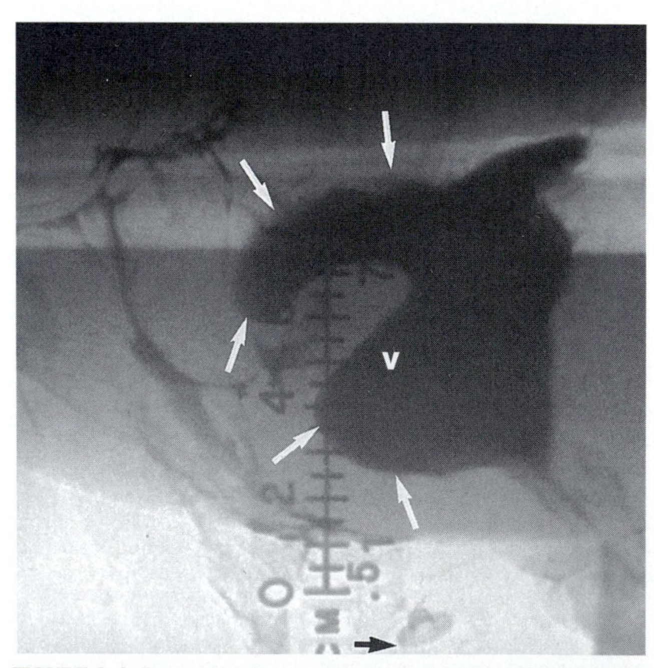

FIGURE 8–9. Rectocele. Arrows show a polylobular-shaped rectocele (arrows) that deforms the contrast-filled vagina (V). The perineal body (arrowhead) is marked exteriorly.

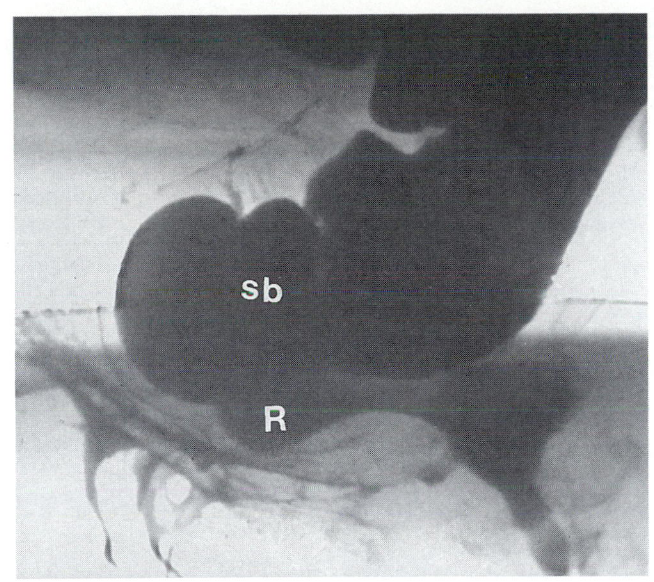

FIGURE 8–10. Enterocele and rectocele. Although the predominant abnormality is an enterocele (SB), a moderate-sized rectocele (R) that retains contrast material after the rectum has been emptied must not be overlooked or surgical treatment may be misguided.

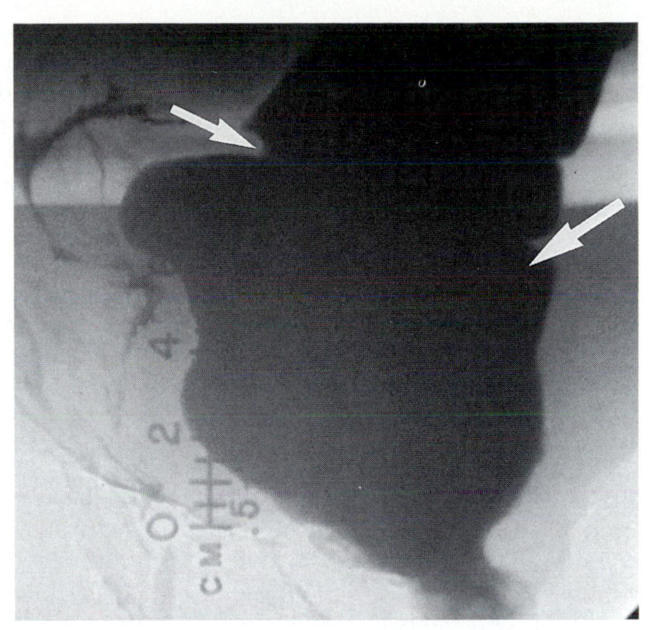

FIGURE 8–12. Rectal intussusception. Infolding of the mucosa and rectal muscles (arrows) continued during this evacuation study until a band of intussuscepted tissues narrowed the rectum.

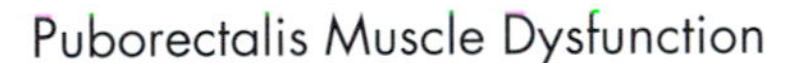

Puborectalis Muscle Dysfunction

Although anal manometry and electromyography provide a specific mapping of the sphincter muscle, fluoroscopy of the pelvic floor can provide an overall pictorial assessment of its function. With normal muscle activity, the puborectalis muscle should contract when the patient squeezes her pelvic muscles, making the angle between the anus and rectum more acute than at rest. With attempts at defecation, the anorectal angle should become more obtuse, allowing the contents of the rectum to be evacuated. When the puborectalis muscle does not relax, the angle between the anus and rectum either remains acute or may become more so.[12,13] Attempts at straining to evacuate the rectum will keep the angle closed and do not permit defecation. These findings can be seen during fluoroscopy (Fig. 8–13).

CLINICAL EXPERIENCE

We reviewed our experience with four-contrast defecography performed on 62 women who presented

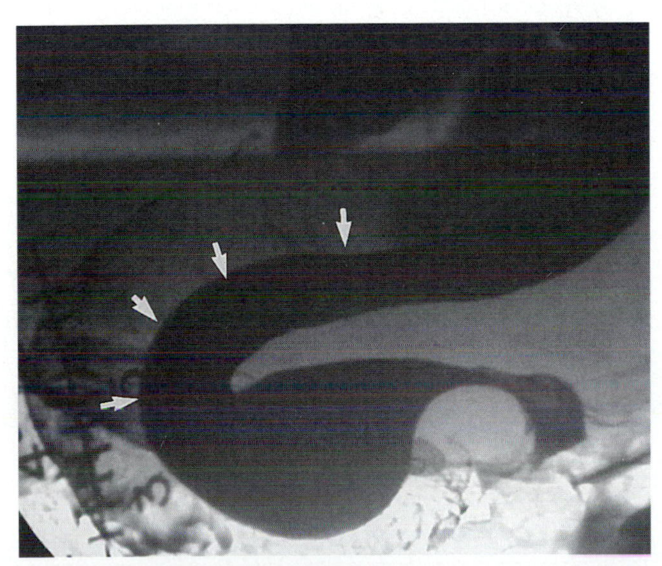

FIGURE 8–11. Sigmoidocele. Arrows outline a portion of the distal colon that is redundant and causes pressure deformity on the vagina. Without radiographic examination, this defect could be clinically mistaken for an uncomplicated rectocele. The true course of the colon and its implications for treatment would not be elucidated without dynamic fluoroscopy of the pelvis.

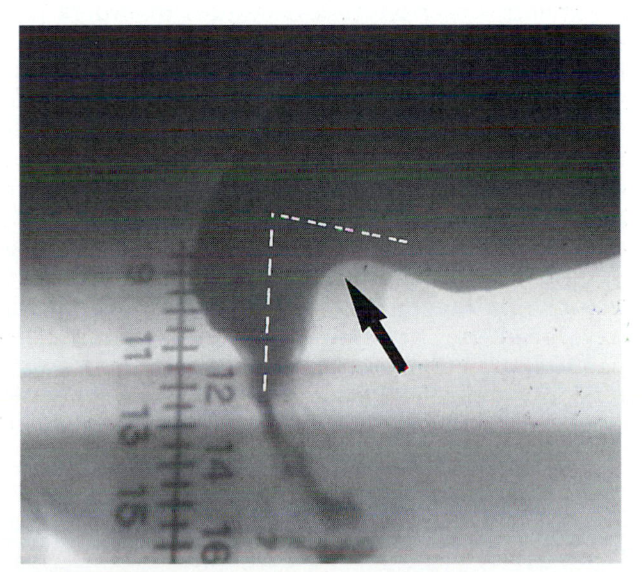

FIGURE 8–13. Incomplete relaxation of the pelvic muscles. Despite vigorous attempts to empty the rectum, this patient could not evacuate the rectal contrast material. Note that the anorectal angle is acute and the pelvic muscles (arrow) remain contracted despite attempts at defecation.

with various coexisting symptoms, such as obstructed defecation or constipation in 25 patients, vaginal prolapse in 44, urinary difficulty in 51, and pelvic pain in 13. Physical examination diagnosis included cystocele in 43, enterocele in 25, rectocele in 32, and rectal prolapse in 1. Prolapse defects were graded as follows: grade 1—above the introitus; grade 2—extending to the introitus; and grade 3—below the introitus.

Four-contrast defecography changed the diagnosis in 46 (75%); 26% of presumed cystoceles, 36% of enteroceles, and 25% of rectoceles were not present on defecography. In contrast, when physical examination was negative for these defects, 63% of patients were found to have cystoceles, 46% enteroceles, and 73% rectoceles on four-contrast defecography. For grade 2 or 3 posterior vaginal eversions, physical examination was accurate in only 61%; in the remainder, the diagnosis was either changed completely or additional unsuspected abnormalities were found (Table 8–1). Physical examination of large anterior defects was more accurate, with 74% of patients being correctly diagnosed.

Our results confirm that large prolapse defects, especially posterior, alter the anatomy enough that physical examination alone may be inaccurate. Fluoroscopic evaluation has proven beneficial in determining the exact nature of the defect. Urinary contrast material is not routinely given for patients with obstructed defecation or constipation; we do recommend giving it when urinary tract symptoms or grade 2 or 3 posterior eversions are present, because cystoceles are frequently also found in these instances.

TABLE 8–1. The Effect of Defecography on the Diagnosis of Patients with Grade 2 and 3 Posterior Vaginal Eversions (*n*=28)

Physical Examination Diagnosis	*Defecography Diagnosis, n(%)*		
	Diagnosis Confirmed	**Diagnosis Changed**	**Additional Findings**
Only rectocele (*n*=13)	8(62)	3(23)	2(15)
Only enterocele (*n*=9)	3(33)	3(33)	3(33)
Both (*n*=6)	6(100)	0	0

SUMMARY

Patients who have pelvic support disorders present with complex physiologic and anatomic problems. Logical and complete evaluation by meticulous, site-specific physical examination, electrophysiologic testing of the urinary tract, and anal manometry is valuable for evaluation. Radiologic visualization of the pelvic floor also has become extremely helpful. Dynamic fluoroscopy permits visual assessment of the interrelationships between the urethra and bladder, the vagina, small bowel, rectum, and anus. Although other modalities such as ultrasound and MRI have been used to supplement investigation of the pelvic floor, we have found that dynamic fluoroscopy reflects the physiologic state of the patient in her everyday life and can yield information concerning pelvic structures that may not be as easily obtainable by other methods.

REFERENCES

1. Kelvin, FM and Stevenson, GW: Radiologic investigation. The anorectum and vagina. In Benson, JT (ed.): Female Pelvic Floor Disorders: Investigation and Management. Norton, New York, 1992, pp 70–88.
2. Brubaker, L, Retsky, S, Smith, C and Saclarides, T: Pelvic floor evaluation with dynamic fluoroscopy. Obstet Gynecol 82:1–6, 1993.
3. Brubaker, L and Heit, MH: Radiology of the pelvic floor. Clin Obstet and Gynecol 36:1–8, 1993.
4. Klutke, CG and Raz, S: Magnetic resonance imaging in female stress incontinence. Int Urogynecol J 2:115–118, 1991.
5. Mahieu, P, Pringot, J and Bodart, P: Defecography: I. Description of a new procedure and results in normal patients. Gastrointest Radiol 9:247–251, 1984.
6. Mahieu, P, Pringot J and Bodard, P: Defecography: II. Contribution to the diagnosis of defecation disorders. Gastrointest Radiol 9:253–261, 1984.
7. Wall, LL and DeLancey, JOL: The politics of prolapse: a revisionist approach to disorders of the pelvic floor in women. Perspect Biol Med 34:486–496, 1991.
8. Walters, MD and Newton, ER: Pathophysiology and obstetrics issues of genuine stress incontinence. In Walters, MD, Karram, MM (eds.): Clinical Urogynecology. CV Mosby, St. Louis, 1993.
9. Oettle, GJ, Roe, AM, Bartolo, DCC and McMortensen, MJ: What is the best way of measuring perineal descent? A comparison of radiographic and clinical methods. Br J Surg 72:999–1001, 1985.
10. Lash, AF and Levin, B: Roentgenographic diagnosis of vaginal vault hernia. J Obstet Gynecol 20:427–433, 1962.
11. Kelvin, FM, Maglinte, D, Hornback, JA and Benson, JT. Pelvic prolapse: Assessment with evacuation proctography (defecography). Radiology 184:547–551, 1992.
12. Shorvon, PJ, McHugh, S, Diamante, NE, et al: Defecography in normal volunteers: results and implications. Gut 30:1737–1749, 1989.
13. Karasick, S, Karasick, D and Karasick, SR. Functional disorders of the anus and rectum: Findings on defecography. AJR Am J Roentgenol 160:777–782, 1993.
14. Goeir, R and Baeten, C: Rectal intussusception and rectal prolapse: detection and postoperative evaluation with defecography. Radiology 174:124–126, 1990.

CHAPTER 9

Assessing Colonic Motility and Colon Transit

Amanda M. Metcalf

In the past, investigation of disordered colonic motility was limited to studies that were either anatomic (i.e., nonphysiologic) or those that had a purely research application. As such, a great deal of reliance was placed on information from the history, specifically, the stool frequency reported by patients. Unfortunately, such reports are inaccurate[1] and correlate poorly with actual colonic transit time.[2] Development of colonic transit studies using radiopaque markers has allowed an objective, clinically applicable measurement of colonic transit to be widely available.

The premise of this type of study is that the transit time of fecal material through the colon is in fact the half-life of such material in the colon. Furthermore, this half-life can be measured by monitoring the progress of radiopaque markers through the colon. This technique is directly analogous to monitoring the concentration of a drug in the bloodstream over time to determine the drug's half-life.

The precise technique of administering the test varies among authors[2–4] but all are very similar. An understanding of the underlying concepts allows application of the technique that is most appropriate and convenient for the given situation.

INDICATIONS

Measurement of colonic transit is most appropriate in patients with complaints of intractable constipation that are unexplained by prior routine studies such as endoscopy or contrast studies of the colon. It may also be used to monitor and objectify the results of medical or surgical therapy of constipation.

TECHNIQUE

PATIENT PREPARATION

All contrast material from previous studies should be cleared from the colon several days before the onset of the test. No contrast studies should be scheduled for the duration of the test. Patients should be instructed to consume their usual diet, continue their daily activities, and avoid the use of any laxatives, enemas, or other medications known to alter gastrointestinal motility for the duration of the study. Patients should be taking supplemental fiber (3.4 g of psyllium fiber, b.i.d.).

RADIOPAQUE MARKERS

Radiopaque markers can be obtained commercially (Sitzmarks, Lafayette Pharmaceuticals, Fort Worth, TX) or can be prepared. The commercially available ring-shaped markers are packaged in gelatin capsules in aliquots of twenty per capsule. Occasionally, the markers will not separate upon dissolution of the capsule in the gastrointestinal tract, so that multiple markers move as a single unit. This prevents calculation of the transit time; it can be avoided by having patients open the capsules and separate the rings prior to consumption. Alternatively, markers can also be prepared from radiopaque tubing. Because specific gravity is known to alter the rate of transit of particulate material, the tubing used should have a specific gravity between 1.0 and 1.5 in order to mimic the specific gravity of normal fecal matter. The shapes fashioned should be approximately 6 mm in greatest diameter and easily visible on a plain radiograph.

STUDY PROTOCOLS

All radiographs taken should include the entire abdomen from diaphragm to pubis to ensure that all segments of the colon will be included.

Single Bolus, Multiple Radiographs

Patients are asked to ingest 20 radiopaque markers. Abdominal radiographs are then taken sequentially at 24-hour intervals until all markers are passed.

Triple Bolus, Interval Radiographs

Patients are asked to ingest 20 radiopaque markers at the same time of day for 3 successive days. Abdominal radiographs are then taken on the 4th and 7th study days at the same time, and every 3 days thereafter until the patient has passed all markers or the study is terminated.

Multiple Bolus, Single Radiograph

Patients are asked to ingest either 10 or 20 radiopaque markers at the same time of day for 6 successive days. An abdominal radiograph is then taken on the 7th day.

INTERPRETATION OF ABDOMINAL FILMS

Interpretation of abdominal films consists of tabulating the number of markers identified and assigning the location of these markers to the various segments of the colon; this relies on identifying bony landmarks of the spine and pelvis and gaseous contours of the bowel. In the absence of clear outlines of the colon, markers located to the right of the vertebral spinous processes above a line from the fifth lumbar vertebrae to the pelvic outlet are assigned to the right colon. Markers to the left of the vertebral spinous processes and above an imaginary line from the fifth lumbar vertebrae to the left anterior superior iliac crest are assigned to the left colon. Markers inferior to a line from the pelvic brim on the right and the superior iliac crest on the left are judged to be in the rectosigmoid and rectum (Fig. 9–1). If gaseous bowel outlines clearly show a pelvic cecum or trans-

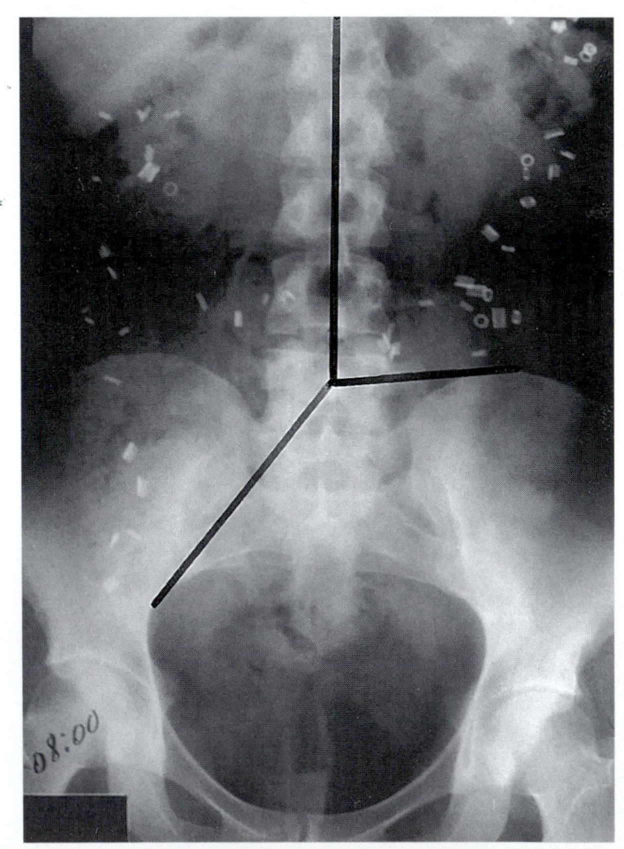

FIGURE 9–1. Segments of the colon as determined by bony landmarks: upper left, right colon; upper right, left colon; lower right, rectosigmoid and rectum. (See text for details.)

verse colon, markers are assigned to be in the anatomic segments based on the gaseous outlines. Previous contrast studies may also be helpful in assigning marker location.

CALCULATIONS

All calculations are based on a simplification of the formula described by Arhan and colleagues for use with a single marker, multiple radiograph technique.[3]

$$\text{Mean transit} = \frac{1}{N}\sum_{i=1}^{j} n_i[\tfrac{1}{2}(t_{(i+1)} - t_{(i-1)})]$$

where N = the number of markers given, n = number of markers present on a film taken at time t_i, $\frac{1}{2}[t_{(i+1)} - t_{(i-1)}]$ = the time interval between successive films, and j = the number of abdominal films taken.

If the time interval between abdominal radiographs is kept constant at 24 hours and the number of markers used is kept at 20, the above formula can be simplified to:

$$\begin{aligned}\text{Mean transit} &= \frac{1}{20}[(n_1 \times 24) + (n_2 \times 24) + \ldots (n_j \times 24)]\\ &= \frac{1}{20} \times 24\,(n_1 + n_2 + \ldots n_j)\\ &= 1.2\,(n_1 + n_2 + \ldots n_j)\end{aligned}$$

where n = the number of markers present on each film and j = the number of films taken.

It is readily apparent that the single marker bolus–multiple radiograph technique provides data at 24-hour intervals on the fate of a bolus of markers in the colon. The multiple-bolus techniques provide the same data but compressed on fewer radiographs. These techniques assume that each bolus of markers moves independently through the colon. Thus, if one gives boluses of markers on three separate days at 24-hour intervals, the radiograph on the 4th day demonstrates the progress of the first bolus of markers at 72 hours, the second bolus of markers at 48 hours, and the third bolus at 24 hours. This solitary radiograph therefore provides the same information as the first three radiographs obtained using a single-bolus technique. A second radiograph on the 7th day provides the same information as the 4th, 5th, and 6th radiographs obtained using a single-bolus technique. Similarly, if one gives boluses of markers for 6 days and then obtains a radiograph, this radiograph will provide data equivalent to seven sequential radiographs obtained after a single bolus of markers. Therefore, the same simplified formula can be used to calculate the transit time, as long as the number of markers given is 20, and the bolus interval is 24 hours. For example, using a single bolus, multiple radiograph technique, the following results are noted:

	Number of Markers			
Film	**Right**	**Left**	**Rectosigmoid**	**Colon**
1	10	6	4	20
2	2	4	6	12
3	0	2	2	4
4	0	0	2	2
5	0	0	0	0
Total	12	12	14	38

Calculated transit is as follows:
Mean right colon transit = 1.2 × 12 = 14.4 hr
Mean left colon transit = 1.2 × 12 = 14.4 hr
Mean rectosigmoid transit = 1.2 × 14 = 16.8 hr
Mean colonic transit = 1.2 × 38 = 45.6 hr

Using a triple bolus, interval radiograph technique, the radiographs demonstrated the following:

	Number of Markers			
Day	**Right**	**Left**	**Rectosigmoid**	**Colon**
4	10	12	12	34
7	0	0	1	1
Total	10	12	13	35

Calculated transit is as follows:
Mean right colon transit = 1.2 × 10 = 12.0 hr
Mean left colon transit = 1.2 × 12 = 14.4 hr
Mean rectosigmoid transit = 1.2 × 13 = 15.6 hr
Mean colonic transit = 1.2 × 35 = 42.0 hr

INTERPRETATION OF RESULTS

It is always prudent to ask patients before the radiographs are taken how and when the markers were actually ingested, what medications they were using, and whether the study period represented a typical time period as far as their bowel habits were concerned. Obviously, if a patient took the markers incorrectly or used laxatives during the study, for example, the results would be uninterpretable and the information obtained not helpful. Table 9–1 shows normal values for comparison.

The inherent day-to-day variability in transit suggests that only major differences from normal should

TABLE 9–1. Normal Values for Comparison of Radiographic Results

	Mean (h)	**95th Percentile (h)**
Right Colon	11.3	32
Left Colon	11.4	39
Rectosigmoid	12.4	36
Total Colon	35.0	68

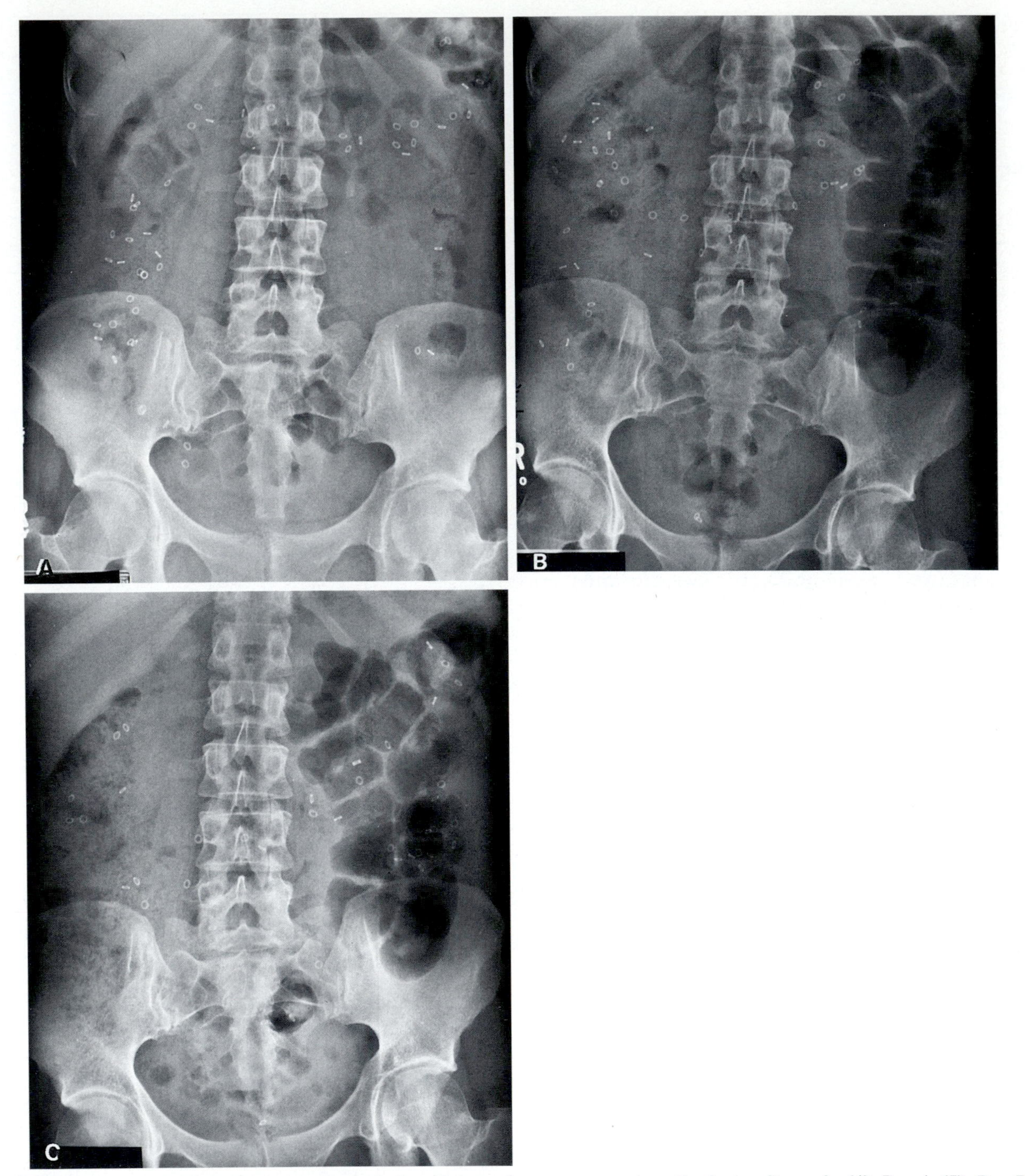

FIGURE 9–2. An example of a colonic transit study in which markers are present on the last radiograph. (*A*), Day 4; (*B*), Day 7; (*C*), Day 10.

be interpreted as a significant finding. In fact, this variability dictates that for transit in a particular segment to be considered delayed, it must be associated with a delay in overall colonic transit. For example, if transit in the right colon was disproportionately faster on the 3rd study day than on previous days, markers may accumulate proportionately in the distal colon, suggesting delayed transit in this segment. In patients with extremely delayed transit throughout the entire colon, it may be necessary to extend the study period to demonstrate the transit time in the rectosigmoid. If few or no markers have passed into the rectosigmoid by the completion of the study, the calculated transit time in this segment may well be inaccurate.

If markers are present on the last radiograph obtained, the true transit time will be at least equal to the calculated transit time and might well be greater.

Several of these points are illustrated by the colonic transit study demonstrated in Figure 9–2. Radiopaque markers are present in all segments of the colon on the last radiograph of the study, making it quite likely that actual transit times are longer than calculated. Calculated transit times are: right colon = 86.4 hours, left colon = 68.4 hours, rectosigmoid = 8 hours, total colon = 162.8 hours. This is clearly an abnormal study with demonstrated delay in both the right and left colon. Because fewer than half the markers had an opportunity to pass through the rectosigmoid by the conclusion of the study, transit in this segment is difficult to assess precisely, but at worst is probably not as abnormal as demonstrated in the more proximal segments.

Several patterns of transit emerge when performing these tests on symptomatic patients. Some patients will have unequivocally normal transit and further work-up may be avoided. Other patients may have hindgut delay, in which transit times in the right colon are normal but markers accumulate in the left side of the colon and rectosigmoid. Such patients usually have defecation disorders demonstrable on other studies, such as internal intussusception of the rectum, nonrelaxing puborectalis, or rectocele. Some patients have delay throughout the entire colon; when not associated with a defecation disorder as mentioned previously, this may be associated with abnormal motility in the remainder of the gut. Small-bowel transit studies and esophageal and gastric motility studies should be ordered in these patients before advising subtotal colectomy. Occasionally, one may see a patient with apparently isolated right-sided delay.

Colonic transit studies are a useful test to assess patients with complaints of disordered motility, and when used appropriately, can allow a logical approach to decisions regarding treatment.

REFERENCES

1. Manning, A, Wyman, K and Heaton, K: How trustworthy are bowel histories? Comparison of recalled and recorded information. Br Med J 2:213, 1976.
2. Metcalf, A, et al: Simplified assessment of segmental colonic transit. Gastroenterology 92:40, 1987.
3. Arhan, P, et al: Segmental colonic transit time. Dis Colon Rectum 24:625, 1981.
4. Bouchoucha, M, et al: What is the meaning of colorectal transit time measurement? Dis Colon Rectum 35:773, 1992.
5. Hoelzel, F: The rate of passage of inert materials through the digestive tract. Am J Physiol 92:466, 1930.

CHAPTER **10**

Endoluminal Ultrasonography of the Anal Sphincters

Jeffrey W. Milsom • Tracy L. Hull

Endoluminal ultrasonography (ELUS) of the rectum, anus, vagina, prostate, and pelvic floor has become a valuable diagnostic tool in the evaluation of patients with pelvic floor disorders. In contrast to conventional external ultrasound, ELUS employs a transducer that is placed directly into a body cavity, usually within millimeters of the region of interest, thereby permitting high levels of resolution and imaging quality with minimal morbidity and patient discomfort.[1] This technique was first used in 1956 by Wild and Reid,[2] who imaged a recurrent rectal cancer by inserting a scanner transanally. Watanabe[3] reported his experience imaging the prostate in 1975. Technical improvements in transvaginal, transurethral, and transrectal scanners have now permitted accurate staging of urologic, gynecologic, and rectal cancers, so that sonography now plays an integral role in the management of these malignancies.[4–8]

Interest quite naturally turned toward imaging the anal canal where defining normal anatomy initially was the primary goal. Studies using cadavers,[9] pathology specimens,[10] and normal patients[11–12] clearly showed that both the internal and external anal sphincters could be separately imaged using standard ELUS probes. Anal ELUS is currently indicated in the assessment of fecal incontinence, evaluation of complex perianal fistulas and abscesses, and staging of anal carcinomas. Management of these conditions may be altered if one has preoperative knowledge of sphincter involvement. This chapter reviews the indications and technique of anal sphincter ELUS.

PRINCIPLES OF ULTRASOUND

Electrical stimulation of a crystal contained within a transducer produces high-frequency sound waves. As the sound waves are reflected by tissue back to the crystal, an electrical impulse is generated and an image is produced. Different tissue densities either allow penetration or produce reflection of the sound waves. For example, sound waves passing through fluid are not reflected, yielding a dark (hypoechoic) image. Therefore, the smooth muscle of the internal anal sphincter (IAS), with a high fluid content relative to the surrounding tissue layers in the anus, appears as a dark hypoechoic layer. The external anal sphincter (EAS), in contrast, is more reflective and produces an image composed of mixed hyperechoic layers (Fig. 10–1). Transducers have a fixed focal length depending on the frequency chosen for the examination. This focal length, in turn, determines depth of penetration by the sound waves; higher frequencies have shorter focal lengths and less tissue penetration.[13]

PERFORMING THE ANAL ULTRASOUND EXAMINATION

EQUIPMENT

The use of ELUS to evaluate anal sphincters is appealing for several reasons. It is a noninvasive imaging study that does not emit radiation. The procedure is usually performed in an office setting, but because the scanner is mobile, imaging can be performed in concert with a surgical procedure in the operating room. The examination is relatively inexpensive, lasts only 10 to 15 minutes, and is well tolerated by most patients.[14] Preparation for the examination is accomplished with a phosphosoda enema given just before the procedure. If a comfortable digital anal examination can be done, no analgesia or sedation is required.

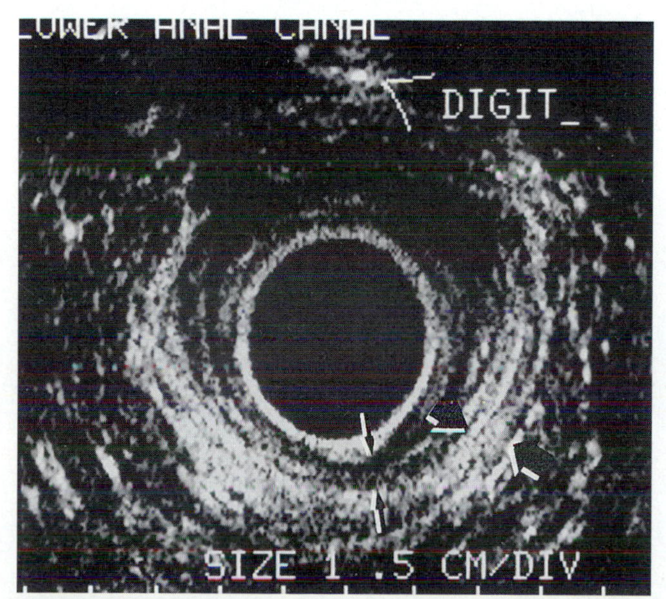

FIGURE 10–1. Endoluminal ultrasound image of a normal anal canal showing the internal (IAS) and external (EAS) anal sphincters; the IAS is delineated by thin arrows, and the EAS by large arrows.

The examination may be performed in any room large enough to accommodate the ultrasound equipment and a standard examination table. The Brüel & Kjær (Nærum, Denmark) scanner type 3535 with a rotating handheld endoprobe (type 1850) has been the instrument used in our clinic. The probe is 24 cm in length; either a 7-MHz or 10-MHz transducer is used. The transducers rotate at 4 to 6 cycles per second, and produce a 360 degree radial image. The 7-MHz probe has a focal length of 2.0 to 4.5 cm and the 10-MHz probe, a focal length of 1.0 to 4.0 cm. The 10-MHz transducer, with its shorter focal length, produces better resolution of superficial structures of the anal canal; we thus prefer to use it when assessing the sphincter.[9]

A lubricated latex balloon inflated with degassed water covers the transducer. This protects the probe and provides effective acoustic coupling. No air must be present between the transducer and the tissue to be examined, because this produces uninterpretable, aberrant images. Many institutions use a hard anechoic plastic cone (diameter 17 mm) filled with degassed water instead of a latex balloon for examination of the anal canal.[15] Use of the cone may avoid the troublesome problem of balloon slippage in and out of the anal canal.

TECHNIQUE

During the examination, the patient is placed in the left lateral decubitus position. The probe is gently inserted 6 to 8 centimeters, or until the transducer is safely above the anal sphincters. In the upper anal canal, the probe is centered in the lumen and slowly withdrawn. Images are recorded within the upper, middle, and lower anal canal; the integrity of the sphincter is assessed. Because the probe may slip out of the anus several times during imaging, the patient must be informed that several reinsertions may be necessary.

ANATOMY

The ultrasonographic layers of the rectal wall correlate well with the histologic layers; these layers descend as distinct entities into the anal canal. Bartram and Burnett[15] defined six sonographic layers of the anal canal:

1. The first hyperechoic layer is the interface of the cone or latex balloon with the tissues.
2. The second layer is hypoechoic (dark) and represents the mucosa.
3. The third layer is hyperechoic and represents the subepithelial tissues.
4. The fourth layer is the internal sphincter, which is hypoechoic.
5. The fifth layer is the hyperechoic longitudinal muscle.
6. The sixth layer shows mixed echogenicity and represents the external sphincter (striated muscle) (Fig. 10–1). Anteriorly its fibers blend into the perineal body in the midanal canal.

Ultrasonographically, the upper, middle, and lower anal canal have distinct characteristics. In the upper anal canal, the external sphincter fuses with the puborectalis, forming a thick posterolateral sling of muscle (Fig. 10–2*A*). In the midanal canal, this sling of muscle merges with the superficial external sphincter. The anococcygeal ligament is visualized as a hypoechoic triangle posteriorly; the vagina is seen anteriorly as an air sac with a hyperechoic lining (Fig. 10–2*B*). In women, the fibers of the external sphincter are not recognizable anteriorly in the upper and middle anal canal; instead, the perineal body is seen anteriorly. The lower anal canal (Fig. 10–2*C*) contains the subcutaneous portion of the external sphincter muscle, whose fibers are complete anteriorly and can be visualized as such. By convention in our practice, when imaging the anal canal, we image each of these three areas.

INDICATIONS

INCONTINENCE

The most common indication for anal ELUS is the assessment of fecal incontinence, in which case disruptions of the internal or external anal sphincters may be identified. Most surgeons would agree that it is helpful to know the nature, location, and extent of sphincter defects in order to plan operative strategy. These defects, whether they are caused by obstetric

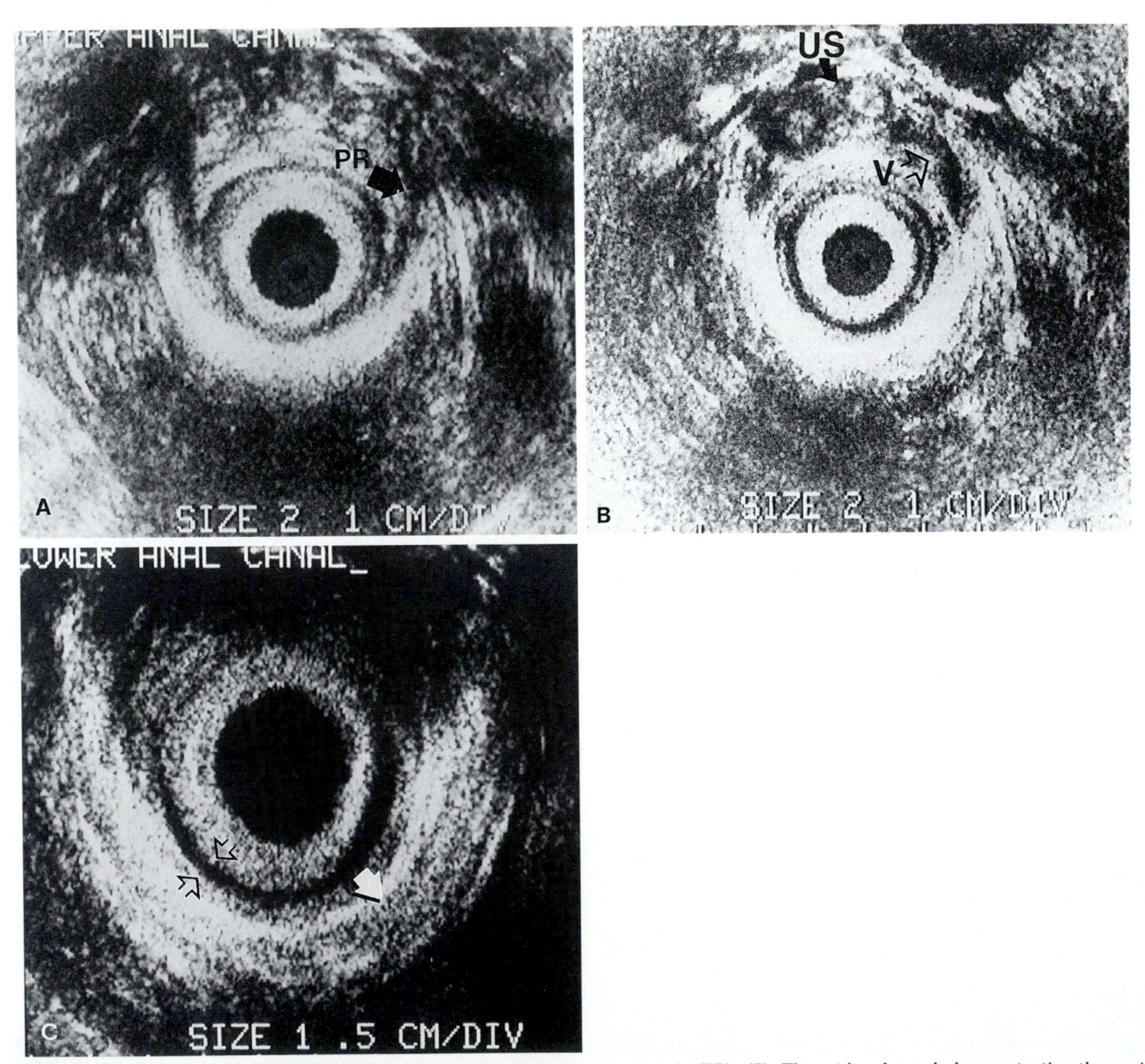

FIGURE 10–2. (*A*), The upper anal canal, demonstrating the puborectalis muscle (PR). (*B*), The midanal canal, demonstrating the vagina (V) and urethral sphincter (US). (*C*), The lower anal canal, demonstrating the internal anal sphincter (open arrows) and the subcutaneous portion of the external anal sphincter (white arrow).

injuries, previous anal surgery, or trauma can be delineated by the 360 degree image provided by ELUS (Fig. 10–3). Sphincter mapping with needle electromyography (EMG) has also been used to localize sphincter defects, but EMG can evaluate only striated muscle, so that the internal sphincter is not assessed. After studying 11 patients with both EMG and anal ELUS, we found ELUS to be considerably less painful and preferable overall to EMG in mapping sphincteric defects.[14] Law and colleagues[16] reached similar conclusions in a study of 15 patients in whom both tests were compared. Correlation between the two techniques was high ($r = 0.960$); but ELUS was better tolerated by patients.

To avoid excessive needle insertions during EMG, Burnett and co-workers recommended ELUS as the initial investigation to precisely locate the sphincteric defect.[17] Needle EMG was then used to confirm the defect in the external sphincter muscle. In her study, 11 of 13 defects found with anal endosonography showed no electrical activity with EMG. Of the two remaining instances, there was one EMG technical failure and the other defect was too deep to reach with the needle. In addition, anal endosonography revealed defects in the internal sphincter in 9 of the 13 patients.

After studying 48 incontinent patients, Nielsen and colleagues[18] concluded that ELUS could be used in place of EMG to detect external sphincter defects. The additional information provided by ELUS regarding the internal sphincter could not be obtained by any other means. Defects or thinning in the external sphincter were detected by ELUS in 22 patients; EMG showed these abnormalities in only 18 patients. The four injuries missed with EMG were located in the middle and upper anal canal, again underscoring the inability of EMG to identify deep defects. Nielsen also found that manometric findings were not affected by the presence of sphincteric defects.

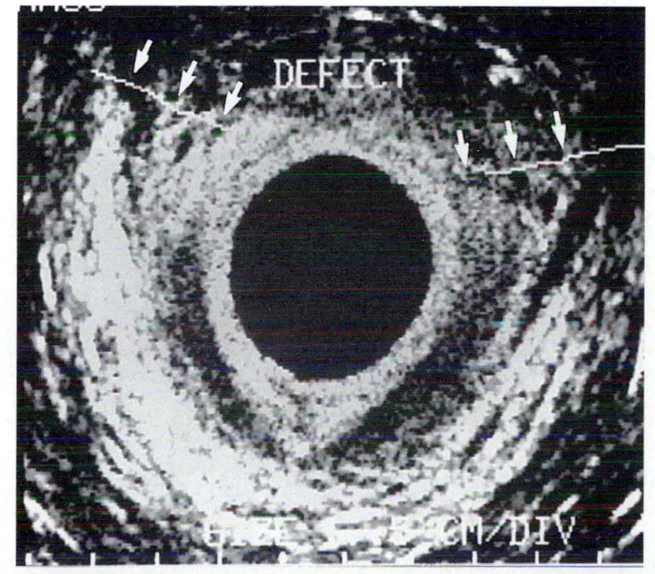

FIGURE 10–3. Defects in the internal and external anal sphincters noted after an obstetric injury. (Arrows mark edges of the defect.)

Using anal ELUS, sphincteric injuries have been identified in incontinent women following childbirth.[19] In a study by Burnett, ELUS was performed in 62 patients with fecal incontinence secondary to obstetric trauma and 18 parous asymptomatic women. In the incontinent group, 56 patients (90%) had defects in the external sphincter, 40 (65%) had defects in the internal sphincter, and 57 (44%) had disruption of the perineal body. There were 37 patients (60%) who had defects in both sphincters. No defects were identified in the control group. Manometry and nerve conduction studies were also performed. In those patients with isolated internal sphincter defects, manometry was abnormal in only 32%. Interestingly, delayed conduction along the pudendal nerves was found in 28 patients and, of these, 19 (68%) also had defects in both sphincters. The study therefore established an important point: incontinence after difficult or complicated deliveries may be due to anatomic disruptions in the sphincter, pudendal neuropathy, or both.

Trauma to the sphincters during anal dilation for anal fissures or hemorrhoids was documented by Speakman and associates.[20] In 12 patients with fecal incontinence following anal dilation, 11 had disrupted internal sphincters and 10 were extensively fragmented. Three also had defects in the external sphincter.

Bartram and Burnett[15] stated that incontinence should be called "idiopathic" only if intact sphincters have been noted after imaging with anal ELUS. In a study of 11 patients initially considered by clinical and anorectal physiologic criteria to have idiopathic incontinence, 4 patients unexpectedly had external anal sphincter defects. In the remaining 7 patients, the external sphincter was intact but a linear relationship was found between the resting anal canal pressure and the thickness of the internal sphincter. Bartram emphasized that although an abnormally thin internal sphincter may adversely affect continence, thickness will normally vary according to patient age. As one ages, smooth muscle is replaced by connective tissue and although the sonographic thickness normally increases with age, the number of functioning muscle fibers decreases. An internal sphincter thickness of 2.0 to 2.5 mm is probably normal in a younger patient but is abnormally thin for an elderly individual and may contribute to her incontinence.

In conclusion, anal ELUS can be an important diagnostic test for the evaluation of fecal incontinence. It is less painful than EMG and gives similar information regarding the external sphincter. It is superior to EMG in identifying deeper defects in the external sphincter, which are inaccessible to the EMG needle. Furthermore, it is the only available study that provides information regarding the internal sphincter. ELUS complements nerve studies and it has been proposed to be the only other test needed besides physical examination to evaluate incontinence.[21] Defects in the internal sphincter may play a greater role than once believed, especially in patients with "idiopathic" incontinence, in whom thinning of the internal sphincter may be a contributing factor.

PERIANAL FISTULAS AND ABSCESSES

Although uncomplicated low anal fistulas can be successfully managed without preoperative imaging studies, occasionally ultrasound may be beneficial in cases of horseshoe fistulas, recurrent fistulas, fistulas or abscesses located proximally in the anal canal, or in patients with perianal pain and suspected sepsis. Using anal ELUS, Schaarschmidt and Willital[22] identified an unsuspected deep ischiorectal abscess in a 7-year-old girl who presented with perirectal pain. Law and colleagues[23] used the procedure to study 22 patients with anal fistulas and prospectively compared results with surgical findings. There was good correlation; ultrasound identified all horseshoe fistulas and 11 of 12 primary tracts. Although 12 patients were clinically felt to have intersphincteric abscesses, only 10 were verified at surgery. The 2 patients incorrectly diagnosed by ultrasound had supralevator extensions at surgery. ELUS failed to identify infralevator (0/2) or supralevator (0/2) abscesses; the researchers felt that these lesions may have been missed because they were deep to the field of view. Of 12 internal openings, 8 were identified.

Cataldo and associates[24] studied 24 patients suspected of having perirectal abscesses. ELUS correctly identified the 19 patients confirmed to have an abscess at surgery. In 63%, anal ELUS identified the relationship between the abscess and sphincter, but only 28% of the internal openings were identified. Cataldo concluded that anal ELUS should be used as an adjunct in the evaluation of complex perianal suppurative disease.

In an attempt to improve the identification of the fistula tract by ELUS, Cheong and co-workers[25] injected hydrogen peroxide into the external opening as an image enhancer. Fistula tracts are hypoechoic, but when injected with hydrogen peroxide, they become brightly hyperechoic, probably due to the nascent oxygen released from the hydrogen peroxide when injected into the tract.

We believe that anal ELUS may be useful in assessing complex and recurrent fistulas (Fig. 10–4). Because these fistulas are difficult to treat, the ease of conducting the ultrasound examination, coupled with the useful information it provides about the relationship of the tract to the anal sphincters, has helped us to plan treatment. As the instruments and techniques become more refined, the accuracy of anal ELUS is likely to improve.

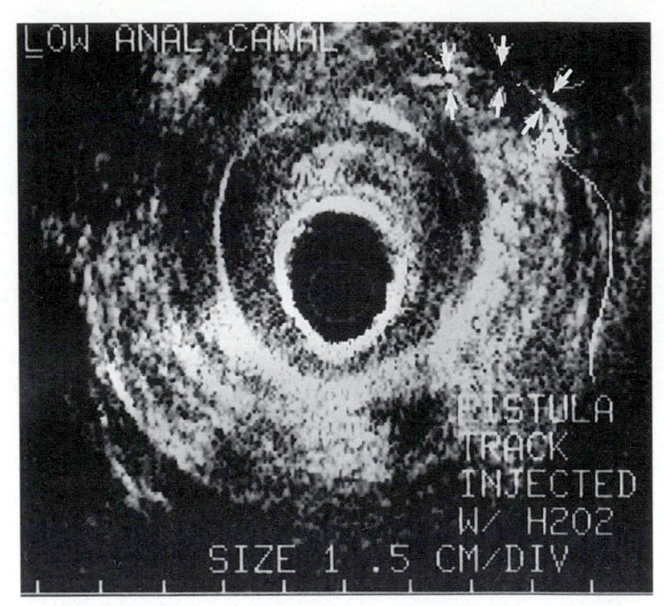

FIGURE 10–4. Complex anal fistula delineated using injection of the tract with hydrogen peroxide (using H_2O_2).

ANAL CARCINOMA

Pretreatment evaluation of anal epidermoid carcinomas using ELUS was first reported by Goldman and colleagues.[26] Fifty patients underwent scanning at the time of diagnosis. Of tumors believed clinically based on digital examination to be confined to the anal sphincter (e.g., T1-2 lesions), two thirds of the carcinomas showed sonographic evidence of muscle penetration (UT3-4). Ultrasound staging also correlated with treatment response; tumors with no or minimal sonographic evidence of muscle invasion responded more favorably to radiation than those with extension beyond the sphincter. Goldman concluded that anal ELUS complemented digital palpation in staging anal carcinoma.

Other authors have confirmed the valuable role ultrasonography may play in staging anal cancers.[27] Assessment of tumor penetration into or beyond the sphincter or into adjacent organs is possible in almost all patients (Fig. 10–5). Accurate assessment of

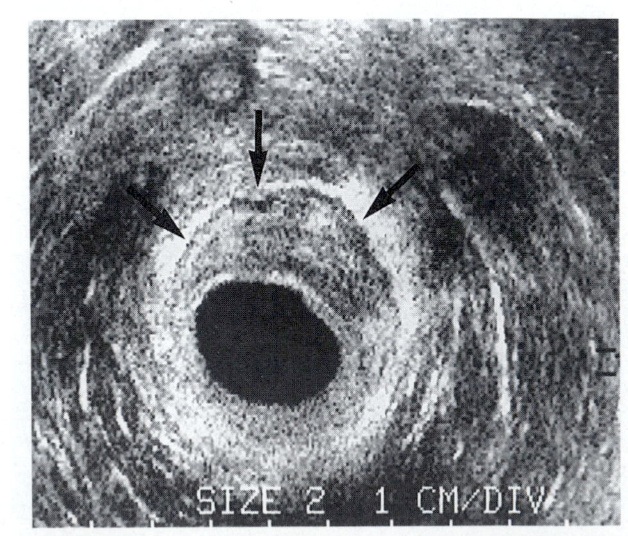

FIGURE 10–5. An anal carcinoma that has penetrated beyond the anal sphincteric musculature (UT3), but does not involve any adjacent organs. (Arrows point to the outer edge of the tumor.)

penetration is important because local excision may be appropriate in selected cases where the tumor is superficial and lacks invasion.

OTHER USES

Anal ELUS may play a role in the evaluation of patients with congenital abnormalities, particularly identification of the sphincter mechanism following operations for imperforate anus.[15]

In patients with obstructed defecation, no correlation has been demonstrated between sphincter size and anal manometry. Patients with obstructed defecation had significantly thicker external sphincter muscles than did healthy controls.[28]

SUMMARY

Anal ELUS is a new diagnostic tool in the assessment of anal pathology. It is extremely useful in the evaluation of fecal incontinence, where it is superior to needle EMG in identifying sphincter defects, especially defects in the upper or mid anal canal, and it certainly is less painful. ELUS should be considered in all patients with significant fecal incontinence, even those patients without prior obstetric injuries or surgical trauma. When imaged with ultrasound, these patients with idiopathic incontinence may prove to have unsuspected external sphincter defects or abnormally thin internal sphincters.

Although most anal fistulas and abscesses may be diagnosed and treated without ELUS, it may have a role in the management of complex or recurrent fistulous tracts. Anal ELUS will prove itself valuable in the staging of anal carcinomas; preliminary results are encouraging. Its ultimate role in the evaluation of anal pathology is likely to become more defined with improvements in the technique and the instrumentation, and as clinicians and ultrasonographers become more familiar with the performance of ELUS.

REFERENCES

1. Mortensen, N: Rectal and anal endosonography. Gut 33:148, 1992.
2. Wild, JJ, Reid: Diagnostic use of ultrasound. Br J Physiol Med 19:248, 1956.
3. Watanabe, H, Igari, D, Tanahashi, Y, et al: Transrectal ultrasonotomography of the prostate. J Urol 114:734, 1975.
4. Gammelgaard G and Holm, HH: Transurethral and transrectal ultrasonic scanning in urology. J Urol 124:863, 1980.
5. Dragsted, J and Gammelgaard, J: Endoluminal ultrasonic scanning in the evaluation of rectal cancer. Gastrointest Radiol 8:367, 1983.
6. Hildebrandt, U and Geifel, G: Preoperative staging of rectal cancer by intraanal ultrasound. Dis Colon Rectum 28:42, 1985.
7. Egender, G, Pirker, E, Rapf, C, et al: Transrectal ultrasonography as a follow-up method in prostatic carcinoma after external beam and interstitial radiotherapy. Eur J Radiol 8:37, 1988.
8. Nakamura, S and Niijima, T: Staging of bladder cancer by ultrasonography: a new technique by intravesical scanning. J Urol 124:341, 1980.
9. Tjandra, JJ, et al: Endoluminal ultrasound defines anatomy of the anal canal and pelvic floor. Dis Colon Rectum 35:464, 1992.
10. Sultan, AH, Nicholls, RJ, Kamm, MA, et al: Anal endosonography and correlation with in vitro and in vivo anatomy. Br J Surg 80:508, 1993.
11. Nielsen, MB, Pedersen, JF, Hauge, C, et al: Endosonography of the anal sphincter: findings in healthy volunteers. AJR Am J Roentgenol 1199:1202, 1991.
12. Nielsen, MB, Hauge, C, Rasmussen, OO, et al: Anal sphincter size measured by endosonography in healthy volunteers. Acta Radiologica 33:453, 1992.
13. Williams, JG: Anal ultrasound in the evaluation of benign anorectal disease. Lecture, Principle of Colon and Rectal Surgery, University of Minnesota, 1993.
14. Tjandra, JJ, Milsom, JW, Schroeder, T, et al: Endoluminal ultrasound is preferable to electromyography in mapping anal sphincteric defects. Dis Colon Rectum 36:689, 1993.
15. Bartram, CI and Burnett, SJD: Atlas of Anal Endosonography. Butterworth-Heinemann, Oxford, 1991, p 1.
16. Law, PJ, Kamm, MA, Bartram, CI, et al: A comparison between electromyography and anal endosonography in mapping external anal sphincter defects. Dis Colon Rectum 33:370, 1990.
17. Burnett, SJ, Speakman, CT, Kamm, MA, et al: Confirmation of endosonographic detection of external anal sphincter defects by simultaneous electromyographic mapping. Br J Surg 78:448, 1991.
18. Nielsen, MB, Hauge, C, Pedersen, JF, et al: Endosonographic evaluation of patients with anal incontinence: findings and influence on surgical management. AJR Am J Roentgenol 160:771, 1993.
19. Burnett, SJD, Spence-Jones, C, Speakman, CT, et al: Unsuspected sphincter damage following childbirth revealed by anal endosonography. Br J Rad 64:225, 1991.
20. Speakman, CTM, Burnett, SJ, Kamm, MA, et al: Sphincter injury after anal dilatation demonstrated by anal endosonography. Br J Surg 78:1429, 1991.
21. Felt-Bersma, RJF, Cuesta, MA, Koorevaar, M, et al: Anal endosonography: relationship with anal manometry and neurophysiologic tests. Dis Colon Rectum 35:944, 1992.
22. Schaarschmidt, K and Willital, GH: Intraanal ultrasound: a new aid in the diagnosis of pelvic processes and their relation to the sphincter complex. J Ped Surg 27:604, 1992.
23. Law, PJ, Talbot, RW, Bartram, CI, et al: Anal endosonography in the evaluation of perianal sepsis and fistula in ano. Br J Surg 76:752, 1989.
24. Cataldo, PA, Senagore, A, Luchtefeld, MA, et al: Intrarectal ultrasound in the evaluation of perirectal abscesses. Dis Colon Rectum 36:554, 1993.
25. Cheong, D, Nogueras, JJ, Wexner, SD, et al: Anal endosonography for recurrent anal fistulas: image enhancement with hydrogen peroxide. Dis Colon Rectum 36:1158, 1993.
26. Goldman, S, Glimelius, B, Norming, U, et al: Transanorectal ultrasonography in anal carcinoma. Acta Radiologica 29:337, 1988.
27. Goldman, S, Norming, U, Svensson, C, et al: Transanorectal ultrasonography in the staging of anal epidermoid carcinoma. Int J Colorect Dis 6:152, 1991.
28. Nielsen, MB, Rasmussen, OO, Pedersen, JF, et al: Anal endosonographic findings in patients with obstructed defecation. Acta Radiol 34:35, 1993.

CHAPTER 11

Electrodiagnostic Assessment: A Diagnostic Adjunct

J. Thomas Benson • Linda Brubaker

Examination of a patient with pelvic floor dysfunction is not complete without a clinical neurologic examination. As discussed in Chapter 4, the physical examination should include a screening assessment of mental status and gait. In addition, Babinski's, patellar, and ankle reflexes should be tested. Lumbosacral sensory dermatome evaluation should be routine. Although not commonly performed with pelvic examination, testing the lower extremities for positional sense (of toes) and vibration perception is necessary to detect neurologic disease affecting the spinal cord. The history should include questions regarding symptoms such as postural hypotension, difficulty with temperature regulation, sweating, or skin blanching disorders. These symptoms suggest neurologic disease affecting the autonomic nervous system.

When the suspicion of neurologic disease is present, electrodiagnostic testing may be used as an adjunct to the history and physical examination. Electrodiagnostic testing increases the clinician's ability to diagnose neurologic disease. Indirect measurements of smooth muscle activity, using, for instance, urodynamics and anal manometry, complement the information gained with history, physical examination, and electrodiagnostic testing.

Certain prerequisites must be fulfilled for safe performance and proper interpretation of electrodiagnostic testing. Clinicians new to neurophysiology are encouraged to work closely with interested neurologic colleagues. In addition, a basic understanding of electricity and electrical safety is imperative. Interested readers may gain the knowledge from various excellent sources.[1] In addition, clinicians must understand some of the cellular mechanisms that allow nerve and muscle to conduct electrical impulses.

Electrodiagnostic testing and monitoring are rapidly developing. Four main categories of testing are particularly useful for pelvic floor evaluation: nerve conduction studies, needle electromyography, tests of sacral reflexes, and, to a lesser degree, somatosensory evoked potentials. This chapter reviews the indications, performance, and interpretation of electrodiagnostic tests useful for pelvic floor evaluation.

ELECTRODIAGNOSTIC EQUIPMENT

Electrodiagnostic testing involves specialized vocabulary and equipment. The goal of these tests is to record spontaneous or stimulated electrical neurophysiologic activity. A great deal of other electrical activity must be "filtered out" to record and interpret meaningful neurophysiologic responses properly. Specific machine parameters are used to *capture* this information. Stimulus parameters which must be selected include stimulus duration (msec), frequency (Hz), and amplitude (μV).

Similarly, recording parameters must be chosen to *capture* an electrical response. This is somewhat analogous to the adjustment of a camera lens, which can alter the focus of a picture that is captured. Recording parameters include filters (which help screen out unwanted electrical activity), gain or sensitivity (which makes responses appear larger or smaller), and sweep speed (which adjusts the time span seen on the screen).

Specific machine settings are recommended for specific neurophysiologic tests. Although these may require adjustment in a variety of clinical settings, the settings used *must* be reported in a complete report.

NERVE CONDUCTION STUDIES

Nerve conduction studies (NCS), among the most common electrodiagnostic tests, are relatively simple to understand conceptually. Briefly put, a nerve conduction time is obtained when a stimulus is given at one point along the nerve and the traveling neural impulse is recorded at a second site. If the traveling neural impulse is recorded along the course of the *nerve*, the response (recorded impulse) is called a compound *n*erve action potential or C*N*AP. More commonly in the pelvis, the traveling neural impulse is transmitted to a muscle. The response is then recorded at this *muscle*, which is responding to the traveling neural impulse. These responses are called compound *m*uscle action potentials or C*M*APs.

Therefore, with nerve conduction studies, the clinician can directly measure conduction. Alternatively, the clinician may measure the time it takes the impulse to travel down the nerve, pass to the muscle, and cause the muscle to respond.

CNAP and CMAP responses have similar characteristics, including latency and amplitude, as illustrated in Figure 11–1. The **latency** is the time interval between stimulus and initiation of response (CNAP or CMAP). The **amplitude** is the magnitude of the response (CNAP or CMAP).

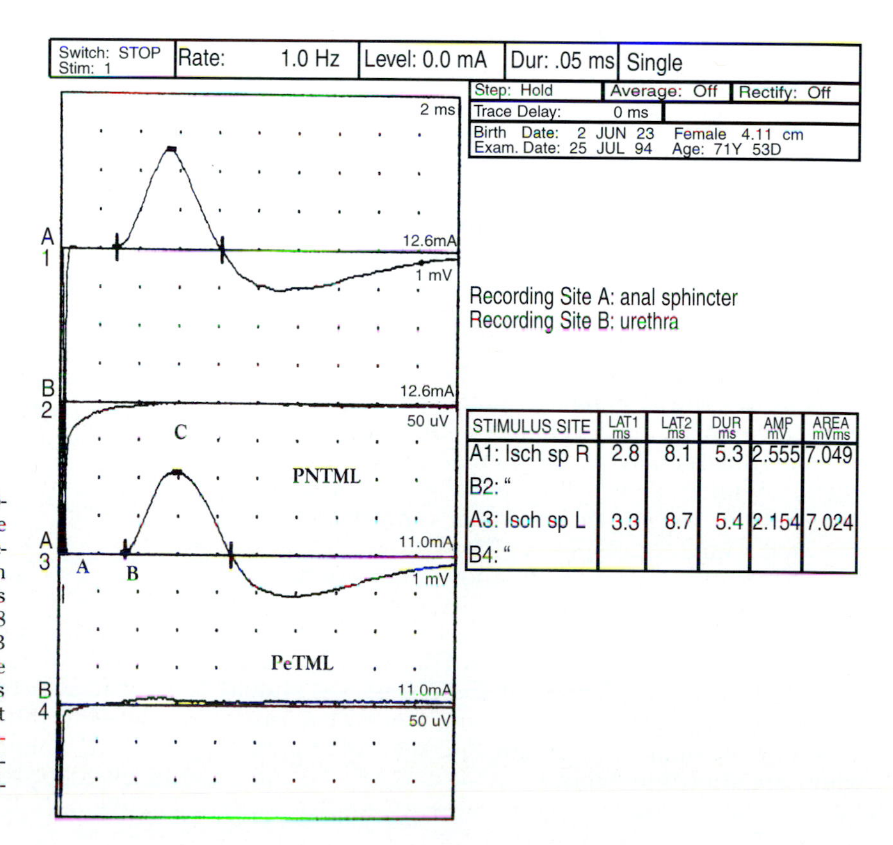

FIGURE 11–1. The compound nerve action potential is recorded following pudendal nerve stimulation. Recordings A1 and A3 indicate responses from the inferior hemorrhoidal branch (PNTML). The segment from point A to point B is the latency of the response (in this depiction, 2.8 msec and 3.3 msec). The distance from point B to point C is the amplitude of the response. The area under the curve can also be calculated, as shown in the data box on the right. In this patient with urinary incontinence, the perineal nerve terminal motor latency (PeNTML) was absent bilaterally, confirming the clinical diagnosis of intrinsic sphincter deficiency.

Conduction along the nerve improves with better myelination and with increasing nerve fiber size. A typical CNAP response is recorded from the largest 15% to 20% of axons in that nerve. Latency of a CNAP response may be prolonged as a result of decreased myelin or loss of axons. The latency of a CMAP also includes neuromuscular junction transmission and muscle contraction. Therefore, in addition to neural disease, CMAP latency may be prolonged by muscular disease or abnormal neuromuscular transmission.

The best response (i.e., largest amplitude) is obtained closest to the responding nerve or muscle. As one moves away from the nerve or muscle, the amplitude of the response decreases.

In the pelvis, CMAPs are more useful than CNAPs because access to the nerve pathway is limited. An important nerve, as discussed in Chapter 3, is the pudendal nerve. CMAPs are widely recorded for this nerve and its innervated muscles.

PUDENDAL NERVE TERMINAL MOTOR LATENCY

Pudendal nerve terminal motor latency (PNTML) studies are growing in clinical importance in the diagnosis and treatment of pelvic floor disorders. The indications for these studies are likely to increase over the next decade.

As reviewed in Chapter 3, the pudendal nerve has three terminal branches: the dorsal nerve to the clitoris, the perineal nerve, and the inferior hemorrhoidal nerve. Terminal motor latency studies may be recorded from both the perineal nerve and the inferior hemorrhoidal branch. In common usage, **pudendal terminal motor latency** refers to the inferior hemorrhoidal branch.

For each of these terminal motor latencies, sites are chosen for placement of the stimulus and recording electrodes. In addition, specific stimulating and recording parameters are selected. Some knowledge of the versatility of electrodiagnostic equipment parameters is useful. This technique was developed at St. Mark's Hospital in London, where the most commonly used electrode is the St. Mark's Pudendal Electrode (Fig. 11–2). This disposable electrode is placed on a glove; the stimulating anode and cathode are then located at the examiner's fingertip, which is placed transrectally at the ischial spine. The transrectal location allows the recording electrode, located at the base of the examiner's finger, to record the anal sphincter response (CMAP).

The resulting CMAP in our laboratory normally has a mean latency of 2.1 ± 0.2 milliseconds in women ages 16 to 35. Normal data on older women are being collected. The amplitude mean is 420 μV, with a range of 200 μV to 750 μV. The right and left nerves should be studied separately, because unilateral abnormalities may be found. Stimulating and recording parameters are shown in Table 11–1.

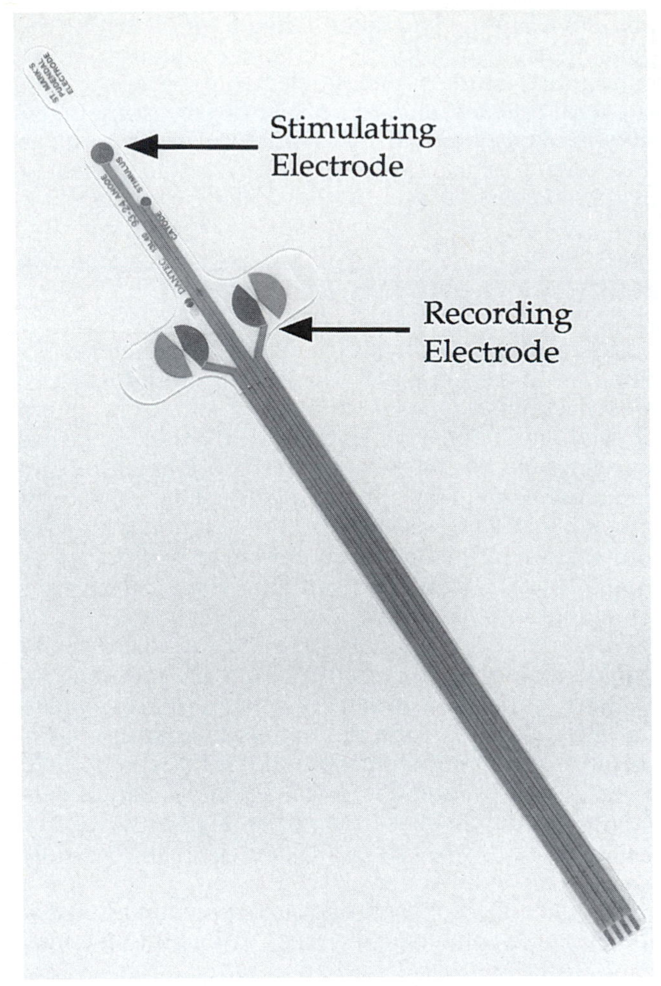

FIGURE 11–2. The St. Mark's pudendal electrode. Note the stimulating anode and cathode at the tip and electrodes at the base, which contact the anal sphincter.

PERINEAL NERVE TERMINAL MOTOR LATENCY

A similar terminal motor latency is recorded from the perineal nerve (PeNTML). The pudendal nerve is stimulated at the ischial spine transrectally, as is done for the PNTML. The response is recorded from the urethral striated sphincter with a ring electrode located on a pediatric Foley's catheter (Fig. 11–3).

The resulting CMAP has, in our laboratory, a mean latency of 2.3 ± 0.3 milliseconds and the laboratory mean amplitude of the positive deflection is 40 μV, with a range of 20 μV to 60 μV. Stimulating and recording parameters are shown in Table 11–1.

CLINICAL APPLICATION

PNTML and PeNTML can be used to evaluate the extent of nerve damage of the pudendal nerve, both as it relates to the external anal sphincter and as it relates to the perineal musculature, particularly the urethral sphincter. PNTML and PeNTML can be used to evaluate the extent of nerve damage caused by

TABLE 11–1. Pudendal Nerve Motor Latency: Parameters for Stimulus and Recording

Parameter	Pudendal Nerve Terminal Motor Latency (PNTML)	Perineal Nerve Terminal Motor Latency (PeNTML)
	Stimulus	
Site	Ischial spine (transrectal)	Ischial spine (transrectal)
Duration (pulse width)	0.05 msec	0.05 msec
Frequency	1.0 Hz	1.0 Hz
	Recording	
Response site	External anal sphincter (St. Mark's electrode)	Periurethral striated sphincter (ring electrode)
Filters		
—High	10,000 Hz	10,000 Hz
—Low	10 Hz	10 Hz
Sweep speed	2 msec	2 msec
Gain (sensitivity)	1 mV	50 μV

vaginal delivery.[2] In a clinically symptomatic patient, there may be a marked abnormality of a terminal branch of the pudendal nerve which persists beyond 6 months following vaginal delivery. Prophylaxis against further damage to the nerve may be strongly considered during subsequent births. Several studies have shown that cesarean section does not cause such damage.[3–5] PNTML is also useful as a predictor of outcome following anal sphincteroplasty. With extensive neuropathic disease, the outcome of surgical therapy, as well as of various medical therapies, is less favorable. PeNTML helps evaluate the extent of urethral competency. It is useful for predicting outcome of therapy for urinary incontinence. These conduction studies have also been used to show the effects of differing routes of surgical therapy for pelvic floor dysfunction.[6]

The latency (time) of these studies measures one parameter of disease, especially reflecting demyelination. Decreasing amplitude of the responses, although not as reproducible and subject to variability, reflects loss of axons. Most pelvic nerve diseases have both demyelinization and axonal loss but in some situations axonal loss is more important in relation to function.

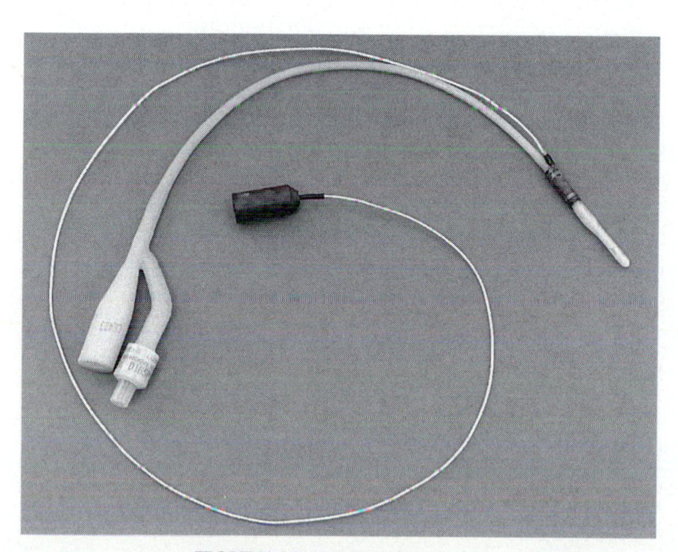

FIGURE 11–3. Ring electrode.

NEEDLE ELECTROMYOGRAPHY (EMG)

This examination places a small needle recording electrode within the substance of a muscle. The activity of the muscle, both at rest and during voluntary contraction, is evaluated. This type of test provides valuable information about the status of the neuromuscular connection and the health of the muscle fibers. Evidence of denervation, with or without reinnervation, may determine the chronicity of a lesion. In addition, evidence for systemic muscle disease can be found.

Various types of needles are used in these examinations. The most common, a concentric needle which has one electrode concentrically surrounding another, is available in disposable 20-gauge to 30-gauge sizes. Special needles such as single-fiber needles, macro-EMG needles, among others, are useful for more specialized forms of needle EMG testing.

Systematic needle electrode examination evaluates insertional activity, spontaneous activity, recruitment patterns, and motor unit action potential (MUAP) configurations. No stimulus is given, because sufficient information is obtained from muscles at rest and during voluntary muscular contraction.

INSERTIONAL ACTIVITY

Insertional activity is observed during and immediately following needle insertion. It represents mechanical damage to the muscle fiber by the needle and subsides within a few seconds. In denervation, insertional activity may be prolonged and may last several seconds. In chronic states with loss of muscle tissue secondary to denervation, insertional activity may be absent.

SPONTANEOUS ACTIVITY

Prior to assessing spontaneous activity, the parameters of the machine are adjusted to increase its sensitivity. At rest, normal skeletal muscle is electrically silent and activation or force is necessary to see motor units. The sphincters are an exception, however, with constant firing of motor units, even during sleep, to allow tone to be maintained. Therefore, normal sphincter activity has electrical potentials without needle movement and with the muscle at rest. When studying the sphincters, these normally firing potentials must be carefully distinguished from abnormal spontaneous activity, which is seen in states of denervation or other conditions causing membrane abnormalities. The most common forms are fibrillation potentials and "positive waves." Another abnormal sphincter activity, "complex repetitive discharges" (CRDs), is seen more often than fibrillations in the urethral sphincter, possibly because CRDs are easier to identify.

For all these parameters the ear is much more helpful than the eye; the examiner must listen as well as watch the oscilloscope.

RECRUITMENT

After evaluating insertional and spontaneous activity, recruitment is assessed. **Recruitment** is the orderly addition of motor units while others, already firing, increase the rate. Normally during exertion, recruitment of motor units is so vast that the EMG pattern of individual MUAPs is no longer recognizable, a so-called "interference pattern." In denervated states or in chronic reinnervation, the recruitment rate may be abnormal, with a reduced number of motor units.

MOTOR UNIT ACTION POTENTIAL CONFIGURATION

The next portion of the needle EMG examination involves examination of the individual MUAP. Parameters of interest are shown in Figure 11–4. With normal healing following nerve damage, adjacent axons attempt to "reinnervate" the muscle fibers. Thus, with reinnervation, each motor unit now supplies a greater number of muscle fibers. The MUAP thus tends to have large amplitude, duration, and number of phases. This occurs because each muscle cell produces its own action potential, which then summates to result in the MUAP.

Unlike neuropathy, in conditions of myopathy, the number of muscle cells in the motor unit is reduced. As a result, the MUAP size (duration and amplitude) is less than normal.

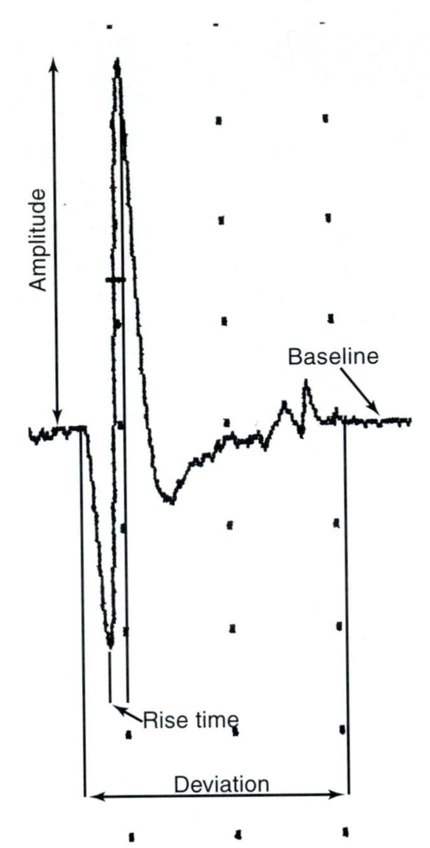

FIGURE 11–4. Motor unit action potential (MUAP) from levator ani. Parameters of interest are duration, amplitude, rise time, and baseline.

Lesion Chronicity

In the first days to a few weeks after injury, the only needle EMG finding is a decreased number of MUAPs, and hence, a correspondingly reduced recruitment pattern. By 3 weeks, fibrillation and positive waves are present, with a persistence of the decreased recruitment. Between 3 to 6 months after onset, changes in the MUAP's shape are seen. If reinnervation has occurred, the MUAPs become complex in shape, showing many different phases or components, compared with the usual triphasic shape. With the passage of several more months, the complex components become incorporated into the more usual configuration. These MUAPs have both increased duration and amplitude however. These findings are seen about 2 years or later after the initial injury and in old or chronic disease. Such findings also indicate completion of any recovery.

SPECIFIC SPHINCTER MUSCLE EXAMINATION

The **external anal sphincter** (EAS) is examined with a 20 mm concentric needle at 27 or 30 gauge. Typically, insertion will occur at 3 o'clock and 9 o'clock, and if "mapping" is being performed, then 10 o'clock, 12 o'clock, 2 o'clock, and 6 o'clock are added. For greater patient comfort, we often employ local anesthetic. EMLA cream (Astra Pharmaceutical Products, Westborough, ME) is applied topically 20 to 40 minutes prior to the study. If desired, additional local anesthetic can be injected, being careful to keep it **intradermal** and to avoid injecting it into the muscle. Twenty MUAPs are collected for morphology analysis. Careful attention to rise time (see Fig. 11–4) is necessary; shorter, steeper rise time indicates proximity to the motor unit. Our laboratory normals for the EAS are listed in Table 11–2. New, computerized quantitative programs, however, reveal smaller amplitudes.

For **puborectalis** examination, a 26-gauge, 45-mm needle is guided into the external anal sphincter at 6 o'clock. The needle then continues through the quiet zone of the inter-sphincteric space before reaching the puborectalis. Normal values are similar to those for the EAS. Alternatively, the pubococcygeus can be approached intravaginally using a 20-mm, 30-gauge needle through the lateral vaginal fornix.

The **periurethral skeletal muscle** is best approached with a 20-mm, 30-gauge concentric needle going dorsal (12 o'clock) to the external urethral meatus, but it can be reached laterally. Insertion to 15 mm to 20 mm is typically required.

CLINICAL APPLICATION

Needle EMG examination helps define the presence or absence of neurologic lesions, distinguishes between upper and lower motor neuron lesions, and evaluates lesion chronicity. Certain subgroups of patients with urinary retention may benefit from needle EMG examination, particularly those in whom specific abnormalities of urethral sphincter musculature are encountered.[7,8]

Surface EMG activity is used in combination with urodynamics and anal manometry and is very helpful in specifying abnormalities associated with decreased cooperative interaction between bladder and urethra or between rectum and anal canal.

Sphincter studies also predict prognosis following surgical and nonoperative treatment of fecal incontinence and constipation. Urethral sphincter EMG is now being studied for its prognostic use in lower urinary tract dysfunction.

TESTING OF SACRAL REFLEXES

Sacral reflexes are frequently tested during physical examination for pelvic floor abnormalities. More precise testing of these reflexes, including quantification, may be done using distinct neurophysiologic pathways. Two clinically relevant sacral reflexes can be tested electrodiagnostically—the bulbocavernosus reflex and the bladder base-to-anal-sphincter (urethroanal) reflex (electromyelography).

TABLE 11–2. Normal Motor Unit Action Potential Parameters for the External Anal Sphincter

Polyphasia: < 15%
Duration: < 6 msec
Amplitude: .15 mV to .5 mV

BULBOCAVERNOSUS REFLEX

The bulbocavernosus reflex can be an important indicator of diseases affecting the cauda equina. A common cause of cauda equina dysfunction is disk disease in the lumbosacral vertebral column. When lumbosacral radiculopathy affects lumbar and S1 nerve roots (centrally located in the cauda equina), an EMG of the affected muscles can assist in evaluation. When disk disease impinges on the S2, S3, or S4 nerve roots, however, EMG studies are less helpful because the mass of paraspinal muscle associated with these nerve roots is not large. For these nerve roots, the bulbocavernosus reflex has particular application.

Technique

This reflex is studied by stimulating the pudendal afferents lateral to the clitoris. The response is recorded at the external anal sphincter. Response parameters of interest include the level of stimulus at which the patient first perceives the stimulus and the latency of both early and late components of the response. The level of first sensation, that is, taken at the first level that the patient perceives the stimulus, is recorded in mAmps. The stimulus used for obtaining the actual response is approximately three times this first sensory level. The afferent (sensory) pathway travels through pudendal cutaneous branches to the principal trunk of the pudendal nerve. Upon reaching the cauda equina, the response goes through the dorsal roots, synapses in the conus medullaris, and exits through the ventral roots. The final motor pathway is the pudendal efferent system to the EAS.

Lateral clitorial stimulation is easily done using a stimulator such as that shown in Figure 11–5. The anode is placed anteriorly (ventrally). The stimulus can be given from either the right or the left side. The response is recorded from needle electrodes that are placed in both the left and right side of the external anal sphincter, allowing recording from either side, thus "lateralizing" the response. This methodology allows localization of a lesion to either left or right afferent or left or right efferent.

Two components to the bulbocavernosus response exist. The mean response latency in our laboratory for the bulbocavernosus reflex is 33.3 ± 3.7 milliseconds for the early response. A delayed response at 60 to 70 milliseconds is frequently present and appears to be more pronounced with suprasacral lesions. The response is usually absent or de-

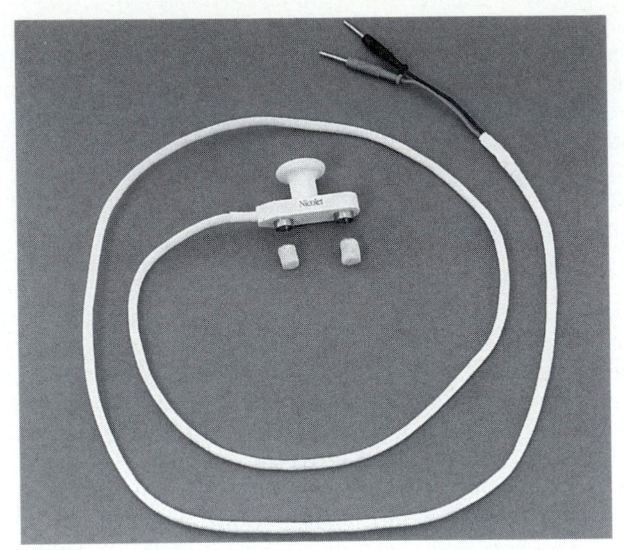

FIGURE 11–5. Stimulator used in testing of sacral reflexes.

layed in lesions of the conus medullaris or cauda equina. In acute lesions, loss of this reflex is an adverse prognostic sign. Chronic lesions are progressive and delay the latency.

Normally the reflex is inhibited during voiding. Although used for evaluation of sexual dysfunction in both sexes, this test evaluates poorly the small nerve fibers that are commonly involved. Autonomic testing may be more sensitive but is not widely available.

Electrical stimulation treatment for urinary incontinence relies upon an intact bulbocavernosus response for effectiveness. Because up to 10% of apparently normal individuals can have an absent clinical bulbocavernous response, determining the presence of the response electrodiagnostically is considered imperative before expecting functional electrical stimulation to be effective in patients without a clinical reflex.

ELECTROMYELOGRAPHY

Electromyelography is a term used by Bradley and co-workers[8] to refer to testing of the urethroanal reflex. This test was developed for evaluation of the pathways for the detrusor and urethra as well as sexual function.[9,10] A stimulus is applied at the proximal urethra with a ring electrode placed around a Foley's catheter (see Fig. 11–3). The afferent pathway carries sensory afferents from the proximal urethra and bladder base. These afferents are small, nonmyelinated fibers which traverse through the pelvic plexus as well as through the hypogastric plexus to the thoracolumbar portions of the spinal cord. The chief pathway, however, appears to be through the pelvic plexus, as verified by effects after epidural block. After synapsing in the cord, the response travels through the pudendal efferent system and is ultimately recorded at the anal sphincter.

As with the bulbocavernosus reflex, the level of the first sensory perception (in mA) is recorded. The reflex is obtained with a stimulus of approximately three times the sensory level. Normal response characteristics include the amplitude (25 mV to 150 mV) and the latency (50 to 80 milliseconds). In the presence of normal supraspinal innervation, this response can also be abolished by volitional relaxation during early voiding. The reflex can be technically difficult to obtain. The response is abolished or diminished in cauda equina injury and is frequently delayed in diabetes. It has been found to be significantly altered or absent in patients with voiding dysfunction following radical pelvic surgery.

Sexual dysfunction can be studied using electromyelography somewhat better than using the bulbocavernosus reflex, because it involves testing of some afferent small-diameter nerve fibers (A delta or C fiber). In patients with a sensory defect, a normal result on electromyelography helps to rule out an afferent problem between the urinary tract and the spinal cord. Normal electromyelography in such patients suggests that the sensory lesion is located either within the central nervous system or within the bladder wall itself. Normal findings in sacral reflex studies, combined with normal sphincter EMG, effectively rule out lower motor neuron disease in this area.

SOMATOSENSORY EVOKED POTENTIALS

Somatosensory evoked potentials (SSEP) are common electrodiagnostic tests that may be useful for evaluation of pelvic floor disorders. SSEPs are responses that are recorded from the central nervous system (brain or spinal cord) in response to stimulation delivered peripherally. SSEP testing is useful in demonstrating normal nerve function, detecting abnormal nerve function, or localizing a problem to a segment of the conductive pathway.[11] The evoked potentials obtained are of very low amplitude (0.1 μV to 20 μV). Because they are buried in the patient's intrinsic "electrical" noise and the environmental noise intrinsic in the machine, they can only be obtained by averaging. The averaging technique records many responses (often hundreds) and allows random electrical "noise" to be distinguished from the actual response, which appears in a "time-locked" fashion. The time response becomes more prominent, whereas "noise" becomes less prominent when many responses are recorded. Because the response can be difficult to obtain reliably, every test must be replicated and controlled.

The response parameters include latencies, which are measured to peak. Typically, abnormal latency is considered to be beyond three standard deviations. The responses obtained from the right and left sides should be compared. An amplitude variance over 50% is considered abnormal.

Pelvic floor SSEP can be stimulated from the pudendal nerve through stimulation at the bladder base. Pudendal SSEPs are obtained by stimulating lateral to the clitoris, allowing right and left sides to be obtained separately. A response may be obtained over cortex L1. Details of electrode placement are described elsewhere.[12] Typically, the first positive cortical peak occurs around 37 to 39 milliseconds.

Bladder-base SSEPs are obtained by stimulating the bladder base with a Foley's electrode. Responses are obtained with electrodes placed over the spinal column as outlined previously. This response is frequently difficult to obtain and its absence may be technical in nature and not necessarily associated with disease. The presence of the response is, however, a strong indication of an intact afferent pathway for the bladder. The latency of this response is about 60 to 70 milliseconds; the delay is presumably due to the slow conduction of the small afferent sensory nerves involved.

CLINICAL APPLICATION

Pudendal SSEPs evaluate the pudendal sensory tract. (They may be useful in selecting patients who will respond to electrical stimulations or transcutaneous electrical nerve stimulation for perineal pain syndromes.) The cortical potentials evaluate spinal transmission and are useful for evaluating proximal pudendal function in urinary and fecal incontinence. In patients with sexual dysfunction who have arousal deficits, the presence of the cortical response helps to separate a psychogenic from a spinal or peripheral origin. The bladder-base SSEPs to the cortex help to exclude a subpontine neurogenic bladder disorder.

AUTONOMIC STUDIES

Dysfunction of smooth-muscle control in different organ systems or of glandular secretions is symptomatic of autonomic neuropathy. Diseases associated with significant autonomic dysfunction include diabetes, amyloidosis, Guillain-Barré syndrome, and Riley-Day syndrome. Minor autonomic dysfunction is generally seen in various types of metabolic diseases such as alcoholism and nutritional deficiencies, and in paraneoplastic neuropathies and toxic neuropathies. There are hereditary sensory and autonomic neuropathies. Autoimmune diseases such as systemic lupus erythematosus and scleroderma may also involve autonomic neuropathies.

Autonomic neuropathy is common in spinal cord disease due to loss of supraspinal influences on sympathetic reflex mechanisms. Clinically, regulation of blood pressure and temperature is impaired; attacks of increased blood pressure and sweating are invoked by external or internal stimuli such as a full bladder.

Electrodiagnostic tests for autonomic dysfunction include orthostatic heart rate recording, sinus arrhythmia testing, and a sympathetic skin response.[10] In orthostatic heart rate testing, electrodes are placed on each palm and the patient's cardiogram activity is recorded. The patient should rise from a supine (baseline) to a standing position. Normally, heart rate increases rapidly, which is maximal at the 15th beat. The heart rate then slows maximally at the 30th beat.

Sinus arrhythmia is studied by recording heart rate activity while the patient is in a reclining position undergoing deep breathing. After 2 to 5 minutes, the patient takes deep breaths at a rate of 6 per minute (5 seconds inspiration, 5 seconds expiration) and the variation in heart rate is expressed as the ratio of the rate during expiration (faster) over inspiration (slower), the E/I ratio. The variation is reduced by aging and is greatly reduced in autonomic neuropathy.

Skin sympathetic response may also be recorded. The effector organ in this test is the sweat gland and recording is therefore done in areas where sweat glands are present, typically the hands and feet. Response occurs spontaneously with sudden emotions or in response to an electrical stimulus. The response can also be obtained over the perineum. The response disappears after autonomic blockade and after sympathectomy. Its exact clinical significance is poorly understood and awaits further study.

Abnormalities of the autonomic function tests in association with peripheral neuropathy in pelvic floor electrodiagnosis may correlate with the degree of axonal involvement. In diabetes the sympathetic skin response has been studied extensively and autonomic involvement is usually suggested by other parameters. Reduction in heart rate variation in the orthostatic test and sinus arrhythmia test is found in a significant number of patients with diabetes. With long-standing diabetes, both peripheral and autonomic nerve function tests become abnormal; the abnormalities are correlated with higher HgbA1C levels and with age and duration of the disease.[13] Because most electrophysiologic testing involves large fibers, autonomic nervous system testing is more difficult. The development of more sophisticated testing for small–nerve-fiber disease is an area of expanding research for the future.

SUMMARY

The use of electrodiagnostic testing for diagnosis of pelvic floor disorders allows investigators to understand the neuromuscular abnormalities associated with incontinence and prolapse. Specific electrodiagnostic testing can be employed to clarify the physiologic disturbance underlying these clinical conditions. In addition, important prognostic information can be obtained, which may lead to the development of novel therapeutic interventions or, perhaps, to refinement of current interventions. Finally, electrodiagnostic testing may help assess potentially deleterious neuromuscular effects of current surgical therapies.

Electrodiagnostic testing holds great promise for both research and clinical care of women with pelvic floor disorders. Motivated clinicians are encouraged to work closely with an interested neurologist in order to gain the competence and insight necessary to perform and interpret these tests.

REFERENCES

1. Barry, DT: Basic concepts of electricity and electrons in clinical electromyography. American Association of Electrodiagnostic Medicine Minimonograph No. 36. American Association of Electrodiagnostic Medicine, 1991.
2. Snooks, SH and Swash, M: Abnormalities of the innervation of the urethral striated sphincter musculature in incontinence. Br J Urol 56:401–405, 1984.
3. Klein, MC, Gauthier, RJ, Robbins, JM, et al. Relationship of episiotomy to perineal trauma and morbidity, sexual dysfunction, and pelvic floor relaxation. Am J Obstet Gynecol 171:591–598, 1994.
4. Sleep, J, Grant, A, Garcia, J, et al. West Berkshire perineal management trial. Br Med J 1984; 289:587–590, 1984.
5. Sleep, J, et al: West Berkshire perineal management trial: three-year follow-up. Br Med J 295(6601):749–751, 1988.
6. Benson JT and McClellan, EJ: Effect of vaginal dissection of pudendal nerve. Obstet Gynecol 82:387, 1993.
7. Fowler, CJ: Pelvic Floor Neurophysiology. In Methods in Clinical Neurophysiology, vol 2. 1991.
8. Bradley, WE, Timm, OW, Rockswold, GL and Scott, FB: Detrusor and urethral electromyelography. J Urol 113:69, 1975.
9. Fowler CJ: Electrophysiologic evaluation of sexual dysfunction. In Low, P. (ed.): Clinical Autonomic Disorders. Little, Brown & Co., Boston, 1993, p 279.
10. Aminoff MJ: Evaluation of autonomic function. In AAEM Didactic Program: Disorders of the Autonomic Nervous System. American Association of Electrodiagnostic Medicine, Rochester, MN, 1990.
11. Van den Bergh, P and Kelly, JJ: The evoked electrodermal response in peripheral neuropathies. Muscle Nerve 9:656, 1986.
12. Benson, JT (ed.): Female pelvic floor disorders: Investigation and management. New York: W. W. Norton, 1992.
13. Ewing DJ, Campbell IW and Clarke BF: Mortality in diabetic autonomic neuropathy. Lancet 1:601, 1976.

CHAPTER 12

Cystourethroscopy

Alfred E. Bent • Anne L. Viselli

Accessibility of the lower urinary tract to endoscopic examination has made cystourethroscopy an integral component in the evaluation of female lower urinary tract dysfunction. Although few data support or refute its routine use, cystourethroscopy may be used to facilitate diagnosis of suspected conditions and to exclude potential coexistent pathology. Urethroscopy and cystoscopy are valuable additions to the gynecologist's diagnostic armamentarium. Information obtained from endoscopic examination may be used alone or, more commonly, integrated with that provided by urodynamic or radiographic evaluation to formulate a management strategy.

HISTORY OF ENDOSCOPY

Early in the nineteenth century, Bozzini introduced endoscopic examination of the female bladder by means of a hollow tube and a candle for illumination.[1] Neither Bozzini nor his invention were well received by the medical community. Development by Nitzke of the compound lens system, originally designed for use in indirect water cystoscopy, and of the incandescent lamp, by Leiter, followed later in the nineteenth century.[2] In 1893, Howard Kelly, director of the first modern gynecologic residency training program at Johns Hopkins University, developed a simple cystoscope used in conjunction with a head mirror. Kelly discovered that when the patient was placed in the knee-chest position, the bladder filled with air, thus allowing visualization of its interior.[3] Using this technique, Kelly was the first to pass ureteral catheters under direct observation. The development of fiberoptics, allowing transmission of high-intensity lighting, and the rod-lens system by Hopkins, using glass rather than air as a transmission medium, propelled modern endoscopy to prominence as a diagnostic tool.[4] These technologic achievements in lighting and optics greatly improved endoscopic visibility and diagnostic accuracy. The 30-degree and 70-degree lenses incorporated into these endoscopes, however, although ideal for viewing the bladder, proved inadequate for viewing the female urethra. Furthermore, the cystoscope's fenestrated sheath permits escape of the infusion medium to the outside until the fenestra is within the distal urethra, thus limiting distension of the distal urethra.[5] The female urethra was consequently often overlooked as a source of significant pathology. In 1973, Robertson developed an endoscope for use in the female urethra incorporating a 0-degree lens and a nonfenestrated sheath, allowing for distension and examination of the distal urethra.[6] Robertson pioneered optics designed to use carbon dioxide as the distension medium. Lenses and optics have since been modified to improve lighting and resolution, but the basic characteristics of the Robertson urethroscope remain essential to proper evaluation of the female urethra.

INDICATIONS

Urologic endoscopy may be done to evaluate the anatomic and functional integrity of the bladder, urethra, and ureters. In addition, material for cytologic and histologic examination may be obtained, and cystourethroscopic techniques may provide access to the upper urinary tract, through the passage of ureteral stents, catheters, and brushes. The many indications for urethroscopy in the female include evaluation of urinary incontinence (particularly if recurrent), obstructive or irritative voiding symptoms, recurrent urinary tract infections, dyspareunia, pelvic pain, hematuria, traumatic injury, and suspected diverticulum, fistula, polyps, condyloma, or ectopic ureter. Besides these, indications for cystoscopy also include evaluation of suspected interstitial cystitis and cervical cancer staging. Some advocate that all patients on whom operative intervention is planned should undergo preoperative cystourethroscopy to prevent serious errors in patient management.[7] Intraoperative cystourethroscopy aids in assessing suture placement, bladder and ureteral integrity, and the response of the urethrovesical junction (UVJ) to anti-incontinence procedures.[8]

CYSTOURETHROSCOPY: GAS VS. FLUID FOR INFUSION

The original Robertson urethroscope was designed to use carbon dioxide as the filling medium. This gas is neat and easy to use and provides rapid distension of the urethra and bladder. It causes mucosal erythema, however, and the rapid bladder distension provided by CO_2 may be uncomfortable for the patient. Painful distension may produce such a stimulus to void that uninhibited detrusor contractions occur, giving the false impression of detrusor instability. Saline solution has the advantage of slower and more physiologic distension, making it useful for the examination of both the urethra and the bladder. In addition, stress testing can be easily performed following bladder filling. The major disadvantage of saline solution is spillage, although the use of towels or specially designed examination tables with pull-out trays minimizes this problem. Visualization is similar through either infusion medium.[9]

CYSTOURETHROSCOPY: FLEXIBLE VS. RIGID INSTRUMENTATION

Cystourethroscopy may be performed with either flexible or rigid endoscopes. In addition to being exceedingly durable, the rigid endoscope has other advantages:

1. Superior optics secondary to the rod-lens system
2. A larger working channel, allowing the passage of accessory instruments
3. A larger lumen for infusion, allowing improved visualization
4. Ease of manipulation and orientation during examination of the bladder

Flexible endoscopes have some well defined advantages over the rigid instruments:

1. Greater comfort for the patient
2. Ease in passing the instrument over an elevated bladder neck
3. The ability to inspect at any angle with deflection of the tip of the instrument[10]

With the exception of the last one, however, these advantages apply to the male patient, in whom the maneuvering required to traverse the length of the urethra and to pass the scope over a bladder neck elevated by prostatic hyperplasia may lead to significant patient discomfort, suboptimal examination, and inadvertent urethral trauma. Flexible endoscopy is therefore almost solely used for examination of the male patient. The equipment and techniques described in this chapter refer to rigid endoscopy.

URETHROSCOPY

EQUIPMENT

The Robertson urethroscope, designed for gas urethroscopy, consists of a sheath and a direct-view telescope swaged onto a handle to which are attached sources of light and gas. This equipment has been modified, but the basic characteristics of the Robertson urethroscope have been preserved. The telescope is composed of a hollow metal cylinder containing a series of solid rod lenses. The objective lens at the tip of the instrument collects the light of the image and transmits the image to the eyepiece through the rod and lens system. The eyepiece of the telescope has an ocular lens that magnifies the image. The urethroscope incorporates a 0-degree (straight-ahead) lens, necessary for viewing both the anterior and posterior surfaces of the urethra. In front of the eyepiece is a light pillar containing and continuous with a fiberoptic bundle within the telescope. The pillar connects to an external fiberoptic light source and transmits light to the visual field.

The urethroscope sheath, unlike that of the standard cystoscope, has a short oblique beak and no fenestra (Fig. 12–1). This design allows distension and proper evaluation of the distal urethra. The caliber of the sheath varies; the size, given in the French scale, refers to the outside circumference of the instrument in millimeters. The 24-Fr sheath should allow comfortable examination in most patients, although a 15-Fr sheath should be available. The sheath incorporates inlet and outlet ports for the infusion medium. For fluid infusion, standard intravenous infusion systems are satisfactory. The telescope is introduced into the sheath and fixed with a watertight lock.

An arthroscope functions well as an operating urethroscope. The arthroscope's offset telescope allows passage of an accessory instrument directly through a central channel to the site of the abnormality.

A camera, high-resolution color monitor, and a video recorder are desirable for documentation, staff education, and patient involvement.

After each procedure is completed, the urethroscope is disassembled and immersed in disinfectant, such as 3.2% glutaraldehyde solution (Cidex Plus 28 day (Surgikos)) for 20 minutes. It is then transferred to a basin of sterile water until ready for use, at which time it is rinsed and gently wiped with a sterile sponge. It is important not to leave the scope immersed in Cidex for longer than 20 minutes, because damage may occur during prolonged soaking. The instrument should be cleaned daily with Alconox detergent and water, rinsed, and placed in dry storage. The scope should be thoroughly cleaned weekly with alcohol and lubricated with super oil.

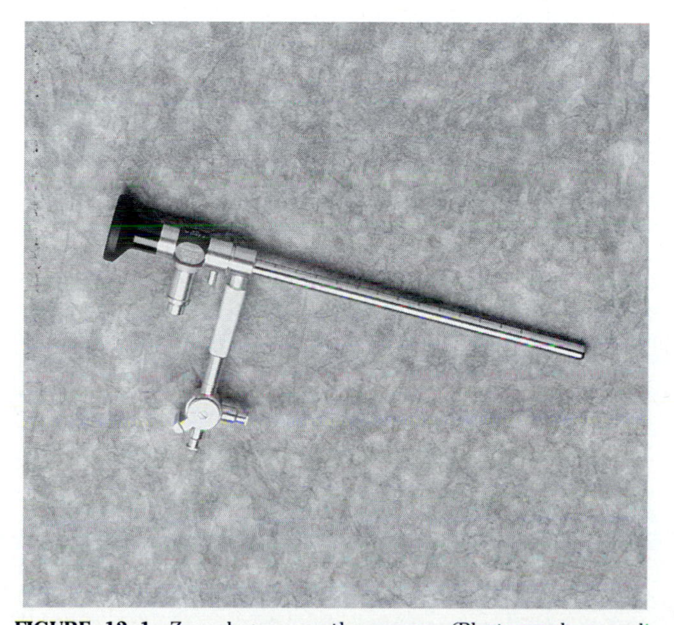

FIGURE 12–1. Zero-degree urethroscope. (Photograph compliments of Karl Storz Endoscopy-America Inc., Culver City, CA.)

OPERATIVE TECHNIQUE

The urethroscope is assembled and connected to the light source, intravenous infusion system, and camera if available. The patient is placed in the dorsolithotomy position, the labia are gently separated and the external urethral meatus is inspected to exclude a local pathologic condition, such as a urethral mucosal prolapse, urethral caruncle, or paraurethral cyst. The meatus is cleansed with an antiseptic solution and, with the sterile water or saline flowing at a rate of 80 to 100 mL/min, the urethroscope is gently introduced through the meatus, with the fluid serving as an obturator. A "no-touch" technique is used to maintain sterility of the instruments.

Urethroscopy is generally well tolerated and is best performed without anesthetic, because an anesthetic, whether topic or by local injection, may interfere with the urethroscopic findings.[11] Local anesthetic agents, such as lidocaine gel, may produce mucosal erythema and give the false impression of an inflammatory reaction. If the urethral lumen is too small to allow the endoscope to pass easily, then either a smaller-caliber sheath should be used or the urethra should be gently dilated. If dilation is necessary, 2% lidocaine (Xylocaine) gel, with or without the addition of 20% benzocaine gel, is applied to the dilator or is inserted into the urethra using a cotton-tipped applicator 5 minutes prior to the procedure. The mucosal erythema resulting from both the anesthetic and the dilation must be considered in the final assessment. Occasionally, a patient will require a bladder pillar block because of marked discomfort at the urethral meatus.[12] If the cervix is in place, 5 mL of a 1% lidocaine solution is injected at the cervicovaginal junction at the 10- and 2-o'clock positions to a depth of 2 mm. In the absence of a cervix, 5 mL of a 1% lidocaine solution is injected at the urethrovesical junction, identified by the balloon of an intraurethral catheter, at the 4- and 8-o'clock positions (Fig. 12–2). To supplement this procedure, 20% benzocaine gel, inserted into the urethra with a cotton-tipped applicator, may be used. Anesthesia for distal urethral biopsy or excision is adequately achieved with local 1% lidocaine injection using a 30-Fr gauge needle.

The angle of insertion maintains the center of the urethral lumen in the middle of the operator's visual field, by either direct observation or video camera. It is essential that the operator observe the urethral mucosa during the initial introduction of the urethroscope, because instrumentation produces erythema. The urethra is only partially distended during the initial introduction because the irrigant flows freely into the bladder. The pleated appearance of the urethral mucosa unfolds ahead of the endoscope as the UVJ is approached. The UVJ appears circular or, more frequently, as an inverted U-shape (Fig. 12–3). When the tip of the urethroscope is at the UVJ, the infusion medium is interrupted and the junction is observed for mucosal abnormalities. Flow is then resumed and

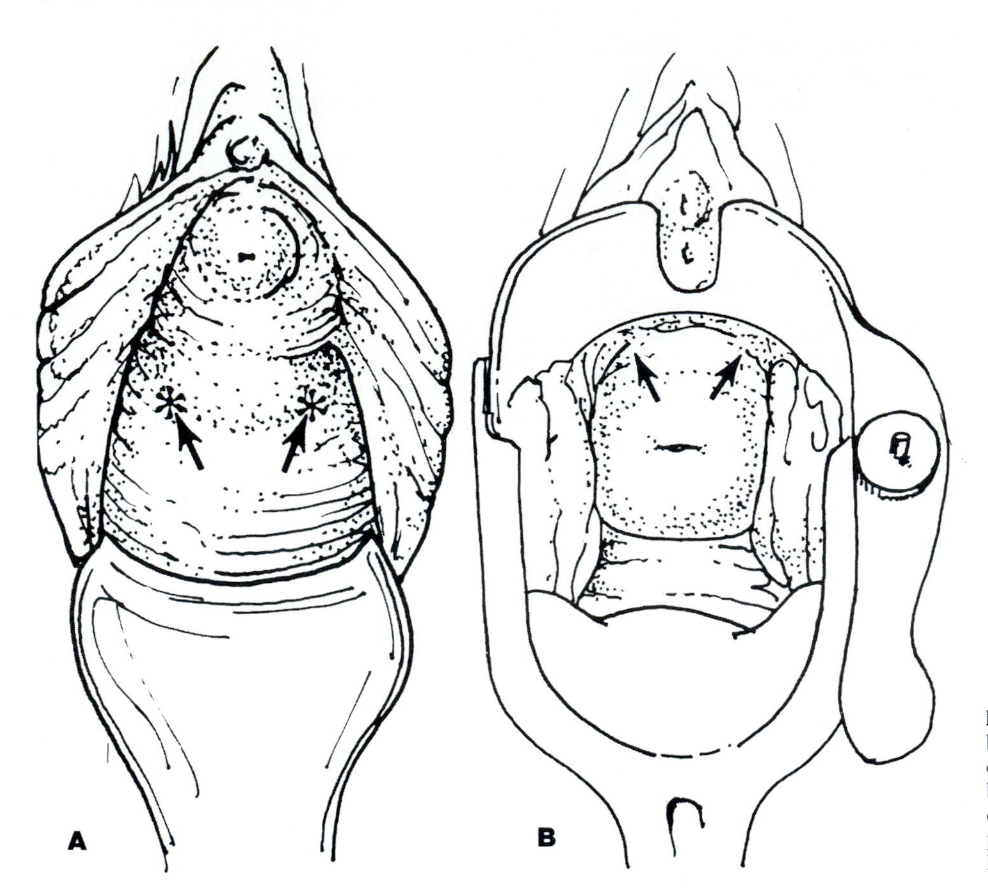

FIGURE 12–2. (*A*), Injection sites for bladder pillar block anesthesia when cervix is present. (*B*), Injection sites for bladder pillar block anesthesia when cervix is absent. (From Ostergard,[12]. Reprinted with permission CV Mosby, St. Louis, MO.)

the urethroscope is passed to the bladder base to view the trigone and the ureteral orifices located at the posterolateral aspect of the bladder. In a few patients, it may be difficult to enter the bladder, even though the instrument passes easily through the urethra. The difficulty occurs at the UVJ, where a mucosal ring catches the tip of the instrument. An index finger placed into the vagina may guide passage of the scope into the bladder.[13] Once the trigone is in view, the scope is rotated 20 to 30 degrees to each side and passed inward along the same axis. The orifice normally comes into view approximately 3 centimeters from the UVJ. The interureteric ridge may be followed in a lateral direction to the other ureteral orifice. If a large cystocele or prolapse obscures the ureteral openings or prevents visualization of the bladder base, a finger is placed in the vagina to reposition the tissues so that the nonvisualized areas may be exposed.

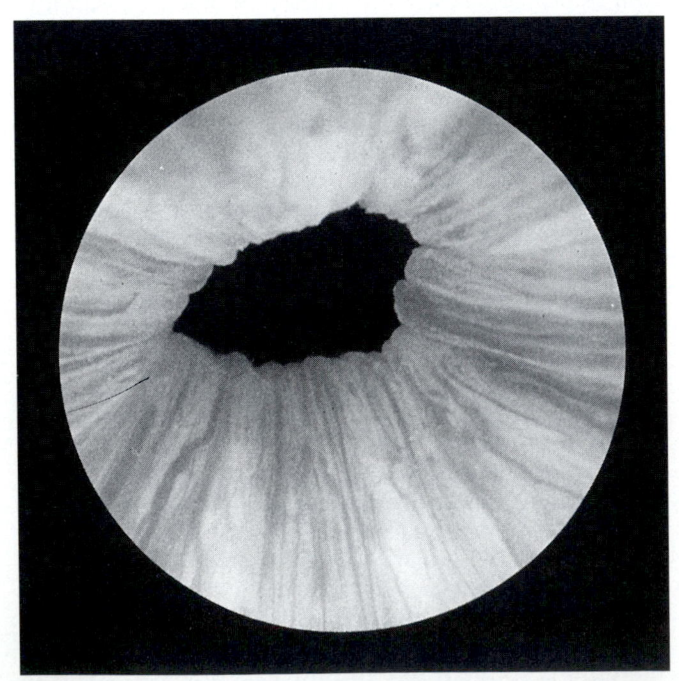

FIGURE 12–3. The urethrovesical junction. (From Schonebeck, J: Atlas of Cystoscopy. Grune and Stratton, Orlando, 1985, p 23, with permission.)

After the expulsion of urine from each orifice is confirmed, dynamic function of the UVJ may be assessed by observing its response to a variety of maneuvers. The urethroscope is withdrawn until the UVJ is about one third closed. The patient it asked to hold her urine and squeeze her rectal sphincter; the response of the UVJ is then noted. Next, the scope is withdrawn until the UVJ is two thirds closed and the patient is asked to perform the Valsalva maneuver and to cough forcefully (2 or 3) times. Again, the response of the UVJ is noted; normally the UVJ should close with minimal descent. After these maneuvers are completed, the urethroscope is positioned so that the UVJ is one third closed.

The bladder is allowed to distend, noting the response of the UVJ to bladder filling, as well as the patient's first sensation of filling, fullness, and maximum cystometric capacity. With the bladder subjectively full, the maneuvers at the UVJ are repeated. The patient is asked to void spontaneously and then to interrupt voiding while the operator observes the response of the UVJ and the bladder to these commands. Finally, with the infusion medium running, the instrument is slowly withdrawn from the UVJ to the external meatus while a finger placed in the vagina compresses the urethra against the endoscope. This allows full distension of the urethra distal to the point of compression. The patient may experience considerable discomfort during this portion of the examination and should be forewarned.

Examination with carbon dioxide gas is conducted in similar fashion, but first sensation is earlier and maximum cystometric capacity is 250 to 300 mL as compared with 350 to 600 mL using saline solution. Rapid infusion of carbon dioxide may provoke detrusor activity.[14]

NORMAL ANATOMIC OBSERVATIONS

Endoscopically, the urethral membrane is gathered in longitudinal folds. One such fold, termed the **urethral crest**, is more prominent than the others and is located along the floor of the urethra. Just inside the urinary meatus, the ostia of ducts draining the periurethral glands may be seen posteriorly, as the infusion medium distends the distal urethra to the high-pressure zone of the midurethra. An intact internal urethral sphincter, composed of coapted urothelium, a rich submucosal vascular plexus and periurethral smooth muscle, and elastic and connective tissue, maintains both passive continence and a margin to continence during stress ("gasket effect").[15] The "gasket effect" of these structures can be evaluated endoscopically with the urethroscope placed in the distal urethra. By interrupting and resuming the flow of the infusion medium, the coaptation of the urethral mucosa and the turgor of the submucosa, produced by the engorged plexus, can be demonstrated. When the urethroscope is in the distal urethra and the flow of the infusion medium has begun, the mucosa will roll away from the tip of the instrument as the infusion pressure exceeds that of the distal urethra.

When the flow is interrupted, the mucosa falls back into place and envelops the tip of the instrument. The obturator effect of the infusion medium is ineffective in separating the mucosa of the midurethra owing to the high resting pressure (on average 75 cm H_2O) generated by the midurethral striated muscle fibers.[15] Midurethral pressure is overcome by the force of the advancing urethroscope. When viewing the midurethra, vascular pulsations may be seen coincident with the heartbeat. The submucosal plexus can be seen glistening through the translucent mucosa, making the urethral interior appear red. As the scope is advanced into the proximal urethra, the infusion pressure again exceeds the urethral pressure and the mucosa rolls away, allowing visualization of the UVJ. The trigone and ureteral orifices may be viewed just inside the UVJ. The trigone, bounded by the ureteral orifices, the interureteric ridge, and the internal urinary meatus, appears as confluent areas of reddened, granular tissue with irregular margins often extending to the ureteral orifices. This characteristic endoscopic appearance, generally referred to as **pseudomembranous trigonitis**, results from squamous metaplasia similar to that found in the vagina and so does not represent a pathologic process. The position of the ureteral orifices on the trigone and their configuration, using the classification described by Lyon, Marshall, and Tanagho should be noted.[16] The orifice may be prominent on endoscopic examination or appear as an inconspicuous slit barely distinguishable from the surrounding mucosa.

ABNORMAL ANATOMIC OBSERVATIONS

Inspection of the external urinary meatus prior to performing the urethroscopic examination may reveal urethral prolapse or urethral caruncle. A urethral prolapse is a circumferential eversion of urethral mucosa through the external meatus. The mucosa is soft, is colored pale pink to red, and is generally asymptomatic. The patient may, however, present with pain and bleeding. Treatment with topical estrogen and sitz baths is usually curative. Redundant mucosa may, in rare cases, require excision.

Urethral caruncle is a benign, polypoid, fleshy growth protruding from the posterior terminal urethra. It consists of connective tissue, blood vessels, and inflammatory cells covered by epithelium. A caruncle is red, measures 0.5 to 1.5 cm and may be asymptomatic or cause pain, bleeding, or both. Because this condition may be confused with urethral carcinoma, a biopsy is often necessary to establish the diagnosis. Estrogen therapy may be attempted initially followed by cryosurgery, laser therapy, fulguration, or excision if a symptomatic caruncle persists.

The operator may encounter resistance when attempting to introduce the urethroscope into the meatus. Stricture of the female urethra almost solely occurs at its terminal portion. Rarely, proximal or midurethral stricture may result from periurethral fibrosis secondary to multiple operative procedures.

Repeated infection of the periurethral glands may lead to abscess formation and cystic enlargement of these glands. Abscess erosion into the urethral lumen results in the formation of singular or multiple diverticula. Virtually all originate from the posterior urethral wall. The ostia may usually be identified on the posterior surface of the middle or distal urethra. If the site of communication between a diverticulum and the urethra cannot be readily identified, digital compression of the urethra by a finger placed in the vagina may cause a copious puff of exudate or pus from the orifice. A thorough urethroscopic examination may identify the diverticular orifice in as many as 90% of patients.[17] Rarely, primary crystallization of urinary salts, due to urinary stasis and stagnation, may lead to stone formation within the diverticulum. Urethroscopy may also aid in locating a suspected urethrovaginal fistula, a postoperative condition complicating 5% to 25% of urethral diverticulum repairs.[18]

The estrogen-dependent internal urethral sphincter, composed of the submucosal vascular plexus and periurethral smooth muscle, as well as elastic and connective tissue, is largely responsible for maintaining passive continence, or resting urethral tone, and provides a margin to continence during stress. Decreased levels of circulating estrogen result in atrophic urethritis, characterized by mucosal pallor, decreased urothelial proliferation and coaptation, and decreased submucosal turgor. Atrophic urethritis may be improved by the administration of systemic or intravaginal estrogen.

Periurethal fibrosis, typically a result of multiple operative procedures performed near the urethra, offers the most profound example of loss mechanisms necessary for continence. On endoscopy, the mucosa is pale and unable to coapt. Devascularization, periurethral scarring, and probable denervation contribute to decreased resting urethral tone and interfere with the mechanisms acting to maintain continence during stress. It is not uncommon for the operator to place the urethroscope in the distal urethra and be able to visualize the entire urethra, from the meatus to the UVJ. Urethroscopy facilitates diagnosis of this "drainpipe" or fibrotic urethra as a cause of incontinence secondary to intrinsic urethral sphincter deficiency.

A variety of urethral tumors may be visualized endoscopically. Urethral condylomata, similar to those found elsewhere in the genital tract, have the appearance of warty, papillary-like excrescences. They are usually localized, broad-based, and have an irregular, often firm epithelialized surface. Urethral fibrous or fibroepithelial polyps appear as small pink or fleshy structures on a slender stalk arising from the posterior urethra. Squamous-cell carcinoma of the distal urethra appears as a solid or a flat, slightly raised lesion with a white, firm epithelial surface. Transitional-cell carcinoma may appear either as individual or multiple fronds on a slender stalk or as solid, sessile lesions. These various tumor types are easily confused and therefore a urethral biopsy, performed under topical or injectable anesthesia, is necessary to establish the diagnosis.

Finally, uncommon ureteral abnormalities may be diagnosed urethroscopically. A ureterocele is a congenital cystic dilatation of the submucosal segment of the intravesical ureter. It is seen endoscopically to bulge into the bladder from its position on the trigone. The ureterocele may be seen to change in size as it intermittently fills and spills urine. The ureteral orifice appears abnormally small in 75% of patients.[19] Because ureteroceles may be associated with ureteral duplication, the operator should look for an ectopic orifice. The upper-pole ureter of a complete ureteral duplication is the source of an ectopic orifice in 80% of patients. In the remaining 20%, a single ureter and collecting system is the source of the ectopy. Approximately a third of ectopic ureters empty at the level of the vesical neck; another third open into the middle and distal urethra.[20] The ureteral orifice that opens into the urethra will often be accompanied by a dilated distal ureter, not to be confused with a ureterocele. Intravenously administered indigo carmine may facilitate locating the ectopic orifice.

ABNORMAL FUNCTIONAL OBSERVATIONS

The UVJ in the stress-incontinent patient appears slack and may close sluggishly and incompletely in response to the hold and squeeze commands and to bladder filling. Varying degrees of UVJ-opening and vesical-neck hypermobility will be observed in response to commands to do the Valsalva maneuver and to cough. In the mildly incontinent patient, a fleeting moment of UVJ opening and closing with little vesical neck descent will be demonstrated. In more symptomatic patients, these maneuvers will cause wide UVJ opening and significant vesical neck descent. In order to assess hypermobility adequately, the operator may need to direct the endoscope downward coincident with the downward movement of the vesical neck as prolapse occurs during straining and coughing. Slowly increasing the intra-abdominal pressure by a slow sustained Valsalva maneuver allows the operator additional time to assess UVJ competence and vesical neck mobility. If stable stress incontinence is present, the UVJ closes and the vesical neck will return to its original position after the strain or cough has ceased.

When performing dynamic urethroscopy, the operator must bear in mind that many factors influence interpretation of the functional integrity of the UVJ and vesical neck. Interpretation is subjective and may therefore vary from operator to operator. Secondly, a change in the patient's position in response to commands, such as lifting the buttocks, may alter the responses observed. Thirdly, some patients may be unable to perform the maneuvers and may actually perform the Valsalva maneuver in response to the hold and squeeze commands. Finally, dynamic urethroscopy is a relatively insensitive and nonspecific predictor of genuine stress incontinence; in response to stressful maneuvers, stress continent patients may demonstrate UVJ opening—vesical neck descent and stress incontinent patients may not.[21,22]

CYSTOSCOPY

EQUIPMENT

The cystoscope consists of a telescope, sheath, and a connecting bridge (Fig. 12–4). The sheath is of varying calibers and is equipped with inlet and outlet ports for irrigation. The cystoscope sheath, unlike that of a urethroscope, is beaked and fenestrated on

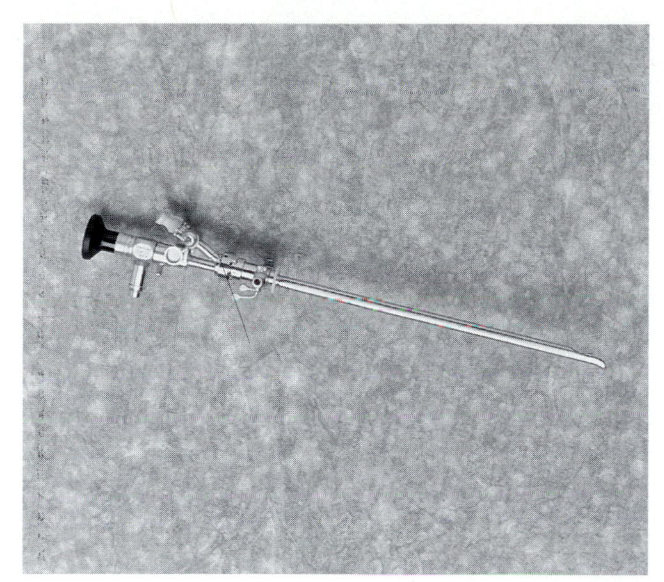

FIGURE 12–4. An assembled cystoscope, showing telescope, sheath, and connecting bridge. (Photograph compliments of Karl Storz Endoscopy, America Inc., Culver City, CA.)

the underside of its terminal portion to accommodate a ureteral catheter deflector. The connecting bridge fits on the end of the sheath with a watertight lock, and may have one or two ports for the introduction of catheters, electrodes, or biopsy forceps. A moveable deflector (Albarran's lever) that extends to the fenestrated portion of the sheath is incorporated into some bridges to manipulate accessory instruments within the bladder. The telescope is introduced into the sheath through the connecting bridge and is fixed with a watertight lock. Telescopes designed for cystoscopic examination incorporate varying viewing angles to allow inspection of all bladder walls. A 30-degree lens (foreoblique) affords best visualization of the base and posterior wall of the bladder; a 70-degree lens is used to view the bladder dome and anterolateral walls (Fig. 12–5). Retroview lenses with a viewing angle of 120 degrees can be used to visualize the anterior bladder neck. A fiberoptic light source and standard intraveous infusion system are again used. Care of the cystoscope is identical to that described for the urethroscope.

OPERATIVE TECHNIQUE

The patient remains in the dorsolithotomy position after the urethroscopic examination is completed. Fluid that was previously infused remains in the bladder. If voluntary voiding was accomplished or if an uninhibited detrusor contraction with significant urinary leakage has occurred, some refilling may be necessary. The 17-Fr cystoscope is assembled and connected to the light source, infusion system, and camera if available. The cystoscope is lubricated with 2% lidocaine gel, supplemented by 20% benzocaine gel or a bladder pillar block in rare cases, and with the irrigant acting as the obturator, the cystoscope is placed through the meatus, and while keeping the bevel end superior and applying pressure against the posterior urethra, passed into the bladder. A 30-degree lens generally provides an adequate view of the bladder unless there is fixation of the UVJ, in which case a 70-degree lens is used. The air bubble located at 12 o'clock in the bladder dome results from the air that escapes from the cystoscope as it is introduced; this is useful to help orient the operator. The bladder walls are systematically examined by moving the scope from the bladder dome to the UVJ along each clock face position, starting at the 12 o'clock position and moving to 4 o'clock and then from 11 o'clock to 8 o'clock. Suprapubic pressure may facilitate examination of the anterior bladder wall behind the symphysis. The cystoscope is then rotated 180 degrees to view the bladder base and trigone. After all bladder walls have been visu-

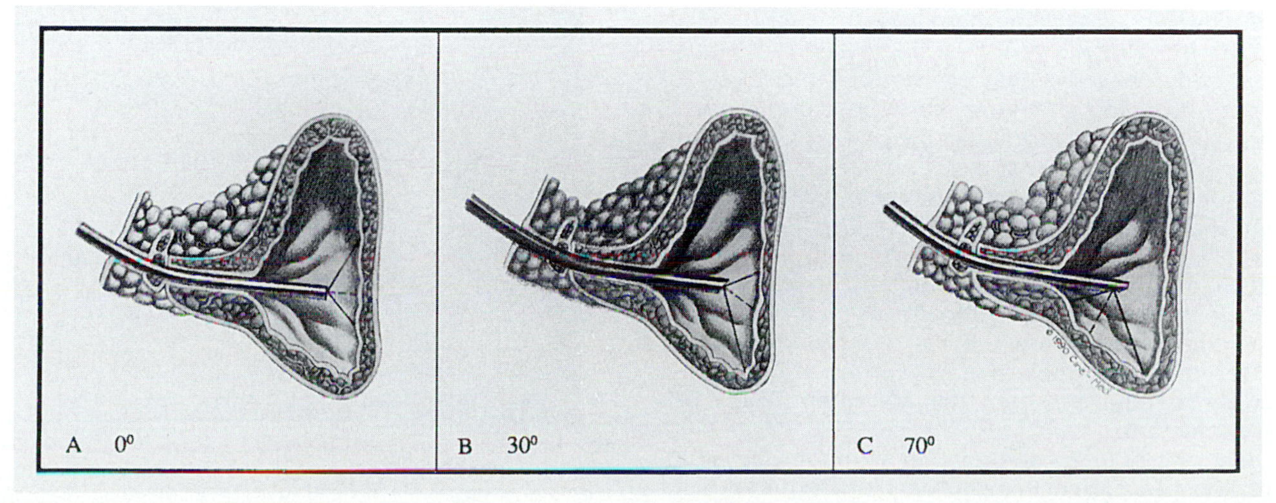

FIGURE 12–5. Viewing angles of the cystoscope. (From American College of Obstetricians and Gynecologists. Urogynecologic Evaluation, Endoscopy, and Urodynamic Testing in the Symptomatic Female. AVL 51. Washington, D.C., ACOG, 1990, with permission.)

alized, the patient's bladder is emptied through the sheath and the cystoscope is removed.

NORMAL ANATOMIC OBSERVATIONS

As the cystoscope is passed through the UVJ, the trigone and ureteral orifices are visualized. The uterus and cervix may be seen indenting the posterior wall of the bladder, producing posterolateral pouches on either side of the midline. The bladder wall is normally colored pale white to pink, with submucosal vessels easily visible through the translucent mucosa. Folds of mucosa, present in the empty or partially full bladder, disappear with bladder distension unless prominent trabeculation is present.

ABNORMAL ANATOMIC OBSERVATIONS

Cystitis, broadly defined, includes all inflammatory abnormalities of the bladder, ranging from common episodes of infectious cystitis to more unusual conditions requiring biopsy for diagnosis. Cystoscopy should be avoided in the presence of known, active bacterial cystitis because of the potential for disseminating causative organisms. Cystoscopy performed inadvertently during an episode of infectious cystitis reveals a varying endoscopic appearance depending upon the severity of the condition. Mild cystitis may be associated with a relatively normal-appearing bladder. Pink to red blotchy patches, marked vessel dilatation, and mucosal edema, evidenced by loss of the submucosal vascular pattern, may be seen in moderate and severe cystitis. Hemorrhagic cystitis may be associated with large confluent mucosal hemorrhages and blood-filled blisters.

Recurrent and chronic infections may be associated with endoscopically identifiable lesions within the bladder. Subepithelial islands of transitional cells may degenerate with central liquefaction to form small, cystic mucosal lesions filled with variable-colored fluid, referred to as **cystitis cystica** and **cystitis glandularis**. The cysts are often multiple, sometimes confluent, and are generally larger in cystitis glandularis. In cystitis cystica, a single layer of transitional cells lines the cyst cavity. Multiple layers of mucus-producing glandular epithelium line the cyst cavity in cystitis glandularis. These lesions, particularly cystitis glandularis, may be masked by marked inflammatory changes and thus be indistinguishable from malignancy. Bladder biopsy is therefore required to confirm diagnosis of cystitis glandularis. Cystitis follicularis, another pattern associated with chronic bacterial cystitis, appears as small white mucosal elevations, shown to be lymphoid follicles, scattered among hemorrhagic areas. No specific therapy is required other than treatment of the primary infection.

Diagnosis of interstitial cystitis is made almost entirely on the patient's symptoms of frequency and urgency and on endoscopic findings observed with repeat bladder distension. On initial inspection, performed under local anesthesia, the bladder may appear normal but occasional blood-tinged irrigant is seen on draining. On repeat filling, performed under general anesthesia due to the patient's inability to tolerate maximal filling while awake, multiple petechial hemorrhages, termed **glomerulations**, and subsequent linear bleeding fissures (Fig. 12–6) and splotchy hemorrhages are observed, as maximum cystometric capacity is reached. In the latter stages of disease, the mucosal surface may be pale with linear scars of earlier lesions and stellate scars radiating from a central ulcer, the classic Hunner's ulcer. Fibrosis of the full thickness of the bladder wall characterizes advanced disease. Early interstitial cystitis, however, may not present with these classic endoscopic findings. Symptoms of frequency and urgency and glomerulations seen cystoscopically on repeat bladder filling characterize an earlier variant of this disease.[23] A biopsy is necessary to distinguish the lesions of interstitial cystitis from carcinoma in situ.

Other less common inflammatory conditions of the bladder, all of which typically cause irritative voiding symptoms with or without hematuria, may be observed endoscopically. Tuberculous cystitis may be associated with mucosal ulcerations and erythematous ureteral orifices. Ureteral involvement with tight stricture formation is a potentially serious complication. Localized or confluent hemorrhagic areas interspersed with fibrotic mucosa characterize radiation cystitis. Hemorrhagic patches may persist years after cessation of radiation therapy. Acute or chronic

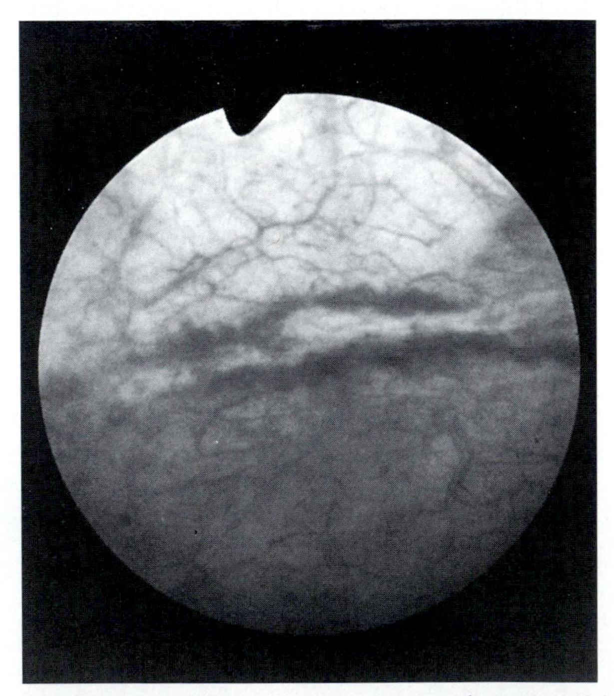

FIGURE 12–6. Linear fissure in bladder mucosa after repeated distension of the bladder. (Bagley, DH, Huffman, JL and Lyon, ES: Urologic Endoscopy; A Manual and Atlas. Little, Brown & Co., Boston, 1985, p 45, with permission.)

cystitis may follow administration of certain bladder toxins, the best example of which is cyclophosphamide. The hemorrhagic cystitis produced by this agent has the endoscopic appearance of diffuse mucosal hemorrhage. Catheter or polypoid cystitis develops in the presence of an indwelling urethral catheter. The resulting inflammatory reaction typically involves the mucosa in direct contact with the catheter balloon and has various endoscopic appearances, ranging from localized or diffuse pseudopapillary edema and submucosal hemorrhages to fibrosis. The inflammatory exudate may coalesce and form a nidus for stone formation. Other intravesical foreign bodies, such as catheter balloon fragments, concrements, and suture material, serve as bladder irritants producing a general or localized inflammatory reaction and an occasional nidus for stone formation.

Bladder calculi develop as a result of urinary stasis secondary to neurogenic bladder dysfunction or outlet obstruction. They also form on abnormal surfaces such as a foreign body or bladder tumor. On endoscopy, the calculi vary greatly in size, shape, and color morphologically. Symptomatic calculi rarely form in the female bladder because outlet obstruction is infrequent and because the female urethra readily permits passage of stones.

Trabeculation is the occurrence of smooth ridges with occasional cellules and sacculations along the bladder wall at maximum cystometric capacity (Fig. 12–7). High intravesical pressure, secondary to anatomic or functional outlet obstruction, or more frequently to detrusor instability, may cause trabeculation. With markedly elevated intravesical pressure, enlargement of a sacculation may occur, giving rise to a bladder diverticulum, an outpouching of bladder mucosa. The necks of diverticula vary in size and are surrounded by a thick muscular band. The interior of a diverticulum should be carefully inspected, because a neoplasm has been found within the diverticulum in approximately 7% of patients.[24]

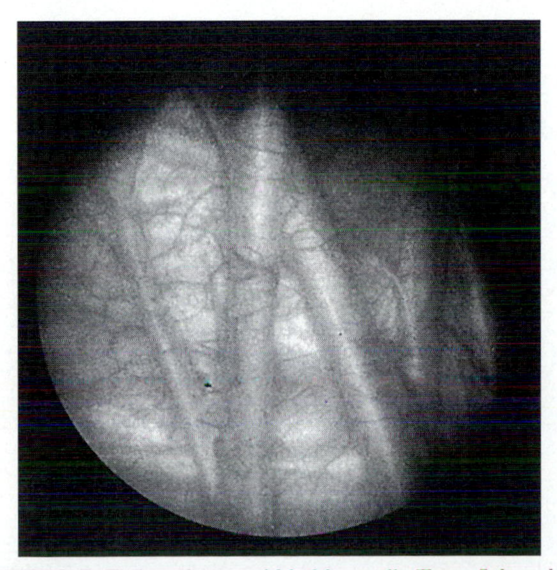

FIGURE 12–7. Trabeculation of bladder wall. (From Schonebeck, J: Atlas of Cystoscopy. Grune and Stratton, Orlando, p 95, with permission.)

Endoscopic inspection remains the major technique for the diagnosis of urothelial tumors. Bladder tumors are commonly located in the lateral and posterior aspects of the bladder wall, often directly lateral to the ureteral orifices, and have a variety of endoscopic appearances. Carcinoma in situ may appear as a nonspecific erythematous area, or more commonly, a patchy, granular, slightly raised, velvety lesion. Among the invasive tumors, the appearance of the lesion correlates well with the grade and often the stage of the tumor. Spherical papillary lesions with a well-defined mass of tumor fronds are usually of a low grade and stage. Other relatively benign lesions appear as flat patches of low-lying fronds on the mucosa. A more solid-appearing, broad-based tumor mass is much more likely to be of a high grade and stage. Blood clots or calculi may form on the surface of urothelial tumors.

In patients suspected of having a vesicoenteric fistula, cystoscopy is the single most useful study in the evaluation. Cystoscopic examination shows the presence of a fistula, commonly on the left bladder wall near the dome, in approximately 50% of patients.[25] Almost all remaining patients will have an inflammatory reaction with bullous edema and papillary proliferation surrounding the fistula site. Rarely, bowel contents may be seen exuding from the fistulous tract into the bladder.

Endoscopic examination of the bladder is likewise essential in the evaluation of a vesicovaginal fistula. The fistula, generally located 2 cm above the trigone on the posterior bladder wall, may appear either as a pinhole opening or a defect several centimeters in diameter. Its endoscopic appearance ranges from edematous, hyperemic mucosa surrounding an intravesical suture in the immediate postoperative period to a smooth defect with normal-appearing mucosa extending to the edges of the fistula in the later stages.

OPERATIVE ENDOSCOPY

Numerous endoscopic procedures may be performed for various conditions of the lower urinary tract. Those operative techniques described here are most often used by the gynecologist or the urogynecologist. Endoscopic treatment of more unusual conditions or conditions requiring greater expertise in operative endourology should more appropriately be referred to the urologist.

A number of mucosal lesions of the bladder and urethra have characteristic endoscopic appearances. Endoscopy, however, serves only to detect the presence and extent of these lesions. Definitive diagnosis requires pathologic examination of a biopsy specimen. Flexible and rigid biopsy forceps are available. The size of the cup and the resultant biopsy are small with the flexible instrument, so multiple biopsies should be taken to avoid overlooking significant pathology. These forceps are generally not strong enough to cut or bite the tissue, but must be withdrawn to amputate the sample. The advantage of these forceps is their flexibility. Using the Albarran's lever and the 70- to 90-degree lens, the instrument may be deflected to biopsy a lesion at an angle away from the forceps. This property makes the flexible forceps particularly useful for biopsy of lesions at the bladder dome. Despite the straight design and rigidity of the rigid biopsy forceps, they can reach most areas in the bladder, with the exception of the dome and the anterior wall. These forceps take a larger sample of tissue, up to 6 mm, and, because of their design, are able to amputate the tissue sharply without crushing it. Bleeding following biopsy of a urethral lesion may be controlled with pressure, silver nitrate, ferrous subsulfate, or electrofulguration. Bleeding following biopsy of a bladder lesion may not need to be treated, although electrofulguration is generally used in the anesthetized patient.

Local injection with 1% lidocaine solution using a 30-gauge needle, supplemented with intraurethral 2% lidocaine gel or 20% benzocaine gel, is adequate anesthesia for urethral biopsy. Intravesical instillation of 50 mL of 4% lidocaine solution with or without a bladder pillar block generally provides adequate anesthesia for biopsy of lesions at the UVJ or within the bladder.

Foreign bodies, except calculi, are best removed endoscopically with instruments designed for this purpose, termed **foreign body** or **grasping forceps**, also available in both rigid and flexible designs. They are similar to biopsy forceps but have serrations or teeth on their jaws to provide a grasping surface.

INTRAOPERATIVE ENDOSCOPY

The potential for ureteral or bladder injury or bladder outlet obstruction during anti-incontinence surgery may be substantially reduced with intraoperative endoscopy. Ureteral kinking or ligation, bladder perforation, and more commonly, some degree of bladder outlet obstruction, due either to incorrectly placed suspension sutures or overcorrection by placing excessive tension on the suspension material, occasionally complicate anti-incontinence procedures. Incorrectly placed sutures may even exacerbate incontinence by "tenting open" the vesical neck, thus preventing its normal response to stressful maneuvers. Operative cystoscopy ensures accurate identification of the vesical neck for suture placement.[26,27] After the suspension material is passed through the retropubic space, cystoscopy should be performed to ensure that the bladder has not been perforated and that the ureters are patent while placing tension on the suspension material.

Overdistension of the bladder may prevent the egress of urine from the orifices. If this appears to be the case, the bladder should be partially drained and endoscopy repeated. Intravenous injection of indigo carmine may aid in assessing ureteral patency. After ureteral and bladder injury have been excluded, tension is again placed on the suspension material while observing the response of the UVJ. Q-tip testing (see Chapter 5) may be used in conjunction with the endoscopic assessment of vesical neck elevation to determine the amount of tension to place on the suspension material.

If urine is not ejaculated from the ureteral orifice despite bladder emptying, it may be necessary to catheterize the ureter to evaluate patency. A variety of types of ureteral catheters is available, the most commonly used of which is the whistle-tip catheter.[28] This catheter is straight and has an opening at its sharp beveled tip and on its side. The equipment necessary for ureteral catheterization depends upon the degree of difficulty the operator expects to encounter. A 30-degree telescope with a simple one- or two-port catheterizing bridge suffices for simple, straightforward catheterization. A 70- to 90-degree telescope with an Albarran's lever, used for deflecting the catheter at an angle away from the cystoscope, is necessary for more difficult catheterizations. The procedure is similar, however, regardless of the equipment used. The catheter is initially aligned in the same plane as the anticipated course of the intramural ureter. It is then advanced along the floor of the orifice and into the lumen with the deflecting arm directing the tip. It is then passed proximally to the desired position. Marked buckling of the catheter indicates

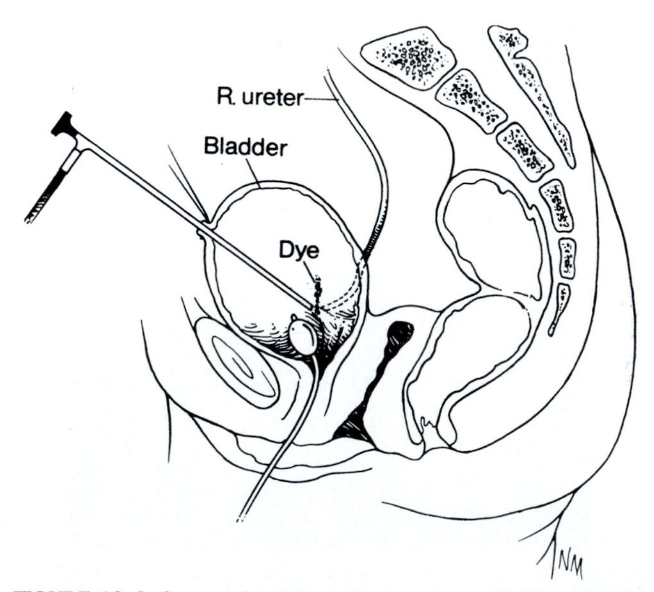

FIGURE 12–8. Suprapubic teloscopy to assess bladder integrity and ureteral patency. (From Timmons,[29] with permission.)

obstruction, tortuosity, or kinking of the ureter. The suspension suture or sling material may need to be removed and replaced.

Suprapubic teloscopy (Fig. 12–8) is a simple method for intraoperative assessment of ureteral patency and bladder integrity during abdominal procedures.[29] Intraoperative transurethral cystoscopy is inconvenient during abdominal surgery, because it necessitates closure of the abdomen and transfer of the patient from the supine to the lithotomy position, and if injury is noted, repositioning the patient and reopening the abdomen. A cystoscopic telescope with a 30- or 70-degree lens is inserted through a stab incision in the dome of the distended bladder at the center of a previously placed purse-string suture. After excluding bladder and ureteral injury, the cystoscope is removed and either the purse-string is simply tied or a catheter is placed through the stab incision and brought out through the abdominal wall for suprapubic drainage. This procedure is useful not only for anti-incontinence procedures, but also for any pelvic operation in which the status of the ureters is not absolutely certain.

COMPLICATIONS OF ENDOSCOPY

Although cystourethroscopy is performed with a "no-touch" technique and sterility of the instruments is maintained as much as possible, organisms residing in the distal urethra may be inoculated into the urethra and bladder during the examination. Postoperative bacteriuria has been reported in approximately 5% of patients.[30] It is recommended that prophylactic antibiotics, such as nitrofurantoin 50 mg b.i.d. for 2 days or a suitable alternative, be given to all patients.[8] Patients at risk for developing endocarditis should be given prophylaxis according to American Heart Association guidelines. Patients experiencing postoperative dysuria may be given phenazopyridine hydrochloride (Pyridium) 200 mg every 8 hours for two to three doses. Small disruptions in the urothelium may result in postoperative hematuria, generally lasting 12 hours to 2 days. Some patients may develop unexplained, persistent lower abdominal cramping or bladder spasms requiring treatment with an analgesic agent.

SUMMARY

Cystourethroscopy may be used as a diagnostic tool to assess the anatomic and functional integrity of the bladder, urethra, and ureters. Operative endoscopy permits confirmation of suspected conditions, through biopsy and pathologic examinations, as well as treatment of a variety of bladder and urethral abnormalities. Adequate endoscopic evaluation requires training in the use of the endoscopes. After becoming proficient in endoscopic techniques, the operator may complement the information obtained from the clinical, urodynamic, and possible radiographic evaluation with that obtained at endoscopy. The best approach to the complex problems of the lower urinary tract is one where information obtained from many sources is compiled and analyzed to create a management decision.

REFERENCES

1. Bozzini, P: Lichteiter eine Erfindung zur Anschung Innerer Theile, und krankheiten nebst abbildung. J Pract Arzeykunde 24:107, 1805.
2. Nitzke, M: Eine neue balbachtungs-und untersuchunigsmethods fur harnrohre, harnbiase und rectum. Wien Med Wochenschr 24:649, 1879.
3. Kelly, HA: Bull John Hopkins Hosp November, 1893.
4. Hopkins, H: Optical principles of the endoscope. In Berci G (ed.): Endoscopy. Appleton-Century-Crofts, New York, 1976, p 3.
5. Greene, LF and Khan, AU: Cystourethroscopy in the female. Urology 10:461, 1977.
6. Robertson, JR: Gynecologic urethroscopy. Am J Obstet Gynecol 115:986, 1973.
7. Appell, RA: When is endoscopy a must? (Unpublished material—Presented at the Tenth Annual Houston B. Everett Memorial Course, Baltimore, February, 1993).
8. Bent, AE: Urethrocystoscopy and the gynecologist. Contemporary Ob/Gyn 37:40, 1992.
9. Bent, AE and Ostergard, DR: Urethrocystoscopy. In Sanfilippo JS, Levine RL (eds.): Operative Gynecologic Endoscopy. Springer-Verlag, New York, 1989, p 272.
10. Kavoussi, LR and Clayman, RV: Office flexible cystoscopy. Urol Clin North Am 15:601, 1988.
11. Bent, AE: Urogynecologic evaluation, endoscopy, and urodynamic testing in the symptomatic female (abstr.). Am Coll Obstet Gynecol 1990.
12. Ostergard, DR: Bladder pillar block anesthesia for urethral dilatation in women. Am J Obstet Gynecol 136:187, 1980.
13. Asmussen, M and Miller, A: Examination of the urinary tract. In Asmussen M and Miller A (eds.): Clinical Gynecological Urology. Blackwell Scientific Publications, Oxford, 1983, p 31.
14. McCarthy, TA and Ostergard, DR: Office urethroscopy. In Buchsbaum HJ and Schmidt JD (eds.): Gynecologic and Obstetric Urology, ed. 2. WB Saunders, Philadelphia, 1982, p 100.
15. O'Donnell, P: Endoscopy. In Raz, S (ed.): Female Urology. WB Saunders, Philadelphia, 1983, p 51.
16. Lyon, RP, Marshall, S and Tanagho, EA: The ureteral orifice: its configuration and competency. J Urol 102:504, 1969.
17. Robertson, JR: Urethral diverticula. In Ostergard DR and Bent AE (eds.): Urogynecology and Urodynamics Theory and Practice, ed. 3. Williams & Wilkins, Baltimore, 1991, p 283.
18. Labasky, RF and Leach, GE: Prevention and management of urovaginal fistulas. Clin Obstet Gynecol 33:382, 1990.
19. Aas, TN: Ureterocele: a clinical study of 68 cases in 52 adults. Br J Urol 32:133, 1960.
20. Snyder, HM: Anomalies of the ureter. In Gillenwater, JY, Graynack, JT, Howards, SS and Duckett, JU (eds.): Adult and Pediatric Urology. Chicago, Yearbook Medical Publishers, Inc. 1987, p 1642.
21. Scotti, RJ, Ostergard, DR, Guillaume, AA, and Kohatsu, K: Predictive value of urethroscopy as compared to urodynamics in the diagnosis of genuine stress incontinence. J Repro Med 35:772, 1990.
22. Versi, G, Cardozo, L, Studd, J, et al: The urinary sphincter in the maintenance of female continence. Br Med J 292:166, 1986.
23. Messing, EM and Stamey, TA: Interstitial cystitis. Urology 12:381, 1978.
24. Kelalis, PP and McLean, P: The treatment of diverticulum of the bladder. J Urol 98:349, 1967.

25. Farringer, JL, Hrabovsky, E, Marsh, J, et al: Vesicocolic fistula. South Med J 67:1043, 1974.
26. Mason, JT and Söderstrom, RM: Suprapubic endoscopic evaluation of vesical neck suspension procedures. Urology 6:233, 1975.
27. Robertson, JR: Endoscopic control while performing urethropexy. In Slate WG (ed.): Disorders of the Female Urethra and Urinary Incontinence. Williams & Wilkins, Baltimore, 1982, p 196.
28. Lange, PH: Diagnostic and therapeutic urologic instrumentation. In Walsh, PC, Gittes, RF, Perlmutter, AD and Stamey, TA (eds.): Campbell's Urology. WB Saunders, Philadelphia, 1986, p 510.
29. Timmons, MC and Addison, WA: Suprapubic teloscopy: extraperitoneal intraoperative technique to demonstrate ureteral patency. Obstet Gynecol 75:137, 1990.
30. Richards, B and Bastable, JRG: Bacteria after out-patient cystoscopy. Br J Urol 49:561, 1977.

CHAPTER **13**

Physical Therapy Evaluation of the Pelvic Floor

Rhonda K. Kotarinos • Dee E. Fenner

HISTORY

Physical therapy evaluation, like any clinical assessment, is begun by taking an accurate history and then performing a physical examination. Accurate and systematic recording of information permits future comparisons and assessment of improvement. After this information is obtained, a plan of treatment with specific objectives and goals is established.

When addressing the nature of the symptoms, information is being gathered that provides a basis for objective measurement of change. Questions of behavior specific to incontinence include:

- When do you lose urine?
- How often do you lose urine?
- How much urine do you lose?
- Do you get up at night (and how often)?
- Do you wear protection (what type and how often is the device changed)?
- How often do you urinate each day (frequency and urgency)?
- How have you altered your daily activities because of your problems?

Documentation of progress can be established by the changes in the answers to these questions.

Special questions are asked that relate to the patient's physical well being as a whole, both at present and in the past. These might include:

- How is your general health?
- How has your condition affected your general health?
- Do you have other medical conditions?
- What medication are you currently taking (prescription and over-the-counter)?
- What is your obstetric history?
- What is your surgical history?

The history should focus both on the patient's present complaints and on problems of the same nature in the past. The examiner needs to determine when the current problem started and if there were precipitating conditions. If there had been previous instances of the same problem, when did they start and what was done as evaluation and management at that time? If previous therapy was done, what was its effect? Are symptoms worsening or improving?

PHYSICAL EXAMINATION

Objective examination should include assessment of posture, overall strength, range of motion of the trunk and extremities, an internal pelvic examination to evaluate pelvic floor tissues and muscles, and special tests.

POSTURE

Posture is defined as "the relative arrangement of the parts of the body."[1] A **posture evaluation** assesses alignment of the body relative to a standard. More specifically, a postural evaluation must note asymmetries in the musculoskeletal systems that may have an impact on the patient's symptoms or on the patient's ability to participate in treatment.

Spastic extrinsic pelvic muscles may alter alignment, thereby impairing function of the intrinsic pelvic floor muscles. For example, posterior pelvic tilt, as seen with a flat back posture, causes the inlet to become more horizontal, thereby increasing pressure over the pelvic diaphragm.[2] Information gained from the postural examination directs treatment to associated areas. Range-of-motion evaluation of the trunk and extremities allows documentation of areas where range is either limited or excessive. In either situation, it is important to determine how this problem will affect the patient's symptoms or alter her ability to participate in management of symptoms.

STRENGTH ASSESSMENT

Gross manual muscle testing provides information about the overall strength of the patient. The abdominal and hip girdle muscles are two vital areas of importance when assessing strength; isolating and addressing only the pelvic floor may be a great disservice. Posture, range of motion, and strength all have some impact on the patient's ability to get to and from the toilet.

Abdominal Wall

Abdominal muscles to be addressed include the external and internal obliques, rectus abdominus, and transversus muscles. Their function in trunk motion is well established. Although the transversus has very little involvement in trunk motion, it does act to increase intra-abdominal pressure needed for vomiting, coughing, parturition, urination, and defecation.[3]

Another function of the abdominal muscles is maintaining a rhythmic rise and fall of intra-abdominal pressure during respiration, never allowing undue relaxation or distension of the abdominal wall. Pressure upward from the pelvic diaphragm, down from the thoracic diaphragm, posteriorly from the rectus abdominus, and medially and laterally from the abdominal muscles are four forces that must be maintained in equilibrium.

In normal conditions this equilibrium is provided by the tension of the muscles of the abdominal wall and the pelvic and thoracic diaphragms. When the abdominal wall is relaxed and weakened, it is not capable of providing the tension necessary to maintain this equilibrium. Intra-abdominal pressure will not be distributed evenly within the abdominal cavity, causing increased downward pressure against the pelvic diaphragm.[4] Persistent pressure to muscles and connective tissues can eventually cause weakness.[5] Morgan felt that direct pressure over the pelvic outlet was prevented by the ability of the intact, taut anterior abdominal wall to deflect the pressure back to the lumbar lordosis and sacrum.[6]

Another function associated with the abdominal musculature is the retentive power of the abdomen. This function can be illustrated by the "barrel effect." Consider the abdominal and pelvic cavities in the erect female as a "barrel" filled with a liquid. The top of the barrel is closed by the diaphragm, the sides are represented by the abdominal wall and the back, and the perineum acts as the floor of the barrel. On tapping the barrel with an opening such as the pelvic outlet, nothing happens because of the counteracting influence of the atmospheric pressure. After placing a second opening in the barrel above the level of the first opening, however, the contents escape by their own weight.[7]

Diastasis recti or atrophied abdominal musculature can compromise the abdominal wall sufficiently to create the situation described. Charles Penrose stated in 1908 that the retentive power of the abdomen depends on the strength or rigidity of the abdominal wall.[8] Therefore, it is very important for the abdominal wall to be evaluated for strength and a diastasis recti.

Strength assessment of the abdominal wall is accomplished according to the standard manual muscle testing format. To assess a patient for a diastasis recti, the patient should be supine with her knees bent. The examiner should place fingertips in the midline of the abdomen near the umbilicus. The patient is then asked to raise her head and shoulders so that her scapulae clear the table and her recti contract. As the recti contract, they should shorten and approach the midline. If they do not approach the midline, the examiner notes how many fingers will fit between the medial recti bellies. In this way the examiner measures the extent of their separation. A separation of 1½ to 2 finger widths is considered normal.

At rest, the normal anatomic size of the linea alba ranges from a pencil-thin line below the umbilicus to 1½ to 2 finger widths above the umbilicus. If one palpates a separation of 1½ to 2 finger widths after head lift but feels it move from a resting position wider than 2 fingers, this could also be determined to be a diastasis recti. At least the examiner is aware that during normal activities the patient's abdominal wall is compromised due to the altered point of insertion of the abdominal muscles. Treatment for the abdominal wall must then be based on the patient's strength score and whether or not a diastasis is present.

Hip Muscles

Generalized weakness in the hip musculature may affect the integrity and treatment of the pelvic floor muscles. Hip girdle muscles must be of sufficient strength to get the patient safely to the toilet in adequate time. Furthermore, if the patient's pelvic floor muscles are so weak that strength is not sufficient for an active contraction, strengthening the hip girdle muscles may help through the mechanism known as **cross transfer of training** or **cross education.**[9]

Intrinsic Pelvic Muscles

The physical therapist must assess the pelvic floor muscles with an internal pelvic examination, to establish the patient's condition in relation to normal function and to provide insight into the function of the body as a whole.

Researchers have made many attempts to devise a manual grading scale for the strength of the pelvic floor contraction. Unfortunately, as would be expected, there have been problems with reproducibility. The true importance of this evaluation is to determine whether or not the patient is capable of an isolated active contraction. A manual scale will never be able to measure the functional capability of the pelvic floor muscles when one considers that the muscle must counter the forces of a sneeze, which have been measured to be 100 mph.

The clinician should not only assess the presence of a contraction, but also palpate for differences between left and right. Overall tone of the contractile and noncontractile tissues can also be palpated. The quality of the contraction and the relaxation should also be addressed. Is the contraction slow, jerky, or abrupt?

In addition, release of the contraction should be assessed. Is there a strong, quick, forceful contraction, with a slow, prolonged release? A slowed or incomplete release of the pelvic floor may relate to post-void fullness, post-void leaking, retention, or frequency. One should also note what other muscles contract and if the patient alters her breathing when contracting her pelvic floor.

The pelvic floor has both sphincteric and supportive functions. An easy way to determine adequacy of the sphincter function is to assess the ability to interrupt or deflect the flow of urine. This should only be done for evaluation purposes and not as treatment. Stopping and starting the flow of urine can lead to a disruption of normal voiding reflexes that can cause urinary retention and subsequent urinary tract infections.[10]

Grading of muscle strength by manual assessments has traditionally been made on a zero to normal scale (0–5) (Table 13–1). In applying this scale to the pelvic floor, a **zero** grade would represent no contraction present. A **trace** ($\frac{1}{5}$) grade is defined as the ability to deflect or decrease urine stream but the inability to maintain the change. Muscle strength at a **poor** ($\frac{2}{5}$) grade is the ability of the patient to maintain a deflection of the urine stream or a reduced flow. A **fair** ($\frac{3}{5}$) grade of strength denotes the ability to stop the flow of urine in a gravity-resisted position, such as sitting or standing. A fair grade indicates that the pelvic floor has some ability to satisfy its sphincteric function. It is clinically difficult to distinguish higher levels of strength, until they assume a **normal** grade, with no urine loss or lack of support in any condition, normal or artificial.

OBJECTIVE ASSESSMENT

If an active contraction is palpated, a more sophisticated measuring device can be used to produce an objective measure of strength. One such device is a perineometer. Kegel introduced the perineometer in the 1950s: a pneumatic device with a conical, air-filled vaginal chamber that measured the forces of the pelvic floor contraction in millimeters of mercury.[11]

Ongoing research addresses the need for a pres-

TABLE 13–1. Grading Pelvic Muscle Strength

Grade	Contraction	Clinical Response or Symptoms
0	No contraction	No change in urine flow
1	Trace	Ability to deflect or decrease urine stream but unable to maintain change
2	Poor	Ability to maintain a deflection of the urine stream or a reduced flow
3	Fair	Ability to stop the flow of urine in a gravity-resisted position such as sitting or standing
4	Good	Ability to stop the flow of urine in any position except when stressed under artificial conditions
5	"Normal"	No urine loss or lack of support in any condition, normal or artificial

sure-based perineometer, but investigators still have many obstacles to overcome. The device must be affordable, durable, and able to produce a valid and reliable measurement. The design features of any perineometer must incorporate size, shape, color, texture, and materials to recognize the physical and psychologic needs of the female with a pelvic floor disorder.

For the clinician who wishes to invest in more sophisticated methods of measurement, computerized surface electrode electromyography and pressure perineometers exist. These instruments offer three distinctive advantages over their manual counterparts:

First, computerization provides ease of recording, storing, manipulating, and retrieving data without the risk of human error.

Second, because these instruments record data online in real time, accuracy is ensured because human error in reading displays and recording data is eliminated. Working at the speed of today's personal computers, these instruments record data in time increments too small for the clinician to observe and record manually. Furthermore, marginal deviations in data can be captured that might otherwise go unnoticed by a clinician viewing and recording results manually.

Finally, these instruments are capable of monitoring other muscle groups to observe inappropriate recruitment. Clinicians can use this feature to teach patients how to isolate and recruit only the appropriate pelvic floor musculature when they invoke active contractions.

SUMMARY

A work-up for urinary incontinence, fecal incontinence, or pelvic pain may not be complete without a physical therapy evaluation. Objective evaluation of the muscular support of the abdomen and pelvis is essential before beginning muscle rehabilitation such as Kegel's exercises or cone therapy. With a thorough evaluation, the proper exercises can be chosen and clinical and physical progress to therapy can be assessed.

REFERENCES

1. Kendall, HO, Kendall, FP and Boynton, DA: Posture and Pain. Robert E. Krieger Publishing, Huntington, NY, 1977.
2. Steindler, A: Kinesiology of the Human Body. Charles C Thomas, Springfield, 1970, p 236.
3. Williams, PL and Warwick, R (eds.). Gray's Anatomy, ed 3. WB Saunders, Philadelphia, 1980, p 558.
4. Steindler, A. Kinesiology of the Human Body. Charles C Thomas, Springfield, 1970, p 237.
5. Frankel, VH and Nordin, M: Basic Biomechanics of the Skeletal System. Lea & Febiger, Philadelphia, 1980, p 79.
6. Morgan, CN: The surgical anatomy of the ischiorectal space. Proc R Soc Med 42:189,1949.
7. Gillian, DT: Textbook of Practical Gynecology. FA Davis, Philadelphia. 1908, p 172.
8. Penrose, CB: A Textbook of Diseases of Women. WB Saunders, Philadelphia, 1908, p 100.
9. Hellbrandt, FA: Cross Education: Ipsilateral and contralateral effects of unimanual training. J Appl Physiol 4:136,1951.
10. Wall, LL, Norton, PA and Delancy, DO: Practical Urogynecology. Williams & Wilkins, Baltimore, 1993, p 144.
11. Kegel AH: Physiologic therapy for urinary stress incontinence. JAMA 146:915–917, 1951.

SECTION FOUR

DISORDERS OF PAIN

CHAPTER 14

Lower Urinary Tract Pain

Tamara G. Bavendam

Millions of women present to health-care providers each year with symptoms of pain or discomfort of the bladder or urethra.[1] The etiology of lower urinary tract symptoms ranges from acute bacterial cystitis to pelvic floor myalgia. Sensations arising from the pelvic organs and supporting musculoskeletal tissue are poorly localized and travel through common pathways to the central nervous system. Consequently, afferent nerve impulses can be perceived as originating in the bladder or urethra although they actually originate in the internal abdominal or pelvic organs or in the bony pelvis with its supporting muscle and fascial attachments. In patients with long-standing pain, multiple factors often contribute to the patient's current pain. These factors often have little to do with the original inciting event. To evaluate and treat chronic pain optimally, a multidisciplinary approach is necessary in most clinical settings. An integrated approach to the evaluation and treatment of chronic pain, including somatic, psychologic, dietary, environmental, and physiotherapeutic factors, has been shown by Peters and co-workers[2] to result in better pain control at 1 year than when psychosocial issues are addressed only after the biomedical evaluation and treatment options were exhausted. Rarely will a single health-care provider have all of the skills necessary to serve the patient's needs best.

After obvious and treatable causes are eliminated (e.g., bacterial cystitis, pelvic mass, vaginitis, perianal pathology), the patient and provider are able to take a problem-solving approach to symptom management (Fig. 14–1). After patients are appropriately reassured that nothing is seriously wrong (e.g., cancer), their main goal is to feel better regardless of the source of symptoms. When symptoms are well-controlled, the specific disorder the patient has is moot.

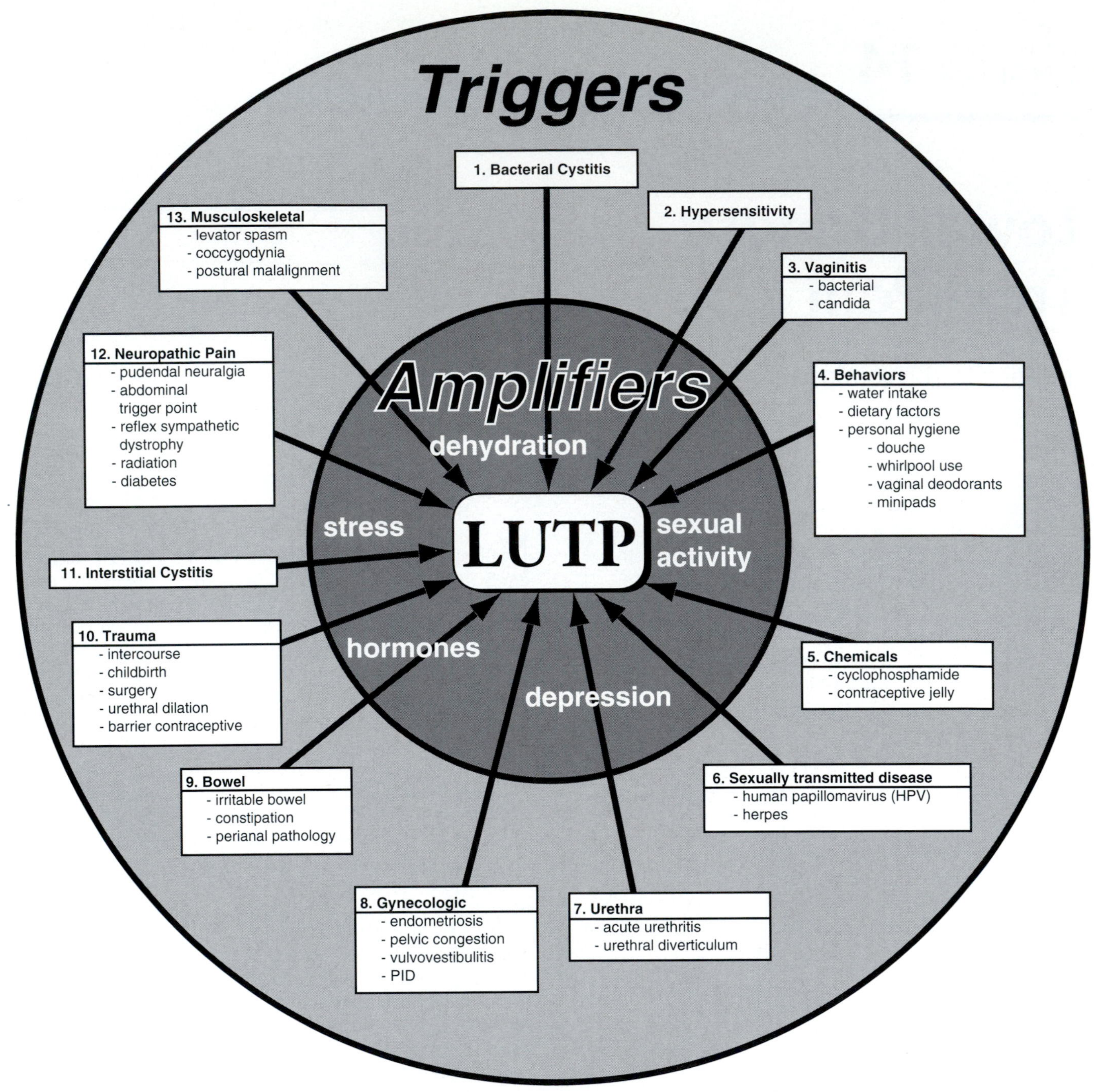

FIGURE 14–1. Factors triggering lower urinary tract pain (LUTP), with potential symptom amplifiers. PID = pelvic inflammatory disease.

LOWER URINARY TRACT FUNCTION

Normal bladder capacity is in the range of 400 to 600 mL. Generally, an initial sense of bladder awareness occurs between 250 and 300 mL, with gradually increasing awareness of fullness and urge to urinate with progressive filling. Within reason, the urge to urinate can be postponed indefinitely through central and peripheral mechanisms—the bladder should never empty without permission. After a desire to empty the bladder occurs, the urethra must relax and stay relaxed while the detrusor generates and maintains a contraction. When the volume in the bladder is less than 200 to 300 mL, the bladder may have difficulty generating and sustaining this contraction. Conversely, without detrusor contraction, the urethra may have difficulty maintaining relaxation.

When there is a source of irritation in or around the lower urinary tract, the urge to urinate may occur at very low volumes (30 to 100 mL). At this low volume, detrusor contraction and outlet relaxation may not be coordinated and urination may be hesitant, slow, and interrupted, with a sense of incomplete emptying. This problem can become exacerbated when the sense of urge is intense or painful at low volumes. The intensity of the urge elicits increased pelvic muscle activity to prevent incontinence, which further exacerbates the difficulty of initiating and sustaining coordinated urination with a low bladder volume. Typically, the inability to void despite a strong painful urge leads to straining to initiate urine flow. Unfortunately, using the Valsalva maneuver to assist with voiding is effective only when outlet relaxation is maintained. Chronic straining against "tight" pelvic muscles can further contribute to voiding dysfunction. Thus, increased bladder sensitivity can become quickly associated with a voiding dysfunction. Regardless of the initial cause of the irritation, the voiding dysfunction can chronically maintain the symptoms.

In general, most women with lower urinary tract pain also note increased frequency of urination. It is helpful to determine what level of bladder volumes signal the urge to urinate and what happens if the signals are ignored. A voiding diary of time and volume of urination over several days and nights is invaluable. A bladder that can hold 600 mL at night but only holds 100 to 300 mL during the day suggests "hypersensitivity" of the lower urinary tract. This situation is different from that of someone who gets up every 2 hours to urinate 100 mL.

The reasons that women do not ignore signals or urgency are important to understand the etiology of the problem. First, there may be a fear of incontinence. Second, holding may be associated with severe pain, aching, or cramping. Third, often the urge sensation is "annoying" enough to impair concentration on other tasks until voiding is complete, even though the urge can be ignored without pain or fear of leakage. Women may also void frequently because they have been told that "holding" after getting an urge can lead to bladder infections. This behavior can lead to voiding progressively smaller volumes out of habit.

When incontinence is the woman's main concern, involuntary detrusor activity is probable. Young women with normal anatomic support may sense pain or discomfort during an involuntary detrusor contraction yet not experience incontinence because the voluntary contraction of strong pelvic floor muscles is able to prevent leakage.[3]

Pain *during* the act of urination is most consistent with acute bacterial cystitis or urethritis. When urine shows no evidence of infection, additional diagnostic considerations should include vulvovaginal inflammation, urethral diverticulum, or, rarely, nonrelaxation of the outlet muscles. Pain *after* urination strongly suggests a muscular etiology; that is, the outlet muscles are relaxed during urination but their activity increases after urination is complete.

PAIN: A CONCEPTUAL OVERVIEW

ACUTE VS. CHRONIC PAIN

Pain is a noxious sensation carried by nerve fibers from the site of tissue injury to the brain. Acute pain is beneficial when it alerts the person to the site of the injury. After injury is recognized and treatment and healing have begun, persistent pain becomes chronic and is no longer beneficial. Chronic pain can severely affect quality of life by decreasing motivation, limiting physical activities, and disrupting sleep patterns.[4] Chronic pain is real, but it does not require the same search for a source as acute pain does. Unfortunately, medical education rarely addresses chronic pain. Most providers and patients alike believe that all pain is acute and that it indicates some underlying serious problem. Evaluations that do not produce specific answers and treatments that do not provide long-term symptomatic improvement or cure can produce excessive anxiety. As patient anxiety increases, so does physician frustration. The doctor-patient relationship erodes; then the patient is off seeking another opinion or "shopping" for a diagnosis.

TYPES OF PAIN

There are three types of pain: somatic, visceral, and neuropathic.[5] **Somatic pain** arises from skin, muscles, and bones. It is rapidly transmitted by fibers to cerebral cortex, where the source of pain is quickly localized, yielding a quick response. Patient descriptions of somatic pain include "sharp," "stabbing," or "throbbing." **Visceral pain** arises from the internal organs and is carried on slower fibers through the limbic system (the center for emotions). The source of pain is poorly localized and is often described in emotional terms such as "awful" or "agony." **Neuropathic pain** is generated in damaged nerve fibers. Its messages, often described as "electrical," "shock-like" or a "painful numbness," are also carried through the limbic system. These descriptions can be helpful in identifying the type of pain, especially in the pelvis, where all three types can coexist. This explains why both visceral and neuropathic pain (with afferent transmission through the limbic system) may present with significant emotional overlay not seen in somatic pain (where the limbic system is bypassed).

TISSUE SENSITIZATION AND REFERRED PAIN

Three basic phenomena of tissue sensitization and referred pain are fundamental to the mechanisms of soft tissue pain without specific identifiable pathology.[6] These concepts are important to understanding and clarifying women's descripton of their pain. The first is the **induction of hypersensitivity of visceral tissue**. This identification requires looking beyond traditional objective data to those factors that mediate pain—the chemicals and neurotransmitters that sensitize nerve endings. Mediators including acid pH, histamine, substance P, and bacterial toxins can transform a normally insensitive organ into an acutely hypersensitive one.[7] Central factors may also trigger mediator release (substance P) from nerve endings.[8] Trauma and disease in tissue may induce sensitivity that persists after healing has occurred.

Referred pain without tenderness is a poorly localized ache without associated hyperesthesia of overlying skin and without soft tissue tenderness in the referral area, such as when low back pain occurs during menstrual cramps. This pain is thought to originate in the dorsal horn where A delta and C fibers from the visceral tissue converge with the same dermatome somatic axons.[7] This convergence-projection phenomenon is not associated with somatic self-generating pain feedback, which will be discussed later in this chapter. Consequently, this pain cannot be blocked by local infiltration of the somatic area to which pain is referred.

Induced referred pain with hyperesthesia and tenderness is associated with somatic self-generating pain feedback. This means that referred soft-tissue pain actually increases sensitivity in the viscera to the same noxious stimulus that initially generated the referred somatic pain. Somatic areas affected by pelvic visceral disease are the abdominal wall, costovertebral angle, and dorsal sacrum.[9] The characteristics of this type of pain are

1. Hyperesthesia of the skin overlying tender areas
2. Tender points within the soft tissue planes, which are sharply tender to palpation and refer pain to characteristic referral areas for that somatic site, which may be in other dermatomes
3. Self-generation and escalation of hyperesthesia and tenderness in both somatic tissue and viscera. Consequently, any normal physiologic function (bladder fullness, ovulation, menses, defecation, coitus, and orgasm) in the pelvis may be perceived as noxious based on somatic self-generating pain feedback. This pain can typically be blocked by injection of a local anesthetic into somatic trigger points, with relief of pain that persists longer than the duration of the anesthesia.

MYOFASCIAL PAIN

Another source of soft tissue pain that can be perceived as originating in the lower urinary tract is myofascial pain, which is generated in hyperirritable spots located within a tight band of skeletal muscle or fascia.[10] Referred pain, tenderness, autonomic phenomena, a self-perpetuating cycle, and reflex spasm in surrounding muscle groups are associated with these points of pain. Tearing, coryza, dizzy spells, and tinnitus are some of the autonomic symptoms that are reported by patients in conjunction with this pain.[11] Muscle pain can lead to inactivity, which further exacerbates the problem. Triggers for myofascial pain include direct trauma to muscles or joints, chronic muscle strain, chilling of fatigued muscles, acute myositis, arthritis, nerve root injury, or visceral ischemia.[12] Myofascial trigger points in the levator and coccygeus muscles can be associated with symptoms of altered lower urinary tract function and pain. It was recognized by Thiele[13] in 1963 that these symptoms are exacerbated before and during menses.

CAUSES OF LOWER URINARY TRACT PAIN

BACTERIAL CYSTITIS

Bacterial cystitis is undoubtedly the most common cause of pain associated with the lower urinary tract. A simple bacterial bladder infection can generally be treated with either a single dose or short (3–5 days) course of antibiotics rather than the 7 to 10 days which has been traditionally recommended.[14] Shorter courses of antibiotics decrease the chances of bowel dysfunction and vaginitis associated with longer courses.

In patients with chronic or recurrent lower urinary tract pain, health-care providers should be careful not to diagnose an infection based on symptoms alone. Doing so leads to much confusion for the patient when the culture results return negative or if symptoms do not resolve with antibiotics. Using nonspecific terminology such as "symptomatic episode" or "bladder inflammation" when the woman presents with symptoms is useful. As soon as the word "cystitis" is used, antibiotics are expected to be necessary for symptom relief. Antibiotics commonly improve symptoms even with a negative urinalysis and culture. One explanation for this occurrence is that all bottles of antibiotics instruct the patient to "drink plenty of water with each dose." After the course of antibiotics is completed, fluid intake returns to normal, which often includes negligible amounts of noncarbonated water; symptoms may thus return because of the hypersensitivity phenomenon discussed below.

LOWER URINARY TRACT HYPERSENSITIVITY

Lower urinary tract hypersensitivity is used to replace terminology such as urethral syndrome, chronic trigonitis, chronic urethritis, and chronic nonbacterial cystitis.[3] It simply refers to an overly sensitive bladder, which can contribute to the cascade of events leading to uncoordinated, low-volume urination; voiding dysfunction; and eventual pain before, during, or after urination. Usually, the pain is worse before or after urination; women will often report that the pain feels different than when they have had a bacterial bladder infection in the past. Explaining these symptoms as similar to a sensitive stomach or to a sore joint, such as tennis elbow, often helps the patient understand that these symptoms are not necessarily caused by an infection. Identifying all potential triggers and eliminating as many of them as possible, while increasing water intake, modifying the diet, and working with pelvic muscle relaxation can alleviate symptoms and minimize the number of symptomatic flareups.

VAGINITIS

Urinary tract pain in women with vulvovaginal inflammation generally occurs during urination, but typically is felt as the urine contacts the external tissues rather than while it passes through the urethra. Often increased frequency of urination is not reported because the woman will avoid urinating in order to prevent pain.

CHEMICAL IRRITATION

Non-oxinyl-9, found in most contraceptive preparations, can cause local irritation in women sensitive to it. In addition, women with allergic sensitivity to latex may report coitally-related lower urinary tract symptoms with the use of diaphragms or condoms.

URETHRAL DIVERTICULUM

Although fairly uncommon, a diverticulum of the urethra should be considered in women with recurrent, culture-proven lower urinary infections, pain during urination, painful coitus, and post-void dribbling.[15] This constellation of symptoms may not be present in all women with diverticula. On physical examination, a sense of suburethral fullness is usually present. "Milking" the urethra may produce purulent secretions. Diagnosis can usually be confirmed on voiding cystourethrogram or cystourethroscopy. Rarely, a double-balloon urethrogram may be necessary. Because this test can be uncomfortable for the patient, however, it is recommended only when strong clinical suspicion cannot be confirmed by the other tests.

LOCAL TRAUMA

Local trauma to the lower urinary tract can be caused by sexual activity, especially when aggressive, prolonged, or without adequate lubrication. Certain positions may be more or less uncomfortable for some women. It is not unusual to have women report partner-specific factors, such as size of phallus, duration of intercourse, or variety of positions associated with their pain. Pain that begins hours or days after intercourse is highly suggestive of neuropathy. Direct pressure on the bladder or urethra caused by a contraceptive diaphragm or cervical cap have been reported by patients to be temporarily related to the onset of the lower urinary tract pain. Changing to a smaller size diaphragm may relieve the symptoms and is recommended particularly in the rare women who are not candidates for other forms of birth control.

Women report onset of symptoms after abdominal or vaginal hysterectomies, bladder neck suspensions, and cystocele repairs, as well as posterior repairs and colorectal and perianal procedures. Mechanism for this pain is not well understood, although it probably represents some form of disruption of the peripheral nerve supply. Urethral dilation represents another form of trauma to the lower urinary tract. Urethral dilations have been standard practice for many years for the treatment of recurrent urinary tract infections, symptoms of obstructive voiding, frequency and urgency of urination, and urinary incontinence. Although there are no conclusive studies of the efficacy and potential harm of this procedure, urologists and gynecologists who specialize in disorders of the lower urinary tract in women commonly accept that its potential for physical and emotional harm far exceeds any potential benefit. Although many women do report temporary symptomatic relief following the dilation, they also report significant pain during the dilation. Because one of the goals of treating a chronic pain syndrome is putting the patient in charge of pain control and breaking the pain cycle, it makes no sense to rely on a treatment method in which the patient is a passive recipient of a painful procedure over which she has no control.

INTERSTITIAL CYSTITIS

Individuals with interstitial cystitis typically report frequency and urgency of urination (urinating as often as every 15 minutes both day and night) as well as suprapubic, perineal, vulvar, or vaginal discomfort before, during, or after urination. The etiology is unknown, nor is there any known cure. Etiologic concepts currently being considered involve infections, vascular or lymphatic obstruction, psychologic factors, glycosaminoglycan alterations, reflex sympathetic dystrophy, toxic urinary agents, and immunologic disorders.[16] With this wide variety of potential etiologic factors, it is not surprising that no intervention is uniformly successful. Often a combination of interventions is required to control symptoms. Pain during or after sexual intercourse is also commonly reported. Diagnosis of interstitial cystitis is currently made based on symptoms, functional bladder data (cystometrogram), and cystoscopic criteria. No specific blood, urine, or bladder-biopsy criteria confirm the diagnosis.[17]

Exact incidence of interstitial cystitis is not known, but its social and economic costs are signficant. Economic costs include direct medical expenses, loss of production due to inability to work, or working at jobs paying wages lower than the national average for women of similar age and educational background. Even more profound are the social consequences: overall decrease in quality of life, increase in suicidal ideation, and inability to function as a parent or to pursue other activities, such as exercise and sex, which are important for overall physical and emotional well-being.

NEUROPATHIC PAIN

Diagnosis of neuropathic pain is rarely considered in women who present with lower urinary tract pain, but it should be considered first in women who describe their pain as "burning" or producing "electric shock-like" sensations. The mechanism of nerve injury may never be known. It can be perpetuated by local trauma, pelvic floor spasm, and repeated injury to the peripheral nerves. Trauma to the pudendal nerve has been attributed to vaginal childbirth and such activities as horseback riding and prolonged cycling.[18] Reflex sympathetic dystrophy[19] has been reported in women with chronic bladder pain. Exposure of the pelvic organs to radiation can damage the blood supply and the nerves, leading to symptoms of lower urinary tract pain.

MUSCULOSKELETAL PAIN

Musculoskeletal pain is probably the most frequently missed diagnosis in patients who present with pain in the pelvis and an altered voiding pattern. Health-care providers are not accustomed to thinking of the pelvic musculoskeletal system as being a source of pain when patients attribute that pain to their internal organs. This pain is typically poorly localized, dull, and aching. Musculoskeletal nociceptors are stimulted by mechanical stimuli (compression or stretching), chemical stimuli, inflammation, and metabolic disturbances. Intrapelvic muscle strain; imbalance between the trunk, hip, and abdominal muscles; poor posture; and strain injuries to abdominal, paravertebral, and gluteal muscles (e.g., by a short leg) can all generate pain localized to the lower urinary tract as well as alterations in voiding function. Abdominal trigger points are believed to arise superficial to the muscles and fascia, but may be influenced and possibly triggered by musculoskeletal abnormalities proximal to the trigger point.[12] A thorough musculoskeletal examination should be considered in all patients with abdominal trigger points that recur in spite of good pain relief with trigger-point injection. Standard physiotherapeutic techniques such as applying heat, cold, massage, and appropriate muscle stretching, strengthening, and relaxation can be effective for this part of the body as well as for the extremities. Their value has been demonstrated in extremely refractory patients with chronic pain; they are now employed early in the management strategy for our patients with lower urinary tract pain.

HISTORY

A complete history is the most important aspect of the initial evaluation of a patient with lower urinary tract pain. A questionnaire filled out by the patient before seeing the health-care provider is invaluable in helping to decipher complex histories; it provides the patient with a vehicle to express anger and frustration. Specific questions to be explored include:

1. *What are your current symptoms?* It is important to obtain specific information about daytime frequency, nocturia, an urgency rating on a scale of 0 to 10, and a pain rating also on a scale of 0 to 10. If symptoms vary, obtain information about when symptoms are at their best and at their worst.
2. *Can you describe your pain?* Ask the patient to be as specific as possible with respect to how it feels and where she feels it. Does the pain vary with how full or empty the bladder feels? Does sexual activity affect the pain? Possible responses include:

   Quality: sharp, burning, heaviness; spasmodic, constant awareness

   Location: suprapubic, vaginal, urethral, lower back, thigh, clitoral

   Relationship to lower urinary tract function: with full bladder, with initiation of urination, during urination, after urination, when urine contacts the external tissues

   Relationship to sexual function: exacerbated or relieved by arousal or orgasm; exacerbated during initial penetration, deep penetration, thrusting; exacerbated after intercourse (immediately or delayed several hours)

   Inquire whether the frequency and enjoyment of sexual activity have been affected, and what has been the impact on the patient's relationship with her partner.
3. *Are symptoms the same 24 hours a day, 7 days a week?* For example, ask if symptoms vary depending on time of day (morning vs. evening) or with physical exercise. Let the patient identify what may be different about asymptomatic vs. symptomatic times.
4. *What were the patient's bladder habits before this problem started?* Find out if hesitancy, a poor, interrupted flow, and a feeling of incomplete emptying are a signficant part of the symptom complex.
5. *Was there a history of infections, frequency, or daytime or nighttime incontinence as a child? If so, were any procedures previously performed, such as meatotomy, urethrotomy, or urethral dilation?* A history of these problems suggests that the patient may have a voiding dysfunction, possibly due to the incomplete matura-

tion of the nerve pathways to the lower urinary tract.

6. *Do symptoms vary with the menstrual cycle?* Women usually report that symptoms are worse between ovulation and menses, particularly 1 to 3 days premenstrually.
7. *Do any of the following exacerbate symptoms?*
   Dehydration: increased physical activity and sweating, or decreased fluid intake
   Dietary factors: coffee, carbonated beverages, acidic foods, juices, spicy foods, sugar, or aspartame
   Physical factors: sitting or standing for prolonged periods, car rides, and lifting
   Emotional factors: stress, anxiety, depression, fatigue, among others
8. *What relieves symptoms?* Common answers include lying down, drinking more water, warm bath or heating pad, cold packs, onset of menses, antibiotics, antispasmodics, relaxation, changing the diet, NSAIDs, phenazopyridine, and prescription pain pills.
9. *What is the patient's normal daily fluid intake?* Ask for the breakdown among the following: coffee (including decaffeinated); carbonated beverages (including seltzers, sparkling water); fruit juices (specifically citrus and cranberry); tea; water; milk; and alcohol.
10. *How were symptoms affected by pregnancy?*
11. *What treatments have been tried and what was the patient's response to treatments?* Specifically, inquire about use of antibiotics, antispasmodics, anesthetics, urethral dilations, bladder instillations, and bladder dilation (office vs. under anesthesia).
12. *What was going on in the patient's life around the onset of the symptom complex?* Common responses include becoming sexually active, having a new sexual partner, using a new form of birth control, suffering hot weather, a low-back or tail-bone injury, a pelvic operation, infection in a pelvic organ, undergoing a minor gynecologic procedure, or developing a perianal process (e.g., fissure, hemorrhoid).
13. *What does the patient think is causing the problem?* Allow the patient to say whatever she believes without discounting anything as ridiculous, impossible or unimportant.
14. *What is the patient's biggest fear about these symptoms?* Typically, women identify the following fears: cancer, an infection being passed back and forth with a sexual partner, possible kidney damage from undiagnosed infection, or that they will never get better or have a normal sexual relationship again.
15. *Does the patient have a history of significant physical, sexual, or emotional abuse that she feels may have some significance to her current symptom complex?* If rapport with the patient has been difficult to establish, it may be better to avoid this question on initial visit.

PHYSICAL EXAMINATION

The examination of patients with lower urinary tract pain includes features not routinely performed. If specific trigger points in the low back or abdomen are identified, these can be injected with anesthetic before proceeding with the pelvic examination.

Following inspection and palpation of the external genitalia, introduce one finger through the introitus, keeping pressure against the posterior vaginal wall. Ask the woman to identify when she experiences discomfort or pain, and whether the discomfort is the same or different from her symptomatic episodes. Initially, palpate the introital muscles circumferentially, then gently introduce the finger to the level of the cervix or vaginal cuff, keeping pressure posterior. Now gradually palpate the levator muscles, following the area of pubic bone, pushing up on the genitourinary diaphragm lateral to the bladder and urethra. This should be done on both sides, observing for symptom reproduction. The lateral pelvic sidewalls are also to be palpated.

The anterior vaginal wall is palpated next. Begin with the urethra just proximal to the meatus and gently palpate toward the bladder neck. The urethra should feel like a midline spongy tube with a "gutter" on either side. The "gutters" may be obscured by a previous anterior colporrhaphy, anterior vaginal wall mass (cyst or infected glands), or urethral diverticulum. Moving superiorly, gently palpate the base of the bladder. A sense of urge to urinate is normal, but a sense of pain, burning, cramping, or aching is not. A bimanual examination is begun by gently putting downward pressure on the suprapubic area while pushing upward on the base of the bladder in the midline with the vaginal finger. Next, move the finger in the vagina lateral to the bladder and push up on the pelvic floor support immediately adjacent to the public bone. Pain in this area is consistent with myofascial pain.

Next, bimanual examination of the uterus and ovaries is performed, again carefully assessing for pain reproduction. When pain is reproduced, return to the same spot with abdominal and vaginal pressure independently to determine whether pain is generated by abdominal or vaginal trigger points or by the tissue in between.

The final part of the internal examination assesses the patient's ability to contract and relax the pelvic floor muscles. This muscle group should be supple and nontender at rest. Circumferential tightening of muscles around the vagina without lifting the buttocks, and immediate relaxation on command should be present.

SPECIFIC TESTING

A voided urinalysis should always be done. Microscopic examination of a spun specimen allows for immediate assessment of hematuria, infection (pyuria), and whether the specimen taken is clean enough to culture. If the specimen appears contaminated with squamous epithelial cells, obtaining an immediate catheterized specimen can eliminate confusion about whether culture results are significant or if the identified hematuria is of urinary tract origin. A catheterized urine specimen may be collected with a small-caliber catheter (12 or 14 Fr.), allowing an accurate determination of the post-void residual (PVR), which may be important in patients with frequency and a feeling of incomplete emptying. Alternatively, PVR can be estimated using ultrasound. A voided urine sample for cytology can be sent as an initial screen to rule out carcinoma in situ of the bladder, which can be present with symptoms of lower urinary tract irritation. Urethral calibration or dilation are not indicated for diagnosis or therapy.

Cystoscopy is rarely indicated as a part of the initial evaluation. During the initial visit, patients expect to find out "what is wrong." Cystoscopies rarely identify the source of the patient's problems and commonly exacerbate symptoms. Normal findings at this point may increase the patient's anxiety rather than provide reassurance: if everything is normal, then why does she feel bad? After the health-care provider has established a rapport with the patient, cystoscopy may offer both parties the necessary reassurance. When hematuria is found, an upper tract evaluation should be done before cystoscopy.

When the initial management approach is not successful, further diagnostic evaluation includes urodynamics to assess neuromuscular function of the lower urinary tract. Uninhibited detrusor contractions occasionally present with spasm and a burning discomfort rather than incontinence due to urgency. Cystoscopy under anesthesia with hydrodistention and bladder biopsies is indicated to look for evidence of interstitial cystitis when the patient does not respond to conservative measures. Hydrodistention brings symptomatic relief in about 30% of women.[20] When cyclic variation exists in the symptoms, dysmenorrhea, or dyspareunia, simultaneous diagnostic laparoscopy can help to identify other potentially treatable cause of the patient's symptoms.

TREATMENT

GENERAL CONSIDERATIONS

Regardless of symptom etiology, treatment always begins with reassurance and education about the structure and function of the lower urinary tract and the interrelationship with the gynecologic, gastrointestinal, and musculoskeletal systems. Anatomic diagrams can be very helpful in gaining patient awareness and acceptance of the concepts being discussed. It is helpful if the patient's spouse or partner also can be present for the discussion to help dispel their myths and fears as well. In cases of very long-standing or severe symptoms, realistic goals for treatment outcome must be established from the outset. A good beginning involves the patient's understanding the interrelationship between mind and body. She must be informed that the evaluation and treatment will not be based solely on her physical organs. Suggesting that her feelings of depression and anxiety are similar to a grief reaction can be helpful. These women grieve for the active, symptom-free life they once had and experience a concurrent sense of loss in all aspects of their lives. This rationale has allowed many women to accept professional psychologic support.

A partnership for symptom control and getting on with life needs to be established. If the goal is to "cure" the disease, the patient is at risk for continual disappointment as one treatment after another fails to bring permanent symptom relief. Patients must also be warned that when they do obtain good symptomatic control, a recurrence of symptoms is likely at some point. The first symptom recurrence generally produces significant fear that the pain syndrome is back and will not go away this time.

The clinician should never fabricate a diagnosis simply to have something to tell the patient. Terminology such as **dysfunction, symptomatic episodes** or **flare-ups** are most accurate and also do not lead to any expectation that antibiotics will help, as they are thought to do by patients with all words that end with "itis." Be sure that all office personnel who will be dealing with the patient understand the importance of terminology. Mixed messages from different personnel fuel fear, frustration, and anxiety.

An authoritarian or paternalistic approach to these women is generally not well received by them. Very few patients resist psychosocial support or physical therapy evaluation and treatment after they understand the rationale for these recommendations. When not covered by health insurance, the cost of psychosocial support can be a deterrent. When this is the case, scheduling short, routine, follow-up visits every 1 to 2 weeks initially with a health-care provider who can listen and provide support can often eliminate the need for frequent phone calls eliciting support.

BEHAVIORAL STRATEGIES

Common sense is important in using behavioral recommendations. Clinical experience suggests that multiple internal and external factors can enhance lower urinary tract sensitivity and contribute to pain and to voiding dysfunction. Dehydration and fluid restriction, for instance, result in concentrated urine, which many women report increases their symptoms. Certain dietary factors also increase bladder sensitivity. Spicy foods, carbonated beverages, and highly acidic foods and beverages such as coffee (even decaffeinated), tea, citrus, cranberry, and tomato juices, as well as chocolate are reported by patients to exacerbate bladder symptoms. *Increasing their water intake* to dilute the urine and "flush" out the lower urinary tract is important. Optimal volume varies, but starting with 4 to 6 glasses of water per day and gradually increasing the level seems to work. Urine passed should be pale yellow; sufficient water intake necessary to maintain urine of this dilution may vary from day to day. Patients must be informed that frequency may actually be worse initially, owing to the increased intake. Pain lessens and urination becomes easier at first, then as it becomes more comfortable to hold larger volumes of urine in the bladder, the frequency will decrease. Bladder holding protocols can be helpful in decreasing frequency after pain is less severe.[21,22] Avoiding specific foods or fluids can also relieve the discomfort.[23] Although the rationale for this is not known, it may be that certain food products act as neuromodulators.

In many women, symptoms are exacerbated between ovulation and menses. Sexual intercourse is a potent trigger for some women in the absence of evidence of bacterial cystitis. Symptoms may start with the onset of sexual intercourse, with a new partner, with a new form of birth control, or with renewed intercourse after a period of abstinence. Stress and anxiety are also commonly reported to exacerbate symptoms. Although it is not always possible to understand or explain why apparent "triggers" should influence lower urinary tract symptoms and function, it does not mean these "triggers" are not real. Recognition of "triggers" provides a means to help the patient manipulate internal and external factors to minimize or prevent symptom flareups. Using a bladder diary periodically to record time and volume of urination can be important in demonstrating improvement to the patient.

Recognizing the potential of voluntary or involuntary pelvic muscle contraction to generate, perpetuate, or exacerbate symptoms is important to the development of self-management strategies. Voluntary pelvic floor relaxation[24] can ease symptoms. Many times patients need instruction in pelvic muscle localization and contraction before they can understand how to relax this muscle group. Techniques that promote generalized relaxation and stress management (e.g., aerobic exercise, distraction) should be used whenever possible. In order for these techniques to be accepted by the patient, these behavioral strategies must be recommended as a valid treatment by the provider. When a patient senses that the health-care provider does not take these recommendations seriously, she is not likely to follow through with them.

PHARMACOLOGIC MANAGEMENT

Many medications can be employed in the treatment of lower urinary tract pain syndromes. Often a combination of drugs can be efficacious. Pharmacologic management can be used even in patients without a confirmed diagnosis of interstitial cystitis. In my practice, however, I do not use dimethyl sulfoxide (DMSO) intravesical instillations unless the patient has findings consistent with interstitial cystitis after cystoscopy with hydrodistention under anesthesia. Sodium pentosanpolysulfate (Elmiron)[25,26] is awaiting FDA approval and is only available on a compassionate use basis from Baker-Nortion Pharmaceuticals (Miami, Florida) for patients who meet the extensive and restrictive research criteria established by the National Institute of Arthritis, Diabetes, Digestive and Kidney Diseases.[27]

Table 14–1 lists the pharmacologic agents most commonly used and the symptoms that may be most helpful in generating a treatment plan. In particular, the use of alpha-blockers (i.e., Prazosin) can be helpful in those rare patients with obstructive voiding symptoms that may be related to nonrelaxation of the urethral smooth muscle.[28] This list of medications should be regarded as indicating general guidelines; in refractory patients, a trial of just one more agent or one more combination may be the key in breaking the pain cycle. Realistic expectations for treatment outcome are necessary, however, and patients must understand that all medications come with a ratio of benefits to side effects that is particular to them and not more widely predictable.

PHYSICAL THERAPY

The addition of a comprehensive physiotherapy evaluation and treatment regimen is invaluable to women with lower urinary tract pain. Four years ago, I began sending our most refractory patients to see physical therapists with a special interest in pelvic floor dysfunction. The success rate with these very difficult symptom complexes was surprising.[29] Gradually, patients were referred earlier and earlier in our treatment sequence, so that currently nearly all patients are referred for physical therapy assessment after their first or second visit. Patients almost universally report that they gain significant, if not total, symptom improvement.

Our practice is to undertake urodynamic evaluations and cystoscopy with hydrodistention under anesthesia only in patients who have failed behavioral and pharmacologic options and physical therapy. The number of hydrodistention procedures has declined from two to four per month to less than one per month since I have been using physical therapy aggressively.

TREATMENTS SPECIFIC TO INTERSTITIAL CYSTITIS

Even patients who present with a confirmed diagnosis of interstitial cystitis may respond well to some of the simple behavioral strategies.

Current treatment of interstitial cystitis is aimed at symptomatic relief through a variety of means including dietary modification; intravesical instillations of various pharmacologic agents including DMSO,[30] hydrocortisone, sodium bicarbonate,[31] heparin,[32,33] oxychlorosene (Chlorpactin),[34] lidocaine,[35] and doxorubicin;[36] and the use of oral agents such as am-

TABLE 14–1. Medications for Treatment of Lower Urinary Tract Pain

Medication	Dosage	Symptom	Sign
		Tricyclic Antidepressants	
• Amitriptyline	10–75 mg @ h.s.*	Sleep disruption; sharp burning, shock-like pain; bladder/urethral burning or constant awareness	Increased pelvic muscle tone; painful bladder
• Doxepin	10–75 mg @ h.s.*		
• Trazodone	50 mg A h.s.		
• Prozac	20 mg po q.i.d.		
		Alpha-blockers	
• Terazosin	1–2 mg @ h.s. (increase to t.i.d. as tolerated and necessary for symptom control)	Hesitancy; slow stream, sense of incomplete emptying. Post-voiding pain and spasm	Abnormal uroflow; ± tender pelvic muscles
• Prazosin			
• Phenoxybenzamine			
		Antispasmodics	
• Oxybutynin	½ T po t.i.d.	Frequency; discomfort with full bladder; severe urgency	Involuntary detrusor contraction on CMG
• Hyoscyamine	*i-ii* po t.i.d.		
• Flavoxate	*i* po t.i.d.		
		Skeletal muscle relaxants	
• Carisoprodol (Soma)	*i* po t.i.d.	Post-voiding pain; dyspareunia	Increased tone of pelvic muscles; pain reproduction with palpation
• Cyclobenzaprine (Flexeril)	*i* po t.i.d.		
• Methocarbomol (Robaxin)	*i* po t.i.d.		
		Anesthetics	
• Phenazopyridine	100–200 mg po t.i.d.	Hypersensitivity; pain during urination; pain localized to meatal area during urination or intercourse	Tender introital area or perimeatal area
• Lidocaine jelly 2%			
• Lidocaine ointment 5%			
		Anticonvulsants	
• Carbamazepine (Tegretol)	200 mg po b.i.d. gradually increase to q.i.d. prn	Neuropathic pain	Sensory deficits (perineum/lower extremity); dysesthesia

*Gradually increase dosage; can use t.i.d. if sedation not a problem

itriptyline,[37] hydroxyzine,[38] nifedipine,[39] and sodium pentosanpolysulfate.[25,26] Other modalities used to treat interstitial cystitis include transcutaneous nerve stimulation (TENS),[40,41] neuromodulation (sacral nerve-root stimulator),[42] surgical enlargement of the bladder (augmentation cystoplasty),[43] substitution cystoplasty,[44] or cystectomy with urinary diversion.[45] Some of the many medication prescribed specifically to this patient population are listed in Table 14–2. These drugs are usually used for other clinical conditions and thus are readily available.

DMSO is FDA-approved for the treatment of interstitial cystitis. It can be used alone or mixed with the other agents previously mentioned. A typical treatment regimen is weekly instillations for 6 to 8 weeks. If good control of symptoms is achieved, treatment can be restarted when symptoms flare up, or a maintenance schedule of instillations every 1 to 2 months can be started. Many patients prefer to learn self-instillation, which allows them to do the treatments when they feel they need them rather than when they can schedule an appointment. Most women have no difficulty learning the technique for self-catheterization and instillation. Bladder infections in this patient population are uncommon and have not been a factor.[46] Women who have significant pain with cathe-

TABLE 14–2. Medications for Treating Interstitial Cystitis

Medication	Dosage	Proposed Action
Amitriptylline	10–75 mg @ h.s.	• Central and peripheral anticholinergic • Block reuptake of norepinephrine and serotonin • Sedative • Analgesic effects
Nifedipine	30 mg q.d. for 2 weeks, gradually increase to 60 mg q.d.	• Decrease frequency and strength of visceral smooth muscle contraction • Suppressive effect on delay-type hypersensitivity
Hydroxyzine	25 mg @ h.s. for 1 week, increase to 50 mg @ h.s. for 1 week, then add 25 mg each morning	• Block neuronal activation of mast cells
Pentosanpoly-sulfate (Elmiron)*	100 mg po t.i.d.	• Reduce bacterial adherence to bladder epithelial cells • Reduce microcrystal adherence • Enhance impermeability of epithelium
Nalmefene†	Not known	• Stabilize mast cell membrane to prevent histamine release

*Awaiting FDA approval; available on compassionate use basis from Baker-Norton Pharmaceuticals, Miami, FL.

†Currently in clinical trials by Baker-Norton Pharmaceuticals, Miami, FL.

terization can place lidocaine jelly into the urethra before catheterization. Some women have severe spasms while the solution is in their bladder. The "cocktail" mixture of the four ingredients listed (Table 14–3) seems to be better tolerated, because it dilutes the DMSO. If the pain experienced during instillation seems to depend on volume, half or a third of the total volume can be used and the rest refrigerated until the next instillation. Some women find that instilling a third of the total volume three times per week works best for them. Table 14–3 lists the supplies and medications my patients use for self-instillation.

TABLE 14–3. Intravesical Supplies for Self-Instillation Using Clean Technique

Supplies
14- or 16-Fr urethral catheter (usually red rubber)
Open-ended syringe
Urine specimen cup (for mixing ingredients)
Water soluble lubricant
Topical 2% lidocaine jelly (optional)
Dimethylsulfoxide Regimen
Rimso 50 (50 mL)
100 mg hydrocortisone (optional)
8.4% (50 mL vial) sodium bicarbonate (optional)
5000 units heparin (optional)
Heparin Regimen
10,000 units heparin
10 mL sterile water

In general, it is best to prepare patients for a 2-month to 3-month trial of any new regimen, because it can take time for the patient to notice improvement. Keeping accurate accounts of frequency, nocturia, pain, and urgency scores in the patient medical records is important. Improvement may be subtle and gradual over time. Nocturia eight times in a night is not normal, but it is an improvement over twelve.

SUMMARY

Evaluation and treatment of women with lower urinary tract pain is both challenging and rewarding. The likelihood of successful symptom management increases exponentially with recognition that the standard biomedical model does not apply to most of these patients. Successful management of chronic lower urinary tract pain requires awareness of all systems that may be involved in generating and amplifying these symptoms, establishment of a partnership with the patient in deciding on treatment strategies, and early recognition of the psychosocial influences on all chronic conditions. The physician is only one of the participants. The clinician must be willing to recognize the importance of health-care providers from other disciplines in order to provide the best care for patients with these often debilitating symptoms.

REFERENCES

1. Krieger, J: Urinary tract infections in women: causes, classification, and differential diagnosis. J Urol 35:4,1990.
2. Peters, AA, van Dorst, E, Jellis, B, et al: A randomized clinical trial to compare two different approaches in women with chronic pelvic pain. Obstet Gynecol 77:740,1991.
3. Bavendam, T: A common sense approach to lower urinary tract hypersensitivity in women. Cont Urol 4:25,1992.
4. Galloway, N: The challenge of painful bladder. In: The Mediguide® to Urology, 1994, p 1.
5. Brookoff, D: Understanding Pain and Pain Medications. Interstitial Cystitis Association, 1990.
6. Slocumb J: Chronic somatic, myofascial, and neurogenic abdominal pelvic pain. J Clin Obstet Gynecol 33:145,1990.
7. Fields, H: Pain from deep tissues and referred pain. In Pain, McGraw-Hill, New York, 1987, p 79.
8. Yaksh, T and Hammond, D: Peripheral and central substrates in the rostrad transmission of nociceptive information. Pain 13:1,1982.
9. Slocumb, J: Neurological factors in chronic pelvic pain: Trigger points and the abdominal pelvic pain syndrome. Am J Obstet Gynecol 149:536,1984.
10. Travell, J and Simons, D: Myofascial Pain and Dysfunction: The Trigger Point Manual. Williams & Wilkins, Baltimore, 1983.

11. Simon, D and Travell, J: Myofascial origins of low back pain. Postgrad Med 73:66,1983.
12. Baker, P: Musculoskeletal origins of chronic pelvic pain: diagnosis and treatment. Obstet Gynecol Clin North Am 20:719,1993.
13. Thiele, G: Coccygodynia: cause and treatment. Dis Colon Rectum 6:422,1963.
14. Reid, G, Bruce, A and Taylor, M: Influence of 3-day antimicrobial therapy and lactobacillus suppositories on recurrence of urinary tract infection. Clin Ther 14:11,1992.
15. Leach, G and Bavendam, T: Female urethral diverticula. Urol 30:407,1987.
16. Ratliff, T, Klutke C, and McDougall, E: The etiology of interstitial cystitis. Urol Clin North Am 21:21,1994.
17. Hanno, PM, et al, (eds) Interstitial Cystitis, Springer-Verlag, London, 1990.
18. Turner, M and Marinoff, S: Pudendal neuralgia. Am J Obstet Gynecol 165:1233,1991.
19. Galloway, N, Gabale, D, and Irwin, P: Interstitial cystitis or reflex sympathetic dystrophy of the bladder? Semin Urol 9:148,1991.
20. Hanno, P and Wein, A: Interstitial Cystitis, Part II. American Urological Association, Houston, 1987.
21. Blaivas, S and Blaivas, J: Successful treatment of sensory urgency and interstitial cystitis with behavioral modification. J Urol 135:189,1986.
22. Parsons, C and Koprowski, P: Insterstitial cystitis: Successful management by increasing voiding intervals. Urol 37:207,1991.
23. Koziol, J: Epidemiology of interstitial cystitis. Urol Clin North Am 21:7,1984.
24. Phillips, H, Fenster, H, and Samsom, D: An effective treatment for functional urinary incoordination. J Behavioral Med 15:45,1992.
25. Parsons, C and Mulholland, S: Successful therapy of interstitial cystitis with pentosanpolysulfate. J Urol 138:513,1987.
26. Mulholland, S, Hanno, P, Parsons, CL, et al: Pentosan polysulfate sodium for therapy of interstitial cystitis: a double-blind placebo-controlled clinical study. Urol 35:552,1990.
27. Gillenwater, J and Wein, A: Summary of the National institute of Arthritis, Diabetes, Digestive and Kidney Diseases workshop on interstitial cystitis. J Urol 143:278,1987.
28. Petersen, T and Husted, S: Prazosin treatment of neurological patients with lower urinary tract dysfunction. Int Urogynecol J 4:106,1993.
29. Bavendam, T, et al: Early experience with physical therapy in the management of pelvic pain in female urologic patients. In: Proceedings, Annual Meeting of American Urological Society, Western Section, 1992, Maui, Hawaii.
30. Perez-Marrero, R, Emerson, L and Feltis, J: A controlled study of dimethyl sulfoxide in interstitial cystitis. J Urol 140:36,1988.
31. Sant, G, and LaRock, D: Standard therapies for interstitial cystitis. Urol Clin North Am 21:73,1994.
32. Perez-Marrero, R, Emerson, LE, Maharajh, DO, et al: Prolongation of response to DMSO by heparin maintenance. Urol 41(Suppl):64,1993.
33. Hanno, P, and Wein, A: Conservative therapy for interstitial cystitis. Semin Urol 9:143,1991.
34. Wishard, W, Nourse, M and Mertz, J: Use of chlorpactin WCS 90 for relief of symptoms due to interstitial cystitis. J Urol 77:420,1957.
35. Asklin, B and Cassuto, J: Intravesical lidocaine in severe interstitial cystitis: case report. Scand J Urol Nephrol 23:311,1989.
36. Khanna, O and Loose, J: Interstitial cystitis treated with intravesical doxorubicin. Urol 36:139,1990.
37. Hanno, P, Buehler, J and Wein, A: Use of amitriptyline in the treatment of interstitial cystitis. J Urol 141:846,1989.
38. Theoharides, T: Hydroxyzine in the treatment of interstitial cystitis. Urol Clin North Am 21:113,1994.
39. Fleischmann, JD, Huntley, HN and Shingleton, WB: Clinical and immunological response to nifedipine for the treatment of interstitial cystitis. J Urol 146:1235,1991.
40. Fall, M, Carlsson, C, and Erlandson, B: Electrical stimulation in interstitial cystitis. J Urol 123:192,1980.
41. Fall, M: Conservative management of chronic interstitial cystitis: Transcutaneous electrical nerve stimulation and transurethral resection. J Urol 133:774,1985.
42. Tanagho, E, and Schmidt, R: Electrical stimulation in the management of the neurogenic bladder. J Urol 140:1331,1988.
43. Smith, R, vanCangh, P and Skinner, DG: Augmentation enterocystoplasty: a critical review. J Urol 118:35,1977.
44. Webster, G and Maggio, M: The management of chronic interstitial cystitis by substitution cystoplasty. J Urol 141:287,1989.
45. Irwin, P and Galloway, N: Surgical management of interstitial cystitis. Urol Clin North Am 21:145,1994.
46. Whitmore, K: Self-care regimens for patients with interstitial cystitis. Urol Clin North Am 21:121,1994.

CHAPTER **15**

Benign Anorectal Conditions

Theodore J. Saclarides • José M. Velasco

Physicians of all disciplines are frequently called on to diagnose and treat benign anorectal disorders. Although hemorrhoids, abscesses, fistulas, and fissures are common conditions, they frequently are overlooked, misdiagnosed, or mistaken for other problems. Establishing the correct diagnosis requires recognizing the significance of pain patterns and thoroughly understanding the regional anatomy.

PAIN PATTERNS

A detailed history of the character, intensity, frequency, and precipitating factors of anorectal pain will often give insight into the underlying disease process. The correct diagnosis may be reached simply on evidence in the history and on physical examination, without the routine use of invasive or expensive tests.

CONSTANT PAIN

Unrelenting anal canal pain associated with a palpable swelling may be secondary to a thrombosed external hemorrhoid, a perianal abscess, or a malignancy invading the anal sphincter. These conditions are generally easily distinguishable from each other by physical examination. A thrombosed hemorrhoid usually has intact epithelium and presents as a purple, spherical subcutaneous mass. A perianal abscess is commonly accompanied by erythema, cellulitis, and intact overlying skin. Epidermoid cancers of the anal canal are hard and usually ulcerating.

A laterally displaced painful swelling (beyond the anal margin) is characteristic of an ischiorectal abscess. Although infected sebaceous cysts or abscesses secondary to hidradenitis may occur in this anatomic region, they are not as frequent.

Constant anal pain without significant external physical findings may herald a deep-seated abscess.

Such abscesses may be located in the intersphincteric plane or in the supralevator space. In these instances, digital examination usually reveals fullness and may itself precipitate further discomfort and tenderness.

EPISODIC PAIN

Pain occurring during and after bowel movements is virtually diagnostic of an anal fissure. The pain may last several minutes or hours before it gradually subsides until the next movement. Deep seated, intermittent rectal pain that is not associated with defecation is probably due to levator spasm. This condition is discussed in detail in Chapter 16.

PATIENT EVALUATION

Common, benign anorectal conditions that cause pain can be easily diagnosed in the physician's office. After the history is taken and the patient has been examined externally, the physician must determine the wisdom of proceeding with a digital or endoscopic examination in the office. The distressed patient who is in extreme pain should undergo evaluation with the benefit of anesthesia, which may be general, regional, or local, based on the surgeon's preference and on individual circumstances. If a digital examination can be performed in the office setting, a circumferential assessment of the rectal wall should include palpation of the rectovaginal septum, levator muscles bilaterally, and the presacral space. Proctoscopy should be performed either at this time or in the operating room during definitive treatment of the problem. Proximal evaluation of the colon using colonoscopy or barium x-rays is performed if symptoms warrant.

An occasional patient presents with pain although physical examintion and proctoscopy fail to identify the source. In these unusual instances, use of computerized tomography or endoanal ultrasound is justified.

HEMORRHOIDS

The submucosa of the anal canal does not form a uniformly continuous ring of thickened tissue. Instead, cushions consisting of blood vessels derived from the superior and middle rectal arteries are concentrated at the left lateral, right anterior, and right posterior quadrants. These vascular cushions are supported and held in place by muscle fibers and connective tissue derived from the internal sphincter and conjoined longitudinal muscle. The prevailing theory regarding the cause of hemorrhoids is that these vascular structures become abnormally dilated or distended, leading to downward displacement, which may be enhanced by destruction of their anchoring connective tissue structures. Hemorrhoids, therefore, are not varicose veins; they are instead normal structures which do not prolapse or bleed unless their supporting tissue deteriorates.[1]

INTERNAL HEMORRHOIDS

Internal hemorrhoids arise above the dentate line and drain into the superior hemorrhoidal plexus. They are classified as follows:

First degree: bleed but do not project beyond the anal canal

Second degree: prolapse externally during straining or defecation but reduce spontaneously

Third degree: prolapse requiring manual reduction

Fourth degree: irreducible

Internal hemorrhoids commonly bleed, more so during periods of constipation. Pain is not a presenting symptom unless the hemorrhoid is complicated by thrombosis, gangrene, or anal fissure. Prolapsing internal hemorrhoids are easily distinguished from rectal prolapse; the former has radial musosal folds, whereas the latter manifests concentric mucosal folds.

Treatment is dictated by the degree of hemorrhoid formation. First- and second-degree hemorrhoids should initially be managed with Sitz baths and with dietary measures to soften stool, reduce straining, and alleviate constipation. If improvement is not seen, a variety of office treatments can be used. These treatments are intended solely for hemorrhoids originating above the dentate line, because they may cause extreme pain if used inappropriately on external hemorrhoids. These measures include sclerotherapy with sodium morrhuate, quinine and urea hydrochloride, phenol, or Sotradecol injected submucosally. Results have been variable; this form of therapy should be limited to small hemorrhoids.[2] Complications include sloughing of tissue, thrombosis, burning, and abscess. Alternately, rubber band ligation and infrared coagulation can be used. Rubber band ligation (Fig. 15–1) is superior to sclerotherapy in that it ameliorates symptoms in 75% to 90% of patients.[3–6] Complications include hemorrhage, pain, external thrombosis, ulceration, and, extremely rarely, sepsis. Infrared coagulation produces results comparable to rubber band ligation, but multiple treatments may be required and the equipment is far more expensive.[7] Persistent symptoms following office treatment generally require surgical hemorrhoidectomy. Even though rubber band ligation may be effective in the treatment of third-degree hemorrhoids, generally third- and fourth-degree hemorrhoids respond best to surgery without attempting the above nonoperative forms of therapy.

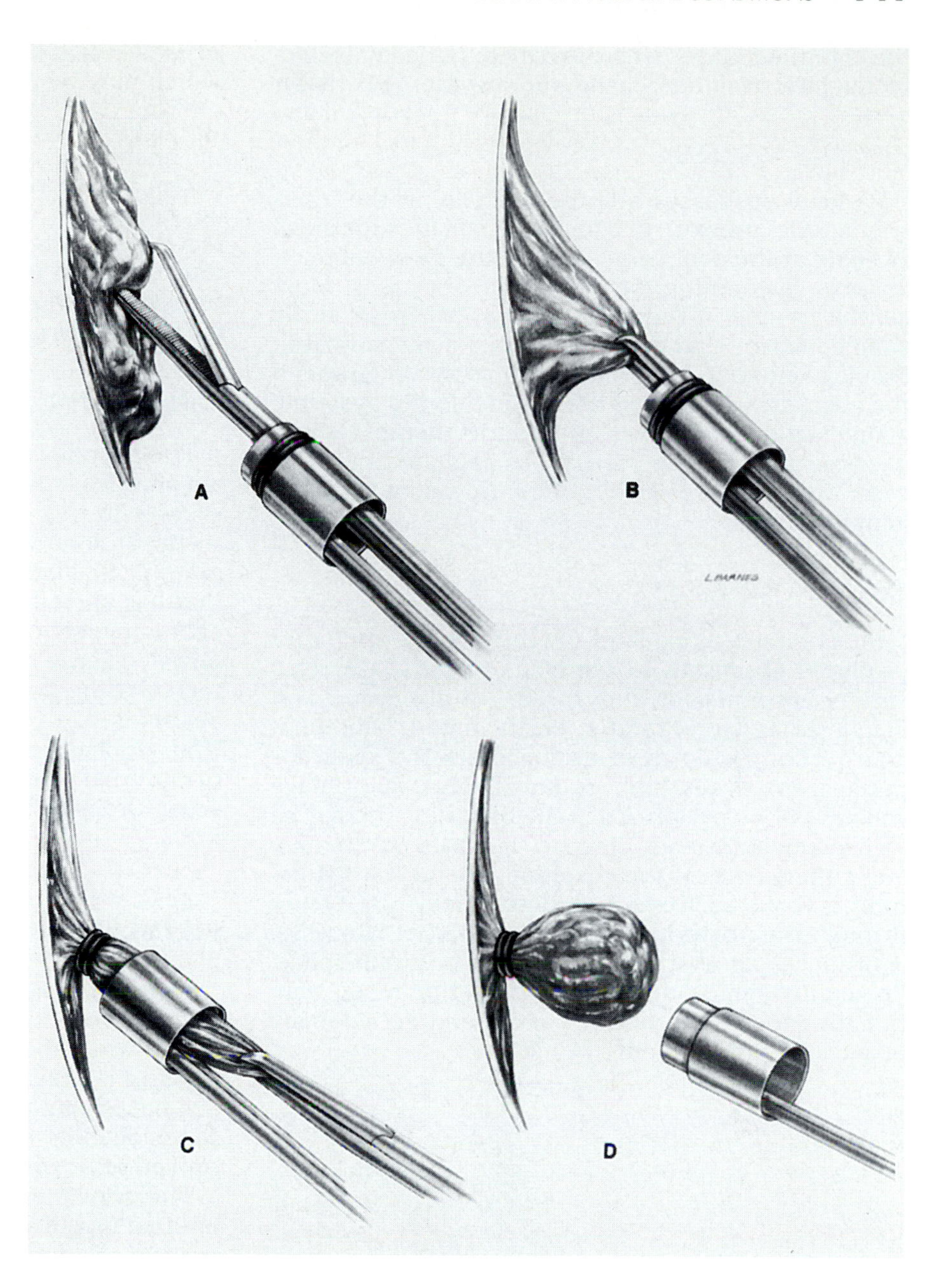

FIGURE 15–1. Rubber band ligation. (*A,B*) Internal hemorrhoid is grasped; (*C*) the applicator is placed over the hemorrhoid and the band released; (*D*) the instrument is withdrawn. (From: Corman ML: Colon & Rectal Surgery, ed. 3, JB Lippincott, Philadelphia, 1993, p 67, with permission.)

EXTERNAL HEMORRHOIDS

External hemorrhoids originate below the dentate line and hence have a similar pain sensation to that of normal perianal skin. As such, they are not amenable to the ambulatory type of treatments used for internal hemorrhoids.

External hemorrhoids produce symptoms of pain (thrombosis), pruritus, and difficulty maintaining hygiene. If the pain warrants surgical intervention, simple incision and drainage is insufficient because the clot may reform; instead, excision of the overlying skin and enucleation of the clot are required. Pruritus and difficulty maintaining hygiene can frequently be managed nonoperatively by simple measures, but surgical hemorrhoidectomy may be indicated for severe, persistent symptoms.

ABSCESSES

Anorectal abscesses may occur secondary to Crohn's disease, trauma, malignancies, radiation, tuberculosis, actinomycosis, or an immunocompromised state. The vast majority of abscesses and fistulas, however, are due to obstruction of the anal ducts and glands. Surrounding the anal canal are 6 to 8 anal glands whose ducts enter the anal canal at the base of the crypts. These glands are located either in the space between the internal and external sphincter or entirely within the internal sphincter.

If the glands become infected, the inflammatory process can then spread in a variety of directions. The clinical presentation and type of pain produced depends on the final location of the abscess. Four presentations have been described: perianal, ischiorectal, intersphincteric, and supralevator (Fig.15–2).

PERIANAL ABSCESS

Perianal abscesses migrate caudally in the intersphincteric groove, producing a small superficial swelling at the anal verge. This is the most common abscess, accounting for 40% to 50% of cases. Most can be treated in the emergency room or office by simple incision and drainage; occasionally, however, drainage must be performed in the operating room if the abscess is large or if the patient shows systemic manifestations of sepsis. Antibiotic therapy is not necessary unless the patient has valvular heart disease, diabetes, prosthetic joints, or a compromised immune system.

ISCHIORECTAL ABSCESS

Infection migrating laterally through the sphincter produces abscesses in the ischiorectal space. This variety accounts for 20% to 25% of abscesses and manifests as large, tender, erythematous, fluctuant areas. The principles of drainage are the same for perianal abscesses, but it is more likely that drainage will have to be performed in the operating room. The incision must be made close to the anal verge to minimize the length of the resulting wound if a fistulotomy is required. If transsphincteric infection occurs through the posterior midline (instead of laterally), it produces an abscess in the deep postanal space. Presenting symptoms include posterior rectal pain radiating to the sacrum or coccyx and occasionally in a sciatic distribution.

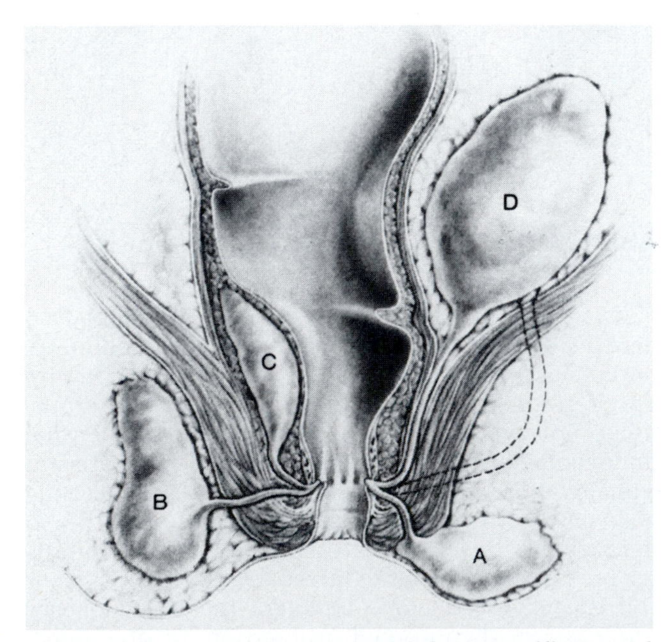

FIGURE 15–2. Classification of anorectal abscesses. (*A*), perianal; (*B*), ischiorectal; (*C*), intersphincteric; (*D*), supralevator. (From: Corman, ML: Colon and Rectal Surgery, ed 3. JB Lippincott, Philadelphia, 1993, p 135, with permission.)

INTERSPHINCTERIC ABSCESS

Infection that dissects upward within the intersphincteric plane produces an abscess cephalad to the anal canal. Although this may not be readily apparent on external examination, its presence should be suspected in any patient with unrelenting deep rectal pain. Digital examination reveals an edematous, fluctuant mass internally. Treatment consists of transanally unroofing the internal sphincter overlying the abscess, thereby providing internal drainage.

SUPRALEVATOR ABSCESS

The supralevator space is bordered by the levator ani muscles below and by the peritoneum above. Abscesses in this region may be secondary to ischiorectal or intersphincteric abscesses that have migrated cephalad, or may be due to pelvic pathology that has spread caudally. Included in this latter category are pelvic inflammatory disease, inflammatory bowel disease, and diverticulitis. Treatment is directed at the primary source within the pelvis. If the absess is due to a cephalad intersphincteric extension, drainage is performed transanally by incising the internal sphincter. If due to a transsphincteric abscess, drainage is performed through the ischiorectal fossa.

FISTULAS

A **fistula** is defined as any abnormal communication between two epithelialized spaces. Many patients with abscesses will subsequently manifest signs of a fistula. In fact, if an abscess wound does not heal completely, or if an abscess recurs in the same location, a fistula is perceived as present until proven otherwise.

The principles of fistula surgery are to identify the internal opening, determine the course of the fistula tract in relation to the sphincter muscle, unroof all tissue between the internal and external opening, and preserve function. Failure to follow these principles may result in recurrent abscesses or incontinence.

The internal opening is identified at surgery by inspecting and carefully probing the tract through the external opening. Goodsall's rule helps identify the probable location of the internal opening, but it is not a substitute for meticulous dissection (Fig. 15–3). This rule states that if the external opening lies anterior to a transverse midline, the fistula tract follows a radial course into the anal canal. If the external opening is posterior, the tract curves to the posterior midline. Exceptions to this rule are those patients with Crohn's disease and those with multiple external openings in the region. If the internal opening is not easily identified after probing the area suggested by Goodsall's rule, the external opening can be injected with a variety of substances that facilitate

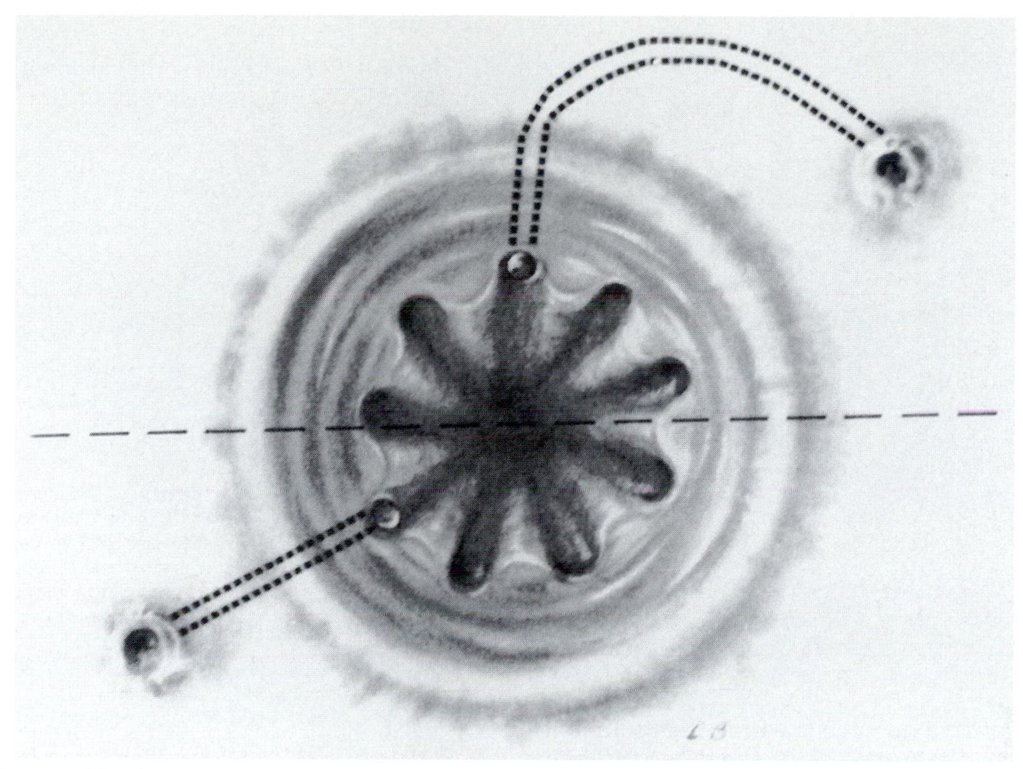

FIGURE 15–3. Course of fistula tracts according to Goodsall's rule. Posterior quadrants are above the dotted line. (From: Corman, ML: Colon and Rectal Surgery, ed 3, JB Lippincott, Philadelphia, 1993, p 147, with permission.)

identification. Included are methylene blue, milk, hydrogen peroxide, betadine, and contrast material such as gastrograffin (in this case, followed by an x-ray).

If the fistula tract courses deep to a substantial portion of the external sphincter, unroofing or division of the tissue may result in incontinence. In these instances, the surgeon has three options:

- Fistulotomy with sphincter reconstruction can be performed
- The internal opening can be covered by advancing a mucosal flap
- A Seton's suture can be inserted

The first two options are probably the domain of an experienced anorectal surgeon, whereas insertion of a Seton's suture is technically easier and probably produces comparable cure rates.

The Seton's suture is inserted through the fistula tract, a loop is formed, and the ends tied together (Fig. 15–4). The suture is progressively tightened over the next several weeks and the sphincter is gradually cut through. This gradual cutting of the muscle is preferable to an abrupt laceration, because fibrosis and inflammatory changes prohibit wide retraction of the muscle edges. As a result, there is less likelihood of incontinence.

INTERSPHINCTERIC FISTULA

High and low types of this fistula are commonly seen. A low intersphincteric fistula originates at the dentate line, courses through the internal sphincter, and passes to the perianal skin. It is treated by simple fistulotomy. A high intersphincteric fistula courses cephalad between the internal and external sphincter, either ending in a chronic abscess cavity or entering the rectum above the dentate line. It is treated by opening the internal sphincter.

TRANSSPHINCTERIC FISTULA

This type of fistula is treated by fistulotomy unless a substantial portion of the sphincter is involved, in which case a Seton's suture is inserted. Rarely, a supralevator extension of this fistula is identified, which is treated by curettage, irrigation, and packing.

SUPRASPHINCTERIC FISTULA

This type of fistula courses cephalad in the intersphincteric plane to the supralevator space, where it passes downward to the ischiorectal fossa and the gluteal skin. Treatment options include mucosal advancement flap, fistulotomy with spincter repair and external drainage, or Seton's division.

EXTRASPHINCTERIC FISTULA

This type of fistula does not originate with infection within the anal canal glands. Instead, it is a consequence of foreign body insertion, impalement injuries, Crohn's disease, or pelvic inflammatory

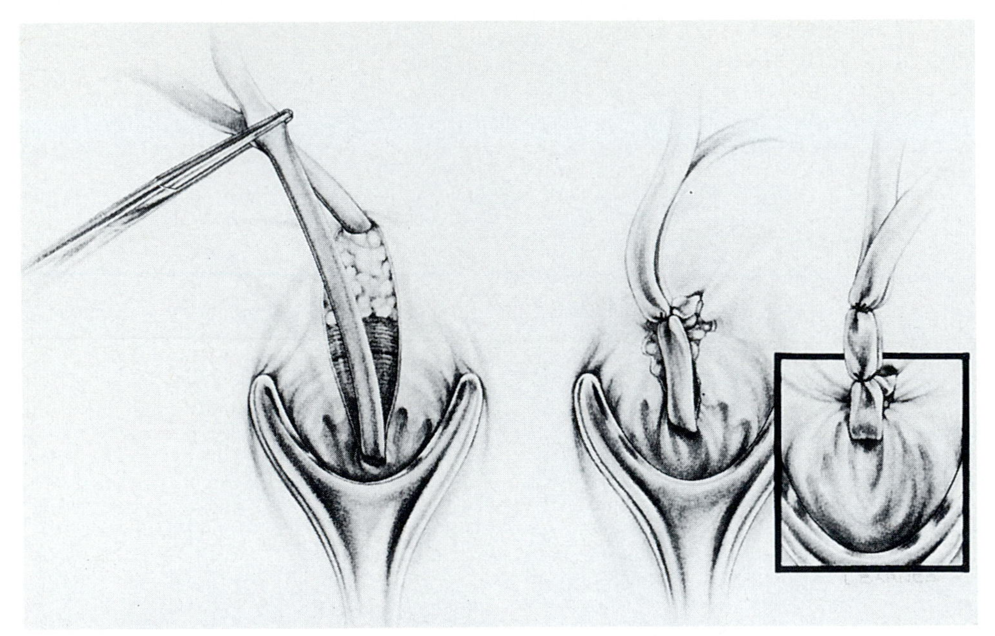

FIGURE 15–4. Seton suture placed within the fistula tract. (From: Culp, CE: Use of Penrose drains to treat certain anal fistulas: A primary operative Seton. Mayo Clin Proc 59:613, 1984, with permission.)

disease. The internal opening is within the rectal mucosa, well above the dentate line; the external opening is on the perianal skin. During its course, the fistula has passed through the levator ani muscle deep to the sphincter muscle. Treatment options are the same for suprasphincteric fistulas. Occasionally fecal diversion is needed if severe disease or tissue loss is present.

ANAL FISSURES

Anal fissures are tears or cuts in the anal canal. They typically cause pain and bleeding during and after bowel movements. Men and women are affected equally. In men, 99% of fissures are located in the posterior midline, and only 1% are found anteriorly. In women, 90% are found in the posterior midline, whereas 10% are found in the anterior region.

Fissures are caused by trauma to the anoderm, usually as a result of passing a hard stool. Fissures may also be a consequence of an acute diarrheal illness, inflammatory bowel disease, syphilis, or tuberculosis; in these instances, the fissure may be located laterally. Most acute fissures will heal, but some will become chronic; this transformation is not a well understood phenomenon and may be related to ischemia.[8]

Physical examination of a chronic fissure frequently reveals a triad of findings: in addition to the fissure itself, one may find a hypertrophied anal papilla within the anal canal and an overhanging external skin tag (Fig. 15–5). This tag is frequently referred to as a "sentinel pile" because it heralds the presence of a fissure at its base. Proctosigmoidoscopy should be performed, although this is usually not possible at the initial consultation due to pain and sphincter

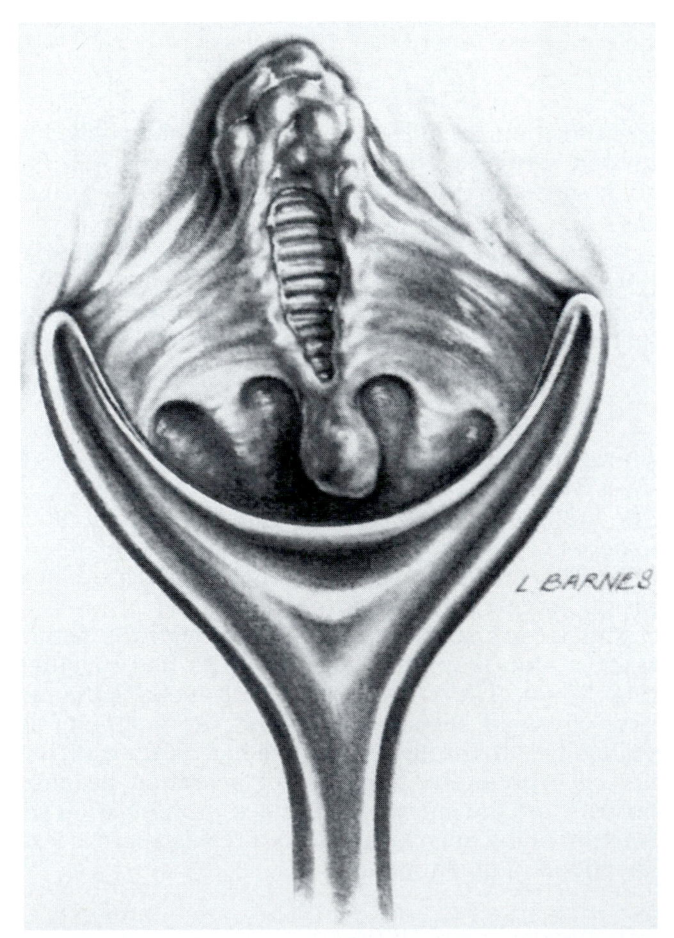

FIGURE 15–5. Chronic posterior anal fissure with "sentinel" pile and hypertrophied anal papilla. (From: Corman, ML: Colon and Rectal Surgery, ed 3. JB Lippincott, Philadelphia, 1993, p 118, with permission.)

spasm. It is usually deferred until the fissure has either healed spontaneously or surgery is performed.

Initial management is nonoperative and consists of Sitz baths, stool softeners, and bulking agents. If symptoms persist after 6 weeks, resolution without surgery becomes increasingly unlikely. Surgical options include sphincter dilation and internal sphincterotomy. Sphincter dilation was widely used in the past and is capable of alleviating pain in most patients, but it may cause an unpredictable amount of sphincter damage, both to the internal and external anal sphincter. Internal sphincterotomy has become the most widely used operation for chronic anal fissure and can be performed in an outpatient setting under a local anesthetic. Complications include abscess formation (2%), temporary fecal soilage (up to 15%), and a nonhealing surgical wound (4%).[9]

SUMMARY

The anorectal conditions discussed in this chapter occur commonly, yet they are frequently misdiagnosed or overlooked. Familiarity with anatomy and an awareness of the pain patterns that accompany these disorders is essential for accurate diagnosis.

REFERENCES

1. Thomson, WHF: The nature of haemorrhoids. Br J Surg 62:542,1975.
2. Alexander-Williams, J and Crapp, AR: Conservative management of haemorrhoids. Part I: Injection, freezing and ligation. Clin Gastroenterol 4:595,1975.
3. Steinberg, DM, Liegois, H and Alexander-Williams, J: Long-term review of the results of rubber band ligation of haemorrhoids. Br J Surg 62:144,1975.
4. Bartizal, J and Slosberg, P: An alternative to hemorrhoidectomy. Arch Surg 112:534,1977.
5. Wrobleski, DE, Corman, ML, Veidenheimer, MC and Coller, JA: Long-term evaluation of rubber ring ligation in hemorrhoidal disease. Dis Colon Rectum 23:478,1980.
6. Gartell, PC, Sheridan, RJ and McGinn, FP: Outpatient treatment of haemorrhoids: a randomized trial to compare rubber band ligation with phenol injection. Br J Surg 72:478,1985.
7. Ambrose, NS, Morris, D, Alexander-Williams, J and Keighley, MRB: A randomized trial of photocoagulation or injection sclerotherapy for the tretment of first and second-degree hemorrhoids. Dis Colon Rectum 28:238,1985.
8. Klosterhalfen, B, Vogel, P, Rixen, H and Mittermayer, C: Topography of the inferior rectal artery: A possible cause of chronic, primary anal fissure. Dis Colon Rectum 32:43,1989.
9. Lewis, TH, Corman, ML, Prager, ED and Robertson, WG: Long-term results of open and closed sphincterotomy for anal fissure. Dis Colon Rectum 31:368,1988.

CHAPTER **16**

Levator Ani Syndrome

William Altringer • Daniel J. Deziel

For over a century conditions characterized by anorectal or perineal pain, such as the levator ani syndrome and proctalgia fugax, have been well recognized but poorly understood clinical entities. The confusion that has accompanied these conditions can be attributed to several factors including a lack of consistent definitions, failure to differentiate functional from organic disorders, and inability to demonstrate physiologic abnormalities consistently enough to explain the clinical manifestations adequately. Although the extent to which these conditions overlap or represent distinct clinical or pathophysiologic syndromes is incompletely settled, certain distinguishing factors have been recognized. This chapter reviews current anatomic, physiologic, and clinical concepts pertinent to understanding these perineal pain syndromes.

LEVATOR ANI SYNDROME

The **levator ani syndrome** is a condition characterized by pain or pressure in the rectum or sacrococcygeal region, presumably by spasm of the levator ani muscles. In a series of reports commencing in 1936, Thiele emphasized levator spasm as a cause of sacrococcygeal pain and comprehensively described the clinical characteristics of afflicted patients.[1,2] He termed this condition **coccygodynia**, however, engendering confusion with coccygeal pain due to skeletal trauma. The designation **levator spasm syndrome** was first coined by Smith in 1959 to describe spasm due to both organic and functional causes.[3]

Among the numerous etiologic factors that have been associated with levator spasm are acute or chronic perineal trauma; anorectal infection; previous spinal, pelvic, or perineal operations; parturition; sexual intercourse; and psychologic stress.[2,4] Local infection has been postulated to result in myositis or reflex spasm of the pelvic muscles. In a series of 324 patients, Thiele noted anorectal infection in 45%, chronic trauma in 32%, and acute trauma in 20%.[2] In contradistinction, Grant and associates were unable to identify a definitive etiologic factor in the majority of their 316 patients.[5] Antecedent anorectal surgery was noted in 17% of their patients and acute trauma in only 2%.

Chronic trauma has been implicated in patients with poor sitting posture, because slumping results in acute angulation of the coccygeal joints and transfers body weight from the ischial tuberosities and posterior thighs to the overflexed coccyx, which has sparse soft-tissue cushion. Symptoms may be precipitated by prolonged sitting, long automobile rides, or repetitive occupational trauma.[2,4]

Typical symptoms consist of dull pain or pressure in the rectum or sacrococcygeal region. The discomfort is described as being situated higher in the rectum than that of common perianal conditions such as thrombosed hemorrhoids, anal fissure, or perianal abscess. Pain is exacerbated by sitting, alleviated by standing or lying, and either unaffected, relieved, or worsened by defecation. Between 10% and 40% of patients also have pain in the gluteal region or thigh, which has been attributed to spasm of the piriformis muscle and pressure on the adjacent sciatic or superior gluteal nerve.[2]

Of affected individuals, 70% to 80% are female, perhaps because of differences in pelvic anatomy such as the larger size of the pelvic muscles and the more posterior position of the coccyx in women. Symptoms are most common between the ages of 40 and 60 years.

DIAGNOSIS

Diagnosis of levator ani syndrome depends upon careful evaluation to exclude other pathology (Table 16–1) and the demonstration of tenderness or spasm of the levator muscles on digital transrectal examination. Careful clinical history, physical examination, proctosigmoidoscopy, and radiologic imaging comprise the basis for detecting most other lesions potentially responsible for causing pain. Among imaging studies, contrast radiography of the gastrointestinal tract, including defecography, can be particularly useful. In addition, computed tomography (CT) or magnetic resonance imaging (MRI) may detect extraluminal pelvic pathology; these tests should, however, be obtained on a selective rather than routine basis.

Anorectal manometry and electromyography have also been proposed as diagnostic tests. West, Abel, and Cutts studied 15 patients with symptoms of rectal pain or pressure consistent with the levator ani syndrome.[6] Most patients complained of constipation as well. Anorectal manometry revealed elevated baseline pressures, internal anal sphincter spasm, and normal reflex relaxation to air. Electromyographic findings of spasm, increased resting activity, and poor phasic contractions correlated with the manometric observations.

The only physical finding of levator ani syndrome is tenderness or spasm of the levator ani musculature when it is palpated during rectal examination. Tenderness in this location may also be caused by deep perianal abscesses; the distinction between these entities rests on chronicity of the symptoms and associated findings such as fever and leukocytosis. The examining finger must be inserted high into the rectal vault. Spasm of the anal sphincter musculature should not be confused with levator ani spasm. The spastic levator ani muscle is felt as a tight band as the finger is swept from a posterolateral to an anterior position. Findings of tenderness or spasm seem to predominate on the left side. The coccyx should also be assessed for direct tenderness or excessive mobility.

TABLE 16–1. Some Identifiable Causes of Perineal and Pelvic Pain

Inflammatory diseases of the pelvis and anorectum
- Cryptoglandular abscess
- Fistula in ano
- Crohn's disease
- Ulcerative colitis
- Ulcerative proctitis
- Radiation proctitis
- Infectious proctitis
- Endometriosis
- Endometritis
- Tubo-ovarian abscess
- Diverticulitis
- Pelvic appendicitis
- Ectopic pregnancy

Mechanical causes
- Internal rectal prolapse
- Descending perineum syndrome
- Urogenital prolapse
- Pelvic surgery
- Anal fissure
- Enterocele

Neoplastic causes: Primary or recurrent tumors, benign or malignant
- Rectum
- Uterus
- Ovary
- Endometrium
- Bladder
- Muscle
- Bone
- Nerve
- Peritoneal metastases

Neurologic causes
- Multiple sclerosis
- Peripheral neuritis and degenerative disease

Orthopedic causes
- Coccygeal trauma—coccygodynia
- Degenerative disease of the lumbosacral spine

TREATMENT

After an appropriately complete investigation excludes other treatable conditions, the therapy for levator ani syndrome involves reassurance of the patient as to the absence of serious pathology and institution of generally simple measures to ameliorate spasm. The patient is educated regarding contributory factors such as poor posture. A doughnut cushion can be used when sitting for long periods.

Warm sitz-baths may be comforting. These should be performed for 20-minute intervals in a bathtub; portable sitz-baths are inadequate, as are heating pads. Pharmacologic therapy of levator spasm has included the administration of muscle relaxants and sedatives, analgesics, anti-inflammatory drugs, and injecting anesthetics or steroids into the levator sling.[2,4]

Digital massage of the spastic levator muscles has been advocated at varying intervals. Thiele recommended that massage be performed 10 to 15 times on each side, repeated daily for 5 to 6 days, and then on alternate days for an additional 7 to 10 days.[2] Massage was the only treatment used on 223 of his 324 patients. Of these patients, 69% were reportedly cured and 23% were improved. Grant, Salvati, and Rubin massaged the affected side 50 times or until tolerance at sessions spaced 2 to 3 weeks apart.[5] Heat and diazepam were also used. Symptom relief was reported in 68% of patients treated with three or fewer sessions and moderate improvement occurred in 19% of patients. Of patients who were successfully treated, 12% experienced recurrent symptoms. Sinaki, Merritt, and Stilwell noted improvement in two-thirds of patients treated with a combination of massage, rectal diathermy, and relaxation exercises.[7]

Electrogalvanic Stimulation

Several uncontrolled reports have found high-voltage electrogalvanic stimulation useful in the treatment of the levator ani syndrome.[8–12] This treatment is based on the principle that stimulation of spastic muscle by low-frequency oscillating electrical current causes fasciculation and subsequent muscle fatigue, thereby eliminating spasm. Suppression of motor neurons or accommodation of central nervous system pathways may also be involved.[9] Treatments are relatively simple and are administered in the office setting. The current is delivered using a hand-held or self-retaining rectal probe, similar to an anoscope, at a frequency of 80 Hz with incremental increasing voltage to 350 to 400 V depending on patient tolerance. Electrogalvanic stimulation is safe, with no significant side effects. Contraindications include pregnancy, presence of a pacemaker, or local malignancy.

Results of electrogalvanic stimulation have been variable, perhaps reflecting differences in patient selection, treatment schedules, definition of outcome, and duration of follow-up (Table 16–2). Sohn, Weinstein, and Robbins were the first to use electrogalvanic stimulation for the treatment of levator ani syndrome.[8] They reported complete symptom relief without recurrence in 50 of 80 patients. There were 15 patients who initially improved but developed recurrent pain within 6 to 30 months. Of 15 patients who did not respond, 6 were felt to have neurologic disease. Nicosia and Abcarian reported complete pain relief in 36 of 45 patients.[9] Using a second course of electrogalvanic stimulation, 5 additional patients with recurrent pain after initial symptom relief were successfully treated. Oliver and colleagues reported the results of electrogalvanic stimulation in 102 patients with levator ani syndrome who were failed by conservative therapy.[10] Good responses occurred in 44 patients, moderate improvement in 25, and poor responses in 33 others. Over one-third of treatment failures were found to have associated pathology, including spinal or neurologic disease, pelvic malignancy, and prostate or anorectal disorders.

Other investigators have had less encouraging results with electrogalvanic stimulation. Athough 60% of patients treated by Billingham and colleagues initially had a good or excellent result, a third of this group developed recurrent symptoms.[11] At an unspecified time of follow-up, only 5 of 20 patients remained symptom-free. Outcome did not correlate with therapy rendered before electrogalvanic stimulation. Similarly, a 28-month mean follow-up of 52 pa-

TABLE 16–2. Electrogalvanic Stimulation for Levator Ani Syndrome

Authors/Year	n	Treatment Schedule	Results: excellent/good (%)	Results: fair/poor (%)	Recurrence (%)	Follow-up
Weinstein, Sohn and Roberts/1982[8]	80	3 1-hour treatments over 3–10 days	81	19	19	6–30 mo
Nicosia and Abcarian/1985[9]	45	15-minute to 30-minute treatments every other day for 1 to 9 treatments	91	9	11	NR
Oliver and colleagues/1985[10]	102	3 1-hour treatments over 10 days	68	32	NR	NR
Billingham and co-workers/1987[11]	20	15-minute to 60-minute treatments for 1–12 treatments	60	40	33	"weeks to months"
Hull and associates/1993[12]	52	3 1-hour treatments over 10 days	43	57	NR	0–71 mo

NR = Not Reported.

tients treated at The Cleveland Clinic demonstrated symptom relief in only 19%.[12] The majority of patients (57%) experienced no benefit.

In summary, no prospective controlled studies have confirmed the efficacy of electrogalvanic stimulation for the treatment of levator ani syndrome. It is, however, a safe and well-tolerated therapy that may have benefit and can be considered for patients with refractory symptoms. It is paramount, however, that patients with symptoms of levator ani spasm be thoroughly evaluated to exclude associated pathology.

Biofeedback

Biofeedback has also been suggested as a treatment for chronic idiopathic anal pain based on demonstration of manometric and electromyographic abnormalities in symptomatic patients. Grimaud and co-workers described manometric and radiologic abnormalities in 12 patients with chronic idiopathic anal pain.[13] Of these patients, 9 also complained of constipation. All had failed medical therapy with analgesics, antidepressants, and local anesthetics. Whether spasm was detected on examination was not reported; colonoscopy was normal. Anal-canal resting pressure was significantly higher than that found in control subjects and in 42% of patients the inhibitory rectoanal reflex was abnormal. Abnormalities demonstrated by defecography included failure of puborectalis relaxation during straining, abnormal perineal descent, internal prolapse, and rectocele. Biofeedback techniques to relax the external and sphincter voluntarily relieved pain in all patients; subsequent manometry confirmed a decrease in the anal-canal resting pressure. At a mean follow-up of 16 months, pain had recurred in one patient. Grimaud and co-workers attribute chronic idiopathic anal pain to contraction of the striated external anal sphincter. Because similar manometric abnormalities and corresponding electromyographic abnormalities have been described by Abell, West, and Cutts in patients categorized as having levator ani syndrome,[6] these same biofeedback techniques can potentially be applied to levator ani syndrome.

PROCTALGIA FUGAX

The term **proctalgia fugax** was introduced by Thaysen in 1935 to describe a condition characterized by episodic, fleeting rectal pain.[14] Although its cause is unknown, it has been attributed to spasm of the levator ani musculature, and thus has been considered a variant of the levator ani syndrome.[15] Other suggested, but likewise unsubstantiated, causes include spasm of the nonstriated anal sphincter, neuralgia, vasospasm, venous stasis, and internal prolapse.[16–18] Examination of patients after or between attacks is generally unrewarding and sparse information is available on patients evaluated while they were experiencing symptoms. An early report describes sigmoidoscopic findings of mucosal edema and erythema and levator tenderness.[19] Manometric studies in two patients suggested that the pain correlated with contractions of the sigmoid colon.[20]

Although proctalgia fugax and levator ani syndrome may share a common pathogenic mechanism, the clinical manifestations are relatively distinct (Table 16–3). Proctalgia fugax most commonly affects young adult males. Survey-based data suggest that it is a common condition; 15% to 20% of individuals may experience symptoms, although relatively few seek medical attention.[16,21] Typical symptoms include localized anorectal pain of abrupt onset and short duration. The pain is described as sharp, aching, or cramping. It persists for less than 10 seconds in 70% of patients and for less than 3 minutes in over 90% of patients.[21] Often no identifiable precipitating factors are evident. In some instances symptoms have occurred at night, following defecation, sexual activity or during times of stress. Symptoms usually abate rapidly and sometimes are relieved by passage of flatus or a bowel movement. Rarely, pain has been associated with autonomic symptoms such as diaphoresis, syncope, or priapism. In most patients, attacks occur a few times a year, although some individuals are troubled by frequent episodes. An association between proctalgia fugax and irritable bowel syndrome has been noted.[16,22] A psychogenic origin has also been theorized.[22] The diagnosis is substantiated only by clinical history and by investigation to exclude other anorectal, gastrointestinal, genitourinary, and pelvic disorders.

Proctalgia fugax requires no specific treatment. Attacks are brief and infrequent and no therapy has been demonstrated to be of prophylactic benefit. As concisely stated by Douthwaite, proctalgia fugax is "harmless, unpleasant, and incurable."[15] Remedies such as muscle relaxants, heat, perineal pressure, and enemas are of questionable benefit. The onset of action of pharmacologic agents is likely to exceed

TABLE 16–3. Comparison of Levator Ani Syndrome and Proctalgia Fugax

	Age	Sex	Pain Character	Pain Location	Pain Duration
Levator ani syndrome	40–60	Female predominance	Dull ache, fullness	Left-sided predominance	Variable
Proctalgia fugax	20–30	Male predominance	Sudden, cramplike	No predominance	Several minutes

symptom duration in most instances. It would seem reasonable to treat any associated irritable bowel symptoms, although no evidence concludes that this will prevent episodic anorectal symptoms.

SUMMARY

The levator ani syndrome and proctalgia fugax are clinical conditions characterized by symptoms of anorectal or perineal pain and pressure. Although the etiology and physiology of these conditions are incompletely understood, spasm of the levator ani musculature is considered a likely mechanism. Patients presenting with these symptoms should be investigated to exclude other treatable gastrointestinal, genitourinary, neurologic, or pelvic conditions. When other diagnoses have been excluded, treatment consists of reassurance and relief of muscle spasm.

REFERENCES

1. Thiele, GH: Tonic spasm of the levator ani, coccygeus and piriformis muscle: Relationship to coccygodynia and pain in the region of the hip and down the leg. Trans Am Proc Soc 37:145, 1936.
2. Thiele, GH: Coccygodynia: cause and treatment. Dis Colon Rectum 6:422, 1963.
3. Smith, WT: Levator spasm syndrome. Minn Med 42:1076, 1959.
4. Salvati, EP: The levator syndrome and its variant. Gastroenterol Clin North Am 16:71, 1987.
5. Grant, SR, Salvati, EP and Rubin, RJ: Levator syndrome: An analysis of 316 cases. Dis Colon Rectum 18:161, 1975.
6. West, L, Abell, TL and Cutts, T: Anorectal manometry and EMG in the diagnosis of the levator ani syndrome. Gastroenterology 98:A401, 1990.
7. Sinaki, M, Merritt, JL and Stillwell, GK: Tension myalgia of the pelvic floor. Mayo Clin Proc 52:717, 1977.
8. Sohn, N, Weinstein, MA and Robbins, RD: The levator syndrome and its treatment with high-voltage electrogalvanic stimulation. Am J Surg 144:580, 1982.
9. Nicosia, JF and Abcarian, H: Levator syndrome—a treatment that works. Dis Colon Rectum 28:406, 1985.
10. Oliver, GC, Rubin, RJ, Salvati, EP, et al: Electrogalvanic stimulation in the treatment of levator syndrome. Dis Colon Rectum 28:662, 1985.
11. Billingham, RP, et al: Treatment of levator syndrome using high-voltage electrogalvanic stimulation. Dis Colon Rectum 30:584, 1987.
12. Hull, TL, Milson, JW, Church, J, et al: Electrogalvanic stimulation for levator syndrome: How effective is it in the long term? Dis Colon Rectum 36.731, 1993.
13. Grimaud, JC, Bouvier, M, Naudy, B, et al: Manometric and radiologic investigations and biofeedback treatment of chronic idiopathic anal pain. Dis Colon Rectum 34:690, 1991.
14. Thaysen, TEH: Proctalgia fugax: a little known form of pain in the rectum. Lancet 2:243, 1935.
15. Douthwaite, AH: Proctalgia fugax. Br Med J 2:164, 1962.
16. Thompson, WG: Proctalgia fugax. Dig Dis Sci 26:1121, 1981.
17. Karras, JD, and Angelo, G: Proctalgia fugax. Am J Surg 82:616, 1951.
18. Ibrahim, H: Proctalgia fugax. Gut 2:137, 1961.
19. Bolen, HL: Spasmodic rectal pain. N Engl J Med 228:564, 1964.
20. Harvey, RF: Colonic motility in proctalgia fugax. Lancet 2:713, 1979.
21. Panitch, NM and Schofferman, JA: Proctalgia fugax revisited. Gastroenterology 68:1061, 1975.
22. Pilling, LF, Swenson, WM and Hill, JR: The psychologic aspects of proctalgia fugax. Dis Colon Rectum 8:372, 1972.

SECTION FIVE

DISORDERS OF FUNCTION

CHAPTER 17

Etiology of Genuine Stress Incontinence

Peggy A. Norton

In the proliferation of literature regarding the evaluation and management of stress urinary incontinence, the etiology of this condition is rarely discussed, because the causative factors have not been clearly defined. In most textbooks, etiology is treated in a single sentence, with references to increased intra-abdominal pressure or childbirth. But how do we explain the tremendous variability seen in response to these factors: the development of stress incontinence in the young nulliparous woman, or the multiparous smoker who remains continent? The etiology of stress incontinence is likely to be multifactorial. *Occasional* stress incontinence appears to be normal in women.[1] Which factors act to exacerbate stress incontinence in women so as to make it a social or hygienic problem for them?

In considering the etiologic factors discussed later in this chapter, the reader should consider the two mechanisms of stress incontinence outlined in Chapter 5. **Bladder-neck hypermobility,** the most common type of stress incontinence in women, results from loss of support by the pelvic floor musculature (which may be caused by muscular or neurologic compromise) and loss of suspension by the pelvic connective tissue in ligaments and fascia. **Intrinsic sphincteric deficiency** arises from loss of the urethral coaption (loss of urethral vasculature, thinning of urethral mucosa, loss of the urethral connective tissue elements, neurologic compromise of the sympathetic smooth muscle, or compromise of the external striated sphincter).

EPIDEMIOLOGY AND POSSIBLE DISEASE MODELS

Although stress incontinence is highly prevalent, surprisingly little research has been undertaken regarding its epidemiology. Several factors might cause stress urinary incontinence, and they may act singly or in combination. Until clinicians clarify the natural history of this condition, it cannot be said whether these factors are predisposing, inciting, or contributing.

Special challenges are present in the consideration of the epidemiology of stress incontinence, one of which is definition. Vigtrup and colleagues[2] reported that 36% of pregnant women in their study experienced stress incontinence, but using the definition of urinary incontinence set forth by the International Continence Society[3] ("loss of urine which is objectively demonstrable and which is a social or hygienic problem"), the prevalence was much lower, only 1.3%. Urinary incontinence is often underreported because of social stigma. This phenomenon has clearly happened in Japanese society, where the problem is underreported but in actuality the prevalence is similar to that in other countries.[4] Researchers who study the family history of incontinence in any culture cannot assume that a mother or grandmother has ever discussed the problem with daughters and granddaughters.

One way to understand the influence of intrinsic and extrinsic factors on disease is to develop a disease model. As risk factors are identified, they must be applied to that disease model. What disease model fits the condition of stress incontinence? One familiar model is that of cancer, in which an inciting factor initiates the process of abnormal growth. Promoting factors then enable these abnormalities to continue to grow. Another possible model is that described by Wilson,[5] whose six principles of teratology might be modified to apply to stress incontinence in this way:

1. Susceptibility to development of stress incontinence depends on the genotype of the individual and the way in which that genotype interacts with the environment.
2. Susceptibility depends on timing of exposure: the postpartum or postmenopause periods may be particularly vulnerable times for patient exposure to exacerbating factors.
3. Factors involved in incontinence act in specific ways (mechanisms) to initiate changes in structures and tissues.
4. The final manifestation of these changes may be structural and functional abnormalities and may produce a spectrum of conditions including genital prolapse, stress incontinence, or anorectal dysfunction.
5. Access of adverse environmental factors to influence disease depends on the nature of that influencing agent: childbirth may initiate changes in many women, whereas work or exercise habits may influence only a few vulnerable women.
6. Manifestations of these changes increase in degree with dosage: with increasing duration or repeated exposure to childbirth, the physician should expect increasing manifestation of the condition.

At present, no disease model for stress incontinence exists. For the purposes of discussion, I will consider risk factors as either *intrinsic or underlying factors* or *extrinsic or environmental factors*. Some factors may have a dual role.

Etiologic factors associated with stress incontinence need substantial clarification supported by conclusive research. It is unfortunate that most of the papers regarding the etiology and risk factors for stress incontinence are retrospective, uncontrolled studies and anecdotal reports. Nevertheless, it is worthwhile to discuss what is known about the possible etiologic factors for stress incontinence to understand more clearly the natural history of this condition. Clinicians await well-designed prospective studies to define the prevalence and risk factors for stress incontinence more clearly.

POSSIBLE INTRINSIC OR UNDERLYING FACTORS

These conditions would predispose a woman to stress incontinence. They would be expected to be heritable, that is, detectable in the family history although with variable penetrance. They would not be expected to be preventable, although their effects potentially could be minimized.

RACE

The role of race is poorly defined. Stress incontinence seems to have a high prevalence in white populations. The prevalence of incontinence seems similar in African-American and white populations in the United States, but there is proportionally more urge incontinence than stress incontinence[6] among African-Americans. Prevalence studies vary greatly because different definitions of incontinence may be used, different age groups may be studied, and cultural differences may affect reporting. Zacharin[7] attempted to measure anatomic differences between Asians and whites that could explain differences in prevalence of stress incontinence. He reported that the fascia of the pelvic structures in cadavers of Chinese women was dense and thick compared with that seen in cadavers of white women.

ANATOMIC DIFFERENCES

Intrinsic anatomic differences have been proposed as one underlying cause of stress incontinence. What is there about the size and shape of the pelvic structures and therefore the levator ani hiatus? DeLancey recorded the anteroposterior diameter of the levator ani hiatus from the pubic symphysis to the perineal body and found that it is greater in women with prolapse and possibly in those with stress incontinence.[8] This effect may, however, result from other factors and may not be predisposing. It is unclear how these anatomic changes might contribute to stress incontinence, but a widened levator ani hiatus may impede pelvic floor closure during times of increased intra-abdominal pressure.

CONNECTIVE TISSUE

Several investigators have studied the role of connective tissue in the etiology of stress incontinence. Keane and colleagues[9] studied nulliparous women with stress incontinence and found an absolute decrease in the total amount of collagen, with a relative increase in the amount of type III collagen. Landon and co-workers[10] found that the rectus fascia of women undergoing surgery for stress incontinence had an absolute decrease in total collagen content compared to continent controls. Kondo and colleagues[11] studied the shear strength of the endopelvic fascia in women undergoing needle procedures for stress incontinence, and found that it was less (weaker) than for continent controls. Norton, Boyd, and Deak[12] did not find abnormal collagen ratios in women with stress incontinence, although the numbers were small. The concept of deficient connective tissue might be one explanation for stress incontinence, but weak pelvic fascia and ligaments might be the result of pelvic floor dysfunction rather than its cause. Based on the work of Paramore[8] and others, DeLancey[8] proposed the model of a boat in drydock to explain the interaction between the pelvic connective tissue suspension and the pelvic floor support. In this model, it may be that the connective tissue (mooring ropes) only fails after the pelvic floor (water) has stopped providing support. The role of connective tissue is most important in bladder-neck hypermobility but also may play a role in urethral mucosa coaption.

NEUROLOGIC ABNORMALITIES

There may be intrinsic conditions that lead to neurologic disorders of the pelvic floor or bladder. One such condition is spina bifida occulta. Because the defect is minimal and affects only the lowest portion of the spinal cord, women with this condition may be asymptomatic for most or all of their lives. The sacral nerve roots may, however, be sufficiently compromised to effect the pelvic floor and bladder. Clinically, these women may be detected as having had a pilonidal cyst, a hairy patch over the sacrum, an odd sacral prominence, or dysmorphic toes (because of the compromise of $S_{2,3,4}$ during development). Occult spinal dysraphism has been associated with detrusor hyperreflexia in several studies.[13] Women with spina bifida present with an open bladder neck and loss of the autonomic adrenergic tone at the level of the bladder neck.[14] The mechanism of stress incontinence in these individuals may represent loss of the external sphincter mechanism.

POSSIBLE EXTRINSIC OR ENVIRONMENTAL FACTORS

Tremendous potential exists for modifying the effects of extrinsic or environmental factors in individuals who are at risk for developing stress incontinence. For example, in these individuals clinicians could focus on improving bowel habits or altering obstetric management.

PREGNANCY AND CHILDBIRTH

Are the processes of pregnancy and delivery two separate processes which act in different ways? Pregnancy may promote stress incontinence in several ways: progesterone relaxation of smooth muscle, changes in connective tissue, pressure of the uterus, and other anatomic changes. Francis[15] reported that in her study of 400 British women, 118 (53%) primigravidae and 150 (85%) multigravidae reported some stress incontinence during pregnancy; however, 49 (42%) of these primiparous women reported occasional loss of urinary control throughout life, similar to the findings of Nemir and Middleton.[1] Stress incontinence may worsen after delivery, but Francis concluded that it rarely appears for the first time after delivery. Surprisingly, Francis found that 90% of women reported dramatic improvement within a few days after delivery, after which they had no incontinence when coughing (38%), whereas 9% continued to be incontinent. The woman who has had stress incontinence before pregnancy is invariably worse during pregnancy, and although it tends to disappear in the puerperium, it recurs with each pregnancy and worsens. Ultimately, it may remain after delivery to become a persistent complaint. Francis concluded that those women who develop stress incontinence in middle age are destined to do so and that pregnancy, rather than parturition, reveals the defect and makes it worse. Allen and co-workers[16] accumulated some compelling evidence that denervation injury to the striated pelvic floor muscles is a major cause of stress incontinence. Recovery occurs in most women within 6 months of delivery, but the damage may be partially cumulative and irreversible. Delivery may cause stress incontinence through denervation (stretch nerve injury), connective tissue injury, or mechanical disruption of muscles and sphincters. The problem of stress incontinence in the nulliparous woman, however, is particularly intriguing. Scott reported that as many as 40% of white nulliparous women have symptoms of stress incontinence.[17]

AGING

The role of aging is intriguing and multifaceted. First, gravity is a constant force whose effects are cumulative over time. Second, subtle but progressive neurologic changes are inevitable results of aging. The loss of estrogen at menopause is an unavoidable fact that may be overcome by estrogen replacement (see discussion later in this chapter). Connective tissue is altered in its cross-linking and reduced elasticity.[18] These factors may affect bladder-neck hypermobility (connective tissue, loss of neuromuscular integrity) and intrinsic sphincteric deficiency (loss of coaption because of reduced urethral vascularity, thinning of urethral mucosa, and again connective tissue alteration and loss of neuromuscular integrity).

HORMONE EFFECTS

Hypoestrogenism is a possible cause of postmenopausal stress incontinence for several reasons. The bladder, urethra, and vagina share a common embryologic source and estrogen receptors are found in the lower urinary tract.[20] Loss of estrogen may affect mucosal coaption of the urethra through decreasing collagen content, decreased vascularity affecting turgor of the surrounding tissues, and thinning of the urethral lining. A recent meta-analysis summarized the effects of estrogen replacement therapy on stress incontinence and found that estrogen subjectively improved stress incontinence in this age group.[21] Many women complain of an exacerbation of their stress incontinence just before menses, which may reflect the smooth-muscle relaxant property of progesterone.

NONOBSTETRIC PELVIC TRAUMA AND RADICAL SURGERY

Trauma to the urethra involving disruption of muscle and nerve is a rare cause of incontinence in women. Benign and radical pelvic surgery may be a more common cause. Women who undergo colpocleisis may develop stress incontinence because the anterior vaginal wall is pulled toward the rectum. One study examined the effect of radical vulvectomy:[22] damage or excision of the distal urethral sphincter was associated with stress incontinence in some women in the absence of bladder-neck hypermobility or intrinsic sphincteric deficiency. Disruption of the terminal autonomic supply and periurethral muscle tone is a well-recognized cause of bladder dysfunction after radical hysterectomy,[23,24] but the usual presentation is urge incontinence.

PULMONARY DISEASE

Conditions exist in which increased intra-abdominal pressure may promote the development of prolapse in women at risk. These conditions include chronic pulmonary diseases such as emphysema, chronic bronchitis, and asthma; ascites or hepatosplenomegaly; and possibly obesity. Smoking is known to be associated with stress urinary incontinence.[25] The effect of smoking may be more than exacerbation through coughing or chronic pulmonary disease; there may also be an effect on the connective tissues of chronic ischemia.

OTHER CONDITIONS OF INCREASED INTRA-ABDOMINAL PRESSURE

Chronic straining or lifting may alter pelvic connective tissue or promote pelvic floor denervation through stretch nerve injury. Women who chronically strain at bowel movements seem especially at risk.[26,27] It has been suggested that the lower rate of prevalence of bowel and pelvic floor dysfunction seen in Asian women may be due to the crouching position used by them for defecation. Equally, exercise patterns involving increased intra-abdominal pressure may contribute to an exacerbation of connective tissue injury or pelvic floor denervation.[28] Although women may have achieved work equity in jobs traditionally held by men, they may be expected to lift excessively heavy loads to the possible detriment of the pelvic floor. Literature is conflicting regarding the role of obesity in stress incontinence, although one study has suggested that weight loss improves the condition in the morbidly obese individual.[29]

DRUG EFFECTS

Medications play a role in the etiology of stress incontinence, perhaps especially in women with an underlying risk factor. Some women taking alpha-blocking agents develop stress incontinence.[30] These women may have an underlying risk factor, and the inhibition of alpha-receptors in the urethral smooth musculature further decompensates the continence mechanism.

SUMMARY

Many factors presented here as extrinsic or exacerbating factors may also play a role as intrinsic or underlying factors. Stress incontinence is likely to be multifactorial, and the interplay between these factors produces the different clinical types of stress incontinence, whether hypermobile, intrinsic sphincteric, or combined. Further prospective studies may describe the factors that place women at risk for stress incontinence, and help clinicians to prevent or ameliorate the condition.

REFERENCES

1. Nemir, A and Middleton, R: Stress incontinence in young nulliparous women. Am J Obstet Gynecol 68:1166, 1954.
2. Vigtrup, L, Lose, G, Rolff, M and Barfoed, K: The symptom of stress incontinence caused by pregnancy or delivery in primiparas. Obstet Gynecol 79:945, 1992.
3. Abrams, P, Blaivas, J, Stanton, S and Andersen, J: The standardization of terminology of lower urinary tract function. Scand J Urol Nephrol 114(suppl):5, 1988.
4. Kato, K, Dondo, A, Okamura, K and Takaba, H: Prevalence of urinary incontinence in working women. Nippon Hinyokika Gakkai Zassh 77:1501, 1986.
5. Wilson, J: Current status of teratology—General principles and mechanisms derived from animal studies. In Wilson, J and Fra-

ser, F (eds.): Handbook of Teratology. Plenum Press, New York, 1977.

6. Bump, R: Racial comparison in urinary incontinence and genital prolapse. Int J Obstet Gynecol 3:267, 1992.
7. Zacharin, RF: A "Chinese anatomy": The pelvic supporting tissues of the Chinese and Occidental female compared and contrasted. Aust N Z J Obstet Gynecol. 17:1, 1977.
8. DeLancey, J: Anatomy and biomechanics of genital prolapse. In DeLancey J (ed.): Pelvic Organ Prolapse: Clinical Management and Scientific Foundations. Clin Obstet Gynecol 36:897, 1992.
9. Keane, D, Sims, T, Bailey, A and Abrams, P: Analysis of pelvic floor electromyography and collagen status in pre-menopausal nulliparous females with genuine stress incontinence. Neurol Urodyn 11:308, 1992.
10. Landon, C, Smith, A, Crofts, C, et al: Biomechanical properties of connective tissue in women with stress incontinence of urine. Neurol Urodyn 8:369, 1989.
11. Kondo, A: Shear strength of the anterior vaginal wall and the rectus fascia: Comparison between women with stress incontinence and those with continence. Neuro Urodyn (in press).
12. Norton, P, Boyd, C and Deak, S: Collagen synthesis in women with genital prolapse or stress urinary incontinence. Neurol Urodyn 11:3, 1992.
13. Khoury, A, Hendrick, B, McLorie, G, et al: Occult spinal dysraphism: Clinical and urodynamic outcome after division of the filum terminale. J Urol 144:425, 1990.
14. Anderson, R: A neurogenic element to urinary genuine stress incontinence. Br J Obstet Gynaecol 91:412, 1984.
15. Francis, WJ: The onset of stress incontinence. J Obstet Gynecol Br Emp 67:899, 1960.
16. Allen, R, Hosker, G, Smith, A and Warrell, D: Pelvic floor damage and childbirth: A neurophysiological study. Br J Obstet Gynaecol 97:770, 1990.
17. Scott, JC: Stress incontinence in nulliparous women. J Reprod Med 2:96, 1969.
18. Norton, P: Histological and biochemical studies. In Benson, T (ed): Female Pelvic Floor Disorders. Norton, New York, 1992.
19. Iosif, C, Batra, S, Ek, A, et al: Estrogen receptors in the human female lower urinary tract. Am J Obstet Gynecol 141:817, 1981.
20. Zuckerman, S: Morphologic and functional homologics of the male and female reproductive systems. Br Med J 2:864, 1936.
21. Fantl, JA, Cardozo, L and McClish, D: Estrogen therapy in the management of urinary incontinence in postmenopausal women: A meta-analysis. Obstet Gynecol 83:12, 1994.
22. Reid, G, DeLancey, J, Hopkins, M, et al: Urinary incontinence following radical vulvectomy. Obstet Gynecol 75:852, 1990.
23. Seski, J and Diokno, A: Bladder dysfunction after radical abdominal hysterectomy. Am J Obstet Gynecol 128:643, 1977.
24. Scotti, R, Bergman, A, Bhatia, N and Ostergard, D: Urodynamic changes in urethrovesical function after radical hysterectomy. Obstet Gynecol 68:111, 1986.
25. Bump, R and McClish, D: Cigarette smoking and pure genuine stress incontinence of urine: A comparison of risk factors and determinants between smokers and nonsmokers. Am J Obstet Gynecol 170:579–582, 1994.
26. Jones, P, Lubowski, D, Swash, M and Henry, M: Relation between perineal descent and pudendal nerve damage in idiopathic faecal incontinence. Int J Colorectal Dis 2:93, 1987.
27. Henry, M, Parks, A and Swash, M: The pelvic floor musculature in the descending perineum syndrome. Br J Surg 69:470, 1982.
28. Nygaard, I, DeLancey, J, Arnsdorf, L and Murphy, A: Exercise and incontinence. Obstet Gynecol 75:848, 1990.
29. Bump, R, Sugarman, H, Fantl, J and McClish, D: Obesity and lower urinary tract function in women: Effect of surgically induced weight loss. Am J Obstet Gynecol 167:392, 1992.
30. Wall, L and Addison, W: Prazosin-induced stress incontinence. Obstet Gynecol 75:558, 1990.

CHAPTER **18**

Nonsurgical Management of Urinary Incontinence

S. Renee Edwards • Linda T. Brubaker

Urinary incontinence is not an all-or-none phenomenon. Many women do not require surgical management of their incontinence. A significant minority of subjectively incontinent women leak urine only under particular circumstances. Another significant minority acknowledges urinary incontinence, but do not feel that it has any adverse impact on their quality of life. Yet another group of women has symptoms or disorders that are not amenable to surgical correction. Finally, surgery to cure urinary incontinence may be unsuccessful or may cause new symptoms. For such women, nonsurgical therapies offer important options for management and treatment of urinary incontinence.

Nonsurgical therapy is readily adopted by healthcare providers who are not trained in the surgical disciplines. Surgical specialists, however, have been slower to adopt the safe, minimally invasive techniques described in this chapter. It is clear that surgical correction of genuine stress incontinence has a higher "cure" rate than simple interventions, but it is also evident that surgical corrections have significantly higher morbidity and cost. The definition of "cure" must include the undesired consequences of the intervention, such as the development of new symptoms.

Many women with urinary incontinence benefit from simpler interventions. The astute clinician should develop skills to identify such opportunities for intervention, which are frequently ascertained during the history and physical examination, as well as during both simple and complex testing. Most patients with urinary incontinence have developed significant awareness of which activities or levels of fluid intake exacerbate their symptoms. During the history, it is frequently helpful to ask which, if any, activities have been reduced or eliminated due to leakage. For example, the competitive tennis player who leaks only when she hits a forceful backhand during the third set of a very difficult game probably does not need "correction" 100% of the time. Simple intravaginal devices may suffice. Alternatively, the woman with mild cognitive impairment and severe urge incontinence may benefit from systemic medication combined with behavioral modifications.

This chapter reviews environmental, behavioral, and muscular changes that may improve urinary control, as well as therapeutic vaginal devices and pharmacologic interventions.

ENVIRONMENTAL INTERVENTIONS

It is not unusual to hear a history of minor incontinence that becomes increasingly more troublesome over a decade. Such a history should raise the physician's awareness that marginally adequate urinary control may be challenged by environmental or functional factors. Many times, patients report slower ambulation and more difficulty with stairs and with fine motor movements, such as those necessary for unfastening clothing. Additionally, impaired vision, including night vision, may make it difficult for the patient to find the toilet in time to prevent unintended urine loss. Several simple interventions may decrease the frequency of "en route" leakage episodes for an individual patient. Women who are awakened from their sleep with a strong urge to urinate, but are not yet actually wet, may have fewer "en route" leakage episodes if the distance to the toilet can be decreased. Some older patients may have slept in the same bedroom for many years. When their urinary control was better, they could awake, go down the hall (or down the stairs) and find the washroom in time. Their lower urinary tract function, however, now no longer allows sufficient time for them to get to that same washroom. Fortunately, some of these patients have an option of moving to a closer bedroom. Others may benefit from a bedside commode or a female urinal (Fig. 18–1). The female urinal is particularly helpful for patients who are able to swing their legs out of bed, but who begin to leak after standing.

Grab bars on the walls and nonskid flooring allow patients to approach the toilet (or commode) confidently, without fear of falling. Easy-to-release clothing facilitates timely voiding. Finally, a toilet seat of appropriate height is critical. Older women may have difficulty sitting on and rising from seats that are too low. Finally, women with difficulty seeing in the dark may benefit from a small night light or series of lights, which can guide them to the washroom.

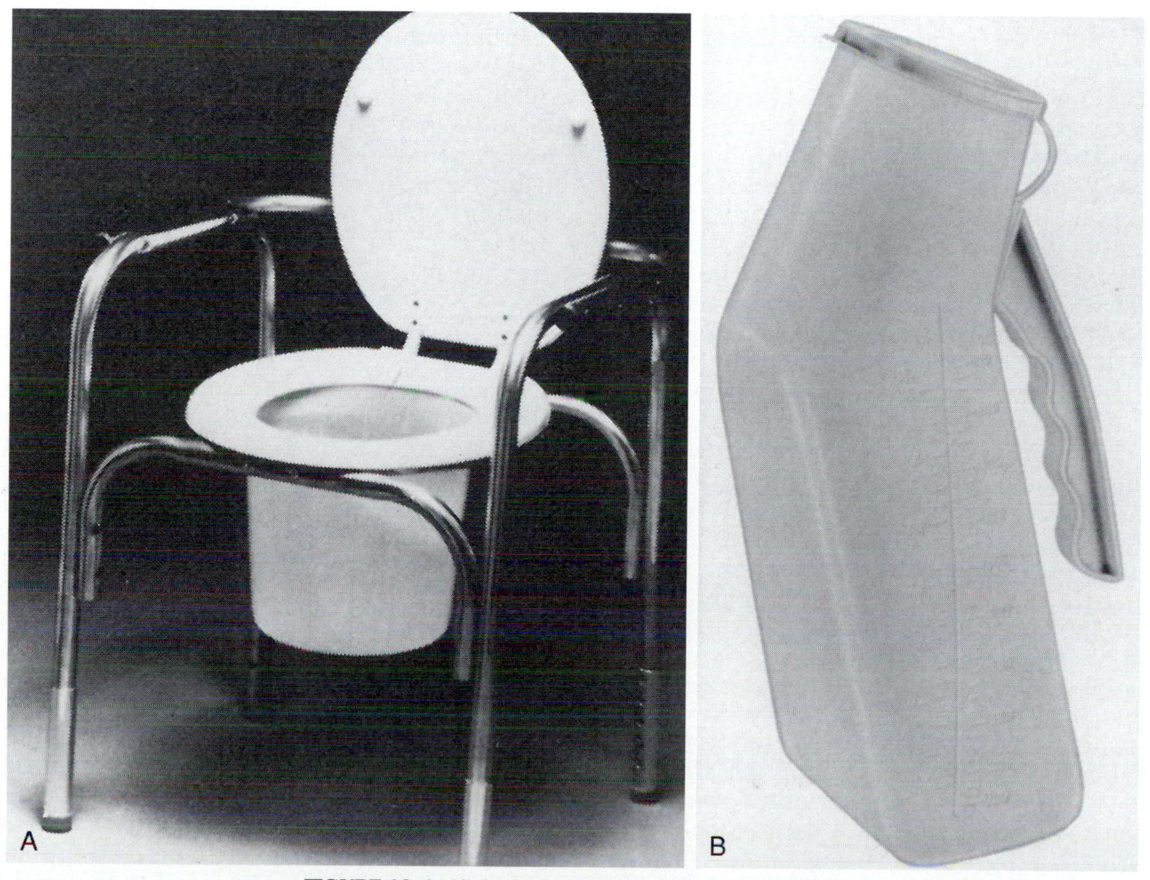

FIGURE 18–1. (*A*) bedside commode; (*B*) female urinal.

BEHAVIORAL INTERVENTIONS

A multitude of behavioral interventions have been described for treatment of urinary incontinence. Although in general these regimens are significantly less efficacious than surgery, they are a first line of therapy for treatment of urinary incontinence because of their low morbidity rates and cost.

TIMED VOIDING REGIMENS

Timed voiding regimens are helpful in women with urge incontinence due to detrusor overactivity. This technique is also useful in certain women with stress incontinence. Timed voiding separates the perception of the need to void from the act of voiding. Fortunately, most patients have a proprioceptive threshold which indicates an upcoming leakage episode. This information can frequently be obtained during the history. Specific questions regarding the consequences of delay may elicit helpful comments such as "If I get an urge and don't answer it right away, I will leak." Keeping a "voiding diary" can indicate the volume that is associated with this urge, although some variation in this volume is typical. Volumes beyond this range tend to be associated with leakage. This can be further corroborated during cystometry when the patient reports her sense of "first urge to void." If additional filling can be continued only briefly, the patient has a very short time before leakage. Alternatively, some patients can delay and tolerate more filling before leakage or detrusor overactivity.

Timed voiding is initiated after an appropriate evaluation as described in Chapter 5. A mutually acceptable voiding interval is selected, typically between 30 minutes and 2 hours. Recommendations can be made after reviewing the voiding diary and verbal history. The patient is then instructed to void "by the clock" and not by her intuition. The patient must be initially successful with this regimen—typically, encouragement is needed. This can be provided with telephone follow-up, if necessary. Those patients with minimal interval between their first urge and the onset of leakage may initially require low-dose systemic medication. The initial interval can be increased (typically at 30-minute increments) approximately every 2 weeks. A voiding diary should be kept to measure progress.

Patients frequently ask two questions:

1. "What if I really have to go 'before my time?'" They should be instructed to use mental distraction techniques and pelvic floor contractions (if they are performed correctly).
2. "What if I don't have to go at the scheduled time?" Patients should be instructed to sit comfortably on the toilet and simply let any accumulated urine flow. It is important, however, not to push urine out without a natural inclination to urinate.

Although timed voiding can be taught by nonphysicians, the physician is cautioned against sending verbal or nonverbal negative signals to the patient, as if implying that timed voiding is a "lesser treatment" or "not really a doctor's job." The physician caregiver is advised to provide the same focus and follow-up as for surgical therapy. Patients must observe the physician's review of any diaries that are brought to the office. A helpful publication is *Staying Dry* by Burgio, Pearce, and Lucco,[1] which reviews this technique in detail and serves to reinforce verbal instructions.

Many variations of this technique have been described. Success rates of approximately 60% are reported. Although the placebo response rate is not known, it may be significant. Given the low morbidity rate and the safety of this technique, however, it continues to be an important first-line therapy for many women with urinary incontinence.

Timed voiding may be useful in long-term–care settings with cognitively impaired residents. Rather than providing flexible intervals, a fixed interval, typically 2 hours, is selected and implemented. Caretakers are encouraged to provide scheduled trips to the toilet every 2 hours during waking hours. Although typically they may resist this "additional work," very quickly it becomes apparent that regular visits to the toilet require less work than cleaning the clothing and body of an incontinent adult. Many of these patients may require wetness protection during sleep, but their perineal skin and general dignity can be preserved during waking hours.

Prompted voiding is a variation of timed voiding that is appropriate for residents with little or no cognitive impairment. Such residents can be "prompted" to go every 2 hours, with a sincere, cheerful offer to assist the resident to the washroom if desired. Certainly reversible causes of urinary incontinence, such as fecal impaction, infection, or delirium should be treated before initiating timed voiding for urge incontinence.

OTHER BEHAVIORAL TECHNIQUES

Other behavioral techniques improve the woman's ability to inhibit her leakage by using pelvic floor muscle contractions. Simple techniques, such as postural changes,[2] have proven beneficial. Many patients acknowledge changes of position such as these. Additionally, biofeedback techniques and pelvic muscle exercises can strengthen the pelvic floor. These are described in detail in Chapter 29. Many times, simple discussion of a strategy for preventing leakage will help. It is not uncommon for patients to report that when they sense an urge to urinate, their initial action is to move immediately toward the nearest toilet. If an inappropriate bladder contraction is occurring, however, the patient is now increasing abdominal pressure, which may make it difficult to avoid leakage. It is useful to counsel the patient to contract the pelvic floor muscles strongly until the greatest urge has passed and then to proceed to the washroom in a controlled fashion. If the urge recurs, she should again stop and strongly control the pelvic floor, thus extinguishing inappropriate bladder contraction. This rudimentary scheme relies on good pelvic floor strength.

DEVICES

INTRAVAGINAL DEVICES

Various intravaginal devices are useful to limit urinary leakage. Patients must be credited with the discovery that one or two tampons in the vagina may reduce stress leakage. This has been confirmed in a well-designed study by Nygaard.[3] Although vaginal diaphragms and vaginal pessaries have been credited with preventing urine loss, no published scientific study has validated it. Anecdotal evidence suggests that in women with minimal to moderate prolapse of the anterior vaginal wall, bladder neck support may be augmented and leakage may be reduced with pessaries. Women with severe prolapse, however, tend to be continent with unreduced prolapse. Replacement of the prolapse with a pessary commonly unmasks the incontinence. It is reasonable to try simple placement of vaginal devices for women with episodic leakage, particularly women who are agile enough to remove and replace the device easily as needed.

CONTINENCE RINGS

Modified pessary-like devices have also been reported. The bladder neck support prosthesis (Fig. 18–2) is a ring with two prongs which selectively elevate the bladder neck.[4] Continence rings are supplied by several U.S. manufacturers. No published studies exist regarding their efficacy. The type of continence ring with an inflatable suburethral balloon

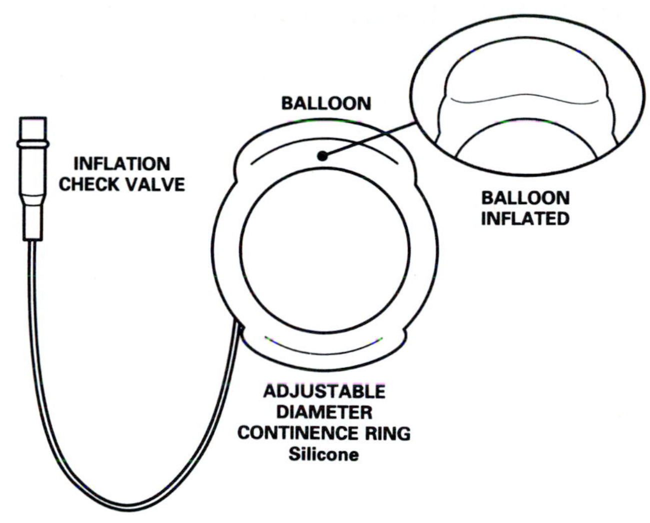

FIGURE 18–3. Continence ring with inflatable suburethral balloon (Cook's continence ring).

(Fig. 18–3) relies on compression of the urethral tissues to prevent leakage. A small, unpublished series did not find this continence ring to be effective when tested urodynamically, however. Unfortunately, the suburethral balloon causes the device to move away from the urethra and leakage continues unchanged. The "firm" incontinence ring (Fig. 18–4) appears more successful. This can be retained by women with mild to moderate anterior wall prolapse. When evaluated urodynamically, this ring appears able to prevent urine loss without adversely impacting voiding function.[5]

EXTERNAL COLLECTING DEVICES

Until recently, external collecting devices for female urinary loss have been unsatisfactory. However,

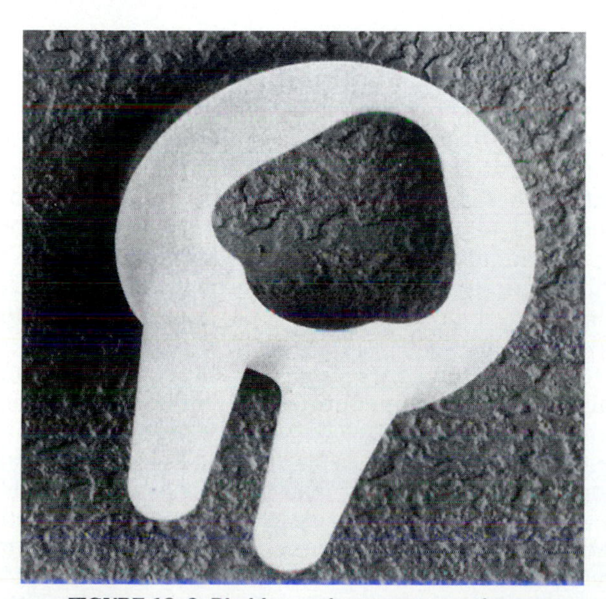

FIGURE 18–2. Bladder neck support prosthesis.

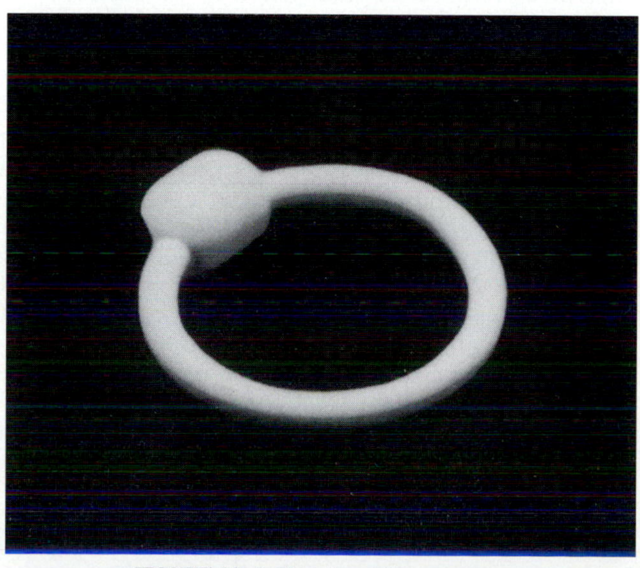

FIGURE 18–4. Firm incontinence ring.

a clever external device recently has been introduced. This is a small, triangular device which is secured to the external tissues over the urethral meatus with a hydrophilic gel. This gel allows easy attachment and removal for normal voiding. The miniguard prevents urine leakage associated with mild to moderate stress incontinence, but cannot hold back large volume urine loss such as that associated with detrusor overactivity or normal voiding.[6]

ELECTRICAL STIMULATION

For approximately 30 years, electrical stimulation has been used to treat urinary incontinence. Although the mechanism of action is not completely understood, two significant mechanisms seem to exist. Electrical stimulations can neurally inhibit inappropriate detrusor contractions through an intact neural pathway. This is the rationale for clinical treatment of detrusor overactivity. Additionally, electrical stimulation of neurally intact muscle can cause hypertrophy of that muscle. Muscle hypertrophy allows strength to be added to the pelvic floor muscles. Pelvic floor strength is associated with decreased leakage due to stress incontinence and an increased ability to inhibit inappropriate detrusor contractions.

At present, the most common form of electrical stimulation for urinary incontinence is transvaginal stimulation. Treatments may be administered with small home devices or larger office units. Typically, a single-patient probe is inserted to an appropriate vaginal depth and current is delivered to the pelvic floor innervation. Although efficacy of transvaginal electrical stimulation for treatment of urinary incontinence is unknown, uncontrolled studies suggest an improvement rate of approximately 60%.[7–9] Ongoing controlled clinical trials will soon determine efficacy levels and placebo response rates.

Transvaginal electrical stimulation is easily initiated in women with urinary incontinence due to genuine stress incontinence, detrusor overactivity, or both. Patients must have intact sacral reflexes, because the neural tissue is stimulated, rather than the muscle itself. There are only a few contraindications to electrical stimulation. Patients with perineal sensory deficits should not be treated until the cause of the sensory abnormality is understood. Such patients may sustain electrical burns if the stimulating electrodes come into contact with the delicate vulvar tissues. Women with cardiac pacemakers (or any other electrical pacing device) are theoretically at risk for inappropriate electrical loops and should not use an intravaginal stimulator. Anecdotal reports exist of such patients using stimulators, but they have been cautiously approached with simultaneous cardiac monitoring. Finally, patients who are reluctant to touch their vulvovaginal tissues and women uncomfortable with electrical implements are poor candidates for these devices.

Electrical stimulator devices vary in their electrical parameters. Unfortunately, little scientific theory guides the relatively empiric use of these settings. Frequencies generally range between 12 and 50 Hz. In general, lower stimulation frequenies are believed to inhibit inappropriate detrusor contractions, whereas higher frequencies are considered appropriate for muscle hypertrophy. Likewise, the rest-work cycle is empiric. Animal studies show that implanted, continuous electrical stimulation of a muscle slowly convert type-2 fibers to the "slower" type-1 fibers.[10] In addition, muscle hypertrophy has been demonstrated in dogs.[11] These physiologic changes have not been equated with strength or reduced clinical leakage, however.

The amount of stimulation necessary for a clinical response is not known. Chronic stimulation with indwelling vaginal devices has been used in European countries. Intermittent stimulation is more common in North America, most often on a schedule of once or twice daily as a 15-minute session for a period of 6 to 12 weeks. These recommendations are quite empiric, however. The literature and clinical observations suggest that suppression of detrusor overactivity occurs within days to weeks, whereas muscle hypertrophy occurs over a longer time.

Electrical stimulation therapy can be continued indefinitely, if desired. If clinical stress incontinence is being treated, however, additional exercises will be necessary to build strength in the pelvic floor muscles. As discussed in Chapter 29, a variety of techniques are available for strength building, some of which are less expensive than long-term electrical stimulation. Alternatively, a significant minority of women seeking treatment for pure or predominant detrusor overactivity report continued remission of symptoms following successful electrical stimulation. The reasons for these clinical observations await scientific study.

PHARMACOLOGIC INTERVENTIONS

The threshold for prescribing systemic medication for treatment of urinary incontinence varies widely among caregivers. The main advantage of drug therapy is that the effects (and side effects) of medication can be assessed quickly. On the other hand, if clinically effective, pharmacotherapy is usually life-long and adds yet another drug to the growing list already so commonly prescribed for elderly patients. It is, therefore, prudent to use the techniques previously discussed before therapy with medications whenever possible.

Unfortunately, there is no therapeutic agent specific for urinary incontinence. The pharmacologic goals of drug therapy are to decrease inappropriate detrusor contractions, to increase urethral resistance, or both. Detrusor contractions are mediated by the autonomic nervous system. Sympathetic stimulation causes bladder contractions, whereas parasympathetic stimulation causes detrusor relaxation. Several classes of drugs, including anticholinergics,

TABLE 18–1. Anticholinergic Medications Prescribed to Reduce Bladder Contractions

Drug	Common Dosage Regimens
Propantheline bromide	15–30 mg b.i.d. or q.i.d.
Hyoscyamine sulfate	0.125 mg q.i.d.
extended release form	0.375 mg b.i.d.
Methantheline bromide	50 mg q.i.d.

antispasmodics, tricyclic antidepressants, and calcium channel blockers, are able to reduce bladder contractions. Anticholinergic medications are most frequently prescribed. Common preparations are listed in Table 18–1. Contraindications to anticholinergic use are important to know. Narrow-angle glaucoma is an absolute contraindication, whereas patients with wide (open) angle glaucoma may receive this medication. A quick physical test to ensure that a patient does not have narrow-angle glaucoma is to hold a penlight lateral to the eye. If the light shines on the lateral nose, they are unlikely to have significant narrow-angle glaucoma. Another relative contraindication is significant constipation, which will invariably worsen.

Anticholinergic medications commonly have side effects, as noted in Table 18–2. Typically, patients are bothered by a dry mouth. With foreknowledge of this side effect and management with sugarless hard candy, most patients are able to tolerate this annoyance. If an effective dose of anticholinergic medication is found, urinary retention should be searched for, because it may be silent. Postvoid residual urine volumes should be periodically assessed.

Initial dosages of anticholinergics should be small to ensure that the patient does not have marked side effects. It is prudent to increase the dosage of medication slowly every several weeks, assessing efficacy and side effects frequently, until a clinically appropriate dosage has been determined.

Antispasmodic agents have also been used to reduce the abnormal activity of the detrusor muscle. Common preparations are listed in Table 18–3. They have the same side effects as the anticholinergic medications.

Imipramine (Tofranil) is a tricyclic antidepressant with both anticholinergic and alpha-agonist properties. It has been used most commonly for urge incontinence but also may have efficacy in stress incontinence. It should be used with caution in elderly patients due to its side effects of orthostatic hypotension and cardiac arrhythmia. Dosage is 25 to 50 mg once to twice a day.

TABLE 18–2. Common Side Effects of Anticholinergics

Dry mouth
Constipation
Blurry vision
Tachycardia
Urinary retention
Confusion

TABLE 18–3. Antispasmodic Medications

Drug	Common Dosage Regimens
Oxybutynin chloride	2.5–10 mg t.i.d.
Dicyclomine hydrochloride	20 mg t.i.d.
Flavoxate hydrochloride	200 mg q.i.d.

Alpha stimulants are believed to stimulate alpha receptors in the female urethra. Although these receptors have not been demonstrated in human female urethral tissue, human male and animal data suggest that theoretically these medications may be useful. Drugs such as phenylpropanolamine and ephedrine may provide a minor degree of increased urethral tone. This class of medication has been studied in a randomized, cross-over study. A study of postmenopausal women by Ahlstrom and colleagues[12] suggested that although this class of drug is minimally effective if given alone, it becomes more effective if given with estrogen.

The role of estrogen in the treatment of urinary incontinence remains controversial. However, it is frequently an initial intervention because of the common clinical experience that estrogenized lower urinary tract tissues are less friable and less prone to irritative symptoms. From a recent literature review, Fantl and co-workers[13] concluded that estrogen has a limited but probably beneficial effect on lower urinary tract function.

Although other classes of drugs have been suggested as treatment for urinary incontinence, good evidence for their efficacy is lacking and such medications should be considered experimental for treatment of urinary incontinence.

SUMMARY

Many women with urinary incontinence may be significantly helped by nonsurgical therapies, either alone or in combination with a surgical treatment. It is not unusual for a woman to benefit from more than one nonsurgical therapy, such as timed voiding as well as low-dose anticholinergic medication. Conscientious listening and keen diagnostic skills can alert the clinician to many of the patients who may benefit from these techniques. Additionally, when surgery provides a suboptimal outcome, these nonsurgical options may offer additional improvement for the incontinent woman.

REFERENCES

1. Burgio, KL, Pearce, KL and Lucco, AJ: Staying Dry: A Practical Guide to Bladder Control. Johns Hopkins University Press, Baltimore, 1990.

2. Norton, P and Baker, J: Postural changes can reduce leakage in women with stress urinary incontinence. Obstet Gynecol 84:770–774,1994.
3. Nygaard, I: Treatment of exercise incontinence with mechanical devices. Int Urogynecol J 3:268,1992.
4. Davila, GW and Ostermann, KV: The bladder neck support prosthesis: a nonsurgical approach to stress incontinence in the adult woman. Am J Obstet Gynecol 171:206–211,1994.
5. Brubaker, LT: unpublished dissertation.
6. Harris, T: External urethral barrier for urinary stress incontinence: A multicenter trial. Int Urogynecol J 6:377,1994.
7. Fall, M and Lindstrom, S: Electrical stimulation: A physiologic approach to the treatment of urinary incontinence. 18:383–407,1991.
8. Kralj, B: The treatment of female urinary incontinence by functional electrical stimulation. In: Ostergard, DR and Bent, AE (eds.): Urogynecology and Urodynamics, ed 3. Williams & Wilkins, Baltimore, 1991, pp 508–517.
9. Plevnik, S, Janez, J and Vodusek, DB: Electrical stimulation. In Krane, RJ and Siroky, MD (eds.): Clinical Neuro-urology, ed 2. Little, Brown & Co., Boston, 1991, pp 559–571.
10. Russell, B, Wenderoth, MP, Goldspink, PH, et al: Remodeling of myofibrils: subcellular myosin chain protein and RNA distribution. Am J Physiol 262:Reg Int Comp Physiol 31:R339–R345,1992a.
11. Bazeed, MA: Effect of chronic stimulation of the sacral roots on the striated urethral sphincter. J Urol 128:1357–1362,1982.
12. Ahlstrom, K, Sandahl, B, Sjoberg, B, et al: Effect of combined treatment with phenylpropanolamine and estriol, compared with estriol treatment alone, in postmenopausal women with stress urinary incontinence. Gynecol Obstet Invest 30:37–43,1990.
13. Fantl, JA, Cardozo, L, McClish, DK, et al; Estrogen therapy in the management of urinary incontinence in postmenopausal women: A meta-analysis. First Report of the Hormones and Urogenital Therapy Committee. Obstet Gynecol 83:12–18,1994.

CHAPTER 19

Genuine Stress Incontinence: Traditional Surgical Management

W. Glenn Hurt

Surgical treatment of genuine stress incontinence dates from the early twentieth century, when periurethral slings were fashioned from various muscles and fascia.[1–6] A wide variety of natural and synthetic materials have been used to create periurethral slings. More recently, the length of the sling has been reduced by some surgeons to a mere suburethral patch, using many of the same materials or buried portions of the anterior vaginal wall.[7] These patches are suspended from their corners by permanent sutures to the fascia of the anterior abdominal wall.

In the same era, others treated urinary incontinence by suturing the anterior vaginal wall or other tissues at the neck of the bladder.[8–10] In 1949, Marshall, Marchetti, and Krantz[11] shifted emphasis from the more popular vaginal surgical approach to the abdominal surgical approach by their description of an abdominal retropubic urethropexy. Their procedure was equally suitable for the treatment of primary, persistent, or recurrent stress urinary incontinence. The Marshall-Marchetti-Krantz procedure or one of its modifications, principally Burch's procedure[12] as described in 1961, is now considered by many to be the standard criterion for measuring the success of other operations for treating anatomic stress urinary incontinence.

Using the principles of treatment common to sling and abdominal retropubic urethropexy procedures, in 1959 Pereyra[13] described the first transvaginal retropubic "needle" urethropexy. He and others subsequently improved upon this procedure, which has now become successful and very popular.

Over 150 different surgical procedures have been described for the treatment of genuine stress incontinence; modifications continue to be developed. The large number of differing procedures indicates that no single type of procedure will cure all patients. Surgeons who operate to cure genuine stress incontinence must be adept in using several different procedures. Based on the clinical findings in each individual patient, the surgeon must select the procedure or combination of procedures that will be most likely to cure the condition.

As a rule, the first surgical procedure performed is most likely to cure a patient's incontinence and have the fewest complications. Failure rates of subsequent procedures rise in proportion to the number of repeated procedures. For this reason, a thorough preoperative evaluation is mandatory, with attention to preoperative care and selection of the best procedure, which should be carefully executed. Postoperative care should be directed toward minimizing complications and ensuring the long-term success of the operation.

GOALS OF SURGICAL MANAGEMENT

From a surgical standpoint, two types of genuine stress incontinence exist. Anatomic genuine stress incontinence is due to hypermobility of an otherwise adequate urethral sphincteric mechanism. It is treated surgically by elevation and stabilization of the urethrovesical junction. Genuine stress incontinence may also be due to urethral sphincter dysfunction resulting from a damaged sphincteric mechanism. This type of stress incontinence is treated surgically by compression and coaptation of the damaged sphincteric mechanism.

Fortunately, most pure genuine stress incontinence is of the anatomic type. The goals of surgical management for anatomic stress urinary incontinence are:

1. To elevate and maintain the proximal urethra and urethrovesical junction in a retropubic position during sudden increases in intra-abdominal pressure.
2. To allow posterior rotational descent of the trigone and base of the bladder during sudden increases in intra-abdominal pressure.
3. To preserve compressibility of the urethra.
4. To preserve integrity of the urethral sphincter mechanism.

Genuine stress incontinence due to urethral sphincter dysfunction usually results from previous surgical attempts to cure urinary incontinence. Surgical management of this kind of genuine stress incontinence aims either to increase the resistance of the outflow tract with relief of the resistance in order to void, or to divert the urinary flow.

SELECTION OF OPERATIVE PROCEDURE

If the patient's genuine stress incontinence is caused by a significant cystourethrocele, an operation that successfully corrects the cystourethrocele may correct the incontinence. A suburethral plication or anterior colporrhaphy of the Kelly[9] or Kelly-Kennedy[10] type is still performed frequently as the initial procedure for the treatment of stress urinary incontinence. As routinely performed, however, these operations, as well as paravaginal repair,[14] are limited in the degree to which they elevate the urethrovesical junction. To overcome this deficiency, some surgeons have modified their anterior colporrhaphy so that it has become basically a vaginal retropubic urethropexy.[15] Others have augmented their abdominal paravaginal repairs with sutures suspending the urethrovesical junction bilaterally to the iliopectineal (Cooper's) ligaments.[16] Anterior colporrhaphy and paravaginal repair procedures are primarily designed to correct a cystourethrocele, which should be the primary indication for their use unless future clinical trials support use of these procedures for treatment of stress urinary incontinence.

Surgical literature reveals that the operative procedure most likely to cure purely anatomically-derived genuine stress incontinence, whether primary, persistent, or recurrent, is an abdominal retropubic urethropexy with colposuspension of the Marshall-Marchetti-Krantz or Burch type. These procedures are most successful in patients with hypermobility of the urethrovesical junction, when vaginal tissues are of good quality, and when vaginal caliber and depth are adequate.

Although the outcome of abdominal retropubic urethropexy and colposuspension is considered the standard criterion by which the results of other operative procedures are measured, in some circumstances other procedures to regain incontinence should be used. For instance, with significant pelvic organ prolapse when the surgeon wishes to use a vaginal reconstructive procedure, a vaginal "needle" urethropexy and colposuspension of the modified Pereyra or Raz type is a reasonable alternative that may produce a comparable rate of cure in selected patients. As with abdominal retropubic procedures, these operations are most successful when vaginal tissues are of good quality, when hypermobility of the urethrovesical junction is present, and when the vagina is, or can be made to be, of adequate caliber and depth. I prefer to use one of the "needle" procedures if there is significant pelvic organ prolapse with "occult" or clinically significant stress urinary incontinence.

Suburethral sling operations are highly successful in curing genuine stress incontinence but are associated with significant postoperative complications and voiding difficulties.[17] For this reason, many surgeons reserve them for women with persistent or recurrent genuine stress incontinence, and for those with urethral sphincter dysfunction. Recent modifications in the sling procedures have reduced the incidence of these problems, however, so that some surgeons are using them to treat patients with primary and uncomplicated genuine stress incontinence. I prefer to reserve the suburethral sling procedure for women with scarred, foreshortened, and somewhat immobile vaginas; those with a low-pressure, immobile urethra; or those with a damaged urethral sphincter mechanism.

PREOPERATIVE CARE

Preoperative evaluation of women with urinary incontinence must be sufficiently detailed to determine precisely its cause or causes. As a minimum requirement, women who have never had surgery for urinary incontinence need the following:

- A diary to document the severity of the urinary condition
- A general history and physical examination
- A neurologic examination
- A detailed pelvic examination
- Determination of postvoid urinary residual
- A urine test for infection, documenting sterile urine
- Assessment of urethrovesical junction mobility
- Visualization of the involuntary loss of a spurt of urine from the external urethral meatus at the acme of stress caused by the Valsalva maneuver (i.e., cough)
- Cystometry to rule out detrusor instability and to determine bladder capacity.

If, based on such an evaluation, the incontinence is determined to be genuine stress incontinence, if there is hypermobility of the urethrovesical junction, and if the patient's symptoms warrant surgery, it is reasonable to schedule surgery when her general medical condition is optimum.

Patients who have persistent or recurrent urinary incontinence following surgery to correct the problem are better served by having an in-depth evaluation, which might include multichannel subtracted urethrocystometry, urethroscopy, imaging studies, and consultation with a urogynecologist.

In the past, many physicians have used evidence of pelvic organ prolapse, rather than the demonstration of urinary leakage, to diagnose genuine stress incontinence. Although the two conditions commonly coexist, they should be thought of, and treated as, separate entities. When stress testing is undertaken to demonstrate genuine stress incontinence, a pelvic examination should be made to determine if there is any pelvic organ prolapse with the patient in the lithotomy, sitting, and standing positions. If prolapse is found, then other weaknesses within the pelvic support system should also be corrected when operating for genuine stress incontinence. All too often, a patient who is cured of her anatomic genuine stress incontinence by elevation and stabilization of the urethrovesical junction then develops a symptomatic cystocele, uterovaginal prolapse, vaginal vault prolapse, enterocele, or rectocele that requires a subsequent operation.

In general, all continence surgery should be deferred until childbearing has been completed. Hypoestrogenic patients should receive an appropriate regimen of estrogen replacement therapy to improve the integrity of their pelvic tissues, unless some contraindication to its use exists. Women should schedule continence surgery at a time that will permit a period of postoperative convalescence and pelvic rest, in order to allow the repositioned tissues to heal without undue stress.

VAGINAL PROCEDURES

ANTERIOR COLPORRHAPHY

The patient is anesthetized, placed in the lithotomy position, and prepared and draped for vaginal surgery. A Foley catheter (14 Fr or 16 Fr) is inserted transurethrally into the bladder, its balloon is inflated, and its open end is connected to straight drainage. If the surgeon chooses to use a suprapubic catheter for postoperative bladder drainage, it may be inserted at this time or at the end of the operative procedure.

A dilute vasoconstrictive solution (vasopressin 20 units in 50 mL sterile normal saline or epinephrine 1:200,000) or normal saline solution may be injected beneath the anterior vaginal wall as a method of "hydrodissecting" the vesicovaginal space and reducing blood loss. The entire thickness of the anterior vaginal wall is incised from within 1.5 cm of the external urethral meatus to the vaginal apex. The vesicovaginal space is dissected bilaterally to the pubic rami.

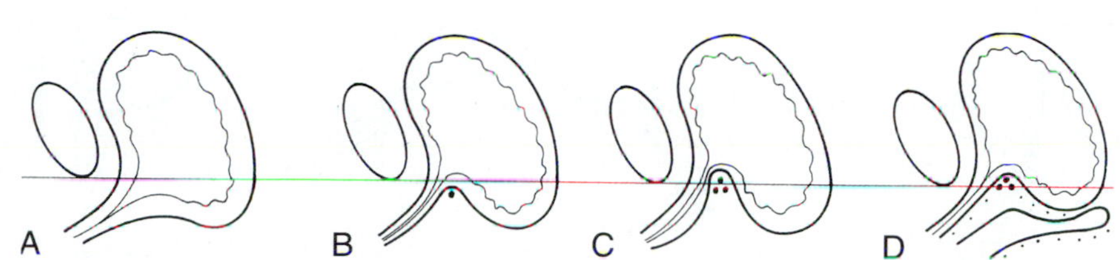

FIGURE 19–1. Anterior colporrhaphy for the treatment of anatomic stress urinary incontinence (lateral view). (*A*) Typically the urethrovesical junction is below the inferior margin of the pubic symphysis and the proximal urethra is somewhat dilated. (*B*) The initial, apical suture plicates the ends of the pubourethral ligaments and pubocervical (endopelvic) fascia beneath the urethrovesical junction. (*C*) Two plicating sutures are placed directly below the first suture. Three plicating sutures may be placed below the second two sutures to further elevate the urethrovesical junction and create a differential wedge of support below it. (*D*) Attention is then directed to correcting any urethrocele, cystocele, or rectocele. (Reprinted from Hurt, WG: Stress urinary incontinence. In Singleton, HM, and Hurt, WG (eds.): Postreproductive Gynecology. Churchill Livingstone, 1990, New York, p. 446, with permission.)

The vaginal ends of the pubourethral ligaments and the pubocervical (endopelvic) fascia are sutured beneath the urethrovesical junction, 4 to 5 cm from the external urethral meatus, with horizontal mattress sutures of permanent or delayed-absorbable material. This apical suture is undersewn by two mattress sutures similarly placed, and often by a third layer of three mattress sutures, to provide a wedge of tissue that elevates and differentially supports the urethrovesical junction (Figs. 19–1 and 19–2). Any defect in the pubocervical fascia beneath the proximal urethra is repaired by interrupted horizontal mattress sutures. Any cystocele is repaired by placing one or two vertical layers of interrupted delayed-absorbable or permanent horizontal mattress sutures placed to approximate the pubocervical fascia. Care must be taken to avoid "undercorrecting" the elevation of the urethrovesical junction or "overcorrecting" any cystocele, either of which may cause postoperative urinary incontinence.

The cut edges of the anterior vaginal wall are appropriately trimmed and then approximated in the midline with interrupted delayed-absorbable sutures.

A modification of an anterior colporrhaphy exists which is, in fact, a vaginal retropubic urethropexy.[15] A delayed-absorbable suture on a stout needle is placed deeply and parallel to the urethra so as to incorporate the periosteum of the retropubis on one side of the urethra; the needle is recovered and the suture brought beneath the urethra before it is placed in a similar fashion on the opposite side; its ends are tied. The first of these sutures is reinforced with a second suture placed in a similar fashion just outside of the first and tied. This suture placement is designed to elevate further the urethrovesical junction and to "tighten" the urethra. A single case series suggests that this procedure is superior to the standard anterior colporrhaphy in curing primary genuine stress incontinence.

NEEDLE URETHROPEXY WITH COLPOSUSPENSION

Many modifications of the original needle urethropexy have been described (Fig. 19–3).[18,19] Some surgeons place their sutures within the paraurethral endopelvic fascia on either side of the proximal urethra (modified Pereyra's); others reinforce the paraurethral endopelvic fascia by placing synthetic bolsters on either side of the proximal urethra (Stamey's); others place a helical suture within the endopelvic fascia on either side of the proximal urethra and also incorporate one or two bites of vaginal wall within each helical suture (Raz's);[20] and others place all of their paraurethral suspending sutures within the anterior vaginal wall on either side of the bladder neck (Muzsnai's).[21]

These modifications have been made to overcome the two major problems of the "needle" procedures: (1) pull-through of the suspending sutures from the paraurethral endopelvic fascia; and (2) pull-through of the knotted ends of the suspending sutures through the anterior abdominal aponeurosis. I prefer to use the Raz[20] or Muzsnai[21] modifications of the "needle" continence procedures.

The patient is anesthetized and placed in Allen's universal stirrups (Allen Medical Systems, Bedford

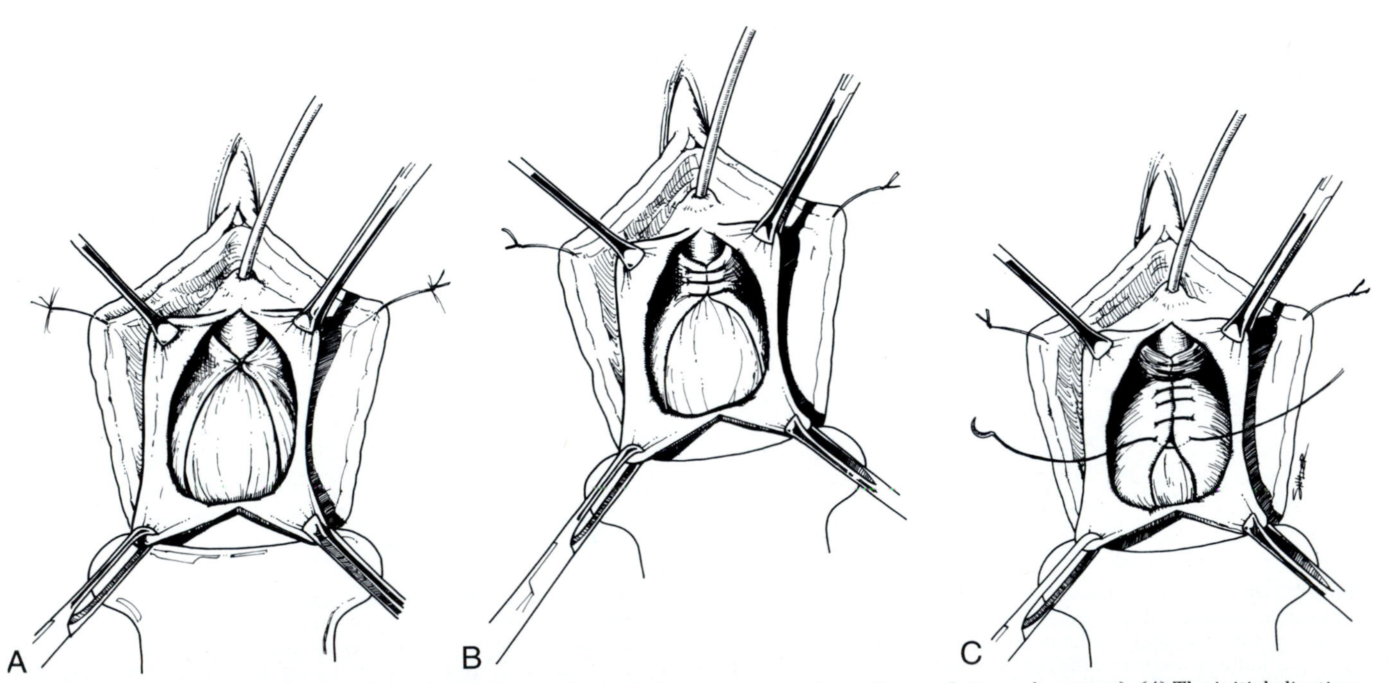

FIGURE 19–2. Anterior colporrhaphy for the treatment of anatomic stress urinary incontinence (suture placement). (*A*) The initial plicating suture is placed directly beneath the urethrovesical junction. (*B*) Two plicating sutures are placed directly below the first suture. (*C*) Plicating sutures are used to correct any significant pubocervical (endopelvic) fascial defect below the urethra and bladder.

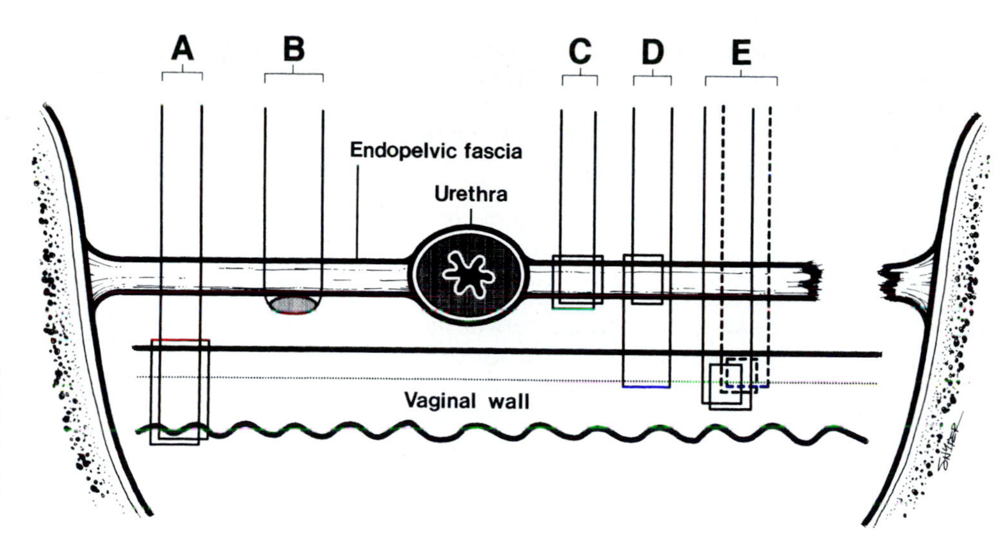

FIGURE 19–3. Needle urethropexy-colposuspension procedures. (*A*) Gittes's. (*B*) Stamey's. (*C*) Modified Pereyra's. (*D*) Raz's. (*E*) Muzsnai's. Modified from Illustrated Medicine, vol 2, No. 3, MP Partners, with permission.

Heights, Ohio 44146) in a modified lithotomy position. She is prepared from the umbilicus, over the perineum, within the vagina, and to midthigh, then draped with a laparoscopy-type drape that allows surgical access through separate openings to the lower abdomen and the vagina. A Foley catheter is inserted transurethrally into the bladder, its balloon is inflated, and its open end is connected to straight drainage.

The procedure begins as for an anterior colporrhaphy, with use of a vasoconstrictive solution, incision of the anterior vaginal wall, and dissection of the vesicovaginal space. Metzenbaum's scissors are used to separate the endopelvic fascia at its attachment to the medial edge of one pubic rami. The surgeon's index finger is then inserted deeply into the retropubic space, at the level of the urethrovesical junction and at a 45-degree angle through the opening between the detached endopelvic fascia and pubic rami. The finger is swept medially to dissect the retropubic space. The same procedure is performed on the opposite side of the urethra. The end of a surgical scalpel, opposite the blade, is inserted into the area of dissection; the blade is then rotated outward against the vulva and pubic rami. This procedure causes the end of the scalpel handle within the retropubic space to gather up the paraurethral endopelvic fascia. A monofilament permanent suture on a taper needle is passed at least three times in a helical fashion, incorporating the detached edge of the endopelvic fascia, which is lateral and adjacent to the urethrovesical junction. An additional bite or two of the underlying anterior vaginal wall is included in the suture helix, the needle is removed, and the long ends of the suspending suture are tagged with a small clamp. A similar suture is placed within the endopelvic fascia and anterior vaginal wall on the opposite side of the urethrovesical junction.

A small transverse incision is made in the skin of the lower abdomen just above the symphysis pubis. The subcutaneous tissues are dissected to the abdominal aponeurosis. With approximately 50 mL of indigo-carmine-colored saline solution in the bladder, the surgeon's index finger is passed through the vaginal incision into the retropubic space up to the dorsal surface of the rectus muscle on one side of the urethrovesical junction. A suture ligature carrier is passed with the opposite hand through the abdominal incision, abdominal aponeurosis, and rectus muscle to come in contact with the tip of the finger in the vagina, approximately 2 cm lateral to the midline. As the finger is withdrawn from the vagina, the tip of the ligature carrier follows it through the retropubic space and into the vaginal field. Both ends of the suspending sutures on that side of the urethrovesical junction are fed into the ligature carrier, and the ligature carrier and suture ends are withdrawn through the abdominal incision. The ends of the suspending sutures are tagged outside the abdominal incision. The same procedure is performed on the opposite suspending suture.

A taper needle is threaded onto one arm of one suspending suture; that end of the suture is then passed back through its initial perforation in the abdominal fascia, some distance beneath the aponeurosis and brought back through the aponeurosis at least 2 cm above and slightly lateral to its original puncture site. The same procedure is performed on the opposite suspending suture.

The ends of the suspending sutures on either side of the midline are tied to themselves to elevate the urethrovesical junction and anterior vaginal wall. The ends of the sutures may then be tied across the midline to further secure them to the anterior abdominal aponeurosis. The abdominal incision is closed.

If there is a significant cystocele, the pubocervical fascia is sutured in the midline with interrupted delayed-absorbable or permanent mattress sutures. Care is taken not to "overcorrect" the cystocele, because this may cause postoperative urinary incontinence. The medial edges of the anterior vaginal wall incision are trimmed and then approximated with interrupted delayed-absorbable sutures. When performing a urethropexy with colposuspension, it is very important to repair all additional pelvic support defects. A transurethral Foley catheter or a suprapubic bladder catheter may be used for postoperative bladder drainage.

SUBURETHRAL SLINGS

Traditionally, suburethral slings have consisted of the passage of a long suspending strap of fascia or synthetic material beneath the urethra and bilaterally up through the retropubic space (i.e., space of Retzius), with the ends of the strap passing through and being sutured to the anterior surface of the abdominal aponeurosis on either side of the midline just above the symphysis pubis[17] (Fig. 19–4).

The patient is anesthetized and her legs are placed in Allen's universal stirrups in a modified lithotomy position. The lower abdomen, perineum, vagina, and upper thighs are prepared and draped with a laparoscopy-type drape that allows the surgeon access to the lower abdomen and the vagina. A Foley catheter is inserted transurethrally into the bladder, its balloon is inflated, and its open end is connected to straight drainage.

As already stated, a dilute vasoconstrictive solution may be injected. A midline incision is made through the full thickness of the anterior vaginal wall from within 1.5 cm of the external urethral meatus to just above the urethrovesical junction. The vesicovaginal and retropubic spaces are dissected as they are for a vaginal "needle" urethropexy with colposuspension. A trapezoidal patch of fascia is fashioned to lie bilaterally beneath the proximal urethra and urethrovesical junction and the urethra.

A lower abdominal incision is made, just as it is for a "needle" urethropexy with colposuspension. A long permanent suture is passed vaginally through the distal paraurethral fascia and the distal corner of the suburethral fascial patch. A second long permanent suture is passed vaginally through the paraurethral fascia at the level of the urethrovesical junction and the corner of the suburethral fascial patch beside it. The ends of each of these sutures are drawn through the retropubic space by two passings of a ligature carrier placed so as to bring the distal suture's ends out just above the pubic bone and the second suture's ends out approximately 4 cm higher. Two sutures are placed in the paraurethral fascia and suburethral sling; their ends are retrieved through the retropubic space in a similar fashion on the opposite side of the urethra. Traction on the ends of the ipsilaterial suspending sutures on either side of the urethra draws the suburethral sling into place. Several simple delayed-absorbable sutures are placed to secure the upper and lower edges of the suburethral sling to the underlying tissues. The long ends of the ipsilateral suspending suture are tied to themselves in a vertical manner across the fibers of the anterior abdominal aponeurosis. No effort is made to elevate the urethrovesical junction. The sling should lie, without tension, just below the proximal urethra and the urethrovesical junction. If the sling is tied under tension in an attempt to elevate the urethrovesical junction, it is likely to obstruct the bladder outlet.

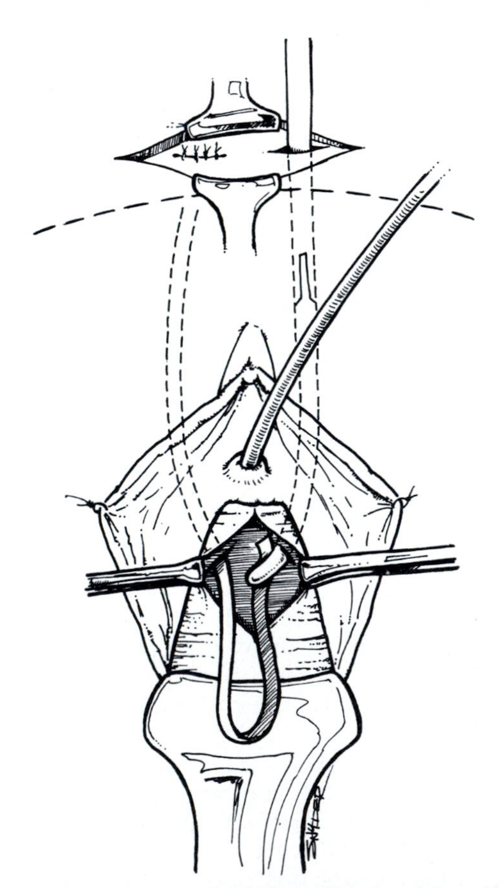

FIGURE 19–4. Long suburethral sling. (Reprinted from Hurt, WG: Stress urinary incontinence. In Shingleton, HM, and Hurt, WG (eds.): Postreproductive Gynecology. Churchill Livingstone, New York, 1990, p. 457, with permission.)

ABDOMINAL PROCEDURES

URETHROPEXY WITH COLPOSUSPENSION

The patient is anesthetized and positioned in Allen's universal stirrups in a low lithotomy position with legs extended, slightly elevated, and abducted. The lower abdomen, perineum, vagina, and upper thighs are prepared and draped and a Foley catheter is inserted, as for a suburethral sling procedure.

The operation is performed through a lower midline or transverse abdominal incision. If there is an indication for intra-abdominal pelvic surgery, it is completed, the pelvis is reperitonealized, and the cul-de-sac is obliterated by midline plication of the uterosacral ligaments or the placement of Moschcowitz's[22] or Halban's[23] sutures. The anterior parietal peritoneum is approximated with running delayed-absorbable suture.

The medial edges of the rectus muscles are retracted with a self-retaining retractor (Fig. 19–5). The loose areolar tissue of the retropubic space is dissected from the posterior surface of the pubis. Approximately 50 mL of indigo-carmine-colored sterile saline solution are injected through the Foley catheter into the bladder. The catheter is clamped to retain the dye within the bladder. The surgeon places the first two fingers of his nondominant hand into the vagina. With upward pressure on one finger, the vagina is elevated at the level of the urethrovesical junction and a peanut gauze in a Kelly clamp is used to displace the bladder medially within the retropubic space from over the elevated fibromuscular wall of the vagina. Any loose fat is removed. A permanent suture on a Mayo (No. 5) tapered needle is passed twice through the entire thickness of the anterior vaginal wall 1.5 to 2 cm lateral to the urethrovesical junction. The needle is removed from the suture and the free ends of the suture are tagged with a small clamp. A second permanent suture is passed through the entire thickness of the anterior vaginal wall 1.5 to 2 cm lateral to the first suture and tagged in a similar fashion. Two permanent sutures are placed and tagged in similar locations on the opposite side of the urethrovesical junction. Following the placement of all four sutures, their clamps are grasped and elevated to determine the security of their placement and the subsequent location of the suspended urethrovesical junction. A Mayo taper needle is then threaded in a sequential fashion on each end of the tagged sutures, and the ends of the sutures are placed through the corresponding iliopectineal (Cooper's) ligament at a point above and slightly lateral to their location within the anterior vaginal wall. Following placement of the suture ends through Cooper's ligaments, the ends of each suture are retagged with clamps. With the surgeon's fingers elevating the urethrovesical junction to the desired retropubic location, the assistant ties the suspending sutures to maintain the position of the urethrovesical junction. Hemostasis is secured within the retropubic space. If concern about hemostasis exists, a suction drain is inserted and its end is brought out through a separate stab incision in the lower abdomen. The self-retaining retractor is removed, and the

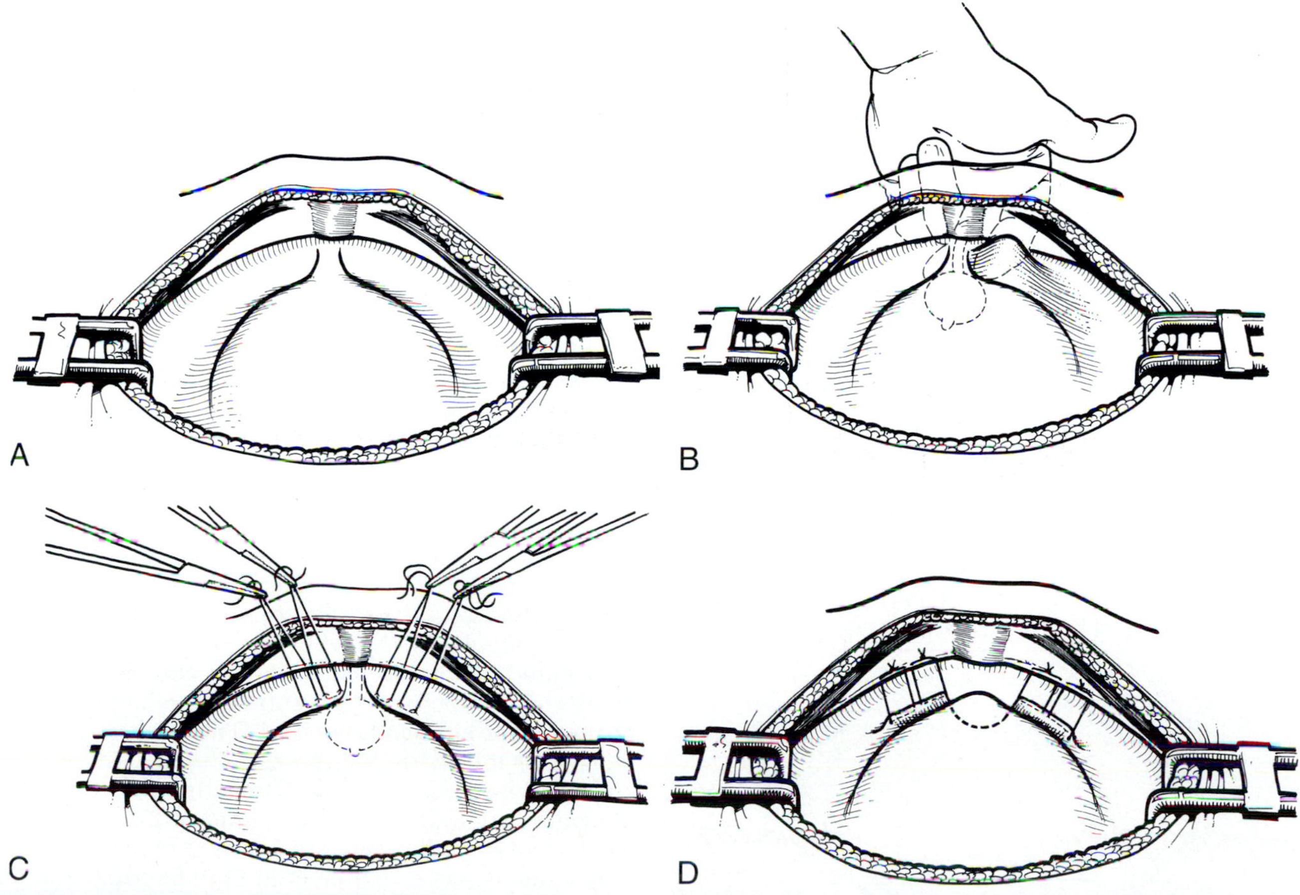

FIGURE 19–5. Abdominal retropubic urethropexy. *(A)* Abdominal wall retracted and retropubic space exposed. *(B)* One finger within vagina elevates vaginal wall next to urethrovesical junction; overlying tissues are displaced medially. *(C)* Figure-of-eight sutures are placed bilaterally through entire thickness of anterior vaginal wall lateral to urethrovesical junction and then directly through Cooper's ligaments (iliopectineal lines). *(D)* Colposuspension is performed by tying suspending sutures; it should elevate, but not obstruct, the urethrovesical junction. (Reprinted from Hurt, WG: Retropubic urethropexy or colposuspension. In Hurt, WG: Urogynecologic Surgery. Aspen, Gaithersburg, MD, 1992, pp. 89–90, with permission.)

medial edges of the rectus muscles may be loosely approximated in the midline with several interrupted delayed-absorbable sutures to prevent development of a ventral hernia. The remainder of the wound is closed in a routine fashion. The transurethral Foley catheter may be used for postoperative bladder drainage or a suprapubic bladder drainage catheter may be inserted and connected to provide straight drainage. If a suction drain was placed in the retropubic space, it may be removed when drainage is negligible. When to begin voiding trials is usually dictated by the surgeon's experience.

PARAVAGINAL REPAIR

The patient is anesthetized, positioned, prepared, and catheterized as for a urethropexy with colposuspension, the same type of incision is used, and any indicated intra-abdominal pelvic surgery is completed in a similar manner. When intra-abdominal surgery has been performed, the paravaginal repair is facilitated by leaving the bowel packed-off into the upper abdomen and by having the medial margins of the rectus muscles retracted by a self-retaining retractor. The retropubic space is dissected most easily and with minimum loss of blood by placing a leading portion of an open 4″ × 4″ gauze pad at the junction of loose areolar tissue and the retropubis. The remainder of the gauze, and additional gauzes, may be advanced with a malleable retractor to separate the areolar tissue from the retropubis.

With the first two fingers of the surgeon's nondominant hand in the vagina, the anterior lateral vaginal sulci are identified and their detachment from the white line (arcus tendineus fascia pelvis) is demonstrated (Fig. 19–6). A longitudinal venous plexus lies along the anterior vaginal sulci just outside the fibromuscular wall of the vagina. Care should be taken during dissection and suture placement not to disrupt this venous plexus or traumatize the obturator vessels and nerves.

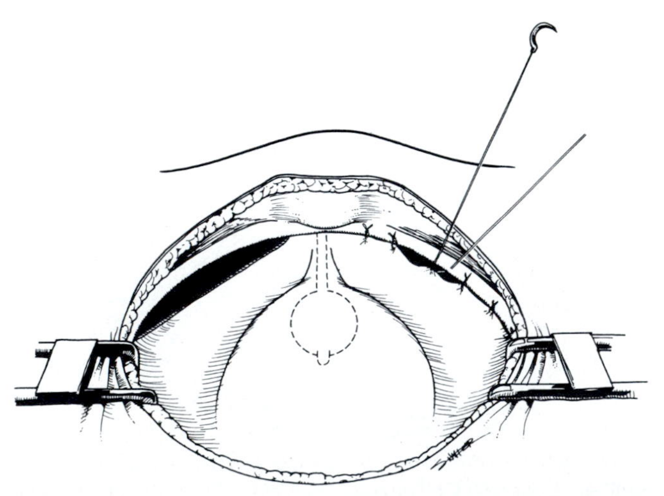

FIGURE 19–6. Abdominal paravaginal repair. (Left side) Separation of the anterior lateral vaginal wall from the white line (arcus tendineus fascia pelvis). (Right side) Reattachment of the anterior lateral vaginal wall to the white line with six to eight simple sutures.

Permanent (2-0) suture on an atraumatic tapered needle is passed around the vascular bundle and through a full thickness of the anterior lateral vaginal sulcus at the level of one ischial spine (Fig. 19–6). The suture is then passed to incorporate the white line of the pelvic sidewall just distal to the ischial spine and tied. A second suture is passed through the full thickness of the anterior lateral vaginal sulcus at the level of the midurethra, around the white line of the pelvic sidewall, and tied. The remaining paravaginal defect is repaired by placing multiple sutures, in a similar fashion, to approximate the anterior lateral vaginal sulcus to the white line. The same procedure is repeated on the opposite side of the pelvis. Hemostasis is secured and, if necessary, a suction drain is placed within the retropubic space. Its end is brought out through a separate stab incision in the lower abdominal wall. Following removal of any abdominal packs and retractors, the incision in the anterior parietal peritoneum is closed, the medial edges of the rectus muscles loosely approximated in the midline, and the remainder of the abdominal incision closed in a routine manner.[16]

The surgeon may choose to leave in place the transurethral Foley catheter or to insert a percutaneous suprapubic catheter. If a suction drain was placed in the retropubic space, it can be removed when little or no drainage is present. The beginning of voiding trials is usually dictated by the surgeon's experience.

COMPLICATIONS OF SURGICAL MANAGEMENT

Complications common to all surgical procedures may result from the patient's medical condition, the anesthetic technique, the skin incision, or concomitant surgical procedures, but these complications are not discussed here. I focus instead on more common intraoperative and postoperative complications that may be associated with continence procedures.

The most common intraoperative complications include direct or indirect injury to the lower urinary tract, pelvic blood vessels, or nerves. The ureters may be angulated, ligated, partially or completely transected, or devascularized. The bladder is more likely to be transfixed by a suture, crushed by an instrument, or surgically incised. The urethra may be incised or indirectly injured as a result of its devascularization or denervation. Detecting and properly managing such injuries at the time of the operation can essentially eliminate subsequent morbidity.

The pelvis has a rich arterial blood supply and an extensive collateral circulation, both of which branch and anastomose about each organ before draining into a pelvic plexus and, eventually, into the iliac veins and inferior vena cava. All branches of the anterior division of the internal iliac artery may be ligated with impunity, but the external iliac artery and its branches must be preserved to avoid jeopardizing the viability of the lower extremities. During retropubic dissections, rupture of the thin-walled venous plexus about the bladder or vagina causes considerable loss of blood. The retropubic space is inaccessible to postoperative evaluation and has no dependent drainage, so the surgeon must secure hemostasis at the time of surgery and, if necessary, place suction drains within the retropubic space to prevent the formation of hematomas. In the presence of vaginal wall sutures, incisions, or dissections, retropubic hematomas may become contaminated by bacteria and can lead to a retropubic abscess that may require postoperative drainage.

Significant postoperative collections of lymph, serum, or urine within the pelvis are rare.

Pelvic nerve injuries associated with continence surgery most often result either from placing patients in the "frog-legged" or lithotomy position or by compressing a nerve by a surgical retractor. The femoral, sciatic, or peroneal nerves are the most likely to be injured by these maneuvers. Dissections and placement of sutures are more likely to injure an obturator nerve or to entrap an ilioinguinal nerve.

When synthetic materials are used in operative procedures, they may cause foreign body reaction or may increase the chance of developing an infectious complication. To reduce the chance of either condition, synthetic materials must be biocompatible, sterile, and of minimum bulk. When synthetic materials are placed within the pelvis, it is best to use antibiotic prophylaxis and a meticulous technique to minimize bacterial contamination of the operative site; the material itself should be carefully excluded from possible sources of infection. If the synthetic materials become a cause of persistent granulations or uncontrolled infections, they may have to be removed.

Osteitis pubis is a rare nonbacterial rarification of bone which appears to result from periosteal trauma. It is said to occur in 2.5% to 3% of patients whose urethropexies are suspended by sutures that incorporate the retropubic periosteum. The condition may be incapacitating for several weeks to months. It may be treated by rest, analgesics, and systemic corticosteroid injections, but it is usually self-limiting. Rarely, a patient may develop osteomyelitis or pyogenic arthritis, or overt bacterial infections that require intravenous antibiotic therapy and possible surgical drainage and debridement.

Urinary tract infections often follow lower urinary tract surgery. Incidence of such infections is reduced if the urine is sterile preoperatively and if the bladder is drained postoperatively by a suprapubic rather than a transurethral catheter. If long-term bladder drainage is needed, clean intermittent self-catheterization is known to be associated with an incidence of infection that is less than half that caused by the use of indwelling catheters. My basic philosophy is to use a transurethral catheter if bladder drainage is expected to be needed for less than 48 to 72 hours, to use a suprapubic catheter if bladder drainage is expected to be needed for longer than 48 to 72 hours, and to discontinue all indwelling bladder catheter drainage as soon as possible if the patient can perform clean intermittent self-catheterization. Antibiotic prophylaxis is not prescribed simply for the mere presence of an indwelling bladder catheter, but symptomatic bladder infections are treated when an indwelling bladder catheter is in place.

In my experience, the incidence of postoperative bladder dysfunction and urinary retention are lowest among patients who have paravaginal repairs or anterior colporrhaphies. It is more frequent with "needle" than with abdominal retropubic urethropexy with colposuspension procedures. It is the greatest problem following one of the suburethral sling procedures. My impression is that efficient postoperative bladder function returns about the same time as bowel function. Therefore, I usually do not start voiding trials until flatus or feces have passed. I discontinue bladder drainage, whether by indwelling catheter or intermittent catheterization, when the patient is comfortable following voiding and her postvoid urinary residual is consistently less than 90 mL. I do not use bethanechol or prostaglandins to hasten the return of an efficient voiding pattern, but I occasionally prescribe warm sitz baths and diazepam if striated muscle spasm is felt to be contributing to a patient's urinary retention.

Detrusor instability may cause urinary incontinence following continence surgery. It is important to know whether the condition was present preoperatively and whether it responded to medical therapy, or if it developed de novo following the operative procedure. Some cases of preoperative detrusor instability are cured by continence procedures, but it is hard to predict who will be cured. Early onset of postoperative detrusor instability may be due to inflammation of the surgical site, a lower urinary tract infection, a foreign body such as a suture within the bladder, or bladder outlet obstruction. If a likely cause is found, it should be treated. Late onset of postoperative detrusor instability is of more concern. If no apparent cause can be found, the condition should be treated with one of the anticholinergic agents (e.g., oxybutynin, propantheline bromide) and bladder retraining drills. Surgical therapy should be a last resort.

RESULTS AND FOLLOW-UP

Review of the surgical literature reveals that Burch's colposuspensions, the best-studied of all retropubic continence procedures and the one reported to have the highest cure rate, fail to cure genuine stress incontinence in 10% to 15% of the patients treated.[24] Another 10% to 15% may develop detrusor instability or voiding difficulties. Galloway, Davies, and Stephenson[25] found that only 22 (44%) of 50

TABLE 19–1. Approximate Cure Rates of Continence Procedures[19]

Procedure	Cure Rate (%)
Anterior colporrhaphy	64
Modified Pereyra's	70
Burch's colposuspension	88

women who had undergone a colposuspension for stress urinary incontinence were dry and free of complications 1 to 6 years after surgery. Cure rates of continence procedures performed with preoperative and postoperative urodynamic studies are summarized in Table 19–1.

Patients who have continence surgery should do everything possible to ensure and preserve a favorable result. They should not smoke, should seek treatment for respiratory disorders, should control their weight, and should avoid recreational and occupational stresses that cause repetitive and often sudden increases in intra-abdominal pressure. Patients going through menopause should receive estrogen replacement therapy, unless they have some contraindication to its use.

REFERENCES

1. Giordano, D: Proceedings of the 20th Congress. Franc. de Chir. 506, 1907.
2. Goebell, R: Zur Operativen Beseiligung der Angebarenen Incontinentia Vesicae. A Gynak Urol 2:187, 1910.
3. Frangenheim, P: Zur Operativen Behandlung der Ankontinenz der Mannlichen Harnrohre. Proceedings of the 43rd Congress. Verh Dtsch Ges Chirurgie: 149, 1914.
4. Stoeckel, W: Uber die Verwendung der Musculi Pyramidales bei der operativen Behandlung der Incontinentia Urinae. Zentralbl Gynakol 41:11, 1917.
5. Price, PB: Plastic operations for incontinence of urine and of feces. Arch Surg 26:1043, 1933.
6. Aldridge, AH: Transplantation of fascia for relief of urinary stress incontinence. Am J Obstet Gynecol 44:398, 1942.
7. Raz, S, Siegel, AL, Short, JL, et al: Vaginal wall sling. J Urol 141:43, 1989.
8. Fothergill, WE: On the pathology and the operative treatment of displacements of the pelvic viscera. J Obstet Gynaecol Br Emp 13:410, 1908.
9. Kelly, HA: Incontinence of urine in women. Urol Cutane Rev 17:291, 1913.
10. Kennedy, WT: Incontinence of urine in the female, the urethral sphincter mechanism, damage of function and restoration of control. Am J Obstet Gynecol 34:576, 1937.
11. Marshall, VF, Marchetti, AA, and Krantz, KE: The correction of stress incontinence by simple vesicourethral suspension. Surg Gynecol Obstet 88:509, 1949.
12. Burch, JC: Urethrovaginal fixation to Cooper's ligament for the correction of stress incontinence, cystocele, rectocele, and prolapse. Am J Obstet Gynecol 82:281, 1961.
13. Pereyra, AJ: A simplified surgical procedure for the correction of stress incontinence in women. West J Surg Obstet Gynecol 67:223, 1959.
14. Richardson, AC, Edmonds, PB and Williams, NL: Treatment of stress urinary incontinence due to paravaginal fascial defect. Obstet Gynecol 57:357, 1981.
15. Beck, RP, McCormick, S and Nordstrom, L: A 25-year experience with 5419 anterior colporrhaphy procedures. Obstet Gynecol 78:1011, 1991.
16. Shull, BL and Baden, WF: A six-year experience with paravaginal defect repair for stress urinary incontinence. Am J Obstet Gynecol 160:1432, 1989.
17. Beck, RP, McCormick, S and Nordstrom, L: The fascia lata sling procedure for treating recurrent genuine stress incontinence of urine. Obstet Gynecol 72:699, 1988.
18. Karram, MM: Transvaginal needle suspension procedures for genuine stress incontinence. In Walters, MD and Karram, MM (eds.): Clinical Urogynecology. Mosby-Year Book, St. Louis, 1993, p 191.
19. Karram, MM: Transvaginal needle suspension. In Hurt, WG (ed): Urogynecologic Surgery. Aspen, Gaithersburg, MD; 1992, pp 61–72.
20. Raz, S: Modified bladder neck suspension for female stress urinary incontinence. J Urol 17:82, 1981.
21. Muzsnai, D, Carillo, E, Dubin, C, et al: Retropubic vaginopexy for correction of urinary stress incontinence. Obstet Gynecol 59:113, 1982.
22. Moschcowitz, AV: The pathogenesis, anatomy, and cure of prolapse of the rectum. Surg Gynecol Obstet 15:7, 1912.
23. Halban, J: Gynakologische Operationslehre. Urban and Schwarzenberg, Berlin and Vienna, 1932.
24. Walters, MD: Genuine Stress incontinence: Retropubic surgical procedures. In Walters, MD and Karram, MM (eds.): Clinical Urogynecology. Mosby-Year Book, St. Louis, 1993, p 203.
25. Galloway, NTM, Davies, N and Stephenson, TP: The complications of colposuspension. Br J Urol 60:122, 1987.

CHAPTER 20

Genuine Stress Incontinence: Innovative Surgical Approaches

Geoffrey Cundiff • Alfred E. Bent

During the last half century, over 100 surgical procedures have been described for the treatment of genuine stress incontinence. The vast majority of these techniques are variations of an anterior vaginal repair, suburethral sling, retropubic urethropexy, or needle urethropexy. These were discussed in Chapter 19. This chapter considers the growing number of alternative and innovative procedures for treatment of genuine stress incontinence.

LAPAROSCOPIC RETROPUBIC URETHROPEXY

BACKGROUND

In spite of the plethora of surgical interventions for genuine stress incontinence, the retropubic urethropexy, as initially described by Marshall and associates and later by Burch, has the most consistent success rate.[1,2] A significant disadvantage of the traditional retropubic urethropexy is the abdominal incision, which prolongs recovery and hospital stay. The laparoscopic retropubic urethropexy mimics an open urethropexy by suspending the urethrovesical junction without a major abdominal incision.

INDICATIONS

Laparoscopic urethropexy may be considered in patients with genuine stress incontinence and hypermobility of the bladder neck. Patients with intrinsic sphincter deficiency should receive alternative therapy.

Laparoscopic urethropexy should be reserved for the primary surgical attempt. Those patients with prior unsuccessful surgery for incontinence will probably benefit more from conventional open surgery. The need for extensive concomitant vaginal surgery can be considered a relative contraindication to the laparoscopic approach, because a needle urethropexy could be performed in these circumstances faster and with fewer incisions. Finally, the physician and patient should be aware that, although the laparoscopic urethropexy appears to mimic the traditional retropubic urethropexy, there are, at present, no prospective data to document the efficacy or longevity of the laparoscopic approach.

TECHNIQUE

Laparoscopy commences with intraperitoneal (or, less commonly, retropubic) insufflation. Common trocar placement includes a 10-mm trocar in the umbilicus, two 10-mm trocars lateral to the rectus muscles and 2 cm medial to the superior iliac spines, and a 5-mm trocar between the pubic bone and umbilicus. Another approach is to use two lower and two higher lateral trocar sites.[3]

A Moschowitz or Halban culdoplasty may be performed before the preperitoneal, retropubic dissection to reduce the occurrence of subsequent enterocele formation.

Using the intraperitoneal approach, the initial peritoneal incision is made 4 to 5 cm superior to the bladder, which permits preperitoneal dissection to the pubic bone. The posterior aspect of the pubic bone is identified, the retropubic space is developed, and Cooper's ligaments are cleared of overlying tissue. The Foley catheter bulb identifies the uretrovesical junction; elevation of the vaginal sulcus with the examiner's finger facilitates the removal of fat as well as suture placement.

As with any laparoscopic procedure, the goals of the laparoscopic approach should not vary from the goals of an open procedure. Thus, two sutures should be placed on each side, with the first 2 cm lateral to the midurethra and the second 2 cm lateral from the urethrovesical junction. The polytetrafluoroethylene suture is initially passed downward through Cooper's ligament using the ipsilateral port (Fig. 20–1). While elevating the periurethral vaginal tissue, a double purchase of near full thickness of the vagina is placed using the contralateral trocar site. The needle is then passed upward through the ipsilateral Cooper's ligament using the middle port.

Sutures are tied down as they are placed, using an extracorporeal technique and a knot pusher, while an assistant elevates the vaginal tissues. As an alternative, Vancaillie and Schuessler use an extracorporeal slipknot technique to attach the paraurethral tissue to the symphysis pubis.[4]

Following bilateral suspension, the retropubic space is irrigated and hemostasis is confirmed. Cystoscopy ensures that the bladder is free of injury or foreign body. The peritoneum can be left open or closed with sutures or clips. Postoperative bladder drainage is accomplished with a transurethral or suprapubic catheter.

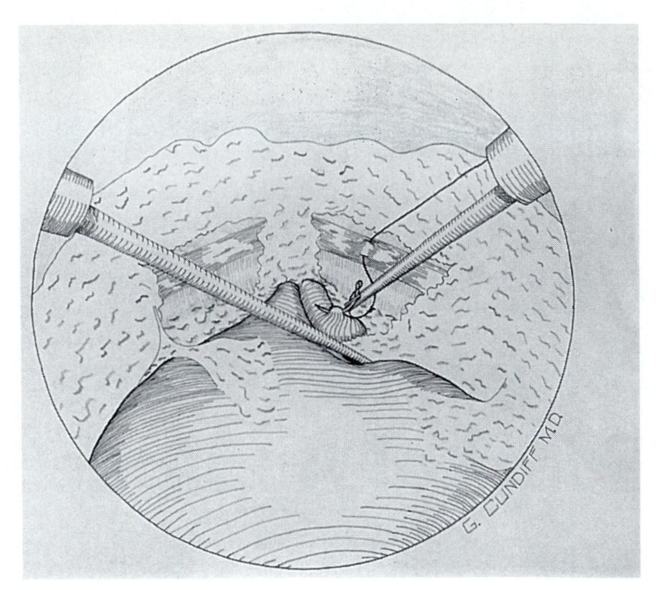

FIGURE 20–1. Laparoscopic retropubic urethropexy. Following dissection of the retropubic space and Cooper's ligaments, with the bladder retracted to the left, the initial suture is passed through Cooper's ligament and the paraurethral fascia, which is elevated by a finger in the lateral vaginal fornix.

COMPLICATIONS AND EFFICACY

The most touted advantage of laparoscopic urethropexy is the shortened recovery period, including promptness of mobilization, discharge from the hospital, and return to work and regular activities. In the absence of proven laparoscopic efficacy and longevity, these advantages are probably overstated, because the success of an operation for urinary incontinence is not related to the brevity of the recovery. In contrast to extirpative procedures, reconstructive retropubic procedures should be followed by recovery time sufficient to permit scarring of the repair in the desired position.

Laparoscopic repair does minimize the patient's postoperative pain, as well as the duration of the hospital stay, but this benefit must offset the increased time and expense in the operating room if it is to be economically viable. A less frequently stated advantage of laparoscopic urethropexy is the ease of dissecting the space of Retzius. The magnification and direct lighting during laparoscopy, as well as the angle of approach, markedly improve the view of this awkward space. The magnified image of the television monitor also facilitates hemostasis and placement of sutures, because vessels can either be avoided or coagulated.[4] The benefit is offset, however, by the challenge of suturing in the retropubic space. This is the rate-limiting step and ultimately determines whether the procedure can be done in a reasonable amount of time in order to make it a viable alternative to the open approach. Moreoever, a steep learning curve exists for any surgeon who attempts to master the technique. Consequently, laparoscopic urethropexy probably belongs in the realm of the practitioner with extensive knowledge of urogynecology and superior skills in operative laparoscopy.

Several small surgical series have reported short-term, subjective success rates of 94% to 100% for a laparoscopic retropubic urethropexy. The tendency to consider the prognosis of a laparoscopic procedure to be equivalent to that of the original operation should be resisted, however; counseling the patient based on this assumption does not represent informed consent. Prospective randomized trials must be completed in order to compare the efficacy, longevity, and economics of a laparoscopic urethropexy to an open urethropexy.

APPROACHES TO INTRINSIC URETHRAL SPHINCTER DEFICIENCY

Genuine stress incontinence due to intrinsic urethral sphincter deficiency requires a partially obstructive surgical repair. As discussed previously, the traditional surgical modality is a suburethral sling. Several different approaches have been developed that attempt to improve the suburethral sling. They include modifications of a traditional suburethral sling, periurethral injections, and an artificial urinary sphincter. These are discussed individually.

SUBURETHRAL PATCH

Background

This modification of a conventional suburethral sling procedure suspends the entire functional length of the urethra and bladder neck, rather than only the proximal urethra. Karram and Bhatia published their experience using a fascia lata patch to suspend the urethra in 10 patients,[5] of whom 9 were objectively cured 1 to 2 years after surgery. The patient considered a failure subjectively improved, although she was noted to have incontinence at cystometric capacity in the standing position. The stated advantage of using fascia lata is that it does not require an extensive abdominal dissection to harvest a rectus fascia patch. Alternatively, synthetic materials, such as Gore-Tex or Marlex, can also be used for the suburethral patch. These materials are easy to obtain but carry the risks of infection and rejection associated with a foreign body.

Technique

Autologous fascia lata patch (5 × 7 cm) is harvested from lateral lower thigh, approximately 4 cm above the patella, and preserved on a moist gauze.

A midline anterior vaginal wall incision is made, extending from just proximal to the urethral meatus to the bladder neck.

After the urethra is exposed, the fascia lata patch is placed so as to overlap the midurethra and urethrovesical junction by about 1 cm. It is affixed to the bladder base and suburethra with 4-0 delayed absorbable suture. Permanent suture is then secured to the lateral aspects of the patch in at least four helical sutures, incorporating the detached paraurethral fascia into each purchase. The helical stitches are carried down past the level of the urethrovesical junction.

Abdominally, a 3-cm transverse incision is made just superior to the pubic symphysis and the fascia is exposed. The helical sutures are transferred and secured abdominally in the manner of a needle suspension. Cystoscopy confirms the integrity of the lower urinary tract. The sutures are tied abdominally and the incisions are closed.

VAGINAL WALL SLING

Juma, Little, and Raz[6] published the results of using a vaginal wall sling to treat 65 patients with intrinsic sphincter deficiency, and reported a success rate of 94%. Of the patients, 45 required intermittent catheterization for a mean period of 6 weeks following removal of the suprapubic catheter, and 8 of these patients developed de novo detrusor instability.[6] Modifications include use of a segment of the anterior vaginal wall for the suspension and an inverted A-shaped anterior vaginal incision.

The dissection of the paraurethral fascia proceeds lateral to the two arms of the A. This leaves a segment of vaginal wall, that is, the upper triangle of the A, in place beneath the urethra and bladder neck (Fig. 20–2). After the urethra is freed from its attachments to the pubic bone, permanent sutures are placed in this island of vaginal tissue bilaterally at the level of the urethrovesical junction and at the level of the distal urethra. These sutures incorporate the vaginal wall and paraurethral fascia at the distal end, as well as the pubocervical and urethropelvic ligament at the level of the bladder neck. The sutures are then transferred to a small abdominal incision and secured to the rectus fascia.

The gold standard of surgical therapy for intrinsic sphincter deficiency remains the suburethral sling. Long-term evaluation of the fascial sling reveals cure rates of 84% to 95%, based on objective data. Success rates are slightly lower in patients who have undergone prior incontinence surgery.[7]

PERIURETHRAL INJECTIONS

Background

A less invasive approach to intrinsic sphincter deficiency is the use of bulk-enhancing agents that increase pressure on the urethra and reduce the size

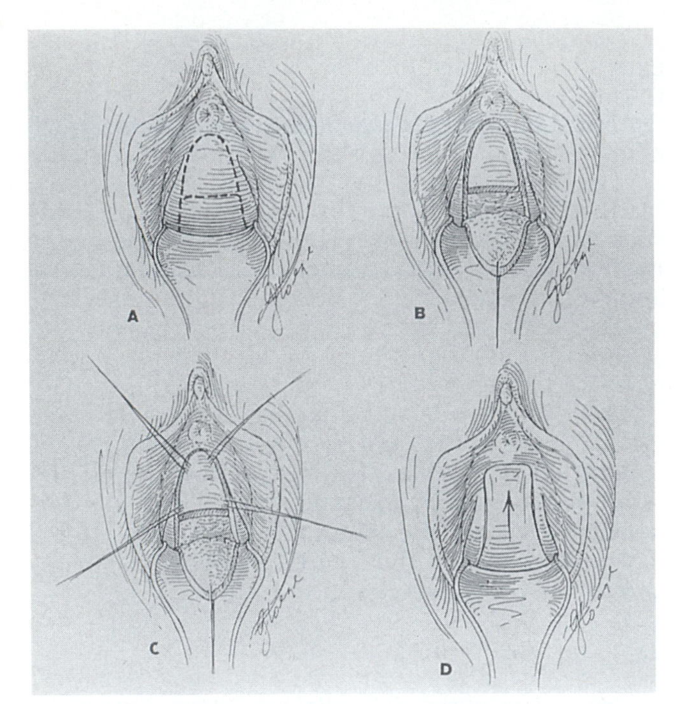

FIGURE 20–2. Vaginal wall sling. *A,* A-shaped incision in the anterior vaginal wall. *B,* Distal triangular island of the anterior vaginal wall serves as suburethral sling and the posterior aspect of incised vaginal mucosa serves as flap of tissue over repair. *C,* Four suspension sutures anchored into sling. *D,* Advancement of flap to cover sling. (From Juma, Little, and Raz: with permission.)

of the urethral lumen, providing resistance to the flow of urine. Currently available materials include Teflon, autologous fat, and collagen.

A highly purified glutaraldehyde cross-linked bovine dermal collagen dispersed in saline is commercially available (Contigen, C.R. Bard) and FDA-approved for treatment of intrinsic sphincter deficiency. Contigen is biocompatible as well as biodegradable. The bovine collagen begins to degrade approximately 12 weeks after injection, but not before eliciting a minimal inflammatory response that causes a replacement of bovine collagen by the patient's own collagen.

Indications

Periurethral injectables should be reserved for patients with intrinsic sphincter deficiency, minimal urethrovesical junction mobility, and normal detrusor activity. Intradermal skin testing is mandatory before collagen use to minimize the possibility of hypersensitivity reactions.

Patients may develop postoperative retention and should be trained preoperatively in intermittent self-catheterization. Repeat treatments are frequently required.

Technique

The patient is positioned in a lithotomy position and prepared and draped for a cystoscopic procedure. A periurethral block is achieved using 1% lidocaine. Urethroscopy and cystoscopy are performed to assess the urethral tissue and surrounding anatomy.

Periurethral approach. If the periurethral approach is to be used, a spinal needle (17-gauge for Polytef and 20-gauge for Contigen) is placed lateral to the urethral meatus at the 4-o'clock position with the needle bevel directed medially. Visualization of the urethral lumen with the urethroscope allows the surgeon to advance the needle to a position just lateral to the urethrovesical junction without breaching the urethral mucosa. A syringe is then attached to the spinal needle and the material injected (Fig. 20–3). Because of its viscous nature, a Lewy syringe or Bruning otolaryngeal injection device is recommended for the Polytef paste. As the material is injected, it can be seen to layer just outside the urethral lumen, causing a bulging into the lumen. Injection should continue until the bulge reaches the center of the lumen. The needle is then removed, reinserted at the 8-o'clock position, and advanced in the same fashion. Injection proceeds until the lumen is almost fully obstructed. This usually requires 7 to 15 mL of material per side. After removing the needle, the patient is helped to a standing position and performs provocative maneuvers to assess the need for further injections.

Transurethral approach. In the transurethral approach, a special delivery system consisting of an endoscope with a cystoscopic sheath and a bevelled needle attachment is utilized. With the endoscope in place, the needle is advanced into the urethral wall and the material injected at a 3-o'clock position and then at a 9-o'clock position. Bulking of suburethral tissue can be directly observed during injections.

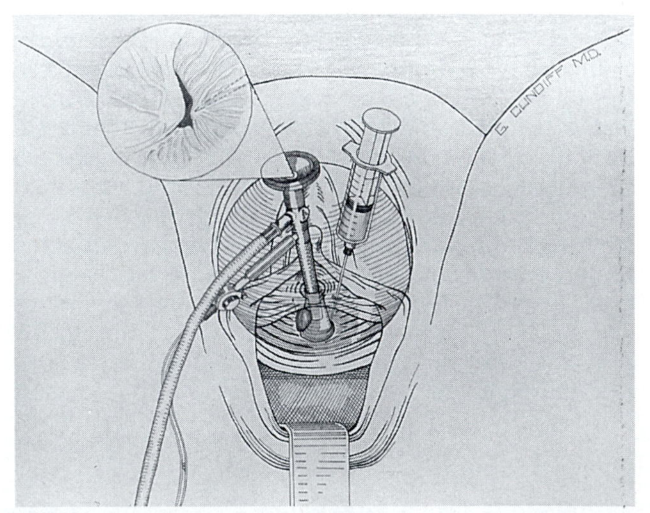

FIGURE 20–3. Periurethral collagen injection. Periurethral approach with cystoscopic view: The right urethral wall passes the midline following the right injection and the bevel of the needle is in the proper location to inject on the left.

Shortcomings of this approach are bleeding from the urethral mucosa, which can obstruct visualization, and extravasation of material into the lumen.

Complications

Periurethral injections are an outpatient procedure, but patients should be assessed for urinary retention. Difficulty voiding should be handled with intermittent self-catheterization, because an indwelling catheter could cause molding of the Contigen or Polytef. Bacteriuria is common following the procedure, leading some clinicians to order a short course of prophylactic antibiotics at the time of the procedure. Postopertive fever is common in patients receiving Polytef and usually resolves after several days. Patients frequently need a second injection to achieve continence; this can be scheduled as early as 1 week following the initial procedure. Carrion and Politano recommend a 4- to 6-month waiting period, because some patients who initially are incontinent after the procedure will become continent after several months.[8]

Efficacy

In a series of 55 women treated with Polytef injections, Carrion and Politano reported a cure rate of 51% with improvement in another 20% and failure in 29%. These patients received an average of 1.8 injections, although the patients who failed generally received fewer.[8] These findings are comparable to those reported by Vesey, Rivett, and O'Boyle in their series of 36 women with stress incontinence.[9] Long-term efficacy is anticipated to be lower with Contigen, because it biodegrades. After continence is achieved with Contigen, 80% of patients remain continent. These results can be improved by eliminating patients with mixed incontinence, because patients with detrusor instability have a significantly lower cure rate.[10] In a multicenter trial of 333 women receiving collagen injections at various sites, no patient had significant anticollagen antibodies nor demonstrated adverse events attributed to immunogenicity.[11] At present, Contigen is the only foreign material approved for periurethral injection to treat intrinsic sphincter deficiency in women. Polytef is not generally used for this indication.

PARAURETHRAL IMPLANTS

Coaptation of the urethral walls may also be achieved with implants. Barrett and colleagues have developed a genitourinary spheroidal membrane and mechanical delivery system for this purpose. The silicone rubber sphere is inserted in the paraurethral space transcutaneously, where it enhances outlet resistance. Placement in six mongrel dogs revealed a mean increase of 16 cm of H_2O in leak-point pressure without device-related complications.[12] Clinical application of this device is under study.

ARTIFICIAL URINARY SPHINCTER

Background

Ideal treatment for intrinsic urethral sphincter incompetence should address the associated incontinence while permitting a normal voiding pattern. Theoretically, these two goals are probably best accomplished by the artificial urinary sphincter.

F. Brantley Scott implanted the first artificial urinary sphincter in June 1972. The device that he employed was developed by a team he headed, in conjunction with American Medical Systems. The original prosthesis underwent significant modifications and improvements to evolve into the model currently in use, the AMS Sphincter 800(AS-800). This elegant example of engineering is considerably smaller and simpler in design than earlier models, yet incorporates features that have lowered the complication rate to an acceptable level.

The AS-800 consits of an inflatable cuff and a pressure-regulating balloon which are both connected, by kink-resistant tubing, to a pump mechanism. The system is filled with fluid at a pressure that is determined by the thickness of the wall of the balloon. The cuff fills automatically so that the pressure of the system maintains the cuff in a closed position. Squeezing the pump moves fluid from the cuff to the balloon; repeated squeezing deflates the cuff. After the cuff is fully deflated, the balloon begins to repressurize the cuff automatically, but a resistor within the pump unit delays refilling of the cuff by approximately 3 minutes, long enough to allow voiding.

Surgical placement of the AS800 can be done from a vaginal or abdominal approach. Implantation includes placing the cuff around the bladder neck, implanting the pump unit within the labia majora, and positioning the pressure-regulating balloon within the abdominal cavity (Fig. 20–4). This arrangement renders the sphincter resistant to stress incontinence, because increases in intra-abdominal pressure are transmitted equally to the balloon, bladder, and cuff, which prevents fluid transfer within the system, thereby maintaining cuff pressure. Continence is maintained even if intra-abdominal pressure is greater than the balloon pressure. In the event of a detrusor contraction with an amplitude greater than that of the balloon pressure, fluid is pushed from the cuff, resulting in urinary loss.

All components are constructed of silicone rubber. The cuff has a 1.5-cm Dacron backing and is coated with Teflon, which makes it 21 times more resistant to wear than silicon alone. After placement around the bladder neck, the cuff is snapped to maintain its cylindric configuration. It is available in graduated diameters with lengths ranging from 4.5 to 11 cm.

The balloon serves as a fluid reservoir but also determines the pressure rendered against the urethra by the cuff. The baseline closing pressure in the cuff is determined by the thickness of the balloon wall. Available balloons range from 51 to 90 cm H_2O. The surgeon's choice of balloon is based on exceeding

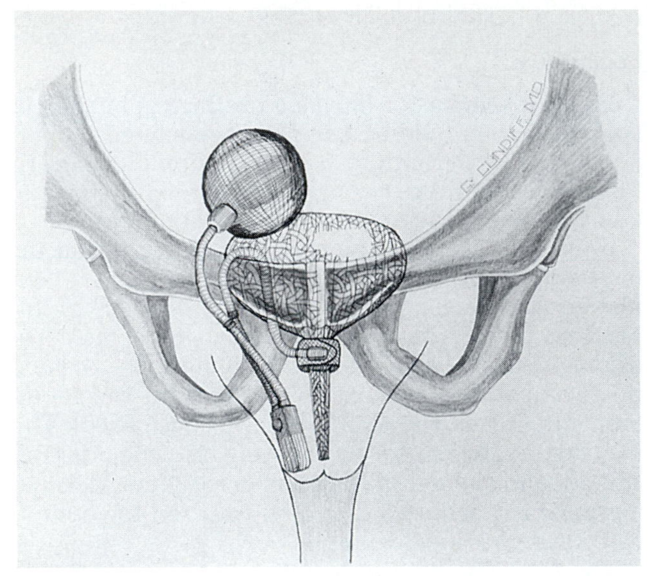

FIGURE 20–4. Artificial urinary sphincter after placement: The cuff surrounds the proximal urethra, the pressure balloon has an intra-abdominal location, and the pump unit is in the subcutaneous tissue of the right labium majorum.

leak-point pressure without exceeding diastolic pressure, which promotes tissue necrosis.

The pump unit includes one-way valves and resistors, which are constructed of stainless steel and encased in silicone rubber. In addition, a raised silicone nipple over a poppet valve controls a deactivation feature that empties the cuff and prevents refilling. This feature was incorporated to permit delayed activation, which facilitates healing in the periurethral tissues and labia immediately following surgery, decreasing the immediate postoperative erosion rate of the sphincter from 18% to 1.3%.[13] Although this feature was originally intended for the surgeon's use, most patients can be instructed in use of the poppet valve, thus giving them control over the length of time the bladder neck is occluded, permitting periodic deactivation.

Inherent within the design are several important safety features. Except with increases in the intra-abdominal pressure, the pressure of the cuff cannot surpass that of the balloon, which is determined by the surgeon at the time of insertion. Nonphysiologic increases in vesical pressure therefore overcome the pressure of the cuff, preventing reflux into the upper urinary tract. Finally, device failure results in loss of cuff pressure so that voiding may continue.

Indications

The artificial sphincter may be considered in patients with intrinsic sphincter deficiency, a stable detrusor with normal compliance and capacity, and a minimally displaced urethrovesical junction. Preoperative bladder capacity should exceed 125 mL. Knowledge of leak-point pressure and voiding pressure help in selecting the appropriate pressure-regulating balloon. The lowest possible cuff pressure that prevents leakage is desired because this lower pressure minimizes the risk of erosion. A pressure just surpassing the leak-point pressure is usually sufficient.

Complications and Efficacy

Engineering improvements have corrected the earlier mechanical problems of the artificial sphincter, and now most problems are secondary to poor selection of patients and faulty surgical technique. The 5-year mechanical reliability rate is more than 90%.[14] Device leakage presents as recurrent incontinence. A kink in the tubing or debris in the system can mimic a leak, but this finding can be differentiated using inflation and deflation radiographs. If surgical revision is planned, it is possible to identify the leak using an ohm-meter. Prolonged tissue compression can cause tissue atrophy beneath the cuff; this may also be confused with a leak within the system. After cross-clamping the tubing to the balloon, the pressure can be measured. Low balloon pressure indicates loss of volume due to leakage, whereas normal pressure reveals tissue atrophy beneath the cuff. Atrophy can be avoided by leaving the cuff in its deactivated state at night.

Infection and erosion are the most serious complications, but fortunately they have decreased significantly since the initiation of deactivation. Erosion generally occurs within the first 12 to 18 months following implantation and is usually associated with pressure necrosis or infection. Infection is commonly due to staphylococcal organisms and is usually subclinical, often without typical signs such as induration or erythema.

Scott reports a 97% continence rate in a series of 37 women with prior failed incontinence surgery.[15] Fishman also reports the highest success rate in this population.[16] Infection and erosion rates, however, are also higher after previous surgery for incontinence. It is not surprising that the removal rates are higher in patients after prior surgery (24%) compared with patients who had not had prior surgery.

Most women with genuine stress incontinence do not require sphincter placement. However, in a small group of carefully selected women with intrinsic sphincter deficiency, the artificial sphincter is an important option for restoration of continence.

SUMMARY

Innovative approaches to genuine stress incontinence attempt to maintain the efficacy of traditional operations while decreasing morbidity.

Several different approaches to treating intrinsic sphincter deficiency were presented; each has its own merits. Although periurethral injectables do not have quite the success rate of some other approaches, they offer the most minimally invasive approach to the treatment of intrinsic sphincter deficiency. The artificial sphincter, at the other extreme, provides the most normal urinary function but is an invasive procedure with significant complications. The suburethral patch provides a more physiologic approach to the standard suburethral sling.

Further clinical trials should help to clarify the proper role of these innovative procedures as alternatives to the proven techniques discussed in the previous chapter.

REFERENCES

1. Bergman, A, Ballard, CA and Koonings, PP: Comparison of three different surgical procedures for genuine stress incontinence: Prospective randomized study. Am J Obstet Gynecol 160:1102,1989.
2. van Geelen, JM, Theeuwes, AG, Eskes, TK, et al: The clinical and urodynamic effects of anterior vaginal repair and Burch colposuspension. Am J Obstet Gynecol 159:137,1988.
3. Liu, CY: Laparoscopic retropubic colposuspension (Burch Procedure). J Repro Med 38:526,1993.
4. Vancaillie, TG and Schuessler W: Laparoscopic bladder neck suspension. J Endourology 6:137,1992.
5. Karram, MM and Bahtia NN. Patch procedure: Modified transvaginal fascia lata sling for recurrent or severe stress urinary incontinence. Obstet Gynecol 75:461,1990.
6. Juma, S, Little, NA and Raz, S: Vaginal wall sling: four years later. Urol 39:424,1992.
7. Horbach, NS: Suburethral sling procedures. In Ostergard, DR and Bent, AE (eds.): Urogynecology and Urodynamics, Theory and Practice. Williams & Wilkins, Baltimore, 1991.
8. Carrion, HM and Politano, VA: Periurethral Polytef injection for urinary incontinence. In Raz, S (ed.): Female Urology. WB Saunders, Philadelphia, 1983.
9. Vesey, SG, Rivett, A and O'Boyle, PJ: Teflon injection in female stress incontinence. Effect on urethral pressure profile and flow rate. Br J Urol 62:39,1988.
10. Lim, KB, Ball, AJ and Feneley, RCL. Periurethral Teflon injection: A simple treatment for urinary incontinence. Br J Urol 55:208,1983.
11. Griffiths, RW and Shakespeare, PG: Human dermal collagen allografts: a three year histological study. Br J Plast Surg 35:519,1982.
12. Barrett, DM, Paruekar, BG, Malizia, AA, Jr., et al: The genitourinary spheroidal membrane: an experimental study of a new percutaneously inserted prosthetic device for the control of urinary incontinence. J Urol 142:1615,1989.
13. Motley, RC and Barrett, DM: Artificial urinary sphincter cuff erosion. Experience with reimplantation in 38 patients. Urology 35:215,1990.
14. Kil, PJ and De Vries, JD: The artificial urinary sphincter in the treatment of incontinence in the female patient. Int Urogynecol J 4:35,1993.
15. Scott, FB: The use of the artificial urinary sphincter in the treatment of urinary incontinence in women. Urol Clin North Am 12:305,1985.
16. Fishman, IJ, Shabsigh, R and Scott, FB: Experience with the artificial urinary sphincter model AS800 in 148 patients. J Urol 141:307,1989.

CHAPTER 21

Urinary Tract Fistulas

Theodore J. Saclarides • Dee E. Fenner

COLOVESICAL FISTULAS

ETIOLOGY

Although the relative frequency of various causes of colovesical fistulas may vary institutionally depending on referral patterns and level of care, the most common cause overall is sigmoid diverticular disease (Table 21–1).[1-8] In fact, colovesical fistula is the most common internal fistula complicating diverticular disease, followed in frequency by colovaginal and colocutaneous fistulas. Males outnumber females in some series by a ratio as high as 6 to 1, lending support to the theory that the uterus may confer a protective effect against this phenomenon. Of those women so afflicted, 50% have had a prior hysterectomy; 83% of women with a colovaginal fistula have previously undergone a hysterectomy.[1]

In the case of sigmoid diverticulitis, fistulization is a late occurrence in the spectrum of changes that accompany this disease. Inflammation ensuing within a diverticulum after occlusion of the diverticular neck leads to bacterial overgrowth, infection, and microperforation. This perforation is usually sealed off by adjacent viscera, but occasionally free perforation into the abdominal cavity, with attendant peritonitis, may follow. A localized phlegmon may progress into a lower abdominal or pelvic abscess which, after adhering to adjacent organs, may fistulize, thereby decompressing the abscess and allowing resolution of the inflammatory focus. Other causes of inflammation-induced colovesical fistulas include inflammatory bowel disease (especially Crohn's disease) and foreign-body perforation.

Pelvic malignancies are a less frequent cause of colovesical fistulas; included are cecal, sigmoid, and rectal cancers, and to a lesser extent, bladder cancers. If these fistulas occur within a "virginal" pelvis, en bloc resection for cure may be attempted. Conversely, the presence of a colovesical fistula in a patient with a history of earlier surgery for these cancers should alert the physician to the possibility of recurrent disease, in which case resection for cure is usually not possible and palliation of symptoms is

TABLE 21–1. Causes of Colovesical Fistulas

Reference	Diverticulitis	Inflammatory Bowel Disease	Colorectal Cancer	Urogenital Cancer	Radiation
Kirsh and co-workers[2]	52%	18%	11%	9%	—
Sarr and co-workers[3]	54%	17%	17%	—	8%
Krco and co-workers[4]	40%	2%	26%	7%	12%
Morrison and co-workers[5]	61%	6%	24%	—	3%
Shatila and co-workers[6]	74%	4%	17%	4%	—
McConnell and co-workers[7]	54%	5%	14%	14%	—
King and co-workers[8]	39%	41%	5%	22%	—

the main goal of therapy. Pelvic irradiation for locally advanced cancers, such as cervical cancer, may cause colovesical fistulas; one must exclude recurrent tumor in these instances before embarking on reconstructive bladder and bowel procedures, which are complicated and carry substantial potential for morbidity due to the unforgiving nature of radiated tissue.

PRESENTATION

Even though intra-abdominal and pelvic conditions are responsible for the overwhelming majority of these fistulas, patients rarely complain primarily of abdominal pain. The reason is that, at this point, inflammation has subsided because of decompression into the bladder. Urinary tract symptoms predominate as a rule, and patients usually complain of cystitis, dysuria, pneumaturia, and fecaluria. They may also have a history of recurrent urinary tract infections unresponsive to multiple courses of antibiotics. Occasionally, urosepsis develops, especially when distal urinary tract obstruction is present. The passage of urine per rectum rarely occurs, presumably because the sigmoid colon is a high-pressure area relative to the bladder and because urine does not flow in this direction.

DIAGNOSIS

Elaborate radiographic and invasive endoscopic tests more often than not fail to conclusively demonstrate a fistula (Table 21–2).[2-6,8] These tests, however, are frequently helpful in indirectly identifying the cause. For example, diverticular disease or inflammatory bowel disease may be seen using a barium enema or during colonoscopy. Assessment should begin with an accurate history and physical examination, during which questions should be asked using everyday language. For example, a patient may not understand or know if she is passing air in her urine, but she will know if her urine stream sputters or hisses. Similarly, she may not perceive stool in her urine, but can tell whether particulate matter is present. If symptoms warrant, further diagnostic testing is justified but surgical therapy should not be withheld because these tests have failed to demonstrate a fistula in a patient whose symptoms are typical in nature.

Cystoscopy

The success of cystoscopy in demonstrating a fistula is variable. Rather than actually visualizing the fistula orifice, one more often sees erythema, inflammation, and bullous edema in the vicinity of the fistula. This procedure is indicated preoperatively in order to exclude the presence of a malignancy, knowledge of which may alter the surgical approach. In the case of diverticular fistulas, the dome of the bladder is usually affected; the trigone is affected if the fistula is caused by recurrent rectal cancer.

Barium Enema

Barium enemas demonstrate the fistula in less than 50% of instances. These examinations are nevertheless helpful in that indirect evidence as to the underlying cause may be obtained. A variation of this procedure is the Bourne test; following a barium enema, a sample of urine is centrifuged and the sample is then radiographed, looking for a barium pellet at the bottom of the tube.[9]

Computed Tomography (CT Scan)

A constellation of findings may be seen during CT scanning of a patient with a suspected colovesical fistula. Included are air within the bladder, a thickened bowel loop in close proximity to a thickened bladder wall, and passage of contrast material between the bowel and bladder. Although CT scans are more sensitive than conventional radiography in delineating the fistula, they usually cannot distinguish among diverticular disease, inflammatory bowel disease, and cancer. This distinction is more easily made by using contrast enemas or endoscopy.

Urologic Radiography

As shown in Table 21–2, cystography and intravenous pyelography are of little value and rarely add to the diagnosis or management of colovesical fistula.

Intestinal Endoscopy

Flexible sigmoidoscopy also rarely identifies a fistula, although this examination is indicated in the assessment of questionable barium enema abnormali-

TABLE 21–2. Diagnostic Yield of Procedures to Detect Enterovesical, Colovesical Fistula

Reference	Barium Enema	Cystoscopy	Cystography	CT Scan	GI Endoscopy
Kirsch and co-workers[2]	32%	88%	56%	11%	6%
Sarr and co-workers[3]	38%	20%	40%	100%	0%
Krco and co-workers[4]	43%	96%	19%	—	0%
Morrison and co-workers[5]	55%	87%	50%	—	—
Shatila and co-workers[6]	29%	75%	42%	—	0%
King and co-workers[8]	34%	57%	—	—	8%

ties, and in distinguishing benign from malignant conditions.

SURGERY

Unless multiple coexisting medical illnesses are present, surgery is advised. In the absence of a bowel obstruction, the colon should be prepared as for any elective resection, namely with an oral lavage solution, cathartics, or enemas. Oral and perioperative intravenous antibiotics are also administered. If the fistula is secondary to a benign process (e.g., diverticulitis, Crohn's disease), a one-stage resection and anastomosis can be done safely and is the preferred surgical option.[3,8,10] A two- or three-stage approach, whereby the fecal stream is temporarily diverted, is rarely necessary. The bladder opening should be curetted and closed if possible; if fibrosis or tension prohibit closure, the bladder is left open and dependent drainage is maintained for 7 to 10 days. The omentum should be placed between the anastomosis and bladder opening to retard refistulization.

If the fistula is secondary to malignant disease or radiation, a one-stage resection is less frequently possible. The extent of local disease instead may dictate fecal diversion alone. In rare cases, an exenteration may be performed, if all cancer can be resected and no evidence of disease beyond the confines of the pelvis exists.

VESICOVAGINAL FISTULAS

Vesicovaginal fistulas are one of the unfortunate obstetric complications of prolonged childbirth. Today, in most developed countries, with active management of labor and the use of cesarean sections for prolonged, complicated deliveries, they are uncommon. Currently, prior gynecologic surgery is the most common cause of fistula formation. In 1988 Lee, Symmonds, and Williams reported a series of 303 patients referred for management of genitourinary fistulas and found that 82% had been caused by gynecologic operations, with more than 50% occurring after total abdominal hysterectomy.[11] Overall, incidence of vesicovaginal fistula following a total abdominal hysterectomy is approximately 0.5 to 1%.[12]

Kursh and co-workers postulated that fistulas producing symptoms during the first 24 to 48 hours after surgery are probably secondary to operative trauma that was unrecognized at the time of the primary procedure. Fistulas that appear 10 to 30 days following hysterectomy may result from devascularization, demuscularization, hematoma with infection, or a misplaced suture that had gradually eroded into the bladder.[13] True delayed fistula formation occurring 30 days or later after the surgery is usually secondary to prior radiation therapy; such fistulas may appear virtually any time subsequent to treatment. In such patients, recurrence or extension of cancer into the bladder must always be considered and evaluated prior to any surgical repair.

PREVENTION

As with most surgical complications, the best treatment is prevention. Prior to hysterectomy, a review of the patient's past medical history, including previous cesarean sections, pelvic inflammatory disease, prior radiation, or history of endometriosis is essential. Surgery should be performed with sharp rather than blunt dissection, especially when separating the bladder from the lower uterine segment and cervix. The uterus should be pulled cephalad, the border of the bladder identified, and the ureters retracted laterally. There should always be wide mobilization of the bladder from the cervix and upper vagina, and the position of the ureters should be monitored frequently. If an injury to the bladder or ureters is suspected, prompt verification is mandatory; this can be accomplished by administering intravenous indigo carmine or by filling the bladder with dye and looking for leakage. With any doubt, the surgeon should either open the dome of the bladder or perform teloscopy and inspect the bladder mucosa for injury. Intraoperative gross hematuria should raise clinical suspicion of a possible injury and should be evaluated accordingly.

DIAGNOSIS

The presence of a vesicovaginal fistula may be evident immediately postoperatively or may not appear for as long as 3 to 5 weeks after surgery. Kursh noted that two thirds of patients complained of excessive abdominal pain, distention, or adynamic ileus.[13] In addition, signs that may indicate trauma to the bladder are gross hematuria, decreased urine output, fever, and bladder irritability. Depending on the size and location of the fistula, the patient may not notice vaginal leakage until after her Foley catheter has been removed, which is generally on the first postoperative day. After that time, any constant wetness, irritation, or leakage from the vagina must be considered as a vesicovaginal or ureterovaginal fistula until proven otherwise.

After a fistula is suspected, complete and thorough evaluation of the urinary tract is warranted. The patient should be examined in the dorsal lithotomy position with a vaginal speculum. Careful inspection should be made of the apex of the vagina, specifically the suture line of the vaginal cuff, where a fistula is most likely to form due to inadvertent incorporation of the bladder into the cuff at the time of closure. This area will be indurated and inflamed; the clinician must be careful to avoid further trauma to the bladder and to avoid widening the fistula. If the fistula is not visualized, the bladder may be filled with 300 mL of methylene blue through a transurethral catheter. Again with direct visualization, dye may be seen leaking through the fistula. If the fistula is still not demonstrated, a tampon may be placed in the vagina and the patient instructed to walk, after which reexamination may reveal dye on the tampon. If the tampon is not stained, one can feel reassured that there is no fistula from the bladder, although this does not rule out a ureterovaginal fistula. Excretory urography is essential to rule out traumatic lesion of either ureter and should always be performed even if a vesicovaginal fistula has been diagnosed by clinical examination, because multiple fistulas may be present. Urethroscopy and cystoscopy are performed to determine the proximity of the fistula to the ureteral orifices.

MANAGEMENT AND REPAIR

When and how vesicovaginal fistulas should be repaired are controversial. The first consideration is timing. It was initially felt that a waiting period of 6 months was mandatory to allow restoration of tissue pliability and resolution of inflammation. The drawback to waiting this long, however, is that most patients continue to be symptomatic, suffering from urinary incontinence and vulvar irritation; consequently they may have social and sexual restrictions. If the tissue is free of infection, inflammation, necrosis, and edema, a waiting period of longer than 6 weeks (during which time dependent bladder drainage is instituted) is not justified. Symmonds has noted that 15% to 20% of fistulas will spontaneously heal during this time, but if healing has not occurred by 6 weeks, further waiting is fruitless.[14]

Early intervention with repair of the fistula as soon as the diagnosis is made has now been reported in several series with good success. Collins noted an 80% primary healing rate of 29 fistulas repaired transvaginally within 2 weeks of the original surgery. He used preoperative steroid therapy,[15] but this is no longer considered essential. Success can still be expected without steroid pretreatment. Blandy and coworkers reported a 100% success rate with an abdominal repair of 25 vesicovaginal fistulas using an open bladder technique and omental flap.[16] The spectrum of currently available antibiotics and the use of small, absorbable, nonreactive suture material have further augmented the success of early surgical repair.

Good surgical principles must be followed. Tancer has stated the optimum time for surgical repair depends on the general condition of the patient, the condition of the tissues surrounding the fistula, and the condition of the urine. The best results are obtained when the patient is not anemic or malnourished, the upper urinary tract is normal, and the urine is sterile. Inflammation and swelling must have resolved.[17]

To obtain a successful repair by any method, the bladder and vagina must be sufficiently mobilized to allow for a tension-free two-layer closure. The fistula tract should be excised. Postoperatively urine must be kept sterile and adequate urinary drainage maintained for 1 to 2 weeks. Suprapubic drainage is preferred, especially if the balloon from a transurethral catheter might lie upon the surgical repair and traumatize the suture line.

Transvaginal vs Transabdoinal Repair

Either a transabdominal or transvaginal repair can be used successfully if the proper surgical principles previously outlined are followed. Obviously, a transvaginal approach is easier and has less danger of morbidity for the patient. Latzko's operation is most commonly used for a transvaginal surgical repair[18] and basically resembles a small colpocleisis.[17]

Principles of the Latzko procedure are as follows. An area of the vaginal mucosa surrounding the fistula is denuded and the pubovesical fascia mobilized. This does not remove the entire thickness of the vaginal wall but only the vaginal mucosa. The first sutures are then placed anteriorly to posteriorly, not from side to side (Fig. 21–1). After the first layer of

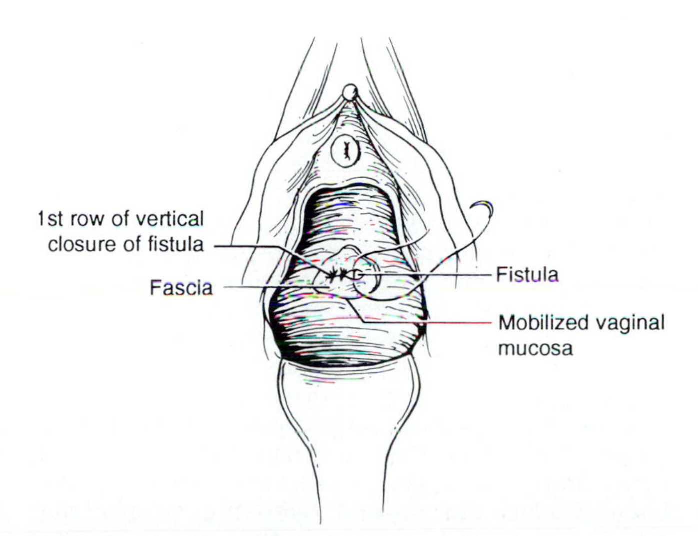

FIGURE 21–1. Latzko's procedure for vaginal closure of a vesicovaginal fistula.

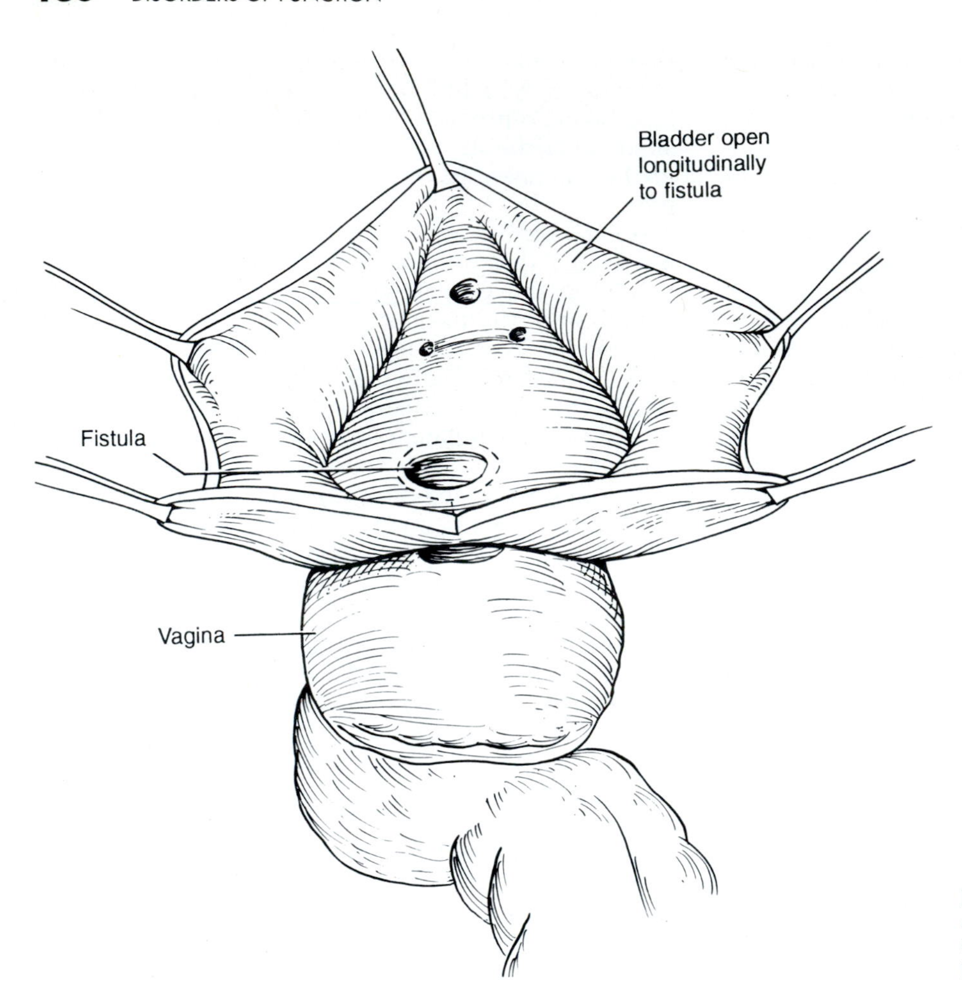

FIGURE 21–2. Transabdominal transvesical approach. Bladder is opened to fistula tract, which is excised. The bladder must be completely mobilized from the vagina.

sutures has been placed, 250 mL of sterile milk or methylene blue are introduced into the bladder through a transurethral catheter and the suture line is inspected for leakage. If extravasation exists, the suture line should be reinforced until a watertight suture line has been created. The second and third layers of imbricating suture lines are then placed. Next, the vaginal mucosa is closed over the repair. As indicated, no attempt is made to excise the fistulous tract during Latzko's procedure. The vaginal mucosa is simply removed from around the fistula and the vaginal wall is used to cover it. In his series of 45 patients, Tancer reported a 93% success rate, with removal of the bladder catheter within the first 3 days. Bladder drainage for 7 to 14 days is generally recommended, however, and the patient is instructed to avoid straining and inserting objects into the vagina for 6 to 8 weeks. Tanzer noted that 3 of 4 primary failures were successfully closed by a second Latzko repair at 8 weeks, and that one fistula had decreased in size and closed spontaneously.[19] Elkins, Delancey, and McGuire reported an 86.5% success rate in the repair of large vesicovaginal fistulas (larger than 4 cm in diameter) using a Latzko closure with a Martius flap. The graft is rotated from the bulbocavernosus muscle and overlying fat pad and placed between the repair and the vaginal mucosa. This flap provides thickness and aids in separating the bladder and vagina.[20]

When adequate transvaginal visualization of the fistula is not possible, an abdominal approach is required. Another indication for a transabdominal approach is a fistula located near the ureteral orifices, in which situation repair may be impossible without reimplantation of the ureter. In general, a low transverse or Pfannenstiel incision is adequate for exposure. The bladder and vagina must be adequately mobilized for the surgeon to perform a layered, tension-free closure. After adequate exposure is obtained, the bladder and vagina are separated using sharp dissection. In 1951 O'Connor and Sokol reported a transabdominal transvesical approach, which allows for wide mobilization of the fistula from the underlying vagina.[21] With this dissection, the bladder dome is opened and the bladder is bisected transversely, carrying the incision to and around the fistula while at the same time excising the scarred fibrous tract. The walls of the bladder are widely mobilized from the underlying vagina and both ureteral orifices are visualized and protected during the dissection and repair (Fig. 21–2). After the tract is excised, the vagina is closed in two layers. Either a peritoneal flap or a pedicle of omentum is brought down and placed between the bladder and the vagina. The bladder incision is then closed in two layers beginning at the apex of the sagittal incision. Wein and Malloy reported a series of 34 patients with high or recurrent vesicovaginal fistulas repaired using this technique; success was achieved in over 90%. They advocate the transabdominal transvesical approach for patients with midvaginal or high vaginal fistulas, narrow vaginas, or concomitant urethral or rectal fistulas. Though no universal criteria have been established for selecting either a transvaginal or transabdominal approach, the surgeon needs to carefully evaluate the patient preoperatively and to assess his or her own surgical skills in choosing the right operation.

Vesicovaginal fistulas are one of the most distressing surgical complications for both patient and surgeon. Careful, sharp dissection and adequate exposure should help prevent them. After being suspected, a thorough evaluation and accurate diagnosis should be made. With careful surgical repair, more than 90% should have a successful outcome.

REFERENCES

1. Kurtz, DI and Mazier, WP: Diverticular fistulas. Semin Colon Rectal Surg 1:93–96,1990.
2. Kirsh, GM, Hampel, N, Shuck, JM and Resnick, MI: Diagnosis and management of vesicoenteric fistulas. Surg Gynecol Obstet 173:91–97,1991.
3. Sarr MG, Fishman, EK, Goldman, SM, et al: Enterovesical fistula. Surg Gynecol Obstet 164:41–48,1987.
4. Krco, MJ, Jacobs, SC, Malangoni, MA and Lawson, RK: Colovesical fistulas. Urology 23:3460–3462,1984.
5. Morrison, PD and Addison, V: A study of colovesical fistulae in a district hospital. Ann R Coll Surg Eng 65:221–223,1983.
6. Shatila, AH and Ackerman, NB: Diagnosis and management of colovesical fistulas. Surg Gynecol Obstet 143:71–74,1976.
7. McConnell, DB, Sasaki, TM and Vetto, RM: Experience with colovesical fistula. Am J Surg 140:80–84,1980.
8. King, RM, Beart, RW, Jr and McIlrath, OC: Colovesical and rectovesical fistulas. Arch Surg 117:680–683,1982.
9. Amendola, MA, Agha, FP, Dent, TL, et al: Detection of occult colovesical fistula by the Bourne test. Am J Roentgenol 142:715–718,1984.
10. Mileski, WJ, Joehl, RJ, Rege, RV and Nahrwold, DL: One-stage resection and anastomosis in the management of colovesical fistula. Am J Surg 153:75–79,1987.
11. Lee, RA, Symmonds, RE and Williams, TJ: Current status of genitourinary fistula. Obstet Gynecol 72:313,1988.
12. Thompson, JD: Vesicovaginal fistulas. In Thompson, JD and Rock, JA, (eds.): Telinde's Operative Gynecology, ed 7. JB Lippincott, Philadelphia, 1992.
13. Kursh, ED, Morse, RM, Resnick, MI and Persky L: Prevention of the development of a vesicovaginal fistula. Surg Gynecol Obstet 166:409,1988.
14. Symmonds, RE: Incontience: Vesical and urethral fistulas. Clinical Obstet Gynecol 27:499,1984.
15. Collins, CG, Collins, JH, Harrison, BR, et al: Early repair of vesicovaginal fistula. Am J Obstet Gynecol 111:524,1971.
16. Blandy, JP, Badenoch, DF, Fowler, CG, et al. Early repair of iatrogenic injury to the ureter or bladder after gynecologic surgery. J Urol 146:761,1991.
17. Tancer, ML: Urologic injuries: Bladder and urethra in complications. Obstet Gynecol Surg.
18. Latzko, W: Postoperative vesicovaginal fistulas: Genesis and therapy. Am J Surg 58:211,1942.
19. Tancer, ML: Observations on prevention and management of vesicovaginal fistula after total hysterectomy. Surg Gynecol Obstet 175:501,1992.
20. Elkins, TE, DeLancey, JO and McGuire, EJ: The use of modified Martius graft as an adjunctive technique in vesicovaginal and rectovaginal fistula repair. Obstet Gynecol 75:727,1990.
21. O'Connor, V and Sokol, J: Vesicovaginal fistula from the standpoint of the urologist. J Urol 66:579,1951.

CHAPTER 22

Constipation: Etiology and Evaluation

Elisa H. Birnbaum

Constipation is one of the most common self-diagnosed and self-treated gastrointestinal disorders in the United States, where an estimated 2% of the population is symptomatic.[1] The financial cost is not insignificant; in 1985 the total market for laxatives in the United States reached $492 million.[2] The concept of "auto-intoxication" was popularized in 1908 by Sir William Arbuthnot Lane, who attributed a multitude of disease states and symptoms to constipation.[3] Many people feel that a daily bowel movement is needed to prevent "auto-intoxication." This misconception contributes to the use and abuse of laxatives. Large studies have shown that normal bowel frequency ranges from three bowel movements per day to three per week.[4–6] It is generally accepted that patients who have fewer than three bowel movements per week are outside the normal range and are considered constipated.[7] Patients may define constipation differently than their physicians, however, and many with normal frequency consider themselves constipated because of straining, incomplete evacuation, painful movements, or dry consistency.[8,9]

Although large surveys suggest that complaints of constipation increase after the age of 65,[1,10–13] 80% to 90% of patients over 60 reported at least one bowel movement per day.[4,14] Confusing the interpretation of these data is the admission of many respondents that they took laxatives frequently.[4] Milne found that only 2% of men and 7% of women over 60 had less than one bowel movement every third day but 38% of the men and 50% of the women surveyed used laxatives.[5] In summary, reports of infrequent defecation may not increase with age, but the use of laxatives does.[6]

ETIOLOGY

Mechanical causes of constipation must be excluded before initiating treatment. In this regard, endoscopy or contrast studies of the colon are used to reveal cancer or obstructing strictures secondary to diverticular disease or inflammatory bowel disease. Sigmoid volvulus rarely causes chronic constipation; instead, it usually presents with abdominal distention and obstipation of short duration. Short-segment aganglionosis (Hirschsprung's disease) is rarely seen and may not be diagnosed until young adulthood.

Constipation may be due to many causes, which are outlined in Table 22–1. Particularly in the elderly, it is often attributed to inadequate fluid or fiber intake, immobility,[6,10,14] and inability to walk to the bathroom.[15,16] Studies have shown that constipated patients have lower stool output and slower transit than normal patients and are not as likely to respond to increases in fiber intake as control patients. Dietary fiber may increase stool weight but its ability to increase stool frequency hasn't been conclusively demonstrated.[17,18] Similarly, the role of increased exercise is controversial; it hasn't shown a consistent effect on large bowel function.[19] Moderate exercise may accelerate transit time but does not significantly affect stool frequency.[20]

Constipation is a frequent side effect of many medications.[12] Aluminum and calcium antacids, diuretics, sucralfate, beta blockers, calcium channel blockers, ganglionic blockers, anticholinergics, opioids, and tricyclic antidepressants are commonly implicated. Many elderly patients take multiple medications, so that there may be an association between the number of medications ingested and symptoms of constipation. Long-term laxative abuse has been implicated as a cause of constipation as well, especially with anthraquinone cathartics.[11]

Metabolic, endocrine, and neurologic disorders may cause constipation. Included are hyperparathyroidism (causing hypercalcemia), hypokalemia, and hypothyroidism. In the latter, breath H_2 excretion tests may show slow small-bowel transit,[21] reversible when treated with hormone replacement. Scleroderma is a systemic disease capable of hindering small- and large-bowel motility by causing neuromuscular atrophy and fibrosis.[22–24] Multiple sclerosis may also cause constipation.[25] Spinal cord lesions or injuries causing paraplegia or quadriplegia may also cause both constipation and fecal incontinence.[26] High spinal cord lesions lead to an overall decrease in motility causing colonic inertia; low cord lesions lead to a loss of inhibitory influences, causing decreased compliance, bowel spasticity, and prolonged left colon transit time.

TABLE 22–1. Causes of Constipation

Lifestyle
Inadequate fiber, fluid intake
Insufficient exercise
Immobility
Medications
Aluminum, calcium antacids
Diuretics
Beta-blockers
Calcium channel blockers
Anticholinergics
Opioids
Tricyclic antidepressants
Mechanical causes
Hirschsprung's disease
Colorectal cancer
Inflammatory bowel disease
Volvulus
Systemic diseaes
Metabolic—diabetes, thyroid disorders
Neuromuscular—scleroderma, multiple sclerosis, spinal cord injuries, tumors
Pelvic floor disorders

Pelvic floor abnormalities should be included in the differential diagnosis of patients with constipation. This group of disorders includes nonrelaxing puborectalis muscle, intussusception, rectal prolapse, rectocele, and the levator ani syndrome. The etiology of these abnormalities is unclear, but it may be related to dysfunction and discoordination of the pelvic floor muscles.[27,28] Rectosigmoid dysfunction may occur in patients with abnormal gastrocolic reflexes.[16,29]

Psychiatric conditions such as depression, dementia, and personality disorders have been associated with constipation.[6,8,14,30–33] Constipation may be a sequela of the medications used to treat these disorders but may also be secondary to faulty toilet habits, poor sensation of feces within the rectum, and inability to walk to the bathroom. Some forms of constipation may be related to psychologically traumatic events such as sexual or physical abuse during childhood.

PATHOPHYSIOLOGY

The pathogenesis of constipation is multifactorial and may be due to reduced number and duration of propulsive movements[34] or neuronal dysplasia of the rectosigmoid.[35] In the latter instances, patients lack pressure receptors in the submucosal layer, so that passive stretching of the bowel wall does not trigger normal propulsive intestinal motility. Long-term laxative abuse (particularly with the anthraquinone cathartics) has been shown to induce toxic degenerative changes in the intramural ganglia and may account for the need for increasing dosage in patients who take these cathartics.[36,37]

Abnormalities within the myenteric and submucous plexuses have prompted investigators to evaluate the role of neuropeptides in constipation. Acetylcholine stimulates contractile activity of colonic smooth muscle,[38] and reduced release of acetycholine has been seen in severely constipated patients,[39] although this finding may have limited clinical usefulness. For example, edrophonium chloride, a strong cholinergic stimulus, does not induce increased motor activity in patients with slow-transit constipation.[40] The anticholinesterase agent neostigmine can increase cholinergic activity in normal patients but it was not able to alter cholinergic activity in patients with severe progressive systemic sclerosis.[23]

Deficiencies in the distribution of other neurotransmitters have also been identified. Lower levels of vasoactive intestinal peptide were found in the enteric plexuses of patients with idiopathic constipation; substance P and neuropeptide Y levels were unchanged in the same patients.[41] Vasoactive intestinal peptide is an inhibitory neurotransmitter; low concentrations of it may allow increased colonic segmentation and decreased motility. An increase in 5-hydroxytryptamine and 5-hydroxyindoleacetic acid has been found in the mucosa and circular muscle in patients with slow-transit constipation.[42]

Although constipation is reported to occur more often in women, constipation symptoms and stool volume and consistency are not associated with specific menstrual phase, parity, or menopausal status.[4,6,7,9–13,43–46] Sex hormones and prostaglandins released from the endometrium have been implicated as potential causative agents of bowel dysfunction, both diarrhea and constipation, during menstruation.[43,47] Peak serum progesterone levels occur in the third trimester of pregnancy but do not correlate with worsening constipation.[48]

Constipation is the most common bowel complaint after hysterectomy and can occur in up to 10% of previously asymptomatic patients.[49] Injury to the autonomic parasympathetic nerves to the left colon and rectum may occur during pelvic surgery and has been implicated as a causative factor in posthysterectomy constipation. An increase in rectal compliance and deficits of rectal sensory function have been demonstrated in women with intractable constipation after hysterectomy.[50] Others have noted an increase in urinary frequency associated with a decrease in bowel frequency after hysterectomy.[51] The development of constipation, however, does not seem to be related to the type of hysterectomy or whether oophorectomy was simultaneously performed.[49,51]

EVALUATION

Increased public awareness that a change in bowel habits may herald the presence of an underlying colorectal cancer has increased the frequency of evaluation and treatment of constipation. Accurate evaluation is critical, because certain forms of constipation may be surgically treated successfully.[52] Initial evaluation should begin with a thorough history and physical examination. Patients should be asked to clarify their symptoms and a detailed bowel history including frequency, ease of evacuation, and consistency should be included. Medical illnesses and all medications taken, both prescription and over-the-counter, should be listed. A digital rectal examination is done to exclude low rectal cancers, anal strictures, rectoceles, and other anorectal abnormalities. Proctosigmoidoscopy may identify a solitary rectal ulcer or anterior erythema that indicates internal intussusception or rectal prolapse. Colonoscopy or barium enema may be helpful in determining a more proximal source of constipation and should be considered, especially if the symptoms are new in onset or blood is present in the stool.

Radiologic and physiologic testing should be considered if symptoms persist despite dietary and medical alterations. The order of testing depends on patient symptoms and physician preference. Colonic transit times are usually performed first if the primary complaint is infrequent defecation. Defecography and balloon expulsion may be more helpful initially if the patient complains of difficulty evacuating stool that is sensed within the pelvis or rectum. Anal manometry and electromyography may be useful if adult Hirschsprung's disease is suspected or if the patient has additional symptoms of incontinence.

To measure colon transit time, the patient must consume a high-fiber diet and refrain from taking laxatives or enemas during the examination period. Noncompliance and diarrhea may give a falsely normal examination. Colonic inertia is probably present if the radiopaque rings are evenly distributed throughout the right, transverse, and left colon by the fifth day. Outlet obstruction, usually due to a nonrelaxing puborectalis muscle or internal intussusception, results in normal transit of the rings to the rectum by the third day. Poor emptying of the rectum, however, results in retention of rings within the rectal ampulla and sigmoid colon, as seen on follow-up radiographs taken on the fifth day. Delayed gastric emptying and prolonged small-bowel transit has been seen in patients with chronic constipation[53] but tests to identify these abnormalities are not routinely performed unless a diffuse motility problem is suspected.

Defecography is used to identify abnormalities of defecation such as intussusception and nonrelaxing puborectalis. Internal intussusception of the rectum can block the anal outlet, resulting in incomplete evacuation of the rectal contents. Full rectal prolapse may be demonstrated by defecography if the patient is unable to reproduce it in the office. Radiologic findings, however, must be interpreted within the context of the clinical presentation.

Anal manometry has limited value in the evaluation of constipation. Resting and squeeze pressures are usually normal unless prolonged straining has caused a stretch injury of the pudendal nerve.[54] Rectal sensation and compliance can be measured manometrically; decreased sensation documented by high minimal sensory rectal volumes may be found in patients with megarectum. The anorectal inhibitory reflex is absent in Hirschsprung's disease and may also be absent in patients with megarectum who require large volume to induce the inhibitory reflex.

Electromyography has not been useful in the evaluation of constipation except in cases of incontinence associated with prolonged straining. Concentric needle electromyographic measurement of puborectalis activity during straining has been proposed as a means of diagnosing nonrelaxing puborectalis.[28] The presence of a needle within the puborectalis muscle may itself cause contraction of the puborectalis muscle during defecation. In addition, paradoxical contraction in disorders other than obstructed defecation limits the usefulness of this test.[55]

Failure to expel a latex balloon filled with 60 to 100 mL of saline or air may be an indicator of disordered defecation.[28] A recent review of patients with nonrelaxing puborectalis muscle revealed that all patients with this cause of outlet obstruction were unable to expel a balloon in the sitting position.[56] Patients who had prominence of the puborectalis muscle demonstrated by defecography and inability to expel a rectal ballon had true disordered defecation.

If underlying psychologic problems are suspected, the patient should undergo a psychologic profile followed by counseling if necessary. The Minnesota Multiphasic Personality Inventory (MMPI) can be used to identify a "neurotic triad" made up of hypochondriasis, depression, and hysteria. This profile pattern may indicate a propensity to manifest psychologic distress as physical symptoms (i.e., somatization). Hypochondriasis and depression were frequently found in constipated patients, and all three symptoms were frequently identified in patients with levator ani spasm.[57] Using the MMPI, Tucker demonstrated that certain psychologic factors were as important as dietary considerations in accounting for variance in stool production.[17]

Patients with normal-transit constipation have been found to have higher psychiatric distress scores than those with slow-transit constipation.[58] It has been suggested that patients with normal-transit constipation may have misperceptions of normal bowel habits and that psychologic counseling may alleviate symptoms of constipation. The Hospital Anxiety and Depression (HAD) questionnaire was used to evaluate patients for chronic constipation before surgical treatment.[30] Patients who had poor surgical outcome had high preoperative HAD scores, suggesting that a more thorough psychiatric assessment before surgery might have been beneficial.

SUMMARY

The cause of constipation is multifactorial, but the treating physician must exclude an obstructing tumor or stricture before embarking on an evaluation specifically intended to diagnose the cause of dysfunctional defecation. In this regard, colonoscopy or contrast colon x-rays are useful. At the very minimum, proctosigmoidoscopy should be done on all patients with a chief complaint of constipation. Colon transit studies and defecography are then used to classify the underlying problem as one of diffuse inertia or pelvic floor outlet disorder.

REFERENCES

1. Sonnenberg, A, and Koch, TR: Epidemiology of constipation in the United States. Dis Colon Rectum 32:1,1989.
2. Rosendahl, I: Laxatives: a drugstore-friendly category. Drug Topics (Sept):48,1986.
3. Lane, WA: Remarks on the results of the operative treatment of chronic constipation. Br Med J 126,1908.
4. Connell, AM, et al: Variation of bowel habit in two population samples. Br Med J 1095,1965.
5. Milne, JS, and Williamson, J: Bowel habit in older people. Geront Clin 14:56,1972.
6. Everhart, JE, et al: A longitudinal survey of self-reported bowel habits in the United States. Dig Dis Sci 34:1153,1989.
7. Johanson, JF, Sonnenberg, A and Koch, TR: Clinical epidemiology of chronic constipation. J Clin Gastroenterol 11:525,1989.
8. Whitehead, WE, et al: Constipation in the elderly living at home: Definition, prevalence, and relationship to lifestyle and health status. J Am Geriatr Soc 37:423,1989.
9. Moore-Gillon, V: Constipation: What does the patient mean? J Royal Soc Med 77:108,1984.
10. Sandler, RS, Jordan, MC and Shelton, BJ: Demographic and dietary determinants of constipation in the US population. Am J Public Health 80:185,1990.
11. Stewart, RB, et al: Correlates of constipation in an ambulatory elderly population. Am J Gastroenterol 87:859,1992.
12. Campbell, AJ, Busby, WJ and Horwath, CC: Factors associated with constipation in a community based sample of people aged 70 years and over. J Epidemiol Community Health 47:23,1993.
13. Hale, WE, Perkins, LL, May, FE, et al: Symptom prevalence in the elderly: an evaluation of age, sex, disease, and medication use. J Am Geriatr Soc 34:333,1986.
14. Donald, IP, et al: A study of constipation in the elderly living at home. Gerontology 31:112,1985.
15. Wald, A: Constipation and fecal incontinence in the elderly. Gastroenterol Clin North Am 19:405,1990.
16. Roe, AM, Bartolo, DCC and Mortensen, NJ: Diagnosis and surgical management of intractable constipation. Br J Surg 73:854,1986.
17. Tucker, DM, et al: Dietary fiber and personality factors as determinants of stool output. Gastroenterol 81:879,1981.
18. Müller-Lissner, SA: Effect of wheat bran on weight of stool and gastrointestinal transit time: a meta-analysis. Br Med J 296: 615,1988.
19. Bingham, SA, and Cummings, JH: Effect of exercise and physical fitness on large intestinal function. Gastroenterol 97:1389,1989.
20. Oettlé, GJ: Effect of moderate exercise on bowel habit. Gut 32:941,1991.
21. Shafer, RB, Prentiss, RA and Bond, JH: Gastrointestinal transit in thyroid disease. Gastroenterol 86:852,1984.
22. Whitehead, WE, Taetelbaum, G, Wigley, FM, et al: Rectosigmoid motility and myoelectric activity in progressive systemic sclerosis. Gastroenterol 96:428,1989.
23. Battle, WM, Snape, WJ, Jr, Wright, S, et al: Abnormal colonic motility in progressive systemic sclerosis. Ann Int Med 94:749,1981.
24. Hamel-Roy, J, Devroede, G, Arhan, P, et al: Comparative esophageal and anorectal motility in scleroderma. Gastroenterol 88:1,1985.
25. Glick, ME, Meshkinpour, H, Haldeman, S, et al: Colonic dysfunction in multiple sclerosis. Gastroenterol 83:1002,1982.
26. Longo, WE, Ballantyne, GH and Modlin, IM: The colon, anorectum, and spinal cord patient: functional alterations of the denervated hindgut. Dis Colon Rectum 32:261,1989.
27. Kuijpers, HC: Application of the colorectal laboratory in diagnosis and treatment of functional constipation. Dis Colon Rectum 33:35,1990.

28. Turnbull, GK, Lennard-Jones, JE and Bartram, CI: Failure of rectal expulsion as a cause of constipation: Why fibre and laxatives sometimes fail. Lancet 1:767,1986.
29. Reynolds, JC, Ouyang, A, Lee, CA, et al: Chronic severe constipation: prospective motility studies in 25 consecutive patients. Gastroenterol 92:414,1987.
30. Fisher, SE, Breckon, K, Andrews, HA, et al: Psychiatric screening for patients with faecal incontinence or chronic constipation referred for surgical treatment. Br J Surg 76:352,1989.
31. Devroede, G, Girard, G, Bouchoucha, M, et al: Idiopathic constipation by colonic dysfunction: relationship with personality and anxiety. Dig Dis Sci 34:1428,1989.
32. Preston, DM, Pfeffer, JM and Lennard-Jones, JE: Psychiatric assessment of patients with severe constipation (abstr). Gut 25:A582,1984.
33. Bleijenberg, G, and Kuijpers, HC: Treatment of spastic pelvic floor syndrome with biofeedback. Dis Colon Rectum 30:108,1987.
34. Bassotti, G, Gaburri, M, Imbimbo, BP, et al: Colonic mass movements in idiopathic chronic constipation. Gut 29:1173,1988.
35. Stoss, F: Neuronal dysplasia: Considerations for the pathogenesis and treatment of primary chronic constipation in adults. Int J Colorect Dis 5:106,1990.
36. Smith, B: Effect of irritant purgatives on the myenteric plexus in man and the mouse. Gut 9:139,1968.
37. Riemann, JF and Zimmermann, W: Ultrastructural studies of colonic nerve plexuses in chronic laxative abuse. Gastroenterology 74:1084,1978.
38. Sarna, SK: Physiology and pathophysiology of colonic motor activity. Dig Dis Sci 36:827,1991.
39. Burleigh, DE: Evidence for a functional cholinergic deficit in human colonic tissue resected for constipation. J Pharm Pharmacol 40:55,1988.
40. Bassotti, G, Chiarioui, G, Imbimbo, BP, et al: Impaired colonic motor response to cholinergic stimulation in patients with severe chronic idiopathic (slow transit type) constipation. Dig Dis Sci 38:1040,1993.
41. Milner, P, Crowe, R, Kamm, MA, et al: Vasoactive intestinal polypeptide levels in sigmoid colon in idiopathic constipation and diverticular disease. Gastroenterol 99:666,1990.
42. Lincoln, J, Crowe, R, Kamm, MA, et al: Serotonin and 5-hydroxyindoleacetic acid are increased in the sigmoid colon in severe idiopathic constipation. Gastroenterol 98:1219,1990.
43. Turnbull, GK, Thompson, DG, Day, S, et al: Relationship between symptoms, menstrual cycle and orocaecal transit in normal and constipated women. Gut 30:30,1989.
44. Hinds, JP, Stoney, B and Wald, A: Does gender or the menstrual cycle affect colonic transit? Am J Gastroenterol 84:123,1989.
45. Kamm, MA, Farthing, MJG and Lennard-Jones, JE: Bowel function and transit rate during the menstrual cycle. Gut 30:605,1989.
46. Wyman, JB, Heaton, KW, Manning, AP, et al: Variability of colonic function in healthy subjects. Gut 19:146,1978.
47. Rees, WDW and Rhodes, J: Altered bowel habit and menstruation (letter). Lancet 1:475,1976.
48. Wald, A, Van Thiel, DH, Hoechsteller, L, et al: Effect of pregnancy on gastrointestinal transit. Dig Dis Sci 27:1015,1982.
49. Prior, A, Stanley, KM, Smith, ARB, et al: Relation between hysterectomy and the irritable bowel: A prospective study. Gut 33:814,1992.
50. Varma, JW: Autonomic influences on colorectal motility and pelvic surgery. World J Surg 16:811,1992.
51. Taylor, T, Smith, AN and Fulton, M: Effects of hysterectomy on bowel and bladder function. Int J Colorect Dis 5:228,1990.
52. Fleshman, JW, Fry, RD and Kodner, IJ: The surgical management of constipation. In Henry, MM (ed.): Baillière's Clinical Gastroenterology. Baillière Tindall, London, 1992, p 145.
53. Van Der Sijp, JRM, Kamm, MA, Nightingale, JMD, et al: Disturbed gastric and small bowel transit in severe idiopathic constipation. Dig Dis Sci 38:837,1993.
54. Snooks, SJ, Barnes, PRH, Swash, M, et al: Damage to the innervation of the pelvic floor musculature in chronic constipation. Gastroenterology 89:977,1985.
55. Jones, PN, Lubowski, DZ, Swash, M, et al: Is paradoxical contraction of puborectalis muscle of functional importance? Dis Colon Rectum 30:667,1987.
56. Fleshman, JW, Dreznik, Z, Cohen, E, et al: Balloon expulsion test facilitates diagnosis of pelvic floor outlet obstruction due to nonrelaxing puborectalis muscle. Dis Colon Rectum 35:1019,1992.
57. Heyman, S, Wexner, SD and Gulledge, AD: MMPI assessment of patients with functional bowel disorders. Dis Colon Rectum 36:593,1993.
58. Wald, A, Hinds, JP and Caruana, BJ: Psychological and physiological characteristics of patients with severe idiopathic constipation. Gastroenterol 97:932,1989.

CHAPTER 23

Medical Management of Constipation

Sheldon Sloan, M.D.

Constipation causes both emotional and financial hardship; estimated pharmaceutical costs exceed $400 million per year.[1] The magnitude of this problem is compounded by the confusion created by the lack of a consistent definition of normal stool frequency. Furthermore, other conditions such as cancer or neurologic or endocrine diseases may masquerade as constipation (Table 23–1). If present, these underlying diseases must be treated, and usually bowel

TABLE 23–1. Causes of Dysfunctional Defecation

Mechanical causes
Luminal (strictures, tumor, diverticulitis)
Extraluminal (tumors, hernias, chronic volvulus)
Muscular (scleroderma, myopathic pseudo-obstruction, myotonic dystrophy, dermatomyositis, amyloidosis)
Rectal (tumors, rectal prolapse, stricture, descending perineum syndrome, rectocele, paradoxical puborectalis activity)
Endocrinologic and metabolic causes
Diabetes mellitus
Glucagonoma
Hypercalcemia (e.g., hyperparathyroidism)
Hypokalemia
Hypothyroidism
Panhypopituitarism
Porphyria
Uremia
Neurologic causes
Peripheral (Hirschsprung's disease, Chagas' disease, neurofibromatosis, autonomic neuropathy, neuropathic intestinal pseudo-obstruction, ganglioneuromatosis, hypoganglionosis)
Central (multiple sclerosis, spinal cord lesions, Parkinson's disease, Shy-Drager syndrome, cerebrovascular accidents, tumors to brain and spinal cord)
Medications causing constipation
Antacids (calcium carbonate, aluminum hydroxide)
Anticholinergics
Anticonvulsants
Barium sulfate
Calcium channel blockers
Iron supplements
Opioids

symptoms will improve. Nonsurgical treatment of idiopathic constipation ranges from behavioral and dietary changes to prescription medications. This chapter outlines the current laxatives available and discusses their pharmacology, dosage, and toxicity. In addition, examples of challenging clinical conditions are presented.

CLASSES OF LAXATIVES

Definitions and classifications of laxatives vary. Although "cathartic" implies a vigorous cleansing of the intestines, this definition has been used interchangeably with "laxative," which has the connotation of a milder response. Depending on the specific medication, the laxative effect is produced either through increased electrolyte secretion, decreased water and electrolyte absorption, increased osmotic pressure within the lumen, or increased luminal hydrostatic pressure. The categories used in this chapter follow the U.S. Food and Drug Administration classification and are listed in Table 23–2.[2]

BULK-FORMING LAXATIVES

Bulk-forming laxatives are nondietary fiber supplements (Table 23–3). These agents decrease whole-gut transit time, lower intracolonic pressure, and produce larger volumes of stool. Additionally, they dilute bile salts that may reduce contractile activity.

Nonstarch plant or fiber polysaccharides are joined by ß1-ß4 linkages and resist digestive breakdown before reaching the colon, where anaerobic bacteria then metabolize the fiber through fermentation. Fiber polysaccharides are subclassified into cellulosic and noncellulosic types. Cellulosic polysaccharides are relatively nonsoluble in water and fermented at only a 50% rate. The more water soluble noncellulosic variety ferments at 90%. The end products of bacterial fermentation are short-chain fatty acids (SCFAs), hydrogen, carbon dioxide, and methane. SCFAs are then metabolized by the colonic mucosa and the liver through the portal circulation; they are important for maintaining local mucosal health and growth. Fiber increases bacterial metabolism and growth, which, in turn, increases fecal bulk and decreases fecal transit time in the colon.

Diet in the Western hemisphere is generally low in fiber; the average citizen of the United States consumes approximately 11 g per day, whereas 20 to 35 g is the recommended amount. Wheat bran is most effective in increasing stool size and weight (5.7 g per additional g of wheat bran ingested), followed, in descending order, by oat bran, beans, mucilage, corn, cellulose, soy, and pectin. Fruit and vegetables are almost as effective as wheat bran in increasing stool weight (4.9 g per gram of ingested fiber). Having been ingested, fiber may prolong gastric emptying; in general, the side effects are more annoying than severe. These include bloating and excess flatulence, which may subside with continued use of the fiber supplement. Dosage may vary depending on the fiber preparation and the severity of the constipation.

TABLE 23–2. Classification of Laxatives

Bulk-forming
Lubricant
Stool softeners
Saline ion laxatives
Hyperosmolar laxatives
Stimulant laxatives
Prokinetic agents
Cleansing laxatives
Opioid antagonists

TABLE 23–3. Types of Bulk-Forming Laxatives

Bran
Methyl cellulose
Psyllium
Sterculia
Wheat husk

LUBRICANT LAXATIVES

Mineral oil is the main active agent in this class; it produces its effect by penetrating and softening the stool. The oil itself is not digested, has minimal absorption, and is an effective agent if used only intermittently; if used chronically, however, potential side effects are possible. This agent should not be used in patients who have difficulty swallowing due to neurologic disorders or esophageal motor abnormalities, nor in those with severe nocturnal gastroesophageal reflux, because aspiration of mineral oil may cause a severe pneumonitis. If used on a chronic basis, mineral oil interferes with the absorption of fat-soluble vitamins (vitamins A, D, E, and K) and may also produce lipoid granulomas in the reticuloendothelial system; formation of these granulomas may be enhanced by the concomitant use of stool softeners. A less serious but still troublesome side effect is leakage of mineral oil past the anal sphincter, thus causing pruritus ani.

Mineral oil in stable emulsions penetrates stool more effectively than nonemulsified oil and may cause less anal soilage. Dosage is 15 to 30 mL orally s.i.d. or b.i.d. Although mineral oil may be given as an enema, this route of administration is best suited for the hospitalized patient.

STOOL SOFTENERS

These laxatives soften stool through a surfactant action that allows water and lipids to mix and permeate the feces.[3] These agents may also inhibit water absorption from the small bowel and colon and may stimulate fluid and electrolyte secretion.[4] Examples are calcium, potassium, and sodium salts of docusate

(Surfak, Dialose, and Colace). These agents may also appear combined with stimulant laxatives in preparations such as Feen-A-Mint, Correctol, Peri-Colase, and Doxidan. Their onset of action ranges from 6 to 72 hours when given orally, and from 2 to 15 minutes as rectal preparations. Side effects include mild abdominal cramping, rashes, and throat irritation. These agents may increase absorption of other medications including phenolphthalein and mineral oil.

SALINE ION LAXATIVES

Saline laxatives contain either a magnesium cation or phosphate anion. Examples include magnesium citrate, magnesium hydroxide, magnesium sulfate, milk of magnesia, Fleet's Phosphasoda, sodium phosphate, and sodium biphosphate. The nonabsorbable ion produces an osmotic effect that increases luminal water content and intestinal peristalsis. Evidence suggests that the magnesium-containing compounds stimulate cholecystokinin release, which may also promote peristalsis.[5] Onset of action is within 6 hours by oral route and within 15 minutes anally; the latter is especially suited for patients with idiopathic megarectum. Frequent use of these medications may cause dehydration and electrolyte abnormalities such as hypermagnesemia, hyperphosphatemia, hypocalcemia, hyperkalemia (when potassium phosphate is used), and hypernatremia (when sodium phosphate is used). Serum electrolytes should therefore be monitored in patients with impaired renal function or in patients with marginal cardiac function, in whom a salt load may precipitate congestive heart failure. Phosphate-containing enemas may also irritate the rectal mucosa and cause proctitis.

HYPEROSMOLAR LAXATIVES

Hyperosmolar laxatives promote peristalsis and cause a net increase in fecal water content. Agents in this group include glycerin, lactulose, and sorbitol. Glycerin is administered solely through the rectum; it not only lubricates the anorectum but also increases fecal water content. Its main side effect is local irritation to rectal mucosa.

Lactulose can be administered either orally or rectally; it increases stool osmolality, because it is a nonabsorbable sugar. In addition, colonic bacteria metabolize lactulose into short-chain fatty acids, which also increase osmolality and intraluminal water. This increased volume stimulates peristalsis and speeds the interval between bowel movements. Lactulose is useful for short-term relief of constipation, but side effects that can discourage patient use include bloating, excessive flatulence, and diarrhea. In patients with chronic liver disease, lactulose is useful in maintaining an acidic pH in the stool, which may lower serum ammonia levels and prevent hepatic encephalopathy. Lactulose can be titrated in increments of 30 mL for the desired number of stools; results may take up to 2 days after oral administration. Lactulose may also be given as an enema in a 25% to 30% solution.

Sorbitol is found in sugarless candy and gum and may cause chronic diarrhea in unsuspecting weight-conscious individuals. Sorbitol is similar to lactulose in that it is a nonabsorbable sugar and reaches the colon as an active osmol. Sorbitol is less expensive than lactulose but has a similar laxative effect. It can be given orally or as an enema in the same concentration as lactulose (25%–30%).

STIMULANT LAXATIVES

Stimulant laxatives, the largest class, include the anthraquinones, polyphenolic agents, castor oil, and dehydrocholic acid. These agents stimulate intestinal motility through increased production of colonic prostaglandins, which decrease water and electrolyte absorption. These agents should only be used for the short-term treatment of constipation, because they are extremely potent.

Anthraquinones

Derived from plants, anthraquinones include aloe, casanthranol, cascara sagrada, and senna. After being ingested, these agents are hydrolysed by colonic bacteria into their active forms, which stimulate colonic peristalsis and induce fluid secretion.[6,7] Although the exact mechanism is not entirely understood, it may be mediated by serotonin and prostaglandins. Anthraquinones have been implicated as a cause of intramural myenteric nerve damage (cathartic colon) in patients with intractable constipation, but this association has not been conclusively proven. Stimulant laxatives can also cause melanosis coli, a condition characterized by increased pigmentation of the colon.[8] Although not pathologic, its presence should alert the clinician to chronic laxative use in spite of patient denial. Senna, an anthraquinone obtained from the plant *Cassia acutifolia* or *Cassia angustifolia*, dates back to Arabian medicine over 1000 years ago. Senna preparations produce their effect within 6 hours. Cascara sagrada, another anthraquinone, is obtained from the bark of the buckthorn tree (*Rhamnus purshiana*), known to be used by native American Indians from California.

Polyphenolic Derivatives

Polyphenolic derivatives include phenolphthalein (Correctol, Ex-Lax) and bisacodyl (Dulcolax, Carter's Little Pills). Active in the small and large bowels, these agents induce a net fluid secretion by increasing mucosal permeability, inhibiting intestinal sodium-potassium adenosine triphosphatase, and stimulating mucosal prostaglandin E release. Onset of action for the oral preparations is from 6 to 12 hours and for rectal administration, 15 minutes to 1 hour. If laxative abuse is suspected, alkalinization of the patient's stool or urine produces a pink color because of the phenolphthalein. Side effects include fluid and electrolyte loss, cramps, rectal discomfort, a lupus-like drug reaction, and Stevens-Johnson syndrome.[9]

Castor Oil

Castor oil is derived from the seed of *Ricinus communis* and was a remedy used by the ancient Egyptians.[10] A potent laxative, castor oil is converted to ricinoleic acid, which acts on the small intestine to reduce net absorption of fluid and electrolytes and to shorten intestinal transit. Its onset of action is slightly shorter than other oral laxatives'.

Dehydrocholic Acid

Dehydrocholic acid is a bile acid capable of producing a mild cathartic effect. It inhibits absorption and at the same time stimulates secretion of water and electrolytes in the colon.[11] Common side effects include abdominal pain, diarrhea, and electrolyte abnormalities. This medication is contraindicated in patients who have intestinal obstruction.

PROKINETIC AGENTS

Prokinetic agents increase cholinergic activity and bowel motility either directly, by stimulating smooth-muscle cholinergic receptors, or indirectly, by inhibiting dopaminergic receptors. Examples of colonic disorders treated with prokinetic agents include idiopathic intestinal pseudo-obstruction, postoperative ileus, scleroderma, and diabetes mellitus. Prokinetic agents are classified by their structure or mechanism of action (e.g., cholinergic agents) (Table 23–4).

Bethanechol

The gastrointestinal tract has M1 and M2 muscarinic cholinergic receptors. The M1 receptors are found in ganglia; whereas M2 receptors are found in smooth muscle. Bethanechol is a cholinergic agonist that binds with the M2 receptors. Experimentally, both the proximal and distal colons are stimulated by bethanechol; when administered to humans, however, the colonic effects of this drug are less well documented. Bethanechol has been used primarily to treat patients with neurogenic bladders, but there is some experience for its use for gastroesophageal reflux disease. Side effects include abdominal cramping, excessive salivation, and diarrhea.

TABLE 23–4. Prokinetic Agents

Mechanism of action	Agents
Cholinergic	Bethanechol Cisapride
Antidopaminergic	Metoclopramide Domperidone
Motilin agonists	Erythromycin
μ-Receptor antagonists	Naloxone Nalmetrene
Serotonergic	Renzapride Zacopride
Other	Somatostatin analog

Metoclopramide

Metoclopramide acts both centrally and peripherally with the nervous system. After crossing the blood-brain barrier, it depresses the chemoreceptor trigger zone within the brainstem, causing drowsiness and lethargy in some patients. The peripheral prokinetic effects are due to augmented acetylcholine activity through the inhibition of dopamine receptors. In the upper gastrointestinal tract, metoclopramide increases lower esophageal sphincter tone and enhances gastric emptying. In fact, its clinical use is primarily as an adjunct in gastroesophageal reflux disease and gastroparesis. In the small intestine, it increases bowel contractions and shortens transit time.[12] Although metoclopramide can stimulate colonic myoelectric activity in both diabetic patients and controls,[13] little information confirms its effectiveness in the treatment of chronic constipation and it should therefore not be used in patients who have shown sensitivity to this medication. Side effects include drowsiness, lethargy, and anxiety; long-term use can cause extrapyramidal side effects such as tardive dyskinesia. Less severe side effects with chronic use include breast enlargement, nipple tenderness, and galactorrhea through the release of prolactin. Metoclopramide is contraindicated in patients taking monoamine oxidase inhibitors, tricyclic antidepressants, sympathomimetics, or phenothiazines, or in patients with seizure disorders or extrapyramidal syndromes.

Cisapride

Cisapride has been used primarily in patients with gastroesophageal reflux disease, but its use is being investigated for other conditions throughout the gastrointestinal tract. Cisapride accentuates release of acetylcholine at the level of the myenteric plexus; it also increases the release of endorphins, motilin, and pancreatic polypeptide and decreases the release of substance P and cholecystokinin. Cisapride has been used to treat slow small-intestine motility seen in postoperative ileus, chronic idiopathic intestinal pseudo-obstruction, and Ogilvie's syndrome. Results have varied. Side effects include headaches, diarrhea, and abdominal cramping.

One of the more promising uses for cisapride is in patients with constipation, where it has been evaluated in several controlled studies. In cases of chronic functional constipation, cisapride has increased stool frequency significantly compared with placebo;[14–16] it has also accelerated colonic transit in patients with colonic inertia.[17] Other studies have shown that cisapride may be beneficial in children with intractable constipation[18,19] and in patients with irritable bowel syndrome.[20,21] Dosage ranges from 5 mg to 20 mg 2 to 4 times a day but should be titrated for the desired effect.

Domperidone

Like cisapride, domperidone has been used primarily for conditions of the upper alimentary tract. Its actions are similar to those of metoclopramide; it is a dopamide receptor antagonist, but unlike metoclopramide, this agent does not cross the blood-brain barrier and therefore it has few central side effects such as drowiness, lethargy, and antiemesis. Actions on the upper alimentary tract include enhanced gastric emptying[22] and motor activity.[23] Use of domperidone in patients with constipation is less dramatic; in two recent controlled trials, no difference was evident in improvement of symptoms, intestinal transit, or frequency of bowel movements in patients with irritable bowel syndrome.[24,25] Although this agent has minimal central nervous system side effects, it may raise prolactin levels, thus causing galactorrhea, gynecomastia, and menstrual cycle irregularities. Other side effects that have been noted with domperidone include diarrhea, increased thirst, headaches, and skin rash. This agent should not be used in patients taking monoamine oxidase inhibitors.

COLONIC LAVAGE

Colonic preparation for surgery, colonoscopy, or radiographic procedures can be achieved by having the patient drink solutions containing polyethylene glycol and sodium sulfate (e.g., Golytely, Colyte). These solutions are not absorbed, so fluid overload is not a concern and they are relatively safe even in patients with renal insufficiency. They should be avoided, however, in patients with a severe bowel obstruction. Their main side effect is a strong catharsis and, if taken late at night, will cause the patient to rest poorly. Studies suggest colonic lavage may be a therapeutic option in patients with intractable constipation[3] and that using only 8 to 16 oz per day will improve stool frequency and consistency.[26]

OPIOID ANTAGONISTS

For patients with narcotic-induced constipation, naloxone, an opioid antagonist, has been helpful. At low doses it has a laxative effect without causing systemic narcotic withdrawal symptoms.[27] Naloxone improves gastric emptying, decreases intestinal transit time, and provides symptomatic improvement in some patients with chronic idiopathic pseudo-obstruction.[28]

GENERAL APPROACH TO THE PATIENT WITH CONSTIPATION

To provide the most effective therapeutic plan for the constipated patient, clinicians must understand the primary pathophysiology; in this regard, a thorough history, physical examination, and appropriate diagnostic tests are essential. First and foremost, obstruction of the colon should be excluded by either radiography or endoscopy. More sophisticated diagnostic techniques such as transit time studies using radio-opaque markers, anorectal manometry, or defecography may later be useful in identifying the underlying cause of constipation.

Treatment of delayed colonic transit and hypomotility should begin with fiber supplementation. This decreases gut transit time, increases stool volume, decreases intracolonic pressure (which may lessen pain), and has an additional benefit of diluting bile salts that can reduce contractile activity. The daily recommended intake of fiber for the relief of constipation is at least 30 g, and because it may have to be taken 2 to 3 times a day, patient compliance frequently becomes an issue. In addition to fiber supplementation, pharmacologic therapy initially with nonstimulant laxatives such as milk of magnesia may be beneficial. If constipation persists, then addition of a stimulant laxative on an intermittent basis may be necessary. Anthraquinones may, however, cause degeneration of intramural ganglia. Cisapride may also be used if the primary underlying pathophysiology is hypomotility. Combination therapy, such as milk of magnesia at bedtime and a glycerin or bisacodyl suppository in the morning, may be used. This may be repeated every 3 to 4 days in order to maintain patient comfort. The available laxatives, their mechanisms of action and side effects are summarized in Table 23–5. Physical exercise is also recommended, because it helps to increase peristaltic activity.

Treatment of patients with slow rectal transit secondary to megarectum (which can be seen in both pediatric and geriatric populations) should focus on facilitating rectal emptying, which, in turn, promotes restoration of rectal tone. This can be accomplished through regular use of osmotic laxatives and habit training, whereby the patient attempts a bowel movement at a regular time each day, usually immediately after breakfast.

In patients with pelvic floor dyssynergia and paradoxical contraction of the sphincter or puborectalis, biofeedback, habit training, or laxative use may be helpful. Biofeedback is accomplished using the visual input provided by anorectal manometry, which teaches the patient to relax the external anal sphincter during straining. Results in the pediatric popula-

TABLE 23–5. Classification of Laxatives, Mechanism of Action, and Side Effects

Class	Examples	Mechanism of Action	Onset	Side Effects
Bulk formers	Fiber Polysaccharides	Decrease transit times Lower intracolonic pressure Increase stool volume	Variable	Bloating Excess flatulence
Lubricants	Mineral oil	Penetrates, softens the stool	—	Interference with absorption of fat-soluble vitamins Aspiration pneumonitis Lipoid granulomas
Stool softener	Docusate salts (Surfak, Colace)	Surfactant action—water and lipoids mix into stool Inhibits water absorption Stimulates fluid secretion	Oral: 6–72 h Rectal: 2–15 min	Cramps Increased absorption of mineral oil
Saline laxatives	Magnesium citrate Milk of magnesia Fleet's phosphasoda	Osmotic effect of magnesium or phosphate ion, increased luminal water and peristalsis	Oral: 6 h Rectal: 15 min	Hypermagnesemia Hyperphosphatemia Hypernatremia Hyperkalemia
Hyperosmolar laxatives	Glycerin Lactulose Sorbitol	Increase fecal water, promote peristalsis Increase stool osmolality	—	Bloating, excess flatulence, diarrhea
Stimulant laxatives	Anthraquinones: cascara, senna Polyphenolic: phenolphthalein, bisacodyl Castor oil Dehydrocholic acid	Stimulates intestinal motility, prostaglandin-mediated Decreased water, electrolyte absorption Increased fluid secretion	Oral: 6–12 h Rectal: 15 min	Melanosis coli Fluid and electrolyte loss Cramps Lupus-like drug reaction Stevens-Johnson syndrome Anthraquinones—degeneration of intramural colonic ganglia
Prokinetic agents	Bethanechol Metoclopramide Cisapride Domperidone	Increased cholinergic activity either directly or indirectly by inhibiting dopamine receptors	—	Cramps, salivation, diarrhea Metoclopramide—lethargy, dizziness, anxiety, extrapyramidal side effects, breast enlargement

tion using biofeedback alone have been encouraging.[29] Biofeedback has also been combined with milk of magnesia therapy, yielding significantly better outcomes than milk of magnesia alone.[30]

Increased segmenting contractions are common in patients with irritable bowel syndrome. In these instances, the use of laxatives other than fiber should be avoided. These patients should be encouraged to exercise. In some cases anticholinergics may be needed; although this may alleviate some abdominal pain, it will not increase frequency of bowel movements.

SPECIAL CIRCUMSTANCES IN MANAGEMENT OF CONSTIPATION

MULTIPLE SCLEROSIS

Multiple sclerosis (MS) is a progressive demyelinating disease of the central nervous system that can attack both sensory and motor pathways. More than half of the patients affected are women; onset of the disease is usually during the third or fourth decade of life. Approximately two thirds of patients have constipation or fecal incontinence.[31] Studies have shown that motor activity of the colon is significantly lower than in normal controls. Colonic motility does not increase after eating (absent gastrocolonic reflex).[32] These patients may also have a highly compliant rectum (megarectum) because demyelination of the conus medullaris can impair fecal sensation.[33] Large volumes of stool may then accumulate in the rectal vault. In a study of 16 patients with MS evaluated initially for urinary complaints, 15 also complained of constipation.[34] Colonic transit time was prolonged in 14 of the 15 patients, with 7 having diffuse slowing and 7 primarily left-sided delay. Based on manometric criteria, 10 patients were found to have anorectal dysfunction.

Therefore MS evidently affects different aspects of defecation, in decreasing the gastrocolonic reflex, decreasing colonic motility diffusely, and diminishing rectal sensation. A thorough investigation would help identify the cause and thus guide subsequent therapy. Initially, the clinician should increase fiber and fluid intake and encourage as much exercise as the patient's condition will tolerate. Additionally, patients should attempt to defecate after meals to use the gastrocolonic reflex; if unsuccessful, a glycerin or bisacodyl suppository may be used from time to time. Because of their potentially damaging effects to the enteric nervous system, chronic use of stimulant laxatives should be avoided. For patients with generalized colonic slowing, cholinergic agents may be tried, but they may cause urinary incontinence. Cisapride may be of value in the patient with prolonged colonic transit, although results are variable.

In summary, MS is frequently associated with constipation, which can occur even in patients who have only mild disease. The approach to therapy is determined by manometric findings, colon transit times, and defecography, which may isolate the problem to one of colonic hypomotility, rectal overcompliance, or pelvic floor malfunction. Treatment that is initially successful but loses its effectiveness may be a sign of worsening MS, and therapy toward the primary disease should also be addressed.

SPINAL CORD INJURIES

Spinal cord injuries may cause bowel dysfunction. The mechanism of constipation varies according to the level of the injury; if above the lumbar vertebra, colonic motility, compliance, and response of the colon to a meal are diminished.[35,36] Spinal cord transection above the fifth thoracic vertebra may lead to autonomic dysreflexia.[37] This reflex, triggered by fecal impaction, can cause severe hypertension and tachycardia, possibly resulting in subarachnoid hemorrhage, cardiovascular accident, and seizures. If the level of injury is lower and includes the cauda equina, the colon becomes more compliant and distended.

Treatment should be individualized and an understanding of the primary injury is essential to define which therapy is most beneficial. Because higher spinal cord lesions may diminish the gastrocolonic reflex, promotility agents such as cisapride may be of benefit.[38] With sphincter or pelvic floor spasticity, rectal distention may be needed to initiate defecation by eliciting the anorectal inhibitory reflex. This can be accomplished either by digital manipulation or by inserting a glycerin suppository.

MEGACOLON

Megacolon refers to conditions associated with a dilated colon. It may be classified by primary and secondary causes. Primary causes include chronic idiopathic intestinal pseudo-obstruction and Hirschsprung's disease; secondary causes are systemic metabolic diseases, medications, and fecal impaction.

Chronic idiopathic intestinal pseudo-obstruction should be suspected when there are recurrent signs and symptoms of intestinal obstruction despite the failure of diagnostic tests to reveal any mechanical cause. There are two forms of this disorder. One results from a visceral myopathy and the other from a visceral neuropathy.[39] The former is associated with other myopathies including megacystis, ophthalmoplegia, and small bowel diverticulosis. The neuropathic form may be associated with other autonomic neurologic abnormalities. In either case, patients may have diffuse gut dysmotility, so esophageal, gastric, and small-bowel motility studies should be done if clinically indicated. Diagnosis is made by a full-thickness biopsy. Treatment is restricted to the use of promotility agents when the expression is mild,[40] but enteral feedings and possibly intravenous hyperalimentation may be needed, depending on the severity and extent of bowel involvement.

Primary megacolon may also be due to Hirschsprung's disease, a congenital disorder characterized by absence of intramural ganglia within the distal colon. Patients with only a very short segment of involvement may not present until early adulthood; more extensive involvement is usually identified earlier in life. In either case, treatment is usually surgical.

Treatment of secondary megacolon depends on the underlying condition. If due to longstanding fecal impaction, disimpaction, improved toileting routine, and the use of gentle rectal laxative therapy (bisacodyl or glycerin suppository, or an occasional enema) may be beneficial.[41] Certain metabolic conditions may also cause megacolon, such as severe hypothyroidism, which produces a state known as **myxedema megacolon**. The colon is primarily affected, but the esophagus, stomach, and small bowel may also be abnormal.[42] Treatment for myxedema megacolon uses thyroid hormone replacement.[43] Other diseases capable of causing megacolon include Parkinson's disease, myotonic dystrophy, diabetic neuropathy, Chagas' disease, porphyria, diabetes mellitus, pheochromocytoma, scleroderma, and amyloidosis, or it may be iatrogenic, caused by medications.

REFERENCES

1. Binder, HJ: Use of laxatives in clinical medicine. Pharmacology 36(Suppl 1):226,1988.
2. Young, FE and Heckler, MM: Laxative drug products for over the counter human use; tentative final monograph. Fed Reg 50:2124,1985.
3. Brandt, LJ: Gastrointestinal Disorders of the Elderly. Raven Press, New York, 1984.
4. Tedesco, FJ: Laxative use in constipation. Am J Gastroenterol 80:303,1984.
5. Donowitz, M: Current concepts of laxative action. J Clin Gastroenterol 1:77,1979.
6. Hardcastle, JD and Wilkins, JL: The action of sennosides and related compounds on human colon and rectum. Gut 11:1038,1970.
7. DeWitte, P and Lemli, L: The metabolism of anthranoid laxatives. Hepatogastroenterology 37:601,1990.
8. Balazs, M: Melanosis coli: Ultrastructural study of 45 patients. Dis Colon Rectum 29:839,1985.
9. Savin, JA: Current causes of fixed drug eruptions. Br J Dermatol 83:546,1970.
10. Brunton, LL: Agents affecting gastrointestinal water flux and motility, digestants, and bile acids. In Gilman, AG, Rall, TW, Nies, AS, et al (eds.): Goodman and Gilman's Pharmacological Basis of Therapeutics, ed 8. Pergamon Press, New York, 1990, pp 914–932.
11. Mekhjian, HS, Phillops, SF and Hofmann, AF: Colonic secretion of water and electrolytes induced by bile acids: Perfusion studies in man. J Clin Invest 50:1569,1970.
12. James, WB and Hume, R: Action of metoclopramide on gastric emptying and small bowel transit time. Gut 9:203,1968.
13. Battle, WM, Shape, WJ, Alavi, A, et al: Colonic dysfunction in diabetes mellitus. Gastroenterology 79:1217,1980.
14. Creytens, G, Velinden, M, Reyntjens, et al: Double-blind study of cisapride in the treatment of chronic functional, non-spastic constipation. Progr Med 43(suppl 1):137,1987.
15. Hernandez, G and Tronosco, G: Double-blind dose response study of cisapride in the treatment of chronic functional constipation. Advances in Therapy 5:121,1988.

16. Müller-Lisner, SA: Treatment of chronic constipation with cisapride and placebo. Gut 28:1033,1987.
17. Krevsky, B, Maurer, AH, Malmud, LS, et al: Cisapride accelerates colonic transit in constipated patients with colonic inertia. Am J Gastroenterol 84:882,1989.
18. Murray, RD, Li, BU, McClung, HJ, et al: Cisapride for intractable constipation in children: observations from an open label trial. J Ped Gastroenterol Nutr 11:503,1990.
19. Staiano, A, Cucchiara, S, Andreotti, ME, et al: Effect of cisapride on chronic idiopathic constipation in children. Dig Dis Sci 36:733,1991.
20. Passeretti, S, et al: Cisapride accelerates total intestinal transit in patients with irritable bowel syndrome associated constipation. Progr Med 43(suppl 1):121,1987.
21. Van Outryve, M, Milo, R, Toussaint, J, et al: Prokinetic treatment of constipation-predominant irritable bowel syndrome: A placebo-controlled study of cisapride. J Clin Gastroenterol 13:49,1991.
22. Albibi, R, Du Bovic, S, Lange, RC, et al: A dose response study of the motor function of the effects of domperidone on gastric retention states in man. Am J Gastroenterol 78:679,1984.
23. Baeyens, R, Boegens, R, Van De Velde, E, and De Schepper, A: Effects of intravenous and oral domperidone on the motor function of the stomach and small intestine. Postgrad Med J 55(suppl 1):19,1979.
24. Lanfranchi, GA, Bazzocchi, G, Fois, F, et al: Effect of domperidone on colonic motor activity in patients with the irritable bowel syndrome. Eur J Clin Pharmacol 29:307,1985.
25. Cann, PA, Read, NW and Holdsworth, CD: Oral domperidone: double blind comparison with placebo in irritable bowel syndrome. Gut 12:1135,1983.
26. Andorsky, RI and Goldner, F: Colonic lavage solution (polyethylene glycol electrolyte lavage solution) as a treatment for chronic constipation: A double-blind placebo-controlled study. Am J Gastroenterol 85:261,1990.
27. Culpepper-Morgan, JA, Inturrisi, B, Portnoy, R, et al: Oral naloxone treatment of narcotic induced constipation: dose response. NIDA Res Monogr 95:399,1989.
28. Schang, JC and Devroede, G: Beneficial effects of naloxone in a patient with intestinal pseudo-obstruction. Am J Gastroenterol 80:407,1985.
29. Wald, A, Chandra, R, Gabel, S, et al: Evaluation of biofeedback in childhood encopresis. J Pediatr Gastroenterol Nutr 6:554,1987.
30. Loening-Baucke, V: Modulation of abnormal defecation dynamics by biofeedback treatment in chronically constipated children with encopresis. J Pediatr 116:214,1990.
31. Hinds, JP and Wald, A: Colonic and anorectal dysfunction associated with multiple sclerosis. Am J Gastroenterol 84:587,1989.
32. Glick, M, Meshkinpour, H, Haldeman, S, et al: Colonic dysfunction in multiple sclerosis. Gastroenterology 83:1002,1982.
33. Taylor, MC, Bradley, WE, Bhatia, N, et al: The conus demyelination syndrome in multiple sclerosis. Acta Neurol Scand 69:80,1984.
34. Weber, J, Grise, P, Roquebret, M, et al: Radiopaque markers transit and anorectal manometry in 16 patients with multiple sclerosis and urinary bladder dysfunction. Dis Colon Rectum 39:95,1987.
35. Glick, ME, Hooshang, M, Haldeman, S, et al: Colonic dysfunction in patients with thoracic spinal cord injury. Gastroenterology 86:287,1984.
36. Aaronson, MJ, Freed, MM and Burakoff, R: Colonic myoelectric activity in persons with spinal cord injury. Dig Dis Sci 20:295,1985.
37. Bell, J and Hannon, K: Pathophysiology involved in autonomic dysreflexia. J Neurosci Nurs 18:86,1986.
38. de Groot, GH and de Pagter, GF: Effects of cisapride on constipation due to a neurological lesion. Paraplegia 26:159,1988.
39. Mayer, EA, et al: A familial visceral neuropathy with autosomal dominant transmission. Gastroenterology 91:1528,1986.
40. Camilleri, M, Brown, ML and Malagelada, J-R: Impaired transit of chyme in chronic intestinal pseudo-obstruction. Correction by cisapride. Gastroenterology 91:619,1986.
41. Read, NW, et al: Impairment of defecation in young women with severe constipation. Gastroenterology 90:53,1986.
42. Bacharach, T and Evans, JR: Enlargement of the colon secondary to hypothroidism. Ann Intern Med 47:121,1957.
43. Batalis, T, Muers, M and Royle, GT: Treatment with intravenous triiodothyronine of colonic pseudo-obstruction caused by myxedema. Br J Surg 68:439,1981.

CHAPTER 24

Constipation: Results of Surgical Therapy

Tracy L. Hull • Jeffrey W. Milsom

Chronic constipation, a physically and socially debilitating disorder, is one of the more frequently encountered problems in medical practice. Symptoms may include inability to evacuate stool secondary to obstructed defecation, abnormalities of the size and consistency of stool making evacuation difficult, or infrequency of passing stool. A chief complaint of "constipation" therefore demands clarification. One proposed definition for **constipation** is straining at stool for more than 25% of the time or having two or fewer stools per week.[1]

Evaluation of a patient complaining of constipation should begin with a thorough history and physical examination to clarify the patient's symptoms and to rule out anorectal pathology, cancer, neurologic or endocrine abnormalities, drug use, and psychiatric disturbances. Flexible sigmoidoscopy or proctoscopy should be performed at the first evaluation. Initial therapy should include a high-fiber diet (up to 30 g fiber per day), increased fluid intake, and stool softeners or mild laxatives. Most patients improve with this conservative approach.

Unfortunately, a small group of patients, primarily young or middle-aged women, fail to respond to these measures.[2,3] This select group requires further evaluation and testing to pinpoint the underlying cause as one of colonic inertia or of pelvic floor outlet dysfunction such as internal intussusception, nonrelaxing puborectalis, or rectocele. These tests include colonic transit study, defecography, barium enema or colonoscopy, anorectal manometry, electromyography, rectal balloon expulsion, biopsy of the rectal wall if there is megarectum, and possibly upper gastrointestinal manometry.

Surgery for constipation was originally advocated by William Arbuthnot Lane in 1908.[4] In truth, careful patient selection is mandatory, because few patients with chronic constipation benefit from indiscriminate surgery. Pemberton, Rath, and Ilstrup prospectively analyzed 277 constipated patients referred to

TABLE 24–1. Surgically Treatable Causes of Constipation

Colonic inertia
- normal size colon and rectum
- megacolon and megarectum
- left colonic dysfunction

Anorectal outlet obstruction
- intussusception
- rectocele

Hirschsprung's disease

the Mayo Clinic over 3 years[5] and found that only 15% were appropriate surgical candidates. Table 24–1 outlines the surgically treatable causes of constipation. The remainder of this chapter focuses on each type of constipation and the surgical options available.

COLONIC INERTIA

NORMAL SIZE COLON AND RECTUM

In patients with debilitating constipation and clearly prolonged colonic transit times, a normal caliber colon and rectum on barium enema, and normal defecography, colon resection may be reasonable. In fact, it is this group of patients who are most suitable for surgery and for whom the outcome is most likely to be successful. In these instances, results of manometry are usually normal. Operative choices include total colectomy with either ileorectal, ileosigmoid, or cecorectal anastomosis. Cecorectal anastomosis may seem ideal, because it preserves the ileocecal valve, but when compared with ileorectostomy, persistent constipation is slightly more frequent,[6] possibly due to dilatation of the cecum over time.[7] Ileosigmoid and ileorectal anastomosis may produce similar results, but at least one clinical series has reported a higher incidence of persistent constipation after ileosigmoid anastomosis.[8] At our institution, we prefer an ileorectal anastomosis, based on better functional results.[9]

When properly selected, more than 70% of patients have had a favorable outcome with surgery.[2,10–12] This is reflected in an improved quality of life and increased frequency of bowel movements. Enthusiasm must be tempered by the fact that new problems may arise during the postoperative period, one of which is diarrhea; up to 30% of patients pass three or more stools per day.[13] Some authors report improvement of diarrhea with time,[5] but others have noted permanently loose stools.[14] Another complication of total colectomy is fecal incontinence; an incidence of 0% to 38% has been reported.[5,7,11]

Despite the entire colon having been removed, constipation may persist in some patients. The need to continue laxatives has been seen in a significant number of patients; Kamm, Hawley, and Leonard-Jones noted that 45% of patients used laxatives after surgery.[15] Vasilevsky and associates reported that 11% continued to require laxatives and 20% used enemas.[10]

Even though constipation is alleviated in many patients, abdominal pain, bloating, and straining may continue to be a problem. Yoshioka and Keighley found no improvement in abdominal distention in 86% of patients who reported this problem preoperatively, but fewer patients (39% vs. 93%) complained of abdominal pain after surgery.[16] Kamm, Hawley and Leonard-Jones reported that 71% of patients continued to experience abdominal pain postoperatively.[15]

Small-bowel obstruction is a potential postoperative complication which may be seen in up to 36% of patients.[3,10,12,16] Many require laparotomy, but in some cases, adhesions do not seem to account fully for the symptoms. This leads to the speculation that perhaps the "obstruction" is only another manifestation of the overall bowel dysmotility seen in patients with intractable constipation.

Patients with a nonrelaxing puborectalis coexisting with colonic inertia probably should not be excluded from consideration for a colectomy; the abnormal pelvic floor outlet should be addressed first, however, and possibly corrected. Kamm, Hawley, and Leonard-Jones found that paradoxical contraction of the puborectalis muscle with straining or the inability to expel a balloon with straining did not correlate with a patient's outcome following colectomy.[15] These results contrast with those reported by van der Sijp and co-workers,[17] who found that all patients unable to expel a balloon before surgery experienced abdominal pain postoperatively and significantly more used laxatives when compared with their counterparts who were able to expel a balloon. Heine, Wong, and Goldberg also found that patients who had nonrelaxing puborectalis muscles preoperatively had suboptimal outcomes. The researchers felt that some predictive value may exist in this finding.[3]

For this group of patients, Pemberton, Rath, and Ilstrup advocate treating the spastic puborectalis with biofeedback as the initial step. They reported findings in 14 patients,[5] 13 of whom learned to evacuate stool spontaneously and were then considered for colectomy. Another 9 elected to have surgery; the reported success rate was similar to patients who had colectomy alone for colonic inertia (no outlet obstruction). Others also believe that the pelvic floor should be addressed initially, because slow-transit constipation may be secondary to obstruction created by an abnormal pelvic floor.[3] If constipation from colonic inertia persists after demonstrating successful relaxation of the puborectalis muscle (generally assessed while straining during electromyography), colectomy can be justified.

Our approach to patients with only slow-transit constipation is to perform a colectomy with an ileorectal anastomosis. If a nonrelaxing puborectalis muscle is detected by preoperative testing, the patient is initially managed with biofeedback. We do not routinely perform preoperative balloon expulsion testing. Patients are told preoperatively that this operation may not improve their constipation and that even if the frequency of movements is increased, pain and bloating may persist. Because diarrhea is a considerable problem for some, patients with marginal manometry (i.e., poor anal sphincter function) are encouraged to avoid anastomosis in favor of a stoma. Many will insist on avoidance of a stoma and in this group intestinal continuity is re-established only after many preoperative discussions have focused on the high probability of incontinence. In fact, all patients (even those with normal anorectal manometry) are warned about the chance for postoperative diarrhea and fecal incontinence. Those with abnormal upper gastrointestinal manometry are offered colectomy but they should be warned that their rate of success may be significantly less than that of patients with normal upper gastrointestinal motility. This is based on the suspicion that a diffuse bowel motility problem may be present and that not only the colon is involved.

MEGACOLON AND MEGARECTUM

In some patients with constipation and delayed transit, a barium enema may demonstrate megacolon or megarectum. Hirschsprung's disease is ruled out by the presence of a rectoanal inhibitory reflex on anometry and by rectal biopsies demonstrating the presence of ganglia. If Hirschsprung's disease has been ruled out, patients with only a megacolon have acceptable results following total colectomy and ileorectostomy.[13] For those with a megarectum (greater than 6.5 cm bowel diameter at the pelvic brim), surgical options are not as clearcut.[18] Before selecting the surgical procedure for these patients, colonic transit time must be determined.

If transit time is normal through the colon in a patient with megarectum, the Soave or Duhamel operation is appropriate.[19] The Soave operation is performed by removing the rectal mucosa, followed by placement of normal proximal bowel within the seromuscular tube and anastomosis to the anus. In the Duhamel operation, the abnormal rectum is left in place; normal proximal bowel is placed in the retrorectal space and the two portions of bowel sutured together beginning at the pelvic floor.

If transit time is prolonged, however, options include an ileostomy or, for young continent patients who wish to avoid a stoma,[20] a proctocolectomy with ileal-pouch–anal anastomosis (an "ileoanal pull-through"). Considerable experience has been gained with the ileoanal pull-through for ulcerative colitis and familial polyposis; this familiarity makes this procedure attractive. In fact, the ileoanal pull-through can be used in patients with refractory constipation following the Soave or Duhamel procedures.

Anorectal myomectomy (extended internal sphincterotomy) has been used to treat pediatric patients with constipation and idiopathic megarectum. Hata, Sasaki, and Uchino reported cure or improvement in 11 patients treated with this approach with follow-up of 1 year or longer.[21] More experience and follow-up are needed with this treatment before it can be uniformly recommended for megarectum in adults, but it nevertheless is an option for patients with short-segment Hirschsprung's disease.

In conclusion, patients with megacolon only and delayed transit can be offered a colectomy with ileorectal anastomosis. If megarectum is found along with megacolon and delayed colonic transit, a proctocolectomy and pelvic pouch procedure may be reasonable. If transit time is normal, patients with megarectum may benefit from a Soave or Duhamel operation, or a pelvic pouch procedure if the first two options have failed. Anorectal myomectomy is still unproven for treating megarectum not associated with Hirschsprung's disease, and more data need to be gathered before that approach can be recommended.

LEFT COLONIC DYSFUNCTION

A select group of patients with constipation demonstrate delayed passage of markers distal to the splenic flexure only. Kamm and associates reported two such patients, in both of whom Hirschsprung's disease had been excluded.[22] A left hemicolectomy with rectal excision was performed in both patients with excellent results. The proximal colon was preserved in an attempt to limit diarrhea. Preston and colleagues found opposite results in five patients who underwent either sigmoid or left hemicolectomy; none were helped by a segmental resection.[7] These patients had delayed transit, but it was not stated if it was segmentally or diffusely abnormal. Thus, the literature on segmental left colonic resection for intractable constipation presents conflicting results. We have no experience in its use in the treatment of constipation.

ANORECTAL OUTLET OBSTRUCTION

NONRELAXING PUBORECTALIS AND PELVIC FLOOR

Nonrelaxation of the puborectalis during straining may produce symptoms of obstructed defecation. Patients generate extreme pressure to have a bowel movement but still find evacuation may not be successful. The puborectalis contracts rather than relaxes when the patient attempts defecation. Results of the colonic transit study may be normal, have delayed passage of markers from the rectosigmoid, or be diffusely abnormal through the colon. Rare patients may also have a dilated rectum visible with barium enema.

Nonoperative treatment should be the initial mode of therapy; one should also address the psychiatric problems of many of these patients.[20] Surgical treatment is not currently advocated; in the past, division of the puborectalis was recommended.[23] Other studies have clearly demonstrated little benefit with this approach; in fact, some patients may be incontinent following division of the puborectalis.[24–26]

Anorectal myectomy, originally intended for diagnosis and treatment of short-segment Hirschsprung's disease, has also been used to treat outlet obstruction without megarectum or Hirschsprung's disease. Pinho, Yoshioka, and Keighly reported long-term results in 57 patients with a median follow-up of 2 years. At 4 months, 62% had improvement, but only 31% demonstrated sustained improvement with longer follow-up.[27] Of patients, 10% were also mildly incontinent.

In conclusion, surgical division of the pelvic floor or sphincter muscles for constipation because of a nonrelaxing puborectalis muscle should probably be of historic interest only. Biofeedback has become the mainstay of treatment.

RECTAL INTUSSUSCEPTION (PROLAPSE)

Internal Intussusception

Difficulty expelling stool can be caused by internal rectal intussusception. This hidden form of prolapse is usually diagnosed only by defecography. Surgical treatment depends upon the severity of symptoms and whether there is co-existing colonic inertia.

Ihre and Seligson used a Ripstein repair (see Chapter 36) to correct the internal intussusception and reported poor results if obstructed defecation was the indication for surgery.[28] McCue and Thomson concurred with these findings, reporting the use of the Ivalon sponge rectopexy to treat internal prolapse and found that dysfunctional defecation persisted after the operation.[29] Roe, Bartolo, and Mortenson reported eight patients who had normal colonic transit times and internal rectal intussusception.[2] Only 3 of 7 had significant improvement in their symptoms at a mean follow-up of 5 months. Two patients with colonic inertia and intussusception failed to improve after rectopexy alone and required a colectomy and ileorectal anastomosis with unknown results.

Berman, Harris, and Rabeler have reported use of the Delorme procedure (rectal mucosal stripping and plication of the muscularis propria) on 21 patients with obstructed defecation. They found that 71% had relief of most of their preoperative symptoms at a mean follow-up of 3 years.[30] No other studies corroborate these results.

Because the results of surgery for internal prolapse are not overwhelmingly successful, caution and judgment must be exercised. This guarded view stems in part from an incomplete understanding of internal prolapse and the degree to which it is responsible for producing symptoms.

External Rectal Intussusception (Prolapse, Procidentia)

Any patient with complete external prolapse and constipation should undergo full evaluation before surgery. In particular, a colonic transit study may help to identify those patients who would benefit from a colectomy. Patients with diffuse slow-transit constipation and external intussusception should be considered for a colectomy with ileorectal anastomosis and rectopexy. Patients with prolapse and normal transit, but with "mild" symptoms of constipation, may benefit from a sigmoid resection with rectopexy.

RECTOCELE

Rectocele can cause severe intractable constipation by sequestering stool and altering the vectors of defecation. Because approximately 80% of normal asymptomatic women may have a rectocele,[31] surgery should be recommended only in those patients in whom symptoms can be confidently attributed to the rectocele.[32] As with other types of constipation, conservative management is attempted first by increasing fiber and water intake, and by adding stool softeners, laxatives, or enemas. If surgery is needed, repair can be performed either transvaginally or transrectally.[33]

SUMMARY

Pelvic floor abnormalities are certainly associated with constipation. Surgery was previously advocated for a "nonrelaxing" puborectalis, but biofeedback is now the treatment of choice. The exact role of surgery for internal intussusception depends on other related factors such as colonic inertia and the severity of the constipation. A rectocele should be repaired only if deemed severely symptomatic, not if it is an incidental finding.

ADULT HIRSCHSPRUNG'S DISEASE

Hirschsprung's disease is a congenital disorder characterized by the absence of ganglion cells in Auerbach's intermyenteric plexus and Meissner's submucosal plexus of the large intestinal wall. Even though congenital, it may occasionally remain undetected until adulthood if the involved segment is short and located in the distal rectum. Radiographic studies usually reveal a dilated colon proximal to the aganglionic bowel, which appears narrow or normal in caliber. It must be differentiated in the adult population from other causes of megacolon: Chagas' disease, volvulus, anorectal obstruction, and central nervous system disorders. Diagnosis is suspected by the absence of the anorectal inhibitory reflex on anal manometry, or by rectal wall biopsy taken 3 cm above the dentate line, showing the absence of ganglion cells. Normal patients may have aganglionosis or hypoganglionic bowel within 3 cm of the dentate line.[34] Diagnosis may be confirmed by histochemical detection of acetylcholinesterase activity.[35]

Surgical options for Hirschsprung's disease vary depending on the length of the aganglionic segment and the surgeon's preference for, and familiarity with, each operation. Either the Duhamel or Soave operation may be performed. Proctectomy with co-

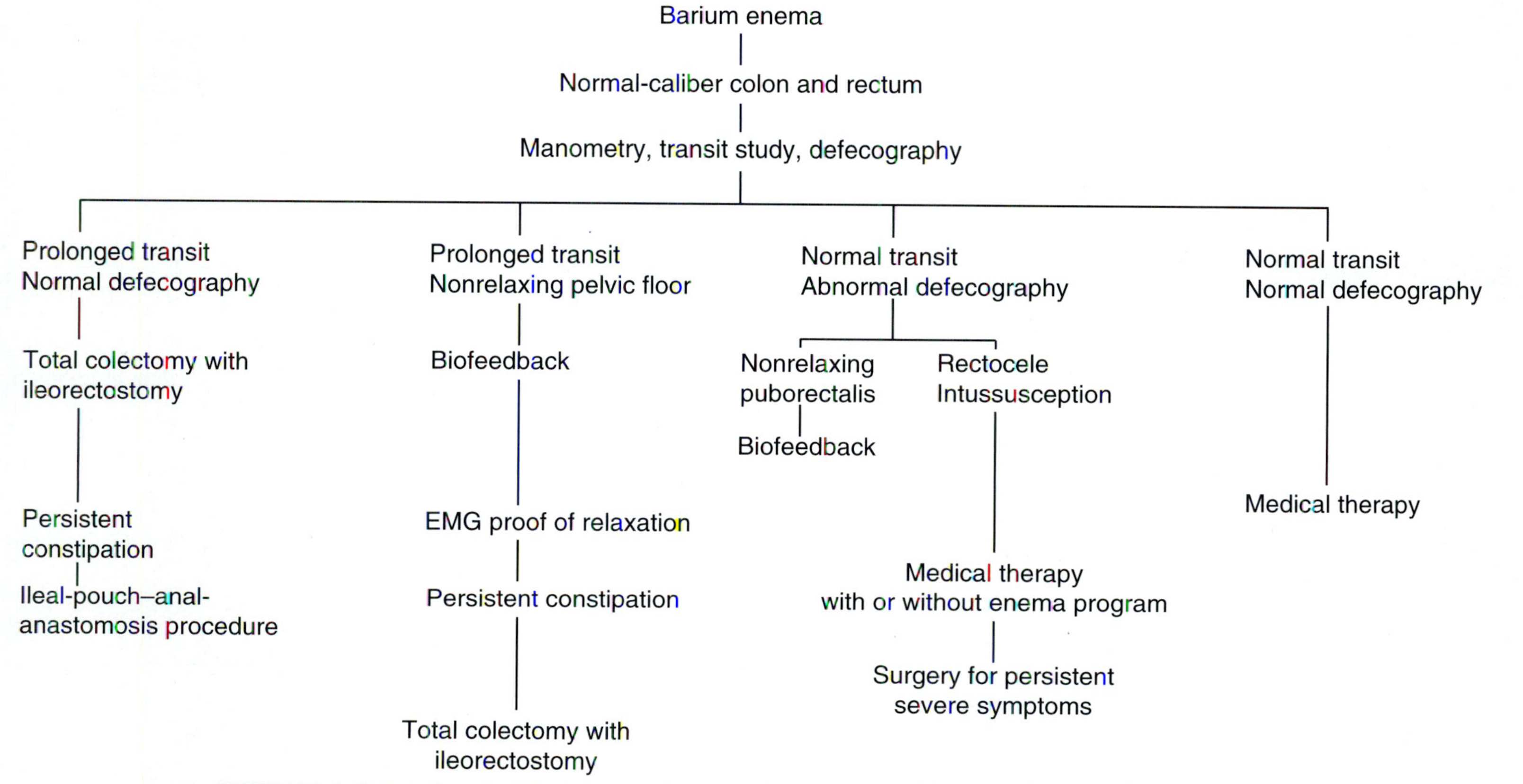

FIGURE 24–1. Choice of surgical therapy to treat constipation in patients with a normal-caliber colon and rectum.

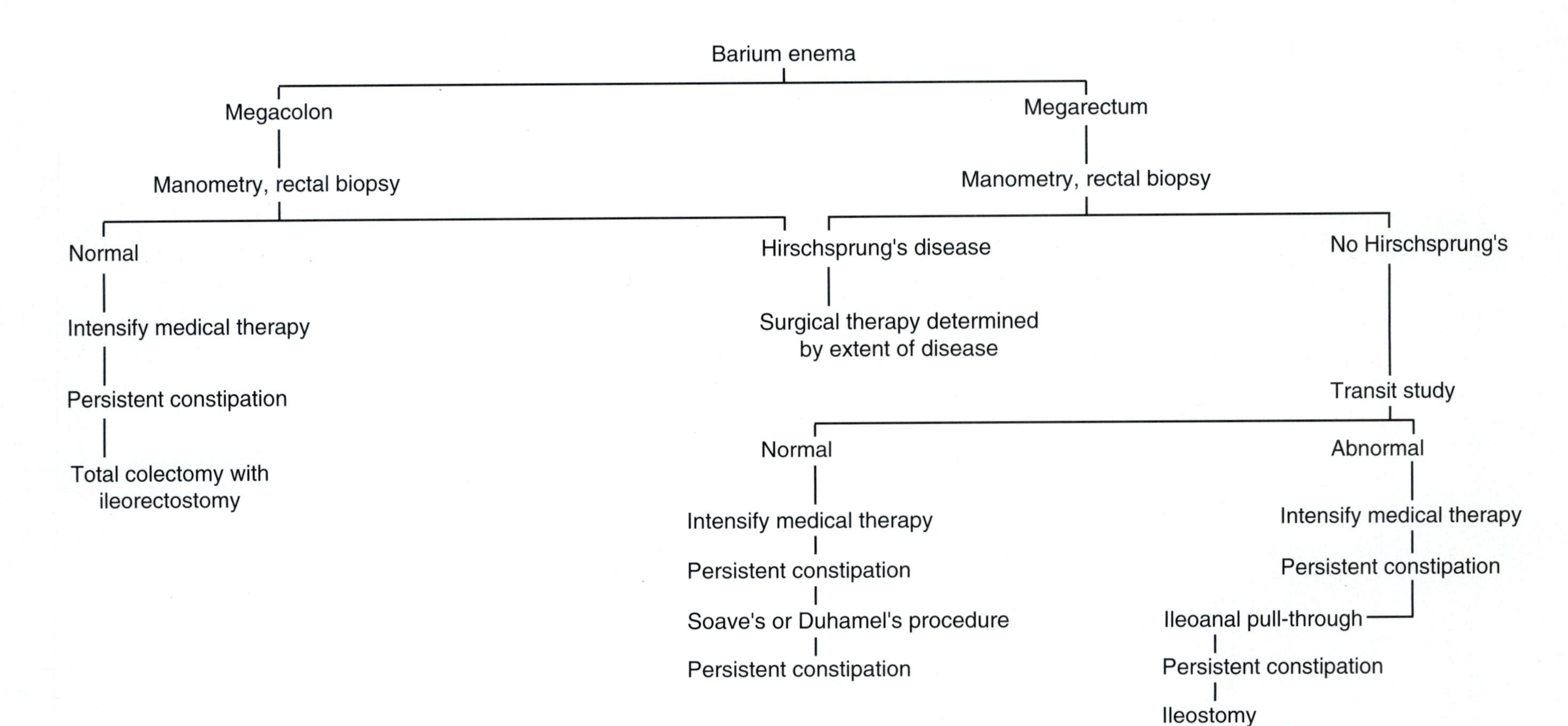

FIGURE 24–2. Choice of surgical therapy to treat constipation in patients with megacolon or megarectum.

loanal anastomosis may be preferred by some surgeons who practice on adult patients, because they are familiar with this procedure for low rectal cancers and the dissection follows similar tissue planes as proctocolectomy with ileoanal pull-through. Short-segment disease is treated by anorectal strip myectomy (internal sphincterectomy).

SUMMARY

Figures 24–1 and 24–2 summarize the surgical approach to patients suffering from intractable constipation. Choice of the most appropriate option for any given patient is based on whether the colon and retum have normal caliber and motility, and whether the pelvic floor facilitates or hinders defecation.

Total colectomy and ileorectostomy are indicated for patients with prolonged colonic transit times, with or without megacolon, who lack pelvic floor abnormalities or megarectum. If constipation persists postoperatively, these patients may undergo proctectomy with ileal-pouch–anal anastomosis to avoid ileostomy.[36,37] Without coexisting puborectalis spasticity, biofeedback should be performed before colectomy; relaxation should be documented before proceeding with surgery if the patient has persistent constipation.

In general, pelvic floor abnormalities should be approached cautiously. A nonrelaxing puborectalis ought not be treated surgically. Furthermore, internal intussusception and rectocele may be incidental findings unrelated to the patient's symptoms.

Surgical options for megarectum depend on whether Hirschsprung's disease is present and whether the patient has abnormal colonic transit times. If Hirschsprung's disease is present, surgical options are chosen based on the length of the aganglionic segment. Internal sphincter myectomy is an accepted procedure for short-segment Hirschsprung's disease but has unproven efficacy for the treatment of outlet obstruction without megarectum. Without Hirschsprung's disease, megarectum with normal transit time is treated by either the Soave or Duhamel procedure. If transit time is prolonged, proctocolectomy with ileal-pouch–anal reconstruction may be performed.

REFERENCES

1. Drossman, DA, Sandler, RS, McKee, DC, et al: Bowel patterns among subjects not seeking health care. Gastroenterology 83:529,1982.
2. Rose, AM, Bartolo, DCC and Mortensen, NJ: Diagnosis and surgical management of intractable constipation. Br J Surg 73:854,1986.
3. Heine, JA, Wong, WG and Goldberg, SM: Surgical treatment for constipation. Surg Gynecol Obstet 179:404,1993.
4. Lane, WA: Chronic intestinal stasis. Br Med J 1:1408,1909.
5. Pemberton, JH, Rath, DM and Ilstrup, DM: Evaluation and surgical treatment of severe chronic constipation. Ann Surg 214:403,1991.
6. Henry, MM: Surgery for constipation. Br Med J 298:346,1989.
7. Preston, DM, Hawley, PR, Lennard-Jones, JE, et al: Results of colectomy for severe idiopathic constipation in women. Br J Surg 71:547,1984.
8. Klatt, GR: Role of subtotal colectomy in the treatment of incapacitating constipation. Am J Surg 145:623,1983.
9. Beck, DE, Jagelman, DG and Fazio, VW: The surgery of idiopathic constipation. Gastroenterol Clin North Am 16:143,1987.
10. Vasilevsky, CA, Nemer, FD, Balcos, EG, et al: Is subtotal colectomy a viable option in the management of chronic constipation? Dis Colon Rectum 31:679,1988.
11. Leon, SH, Krishnamurthy, S and Schuffler, MD: Subtotal colectomy for severe idiopathic constipation. Dig Dis Sci 32:1249,1987.
12. Rex, DK, Lappas, JC, Goulet, RC, et al: Selection of constipated patients as subtotal colectomy candidates. J Clin Gastroenterol 15:212,1992.
13. Coremans, GE: Surgical aspects of severe chronic non-Hirschsprung constipation. Hepatogastroenterology 37:588,1990.
14. Kamm, MA: The surgical treatment of severe idiopathic constipation. Int J Colorect Dis 2:229,1987.
15. Kamm, MA, Hawley, PR and Lennard-Jones, JE: Outcome of colectomy for severe idiopathic constipation. Gut 29:969,1988.
16. Yoshioka, K and Keighley, MRB: Clinical results of colectomy for severe constipation. Br J Surg 76:600,1989.
17. van der Sijp, JRM, Kamm, MA, Bartram, CI, et al: The value of age of onset and rectal emptying in predicting the outcome of colectomy for severe idiopathic constipation. Int J Colorect Dis 7:35,1992.
18. Walsh, PV, Peebles-Brown, DA and Watkinson, G: Colectomy for slow transit constipation. Ann Roy Coll Surg Eng 69:71,1987.
19. Lane RHS and Todd, IP: Idiopathic megacolon. Br J Surg 64:303,1977.
20. Keighley, MRB: Surgery for constipation. Br J Surg 75:625,1988.
21. Hata, Y, Sasaki, F and Uchino, J: Sphincteromyectomy and sphincteroplasty in chronic constipation with megarectum. J Pediatr Surg 23:141,1988.
22. Kamm, MA, van der Sijp, JR, Hawley, PR, et al: Left hemicolectomy with rectal excision for severe idiopathic constipation. Int J Colorect Dis 6:49,1991.
23. Wallace, WC and Madden, WM: Experience with partial resection of the puborectalis muscle. Dis Colon Rectum 12:196,1969.
24. Barnes, PRH, Hawley, PR, Preston, DM, et al: Experience of posterior division of the puborectalis muscle in the management of chronic constipation. Br J Surg 72:475,1985.
25. Kamm, MA, Hawley, PR and Lennard-Jones, JE: Experience of lateral puborectalis division for severe constipation. Gut 28:A1364,1987.
26. Keighley, MRB and Shouler, P: Outlet syndrome: is there a surgical option? J Roy Soc Med 77:559:1984.
27. Pinho, M, Yoshioka, K and Keighley, MRB: Long-term results of anorectal myectomy for chronic constipation. Dis Colon Rectum 33:795,1990.
28. Ihre, R and Seligson, U: Intussusception of the rectum—Internal procidentia: Treatment and results in 90 patients. Dis Colon Rectum 18:391,1975.
29. McCue, JL and Thomson, JPS: Rectopexy for internal rectal intussusception. Br J Surg 77:632,1990.
30. Berman, IR, Harris, MS and Rabeler, MR: Delorme's transrectal excision for internal rectal prolapse. Dis Colon Rectum 33:573,1990.
31. Shorvon, PJ, McHugh, S, Diamant, NE, et al: Defecography in normal volunteers: *Results and implications*. Gut 30:1737,1989.
32. Gordon, PH, Nivatvongs, S: Principles and Practice of Surgery for the Colon, Rectum, and Anus. Quality Medical Publishing, St. Louis, 1992, p 939.
33. Sullivan, ES, Leaverton, GH and Hardwick, CE: Transrectal perineal repair. Dis Colon Rectum 11:106,1968.
34. Wheatley, MJ, et al: Hirschsprung's disease in adolescents and adults. Dis Colon Rectum 33:662,1990.
35. Goto, S, Ikeda, K and Nagasaki, A: Hirschsprung's disease in an adult. Dis Colon Rectum 27:319,1984.
36. Nicholls, RJ and Kamm, MA: Proctocolectomy with restorative ileo-anal reservoir for severe idiopathic constipation. Dis Colon Rectum 31:968,1988.
37. Hosie, KB, Kmiot, WA and Keighley, MRB: Constipation: another indication for restorative proctocolectomy. Br J Surg 77:801,1990.

CHAPTER 25

Fecal Incontinence: Etiology and Evaluation

James W. Fleshman

DEFINITION

Fecal incontinence is defined as the inability to defer the elimination of stool or gas until there is a socially acceptable time and place to do so. Although there are numerous incontinence-grading systems, Miller and co-workers[1] have described a particularly helpful system that incorporates frequency, degree of incontinence, and impact on lifestyle into a rating system, which also has prognostic value.

The frequency of incontinence is an issue that the clinician must address with the patient. Certainly, the patient who reports episodes of gross incontinence occurring daily or several times a week has more inconvenience than the patient who has only a monthly episode of soilage. Quality of life and frequency of incontinence are major factors in determining whether the morbidity of corrective surgery is justified.

ETIOLOGY

OBSTETRIC

The most common iatrogenic cause of fecal incontinence is sphincter damage following vaginal delivery.[2,3] This damage can occur by two distinct mechanisms: (1) mechanical disruption of muscle fibers, and (2) disruption of the innervation to skeletal and probably to smooth muscle.[4] The risk of injury to the anal sphincter rises significantly in women who have midline episiotomies; there is a well-documented threefold to fourfold increase in the incidence of extension of the incision into the anal sphincter and mucosa during delivery.[5] Obstetricians attending the delivery of large infants, anticipating instrumented deliveries, or intent on avoiding third-degree and fourth-degree extensions should consider the use of the mediolateral episiotomy.[6] Alternatively, the modified median episiotomy can be used; although seemingly logical, its clinical usefulness has yet to be reported in a randomized clinical trial.

Recognition of anal sphincter disruption and repair of the sphincter at the time of vaginal delivery appears to prevent overt clinical symptoms of incontinence for most women sustaining such damage. Many patients, however, require secondary sphincteroplasty, which may be performed in the early postpartum months. On the other hand, some women retain fecal continence despite nearly complete disruption of their external sphincter. This may be due to the strength and integrity of the remaining sphincter, combined with adjustments in lifestyle, diet, and hygiene. These women may not present for treatment of fecal incontinence until many years after the obstetrically provoked sphincter disruption.

Neurologic injury may be found by measuring pudendal nerve–terminal motor latencies and using needle electromyographic (EMG) techniques (see Chapter 11). Neurophysiologic testing in this area remains in its infancy and much research is needed to characterize the natural history of neuromuscular injury and repair. Additionally, the relationship of clinical symptoms to documented abnormalities needs to be clarified.

Although fecal incontinence as an obstetric sequela may not be entirely preventable, certain steps can minimize its occurrence. Specific efforts to protect the anal sphincter at the time of vaginal delivery should be considered, particularly when an instrumented delivery or large infant is anticipated. If episiotomy is indicated, performance of a mediolateral episiotomy preferentially protects midline structures.

The likelihood of achieving successful repair of obstetric sphincter injuries can be optimized in a proper surgical setting. Anatomic reapproximation is necssary through the entire longitudinal length of the anal sphincter. Although obstetric texts have traditionally depicted a very distal repair of the sphincter, the entire length of the rectovaginal septum and the perineal body must be reconstructed. Ideally, this requires proper lighting and instrumentation; if these are not accessible in the delivery room, the patient should be transferred to a well-equipped operating room.

PRIOR ANORECTAL SURGERY

Fistula surgery in women, especially in the anterior portion of the anal canal, may result in fecal incontinence, depending on the degree of internal and external sphincter division. Anteriorly, the external sphincter is somewhat thinner and the length of the high pressure zone shorter relative to other quadrants of the anal canal. A good principle to follow therefore is to perform anterior fistulotomy only when the fistula is clearly superficial and incorporates minimal sphincter muscle. If the fistula tract runs deeply through the muscle as the tract courses toward the anal canal, fecal incontinence after anterior anal fistulotomy can be avoided with either a Seton suture or a rectal advancement flap; the latter is also performed for repair of rectovaginal fistulas and is discussed in more detail in Chapter 28.

In most instances, midline division of the posterior fibers of the external sphincter during fistulotomy does not cause major incontinence because the puborectalis is intact. A posterior midline division, however, may cause a keyhole-shaped deformity and troublesome leakage of gas and mucus due to the crevice created by the incision.

Fecal incontinence following hemorrhoidectomy is rare. When incontinence does occur, it may be caused by a loss of anorectal sensation, inadvertent injury to the muscle, or tissue loss caused by infection in the excisional hemorrhoidectomy site. Mucosal prolapse or ectropion may occur following a Whitehead hemorrhoidectomy; this procedure involves a complete circumferential excision of the anal mucosa and anoderm. Soilage after this operation may result from overflow incontinence around a fecal impaction, wetness from the ectropion, or loss of sensation secondary to excision of the transitional zone and sensory mucosa.

TRAUMA

Blunt pelvic trauma or penetrating injuries to the anal canal from impalement or gunshot wounds may cause fecal incontinence due to diffuse tissue loss or trauma to the pudendal nerve.

INFLAMMATORY BOWEL DISEASE

Chronic diarrhea resulting from inflammatory bowel disease or irritable bowel syndrome may render a marginally competent sphincter unable to control gas or stool. Incontinence may be made even worse if the rectum itself is diseased from long-standing Crohn's proctitis; in these patients, rectal compliance and storage capability are abnormally reduced, producing symptoms of intense fecal urgency, anxiety, soilage, and ultimately incontinence. Prior anal surgery for multiple abscesses and fistulas, which may accompany Crohn's disease, may also impair sphincter function.

RADIOTHERAPY

Irradiation for pelvic cancer may cause both decreased anorectal sensation and diminished rectal capacity and compliance. As a result, fecal incontinence is not an unusual complaint, especially after procedures involving partial proctectomy, which diminishes rectal storage even further. The degree of incontinence is proportional to the dose of radiation; the effect of 4,500 R on anal sphincter function appears to be minimal. At doses above this level, however, the rectum may become chronically fibrotic and continence may be impaired.[7] Postoperative irradiation following proctectomy may cause stricturing of the anastomosis as well as fibrosis of the neorectum, which may in turn cause incontinence.

PRIOR COLECTOMY

Loss of the sampling reflex (anorectal inhibitory reflex) and diminished storage capacity may occur in patients undergoing a very low anterior resection of the rectum followed by colorectal or coloanal anastomosis, or following total proctocolectomy with ileal-pouch anal anastomosis. Poor function usually commences soon after surgery, but control may improve over the ensuing months. Occasionally, the anorectal inhibitory reflex is recovered because of either reinnervation of the proximal neorectum or assumption of the distension sensation by the pelvic floor musculature, allowing the reflex to occur.

RECTAL PROLAPSE, RECTOCELE

Rectal prolapse is accompanied by fecal incontinence in 40% to 60% of patients and may be due to stretching of either the internal sphincter by the prolapse or the pudendal nerves as a consequence of chronic straining and perineal descent. Following prolapse repair, continence improves in approximately 50% of patients.[8,9] Anterior mucosal prolapse, considered by some to be a precursor of prolapse, may cause lowered sensation and leakage of mucus. A rectocele may occasionally evacuate retained stool without warning and this may be perceived as incontinence. Similarly, fecal impaction may lead to soilage; chronic rectal distention by retained feces relaxes the internal sphincter, thus permitting stool to pass. Short-segment Hirschsprung's disease may cause similar symptoms of overflow incontinence.

NEUROLOGIC DISEASE (CONGENITAL AND ACQUIRED)

Scleroderma and multiple sclerosis can affect the pudendal nerve-motor unit complex. Scleroderma may initially produce a hypertonic internal sphincter, but with progressive disease, squeeze pressures decline. Multiple sclerosis affects nerves randomly and may involve the pudendal and pelvic floor nerves, causing poor voluntary function. Diabetes-induced peripheral neuropathy results in diminished anal canal sensation and sphincter function.

With upper spinal cord injuries, the anorectal inhibitory reflex is intact, but there is no voluntary control to prevent elimination of the rectal contents as the internal sphincter relaxes in response to rectal distension. Spontaneous rectal evacuation ensues if the internal anal sphincter relaxes simultaneous with a mass peristaltic movement of the colon. Lower spinal cord trauma may injure the peripheral nerve roots of S1-4, which are the source of the pudendal nerve and sacral nerves innervating the pelvic floor. Destruction of the peripheral nerves may result in loss of all voluntary contraction.

EVALUATION

Pretreatment physiologic tests are necessary and helpful for several reasons:

- They may identify the underlying cause of fecal incontinence.
- They may separate patients who are best suited for corrective surgery from those who should undergo nonoperative therapy.
- They may help to inform patients as to the likelihood of benefit from surgery.
- They record a baseline assessment against which post-treatment function can be compared.

OFFICE EVALUATION

All patients who are incontinent should undergo a digital rectal examination and proctosigmoidoscopy to exclude cancer, inflammatory bowel disease, fecal impaction, or stricture. The perineal body should be assessed for thinning of the anterior midline and evidence of a prior midline episiotomy. A bimanual assessment of the thickness of the rectovaginal septum is necessary, because a normal amount of skin may be present even though the underlying anterior fibers of the external sphincter are disrupted or absent. The patient is then asked to squeeze and strain against the finger in the anal canal. The pressure obtained during this maneuver is usually underestimated by the examiner's finger; only a gross determination is possible. An experienced examiner, however, may be able to select the patient who benefits from anterior sphincter reconstruction based solely on the digital rectal examination.

ANAL MANOMETRY

The techniques and instrumentation of anal manometry have been described in Chapter 7. Important manometric parameters include sphincter length, resting pressure, squeeze pressure, anal canal sensation, compliance, and the presence of an anorectal inhibitory reflex. The anterior quadrant is of greatest interest in patients with suspected obstetric injury to the anal sphincter, in which cases both anterior resting pressure and squeeze pressure are usually abnormal. It is also possible to construct a pressure-volume directional curve (known as a vectorgraph), which reflects the functional state of the anal canal in all quadrants. This requires computerized reconstruction of the pressure and volume profiles at rest and during squeezing. A defect may reflect diminished sphincter function in that area.

The minimal sensory volume, an important measurement of anorectal sensation, can be determined by inflating a latex balloon with sequential volumes of air. Diminished sensation may result from a defect in the pudendal nerve or in the sensory rich mucosa of the anal transition zone. The anal canal is also innervated by nerves that respond to vibration, electrical current, and temperature; these sensory parameters may all be evaluated using different techniques and equipment.

Anal manometry can be very helpful in difficult clinical situations. For example, the patient who has had multiple unsuccessful procedures for fecal incontinence and who has undergone fecal diversion before a final attempt at repair should have objective testing to determine whether the sphincter will function properly after reversal of the stoma. For patients in whom an operation is planned that in and of itself may result in incontinence (for example, anal fistulotomy or coloanal anastomosis), it is also appropriate to obtain studies to determine if there is any preoperative impairment.

ELECTROMYOGRAPHY

Several electrodiagnostic tests helpful in detecting neuromuscular injury are reviewed in Chapter 11. The needle EMG traditionally has been used to demonstrate the presence or absence of electrically active muscle fibers, knowledge of which can be used when planning surgical correction of the incontinence. Study of the individual motor unit potentials provides useful information regarding possible prior injury with reinnervation, and quantitative motor unit analysis supplies data regarding motor unit recruitment. Although valuable information is gained

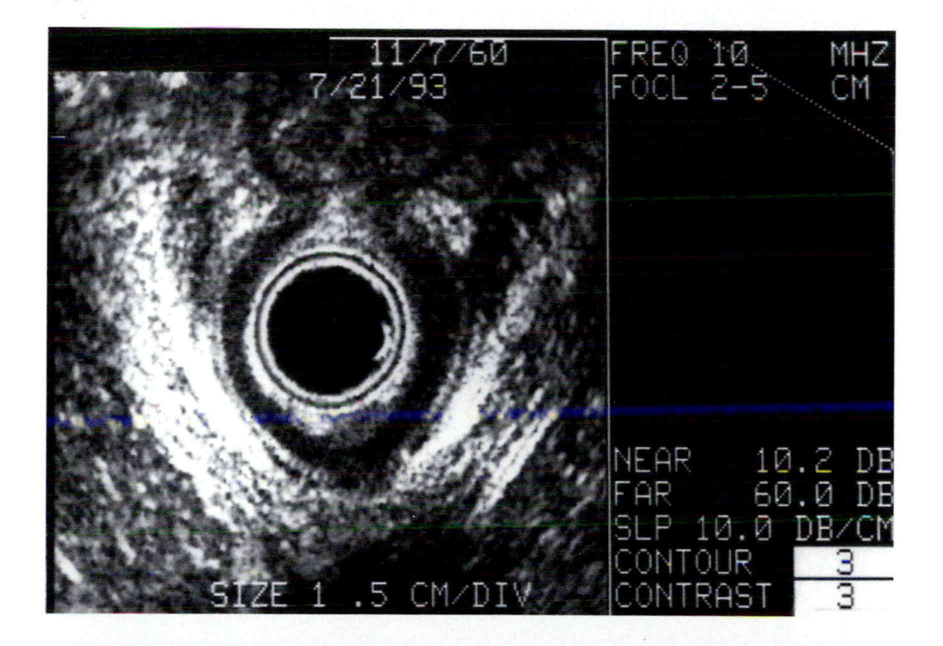

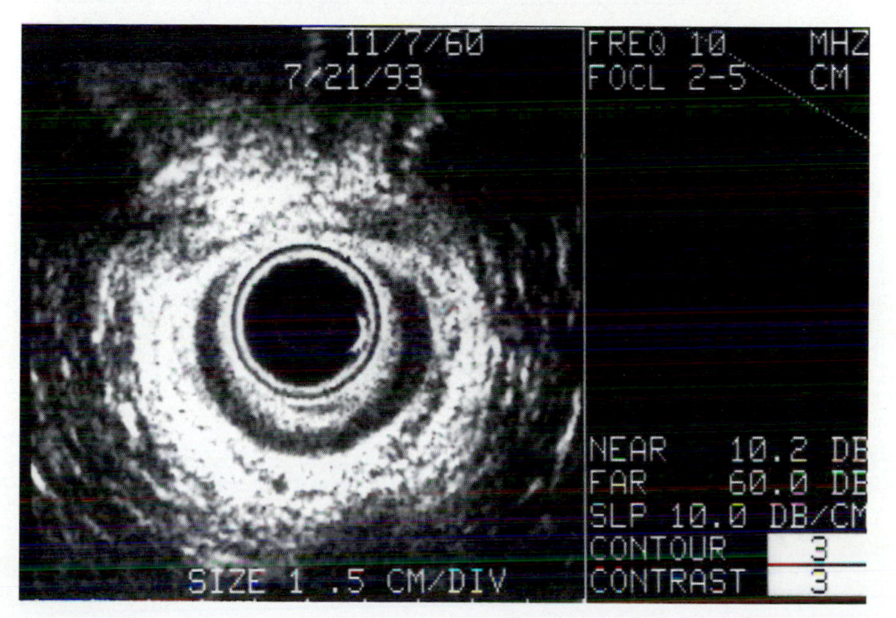

FIGURE 25–1. (*A*) Separation of the internal sphincter at the level of the puborectalis. (*B*) An anterior injury to both the internal and external sphincter; a scar is also present in this location. The patient is positioned so that anterior structures are at the upper aspect of the ultrasound images.

using EMG techniques, localization of muscle can be accomplished using modalities such as anal ultrasound. Such imaging studies are better tolerated by patients.

Pudendal motor latency studies were also discussed in Chapter 11. Significant neuropathy can be present despite a normal pudendal motor latency. Pudendal motor latency depends on the fastest-conducting neural fibers. Although extensive damage may have occurred, if the fastest fibers continue to conduct quickly, motor latency will not change. Abnormal motor latency is generally associated with slowed conduction, either from demyelination or axonal damage.

DEFECOGRAPHY

Defecography is occasionally used to identify or confirm rectal prolapse, internal rectal intussusception, or anterior rectocele as the source of incontinence, soilage, or obstructed defecation. Incontinence evident only during defecography must be evaluated further, because its significance is unclear; frequently it does not correlate with true fecal incontinence. The coexistence of internal intussusception and fecal incontinence may indicate a necessary repair of internal intussusception; this must, however, be decided on an individual basis. In general, defecography should not be used as a first-line test in the evaluation of fecal incontinence, because it is far more useful in the work-up of constipation and obstructed defecation.

TRANSANAL ULTRASOUND

Ultrasound imaging has only recently been suggested as a technique for evaluating the anal sphincter mechanism. Interfaces among muscle layers, fat, and mucosa allow accurate delineation of the anatomy of the anal canal. The Bruel and Kjaer system, with a 10-mHz probe covered by an anal cap, provides a 360-degree cross-sectional picture of the anal canal as the probe is withdrawn from the rectum. Identification and measurement of the internal and external sphincter in all quadrants, measurement of the distance between the rectum and the vagina in the perineal body, and identification of muscle disruption and scarring are all possible. The internal sphincter appears as a hypoechoic, dark ring around the anal canal. The external sphincter is a gray 1½-cm-thick circle outside the internal sphincter with hyperechoic lines throughout (Fig. 25–1). Scarred areas frequently have a featureless, homogenous gray appearance.

SUMMARY

Fecal incontinence is a socially distressing and disabling problem. There are many causes of incontinence, as outlined in this chapter; an algorithm for its evaluation and management is presented in Figure 25–2.

The trauma of vaginal delivery is a significant contributor to female fecal incontinence through me-

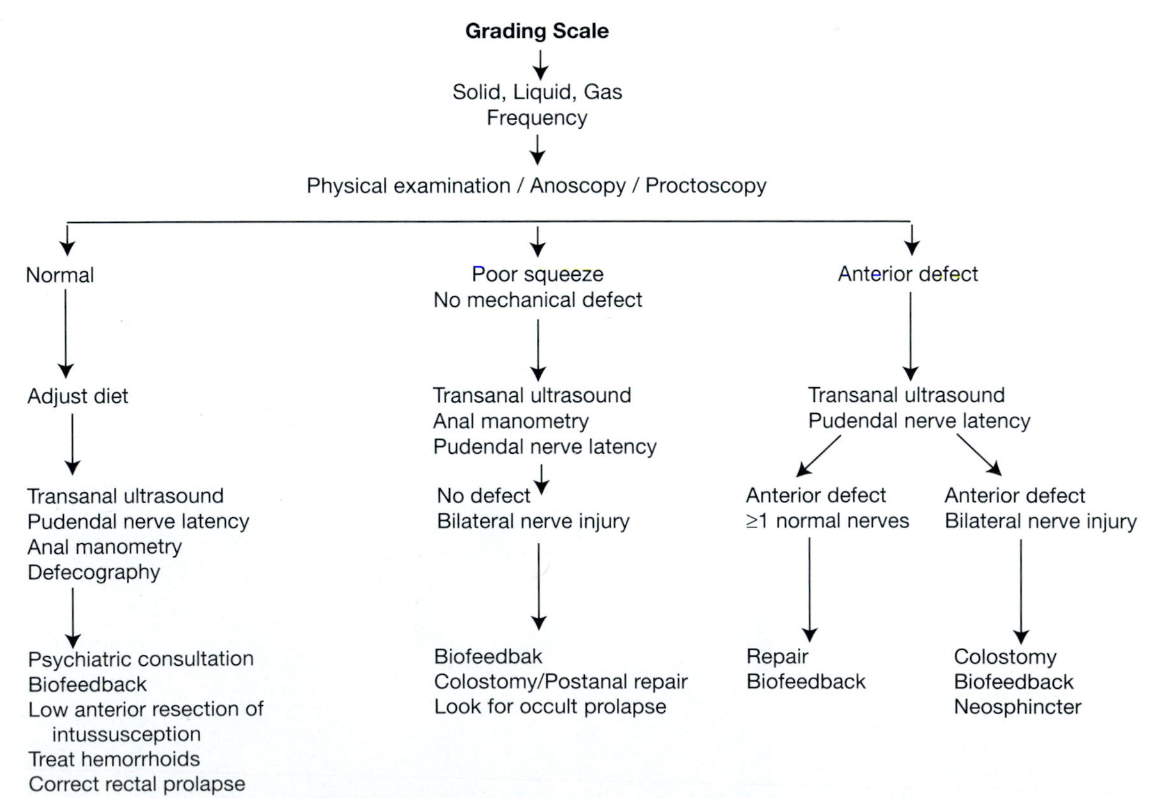

FIGURE 25–2. Algorithm for the evaluation and management of fecal incontinence.

chanical fiber disruption and neuronal injury. Efforts at identification of injury and proper reapproximation of the disrupted anal sphincter are critical for prevention of subsequent fecal incontinence. Women reporting obstetrically provoked fecal incontinence may be simply evaluated for sphincteroplasty using history and digital examination. Ancillary diagnostic techniques are usually needed for patients without a clear antecedent obstetric trauma. Such tests include electrophysiologic evaluation, ultrasound, manometry, and, less often, defecography. Such investigations should be used in concert with the history and physical examination to ensure accurate diagnosis and choice of optimal therapy.

REFERENCES

1. Miller, R, Bartolo, DCC, Locke-Edmunds, JC, et al: Prospective study of conservative and operative treatment of faecal incontinence. Br J Surg 75:101–105, 1988.
2. Fleshman, JW, Peters, WR, Shemesh, EI, et al: Anal sphincter reconstruction: Anterior overlapping muscle repair. Dis Colon Rectum 34:739–743, 1991.
3. Madoff, RD, Williams, JG and Caushaj, PF: Current Concepts: Fecal Incontinence. N Engl J Med 326:1002–1007, 1992.
4. Cornes, H, Bartolo, DCC and Stirrat, GM: Changes in anal canal sensation after child birth. Br J Surg 78:74–77, 1991.
5. Wilcox, LS, Strobino, DM, Baruffi, G, et al: Episiotomy and its role in the incidence of perineal lacerations in a maternity center and a tertiary hospital obstetric service. Am J Obstet Gynecol 160:1047–1052, 1989.
6. May, JL: Modified median episiotomy minimizes the risk of third-degree tears. Obstet Gynecol 83:156–157, 1994.
7. Birnbaum, EH, Myerson, RJ, Fry, RD, et al: Chronic effects of pelvic radiation therapy on anorectal function. Dis Col Rectum 37:909–915, 1994.
8. Parks, AG: Anorectal incontinence. Proc R Soc Med 68:681–690, 1975.
9. Snooks, SJ, Henry, MM and Swash, M: Anorectal incontinence and rectal prolapse: Differential assessment of the innervation of the puborectalis and external anal sphincter muscles. Gut 26:470–476, 1985.

CHAPTER **26**

Fecal Incontinence: Nonsurgical Therapy

Jeannette Tries • Eugene Eisman

THEORETIC BACKGROUND

Biofeedback has evolved from two fields of academic psychology: psychophysiology and learning theory. Psychophysiology provided methods, instrumentations, and the knowledge of the anatomy and physiology required for a clinical understanding of the disorders appropriate for this form of therapy. The initial focus was on the autonomically innervated response systems but, in time, this was broadened to include systems innervated by both branches of the peripheral nervous system. The anal sphincter is an example of such a system.

A major question that arose in the 1960s, in both learning theory and psychophysiology, was whether it is possible to change autonomically mediated responses using operant procedures. Using animals medicated with curare, Miller and DiCara[1] showed that operant procedures could produce bidirectional changes in heart rate, blood pressure, and glandular activity without somatic (striated-muscle) involvement. These findings challenged the view that smooth-muscle learning was possible only through classic conditioning and suggested that clinical disorders, such as elevated blood pressure and cardiac arrhythmias, could be treated with operant procedures.[2] Hence the emergence of the biofeedback field. Miller's work, however, has yet to be satisfactorily replicated, leaving unanswered the possible mechanisms of smooth-muscle learning.[3]

In contrast to the theoretic importance of this question, the significance of the precise mechanism of visceral learning seems to be less critical in clinical applications, because skeletal and visceral responses are often inextricably linked as parts of centrally integrated response patterns.[4] The colon, rectum, and anus provide an ideal example of this interaction; the autonomic and somatic nervous systems both play a vital role in maintaining normal bowel function. Because of this integration, opportunity exists for the use of operant procedures to alter disordered bowel function by conditioning the pelvic floor muscles and external anal sphincter (EAS).

DEVELOPMENT OF BIOFEEDBACK FOR INCONTINENCE

In a critical review of the literature up to 1990 concerning biofeedback for adult fecal incontinence, Enck[5] found 13 clinical studies with design adequate for consideration.[6–18] Of these 13 studies, 12 indicated that biofeedback was superior to conventional therapy. Although the definition of success varied among the investigators, rates of reported improvement ranged from 50% to 90%, with a mean overall success rate of 79.8% among 322 subjects.[5]

Kohlenberg[19] was the first to report the use of operant procedures to improve sphincter strength and reduce incontinence; a 13-year-old boy with fecal seepage and low sphincter pressure was treated with a straightforward training protocol using a water-filled balloon positioned in the anal canal. The patient's efforts were rewarded with money when sphincter pressure was increased. As a result of this training, soiling was reduced but the patient did not become continent.

Engel, Nikoomanesh, and Schuster,[9] using a manometric three-balloon probe,[20] reported what is now considered to be the seminal study of the biofeedback treatment of incontinence. Inflation of a rectal balloon simulated the descent of stool; subjects were then instructed to attend to the sensation of rectal distention and to contract the EAS in response to it. An important feature of the training protocol was the reinforcement of a short-latency (rapid) EAS contraction while maintaining stable intra-abdominal pressure. This biofeedback protocol addressed three factors that contribute to continence: (1) awareness of sensory cues that normally signal impending loss of stool; (2) timely EAS contraction to the perception of distension; and (3) reduction of a maladaptive rise in intra-abdominal pressure, which frequently accompanies EAS contraction and is counterproductive to storage of feces. In other words, sensory discrimination provided by balloon distention reinforced a training response to internal cues that could be applied to daily life.[9] After one to four treatment sessions, four of seven patients achieved continence and two had significant improvement; one patient did not complete therapy. Others[6,10,15,16] have used similar training methods and have obtained comparable outcomes, but these studies did not include control groups.

In a controlled study with geriatric subjects, Whitehead, Burgio, and Engel[18] placed all subjects on habit training and randomly assigned half of them to a sphincter-exercise protocol. After 4 weeks, there was only an 11% reduction in incontinent episodes; no difference was seen in either symptom reduction or sphincter strength as measured with manometry in those subjects who had performed sphincter exercises. Subjects were then given biofeedback training using the protocol established by Engel, Nikoomanesh, and Shuster,[9] with an emphasis on reinforcing sphincter contractions for 10 seconds in response to rectal distention. With the addition of biofeedback, a 77% overall reduction in episodes of fecal incontinence and a significant increase in sphincter strength were obtained. Other controlled studies,[8,11,14,16] using somewhat different protocols, have obtained equivalent rates of symptom reduction with variable improvement in sphincter strength.

RECTAL SENSATION: AN ESSENTIAL FACTOR IN CONTINENCE

An observation made by a number of researchers is that a rapid sphincter response to rectal distention is essential for continence and is dependent on intact sensory discrimination. To demonstrate the importance of rectal sensation, Buser and Miner[6] studied a group of patients with incontinence with delayed perception of rectal distention. A 92% reduction in incontinence episodes was achieved following a protocol that was designed to provide reinforcement for immediate perception of, and EAS contraction to, rectal distention.

Two studies attempted to determine which components of biofeedback training were most effective.[11,14] Using a single-case experimental design, Latimer, Campbell, and Kasperski[11] systematically evaluated sensory discrimination, sphincter strengthening, and sphincter coordination training using a probe with three balloons. Clinical improvement was associated with improved rectal sensation. External sphinter deficits that were identified by pretreatment manometry did not predict an individual subject's response to a specific biofeedback intervention, nor did maximum voluntary squeeze pressure change appreciably following training. In another study using a two-phase cross-over design in which sham sensory training, active sensory training, sphincter coordination training, and sphincter strength training were compared, improvement in rectal sensitivity contributed most significantly to improved continence.[14] Attainment of continence was always associated with improved sensory discrimination in response to rectal stimulation, but not all patients with improved sensation developed continence. Again, however, despite a 76% reduction in the frequency of symptoms of incontinence, manometric indices of sphincter function did not change. The only objective change in anorectal function observed as a result of the biofeedback training was an improved sensory threshold for rectal distention. Given these findings,[11,14] it appears that although adequate sensation of rectal distention is necessary, it is not the only requirement for continence.

The most probable explanation for the lack of objective changes in EAS function is that the biofeedback protocols employed did not systematically reinforce improved EAS contractions in terms of greater amplitude, endurance, and isolation from abdominal contraction. In both studies,[11,14] sphincter contraction was reinforced verbally with only the examiner's using the visual feedback display to guide the patient. It is unlikely that therapist-produced verbal reinforcement alone can provide the kind of precise sensory information that is required to direct and update motor plans that would improve the quality of sphincter contractions, especially where sphincter afferent and efferent activity are compromised by trauma or disease. Similarly, no attempt was made to control for the typically observed increase in intra-abdominal pressure, which can restrict the effectiveness of the sphincter training. Furthermore, strength training was limited to three sessions of 20[14] or 60[11] minutes, hardly sufficient time to strengthen muscles that are weak. Given these limitations, a valid comparison between strengthening procedures and sensory discrimination training cannot be made.

STRENGTHENING THE EXTERNAL ANAL SPHINCTER AND PELVIC FLOOR MUSCLES

Other investigators have focused exclusively on improving EAS control.[13,21] Schiller and co-workers[21] infused the rectum with increasing amounts of saline in a woman who had daily incontinence for liquid stool. The patient received visual and verbal feedback about the amount of solution retained. Rectal capacity improved six-fold and the patient became continent after 1 week of therapy even though diarrhea persisted. MacLeod[13] studied 113 patients with incontinence of varied etiology using an intra-anal electromyographic (EMG) probe. A 63% reduction in incontinence was obtained. The training procedure called for the reinforcement of EAS contractions of greater amplitude and of durations up to 30 seconds. Unfortunately, there was no control for inadvertent abdominal contraction and this may be the reason that the percentage of improvement obtained was smaller than in other studies. Patients were observed for 6 months to 5 years without any report of relapse.

As indicated previously, a number of investigators have found that improved continence is not necessarily associated with improvement in sphincter strength as measured either manometrically or by saline retention test.[11–15,17] This observation indicates that continence is a function of several variables and that each factor may require a specific training method to produce objective change and thus maximize clinical outcome. Studies that did not find appreciable change in sphincter function did not use conditioning methods that enhanced the ability to perform isolated sphincter contractions. Some protocols did not employ direct visual feedback for either sphincter contraction or abdominal substitution. Others did not train patients to sustain sphincter contraction, but rather reinforced only a rapid EAS response to rectal distention. Because feedback was not provided for the specific goal of shaping isolated and sustained EAS contraction, there could be little generalization to a home exercise program which, over time, might have changed muscle strength if appropriate sphincter training had occurred in the laboratory.

When training protocols included direct feedback for improving the amplitude and duration of sphincter contractions while discouraging increases in intra-abdominal pressure, researchers have been able to demonstrate improved sphincter contractility.[18,22] In one study, Chiarioni and colleagues[22] obtained an 85% reduction in incontinence in 14 subjects with chronic diarrhea who were not helped by earlier medical treatment. There was an associated improvement in the ability to sustain an EAS contraction from 19.2 seconds to 38.3 seconds. All nine patients reporting complete resolution of incontinence could sustain a 30-second EAS contraction after treatment. These findings differ from those obtained by Loening-Baucke,[12] who compared two treatment groups drawn from a similar patient population. One group was treated with biofeedback plus conventional medical treatment and the other with conventional therapy alone. Incontinence was reduced by about 50% in both groups. There was no difference between groups in maximum voluntary contraction following training. The disparate outcomes of these two studies were likely due to differences in the training procedures employed. Although Loening-Baucke[12] trained coordinated EAS contraction to rectal distention, no attempt was made to reinforce EAS contraction of sufficient duration to exceed the time required for recovery of internal anal sphincter (IAS) inhibition following rectal distention. It is not possible to evaluate the adequacy of their home-training program because the number of Kegel's exercises per day was not specified. In contrast, Chiarioni and colleagues[22] were careful to reinforce EAS contractions of greater amplitude and duration up to 30 seconds in response to rectal distention and in isolation from abdominal contraction. Subjects were also assigned a vigorous EAS home exercise program to include twenty 30-second contractions, three times per day.

CONFOUNDING FACTORS IN THE LITERATURE

Like many biofeedback applications, those for fecal incontinence employ various "adjunctive" manipulations in conjunction with the operant conditioning of targeted physiologic responses. These adjunctive procedures include bowel or "habit" training, dietary manipulations, and the use of medications. For the most part, these protocols have not been subjected to experimental control. Biofeedback therapy is also likely to be associated with nonspecific beneficial effects due to factors such as

- The attention shown by a concerned health professional to a problem that patients generally do not discuss with others
- The keeping of a symptom diary by the patient over the course of treatment
- The elaborateness of the feedback procedure itself
- The actual instrumenting of the anal canal, which may improve sensory awareness of the area in and of itself.

Most studies have not considered these confounding factors; only two have attempted to control for them to some degree.[12,18] As a result, the degree to which these nonspecific factors and adjunctive procedures contribute to clinical outcome is unknown. Moreover, the treatment protocols used and the causes of the incontinence have varied. Wald and Tunuguntla,[16] who restricted their sample to patients with diabetes mellitus, were the exception.

In summary, the research literature supports the idea that some minimal level of sensitivity to rectal distention is essential for continence and that biofeedback therapy can be effective in improving rectal sensation. The association between measures of EAS strength and clinical outcome, however, has not been consistent. As a result, the degree to which improved strength contributes to continence is unknown. Similarly, the relationship between improved strength and increased sensitivity is not understood. The disparity between obtained changes in sensation compared with sphincter strength seems to be associated with the underlying physiologic mechanisms that a specific biofeedback application alters. On one hand, sensation consistently improves with biofeedback; many studies report improvement after only one treatment session. Because this improvement occurs so rapidly, it appears to be associated with relearning neurophysiologic patterns that are essentially intact but have not been used due to faulty perception. On the other hand, where EAS weakness is the primary contributor to incontinence, short-term training in sensory discrimination and in EAS coordination is unlikely to alter muscle tone or strength sufficiently to modify the condition. Thus, in a patient whose muscles are weak but whose sensation is intact, symptom reduction would depend on changing muscle strength through an extended and well-designed exercise protocol. This approach was clearly demonstrated by Chiarioni and colleagues[22] in patients with diarrhea and incontinence, where the focus of therapy was on not only improving the coordination of the EAS response to distention but also increasing the strength of the EAS. It would seem, therefore, that it is not only possible, but also desirable, to include a well-designed protocol for EAS strengthening in any program for biofeedback treatment of fecal incontinence.

SUMMARY OF REPORTED FINDINGS AND CLINICAL OBSERVATIONS

The goal of most biofeedback protocols for fecal incontinence is to reinforce sensory discrimination and coordinate EAS contraction in response to rectal

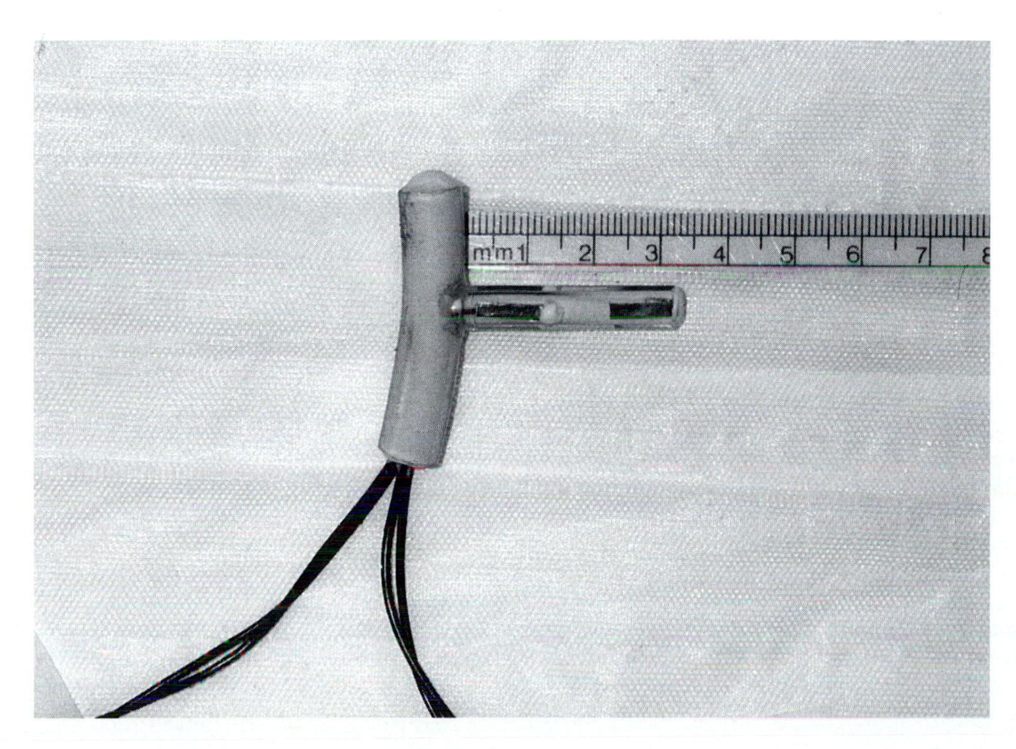

FIGURE 26–1. The multiple electrode anal probe, which measures surface electromyographic activity from two sites within the anal canal. Two bipolar electrodes adjacent to the T-handle measure subcutaneous external anal sphincter (EAS) activity whereas the proximal pair record activity from the deeper EAS and puborectalis muscles. The T-handle remains external to the anal verge when the probe is positioned.

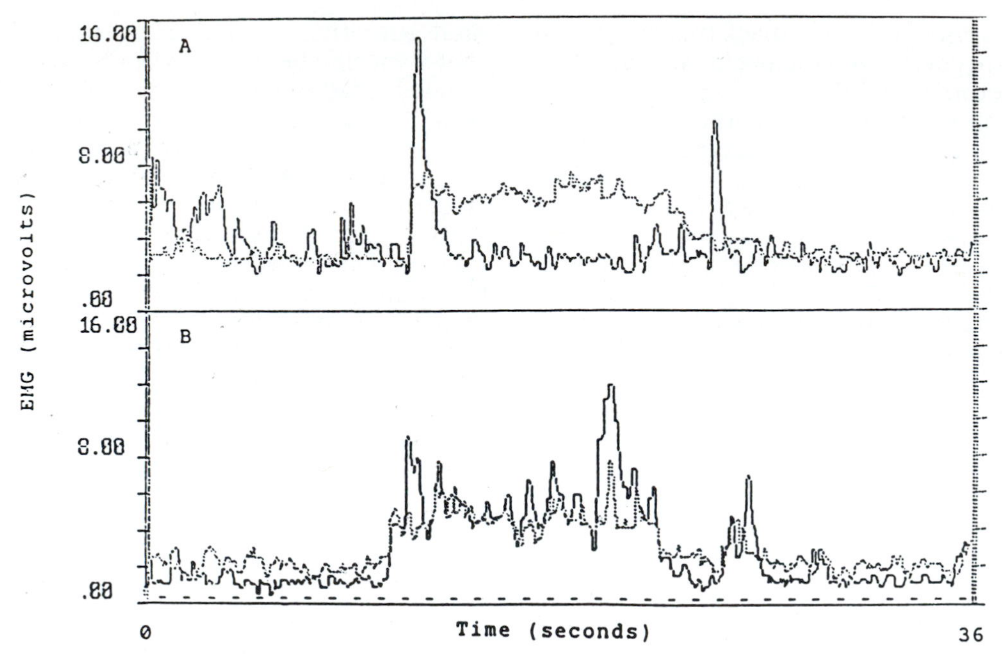

FIGURE 26–2. Two electromyographic (EMG) recordings of a maximum voluntary external anal sphincter contraction over 10 seconds, taken from a 57-year-old woman with urinary and fecal incontinence (*A*) on the date of her initial biofeedback evaluation and (*B*) weeks later at discharge. The darker line is a recording of muscle activity from the proximal anal canal; the lighter line records distal anal canal activity. Note that on the initial evaluation (*A*), proximal EMG activity level decayed within 1 second of initial recruitment but the distal measures were sustained over the 10-second contraction. At discharge (*B*), proximal EMG can be maintained at a stable amplitude for the duration of the contraction. This change in EMG covaried with improvement in external anal sphincter and internal anal sphincter Schuster's balloon pressure measurements and was associated with a clinically significant reduction in symptoms. Because rectal sensation was intact at the beginning of treatment, improvement in puborectalis contraction probably contributed most to clinical improvement because overall, both EMG and pressure amplitudes remained less than normal at discharge.

distention. These procedures have resulted in significant clinical improvements that have been associated with objective improvement in sensory thresholds. When the training procedures have specifically reinforced quantitative and qualitative changes in EAS contraction in terms of amplitude, endurance, and isolation from abdominal contraction, objective improvement in EAS strength has also been reported.[18,22] To date, there have been insufficient data to determine the degree to which patients benefit from both sensory discrimination training and strengthening protocols. The most judicious approach, therefore, is to use operant procedures to normalize all aspects of anorectal function that are found deficient through manometric and EMG evaluation.

The best method of strengthening pelvic floor muscles has yet to be demonstrated. For example, Chiarioni and colleagues[22] observed that improved continence was more closely associated with endurance than with the amplitude of the voluntary EAS contraction. All patients who could sustain an isolated EAS contraction beyond 30 seconds became continent regardless of the actual amplitude of the contraction. It may be the case, therefore, that reinforcement of a rapid EAS response to rectal distention without conditioning endurance for contraction will not potentiate the tonic fibers of the EAS and puborectalis muscle.

One report demonstrated that integrated surface EMG can differentially measure striated muscle activity at multiple sites within the anal canal.[23] Activity within the distal anal canal stems primarily from contractions of subcutaneous EAS fibers; proximal activity serves as a relative index of muscle contractions generated by the deep EAS and puborectalis muscle[23] (Fig. 26–1). Diminished proximal anal canal muscle activity with voluntary contraction therefore represents weakness of the puborectalis. In these instances, it would be desirable to reinforce more specifically contraction of the deeper muscles and to condition a sustained contraction. This differential assessment may have some clinical advantages over a single pelvic-floor measure, especially where the deeper levator ani muscle has been weakened through partial denervation injury or by other causes (Fig. 26–2).

BIOFEEDBACK TREATMENT GOALS FOR FECAL INCONTINENCE

A description of specific biofeedback training procedures is beyond the scope of this chapter; the reader should consult another source for a more detailed description of procedures used for fecal incontinence.[24] Several training goals should be included in any biofeedback application for fecal incontinence.

After identifying the functional anorectal abnormalities with manometric and EMG methods separately or in combination, biofeedback goals to improve bowel dysfunction generally include shaping:

1. Sphincteric contractions for greater amplitude and improved duration in isolation from abdominal or gluteal contraction and associated elevations in intra-abdominal pressure
2. Sphincteric contractions with short response latencies and immediate recovery to baseline after voluntary contraction ceases
3. Heightened perception to lower levels of rectal distention, which is paired with immediate external anal sphincter contraction as the internal anal sphincter relaxes
4. Sphincteric inhibition below resting baseline concurrent with appropriate elevation in intra-abdominal pressure during the defecation maneuver
5. Reduction of chronically elevated striated sphincter muscle activity, when present

SUMMARY

Although biofeedback treatment for fecal incontinence is clearly effective, the mechanisms that contribute to clinical improvement are not readily understood beyond biofeedback therapy's potential for improving rectal sensation. Further research is needed to determine the most efficient strengthening procedures for the EAS and pelvic floor muscles and also to decide when sphincter relaxation training should be included in biofeedback protocol. Moreover, there has been little investigation of the role of the striated muscles in the mediation of disordered smooth-muscle activity (e.g., irritable bowel syndrome) and the degree to which this mediation can be altered with operant procedures. Research seeking greater resolution of these issues will certainly improve the quality of life for many women.

REFERENCES

1. Miller, NE and DiCara, LV; Instrumental learning of heart rate changes in curarized rats: Shaping and specificity to discriminative stimuli. J Comp Physiol Psychol 63:12–19, 1967.
2. Perski, A, Engel, BT and McCroskery, JH: The modification of elicited cardiovascular responses to operant conditioning of heart rate. In Cacioppo, JT and Petty RE (eds.): Perspectives in Cardiovascular Psychophysiology. Guilford, New York, 1982, p 296.
3. Bower, GH and Hilgard, ER: Theories of Learning, ed 5. Prentice-Hall, Englewood Cliffs, NJ, 1981, p 259.
4. Miller, NE: Biofeedback and visceral learning. Annu Rev Psychol 29:373–404, 1978.
5. Enck, P: Biofeedback training in disordered defecation: A critical review. Dig Dis Sci 38:1953–1960, 1993.
6. Buser, WD and Miner, PB: Delayed rectal sensation with fecal incontinence. Successful treatment using anorectal manometry. Gastroenterology 91:1186–1191, 1986.
7. Cerulli, MA, Nikoomanesh, P and Schuster, MN: Progress in biofeedback conditioning for fecal incontinence. Gastroenterology 76:742–746, 1979.
8. Enck, P, Kranzle, U, Schwiese, J, et al: Biofeedback training in fecal incontinence. Dtsch Med Wochenschr 113:1789–1794, 1988.
9. Engel, BT, Nikoomanesh, P and Schuster, MM: Operant conditioning of rectosphincteric responses in the treatment of fecal incontinence. N Engl J Med 290:646–649, 1974.
10. Goldenberg, DA, Hodges, K, Hershe, T and Jinich, H: Biofeedback therapy for fecal incontinence. Am J Gastroenterol 74:342–345, 1980.
11. Latimer, PR, Campbell, D and Kasperski, J: A components analysis of biofeedback in the treatment of fecal incontinence. Biofeedback Self Regul 9:311–324, 1984.
12. Loening-Baucke, V: Efficacy of biofeedback training in improving faecal incontinence and anorectal physiologic function. Gut 31:1395–1402, 1990.
13. MacLeod, JH: Management of anal incontinence by biofeedback. Gastroenterology 93:291–294, 1987.
14. Miner, PB, Donnelly, TC and Read, NW: Investigation of mode of action of biofeedback in treatment of fecal incontinence. Dig Dis Sci 35:1291–1298, 1990.
15. Riboli, BE, Frascio, M, Pitto, FM, et al: Biofeedback conditioning for fecal incontinences. Arch Phys Med Rehabil 69:29–31, 1988.
16. Wald, A and Tunuguntla, AK: Anorectal sensorimotor dysfunction in fecal incontinence and diabetes mellitus: Modification with biofeedback therapy. N Engl J Med 310:1282–1287, 1984.
17. Wald, A: Biofeedback therapy for fecal incontinence. Ann Intern Med 95:146–149, 1981.
18. Whitehead, WE, Burgio, KL and Engel, BT: Biofeedback treatment of fecal incontinence in geriatric patients. J Am Geriatr Soc 33:320–324, 1985.
19. Kohlenberg, JR: Operant conditioning of human anal sphincter pressure. J Appl Behav Anal 6:201–208, 1973.
20. Schuster, MM, Hookman, P, Hendrix, T and Mendeloff, A: Simultaneous manometric recording form of internal and external anal sphincter reflexes. Bull John Hopkins Hosp 116:79–88, 1965.
21. Schiller, LR, Santa Ana, C, Davis, GR and Fordtran, JS: Fecal incontinence in chronic diarrhea. Report of a case with improvement after training with rectally infused saline. Gastroenterology 77:751–753, 1979.
22. Chiarioni, G, Scattolini, C, Bonfante, F and Vantini, I: Liquid stool incontinence with severe urgency: Anorectal function and effective biofeedback treatment. Gut 34:1576–1580, 1993.
23. Eisman, E and Tries, J: A new probe for measuring electromyographic activity from multiple sites in the anal canal. Dis Colon Rectum 36:946–952, 1993.
24. Tries, J, Eisman, E and Lowery, SP: Biofeedback therapy for fecal incontinence. In Schwartz, M (ed.): Biofeedback: A Practitioner's Guide, ed 2. Guilford, New York, 1995.

CHAPTER 27

Fecal Incontinence: Surgical Therapy

Steven D. Wexner • Stephanie L. Schmitt

Fecal incontinence is a complex problem with a multifactorial etiology. The multitude of procedures that have been devised to treat this disorder reflects its many causes and complex physiology. Currently available surgical therapeutic alternatives form the basis of this chapter.

Initially, fecal continence was thought to have been primarily contingent on maintenance of an acute angle between the anal canal and rectal vault, producing, in essence, a flap-valve mechanism.[1] It was proposed that with the contraction of the pelvic floor muscles with or without increased intra-abdominal pressure, the anterior rectal wall formed a flap and "covered" the top of the anal canal, providing continence. Other studies by Bannister, Gibbons, and Read[2] and Bartolo and associates[3] have shown that the mechanisms of continence are more complex, particularly in that continence is maintained by the integrated action of the external and internal anal sphincters, the puborectalis, the levator plate, and intact sensory pathways.

Surgical procedures used to treat incontinence can be distinctly categorized: direct repair of the external anal sphincter defect,[4,5] posterior plication of the levator ani muscle,[6–8] and encirclement of the anal canal either with synthetic material[9,10] or by nonsphincteric muscle transposition.[11–24] Other innovative techniques developed include combinations of the above procedures (total pelvic floor repair) and artificial sphincter implantation.[22–24]

PREOPERATIVE ASSESSMENT

Evaluation of the patient with fecal incontinence must include a thorough history, which may disclose the etiology of the underlying problem. Information regarding the frequency, duration, and severity of incontinence, impact on lifestyle, and the need for protective absorbent pads should be obtained.[25] Underlying neurologic disease may become evident by asking about it. A history of dietary habits and current medications may reveal a straightforward cause and easy solution.

A thorough anorectal examination including visual inspection and palpation of the perineum should be undertaken to detect defects in the sphincter mechanism; this is aided by synchronous vaginal and rectal digital examination. Obstetric injuries may cause anterior displacement of the anus as well as attenuation of the perineal body. Evidence of neurologic disease, such as abnormal perineal descent or a patulous anus, should be sought. In addition, proctosigmoidoscopy is recommended to exclude neoplasms or proctitis as a cause of incontinence.

For patients with obvious sphincter injuries and incontinence historically related to a specific iatrogenic or traumatic cause, most surgeons elect to forgo physiologic investigation. In such instances, surgery is promptly recommended to the patient. Testing is most certainly indicated in complex cases; the information obtained from anorectal manometry, electromyography, pudendal nerve terminal motor latency, and anal ultrasound will aid in selecting operative or nonoperative treatment. In cases of idiopathic incontinence, more extensive testing may be required, including anal mucosal electrosensitivity, cinedefecography, and single-fiber electromyography.

Some studies have investigated the ability of preoperative neurophysiologic tests to predict a successful surgical result. In the study by Laurberg, Swash, and Henry of women with incontinence secondary to obstetric trauma, normal preoperative pudendal-nerve motor latency correlated with a good or excellent outcome in 80% of patients. Of those with prolonged pudendal conduction, in contrast, only 11% had an excellent result. Wexner, Marchetti, and Jagelman also noted a correlation between subjective functional postoperative results and objective physiologic assessment.[27]

For sphincter injuries due to obstetric trauma, prompt recognition is essential; the ideal time for repair is at the time of injury. If the repair fails, a waiting period of weeks to months is indicated to allow fibrosis to occur as well as resolution of swelling and infection; this approach optimizes potential for successful repair at a later date.

ISOLATED SPHINCTER DEFECTS

Corrective surgery is most likely to be successful when incontinence is secondary to an isolated sphincter defect. Previous operations for fistulas or hemorrhoids and obstetrical trauma are the most common causes of surgically correctable fecal incontinence.[28] Sphincteroplasty may be accomplished with either a direct end-to-end apposition of the severed muscle edges or by an overlapping technique.

DIRECT-APPOSITION SPHINCTER REPAIR

The technique of direct-apposition sphincter repair involves mobilization of the external anal sphincter and excision of the scarred tissue. The divided ends are then directly reapproximated (Fig. 27–1). Becaue of suture-line disruptions, results are poor with this technique; emphasis is now placed on overlapping sphincteroplasty.[25,26,28–34]

OVERLAPPING SPHINCTEROPLASTY

Technique

All patients are given a full mechanical and oral antibiotic bowel preparation. Parenteral broad-spectrum antibiotics are administered on-call to the operating room. An indwelling bladder catheter is inserted after the induction of anesthesia. The patient is then positioned on a Kraske roll in the prone-jackknife position. Alternatively, the lithotomy position may be used. Benzoin is applied to the buttocks, which are then taped apart.

A solution of 0.25% bupivicaine and 0.5% lidocaine with 1:400,000 units of epinephrine is used to achieve a circumanal and bilateral pudendal nerve block. Alternatively, spinal, caudal, or general anesthesia can be given. A curvilinear incision with an arc of 180 to 200 degrees is made approximately 0.5 cm caudal and parallel to the outer edge of the anal verge. Care should be taken to avoid damage to the pudendal nerve, which inserts posteriorly into the sphincter (Fig. 27–2). Scar tissue found between the laterally displaced ends of the external sphincter is dissected to the level of the anorectal ring and the levator ani muscles. Dissection proceeds laterally until the external anal sphincter is sufficiently mobilized. Anteriorly, care must be taken to separate the scar from

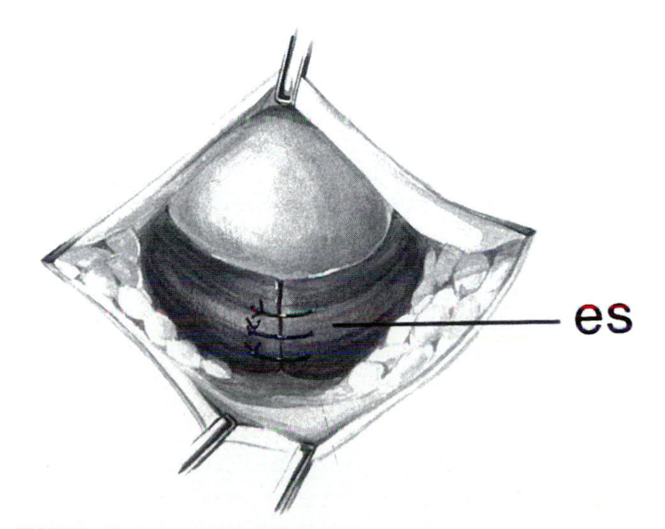

FIGURE 27–1. Technique of direct apposition of the external anal sphincter after excision of scar tissue. *es* = external [anal] sphincter. (Reprinted from Cherry and Greenwald[29], p 114, with permission.)

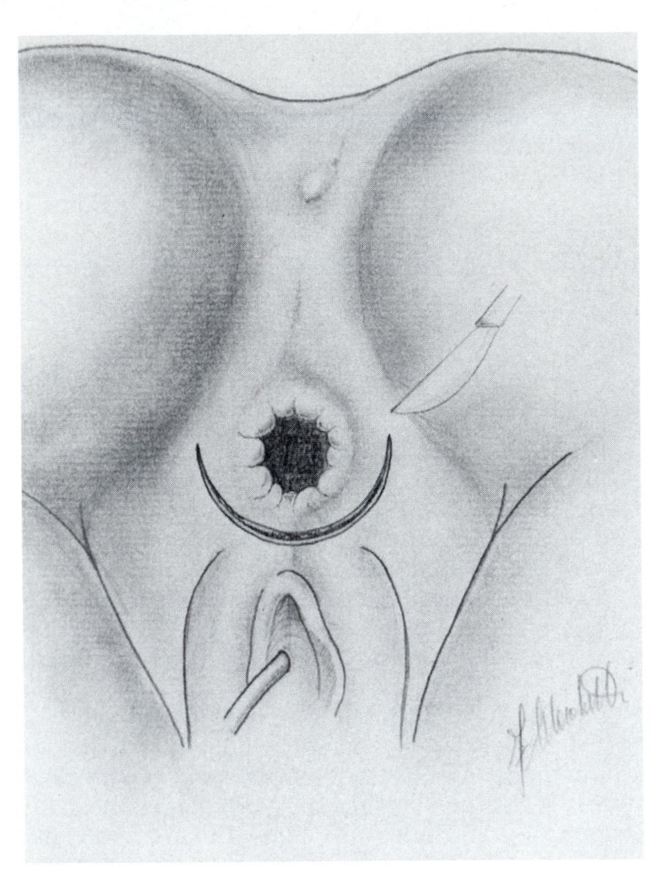

FIGURE 27–2. The incision for sphincteroplasty is performed 0.5 cm outside the anal verge and is limited to an anterolateral 200 degree arc. (Reprinted with permission from Wexner, Marchetti, and Jagelman,[27] © American Society for Colon and Rectal Surgeons, with permission.)

the posterior vaginal wall without entry into the vagina itself. The intersphincteric space is then mobilized from lateral to medial to the area of the midline scar. Consequently, the external and internal anal sphincters are separated. At this point, if the external anal sphincter is in continuity, it is sharply divided through the midportion of the fibrotic midline scar; the scar itself should not be excised. The levator ani muscles are then apposed with interrupted 4-0 polyglactin sutures. Next, the internal anal sphincter is separately plicated with a series of interrupted 4-0 polyglactin sutures (Fig. 27–3). These sutures should be placed laterally sufficient to achieve a snug repair, as judged when the surgeon's contralateral index finger is placed in the anal canal. The ends of the previously divided external anal sphincter are then tightly overlapped and sutured together with interrupted 4-0 polyglactin mattress-type sutures (Fig. 27–4). Lateral and anterior aspects of the wound are closed in a V–Y manner to increase the anovaginal distance. The central portion of the wound is left open (Fig. 27–5).

The patient is instructed in the use of a water-spray bottle to optimize perianal hygiene and is then maintained on constipating medications, parenteral broad-spectrum antibiotics, and a clear liquid diet for the first 2 postoperative days. On the third day, a normal diet is permitted. The bladder catheter is then removed and the parenteral antibiotics discontinued. Psyllium dietary supplements and a 1-week course of oral metronidazole are begun. The wound usually heals within 4 to 6 weeks.

Results

The largest series of overlapping sphincter repairs for acquired fecal incontinence was reported by Fang and co-workers.[4] Among 17 males and 62 females, incontinence was due to obstetric trauma (54%), noniatrogenic trauma (34%), and rectal prolapse (3%). Results were excellent in 58% and good in 31%. Although the wound was left open, only a 2% incidence of wound infection occurred. None of the patients underwent diverting colostomies.

Flesham and associates[30] reported 55 women who underwent overlapping sphincteroplasty for fecal incontinence. The cause of the incontinence was obstetric injury in 48 and prior fistulotomy in 7. Results were excellent in 50% (continent of solid, liquid, and gas), 22% were incontinent of only flatus, 22% were incontinent of both flatus and liquid stool, and 6% continued to be completely incontinent. All wounds

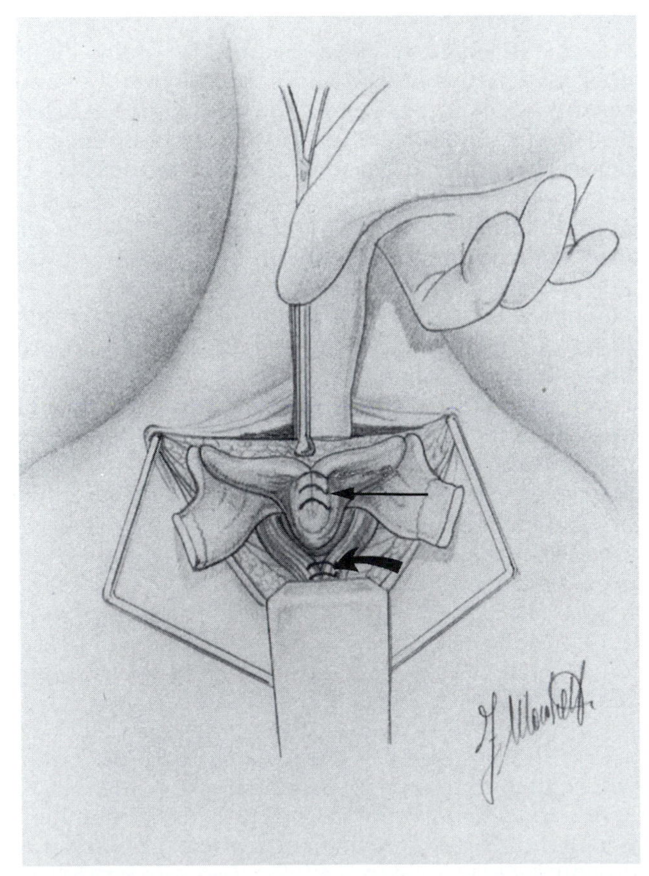

FIGURE 27–3. Internal anal sphincter imbrication (straight arrow). Note levator ani plication (curved arrow). (Reprinted with permission from Wexner, Marchetti, and Jagelman,[27] © American Society for Colon and Rectal Surgeons.)

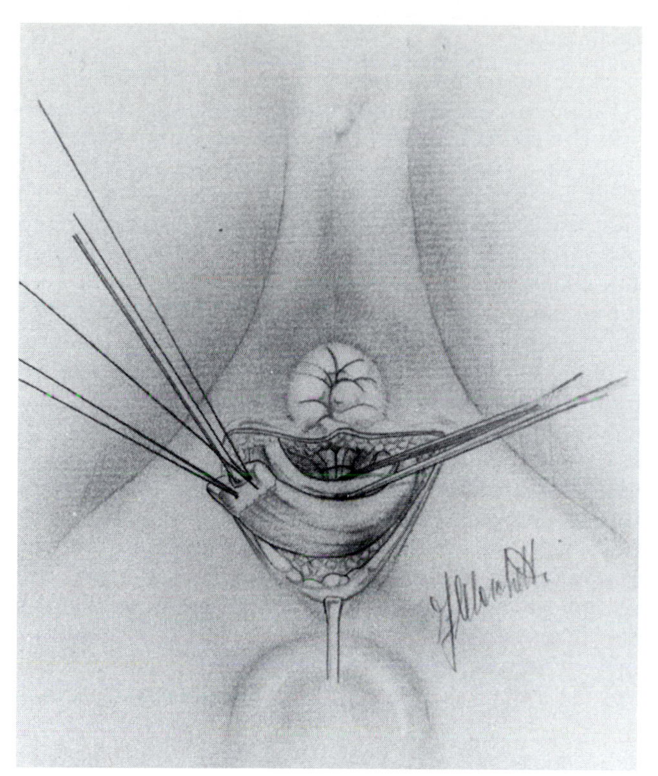

FIGURE 27–4. The overlapping repair of the divided external anal sphincter. (Reprinted with permission from Wexner, Marchetti, and Jagelman,[27] © American Society for Colon and Rectal Surgeons.)

were closed and perianal drains were placed in 33 of the patients. Wound infections developed in 5 of the 22 patients (22%) in whom a drain was not used and in only 3 of the 33 patients (11%) in whom a drain was used. Wound infection did not adversely affect surgical success. Concomitant colostomies were not performed in any patients.

Ctercteko and co-workers[31] reported a retrospective analysis of 44 patients who underwent overlapping sphincteroplasty. Incontinence was due to obstetric injury in 41%, iatrogenic injury in 34%, noniatrogenic trauma in 18%, and neurogenic causes in 7%. A third of patients underwent a diverting stoma. Satisfactory results occurred in 81% of patients, which included complete continence of liquid and solid stool (54%) or incontinence of only liquid stool (27%). Wound infections occurred in 24% of patients. Statistically significant differences in postoperative continence existed according to age (> 45 years), length of incontinence preoperatively, and number of previous attempts at repair.

Wexner, Marchetti, and Jagelman[27] reported a homogeneous prospective series of 16 incontinent women with anterior sphincter injuries secondary to obstetric trauma in 15 patients and fistulotomy in 1 patient. Anterior overlapping sphincteroplasty (as described elsewhere in this chapter) was performed in all patients; none underwent diverting stomas. Preoperative evaluation of all patients included anorectal manometry, electromyography, and pudendal nerve terminal motor latency assessment. Preoperative and postoperative manometry and functional evaluation were performed. Subjective functional improvement correlated with objective physiologic improvements. Excellent or good results were reported in 76% of patients, fair results in 19%. Central portions of the wounds were left open. There were no postoperative wound infections. Although preoperative pudendal neuropathy correlated with suboptimal outcome, advanced age did not. Of the 3 patients reporting, only 2 had fair results with bilateral prolongation of the pudendal nerve terminal motor latency; the only poor result occurred in an insulin-dependent diabetic. It was concluded that pudendal-nerve terminal motor latency was the most significant predictor of outcome after sphincteroplasty. The same conclusion has been reached by other investigators.[17]

IDIOPATHIC-NEUROGENIC FECAL INCONTINENCE

The advent of anorectal physiologic testing, especially electromyography, has permitted a more accurate categorization of the individual causes of incontinence. When specific causes have been ex-

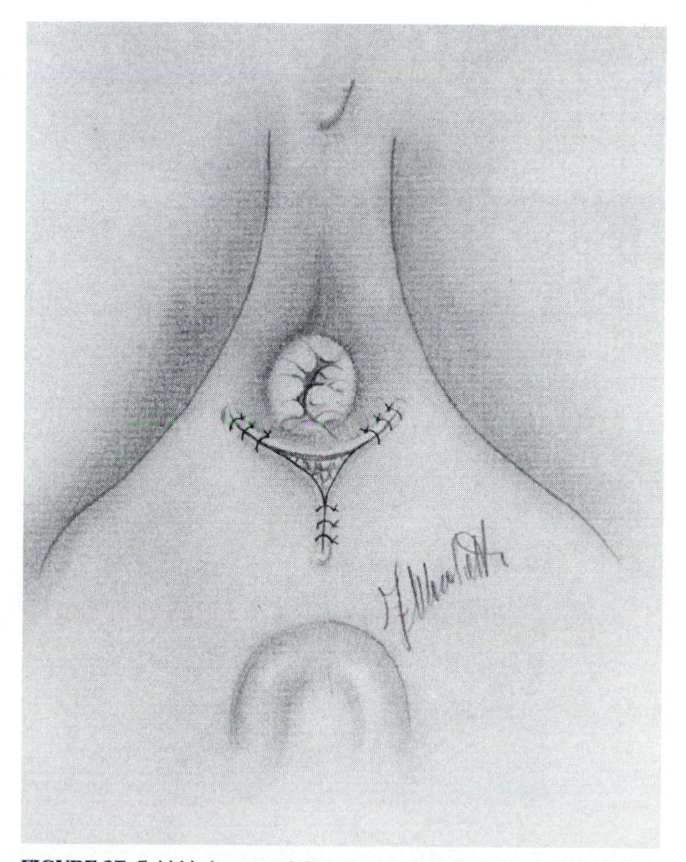

FIGURE 27–5. V-Y closure of the wound, leaving the central portion open. (Reprinted with permission from Wexner, Marchetti, and Jagelman,[27] © American Society for Colon and Rectal Surgeons.)

cluded, such as iatrogenic injuries, prolapse, and pudendal or autonomic neuropathies, this form of incontinence should be termed **idiopathic**. **Neurogenic incontinence** results from denervation of the pelvic floor and has been associated with perineal descent, a more obtuse anorectal angle, and shortening of the anal canal on defecography. Many patients who would have formerly been labeled as having "neurogenic" incontinence are now known to have "idiopathic" incontinence.[27] The reverse is also true.[33,34] In either case, sphincter imaging with anal ultrasound should be done to exclude an occult sphincter injury as the cause of incontinence. Only if the sphincter is anatomically intact should the incontinence be diagnosed as neurogenic or idiopathic.

POSTANAL REPAIR

Postanal repair, first described by Alan Parks, was designed to correct the above anatomic defects, which were thought to result from sphincter denervation.[6] Postoperative continence was achieved in 80% of patients in the early reports.[6,7]

Technique

After induction of either a general or regional anesthetic, an indwelling bladder catheter is inserted and the patient is placed in the prone jackknife position on a Kraske roll. An inverted V-shaped incision is performed approximately 5 cm posterior to the anal verge. Skin and subcutaneous tissues are detached from the underlying sphincter mechanism. The dissection is then performed in the intersphincteric plane, with separation of the internal and external anal sphincters. This mobilization is continued cephalad to the level of Waldeyer's fascia, at which point the levator ani muscle complex is seen.

Interrupted sutures are then placed through the two limbs of the iliococcygeus muscle (Fig 27–6), which cannot be overlapped or even apposed due to the distance between them. Instead, the sutures are tied without tension to form a lattice to support the posterior rectal wall. Interrupted sutures are then placed in the two limbs of the pubococcygeus muscle; it may be necessary to form the lattice posteriorly, whereas anteriorly the lack of tension allows apposition of the muscle. Finally, the puborectalis

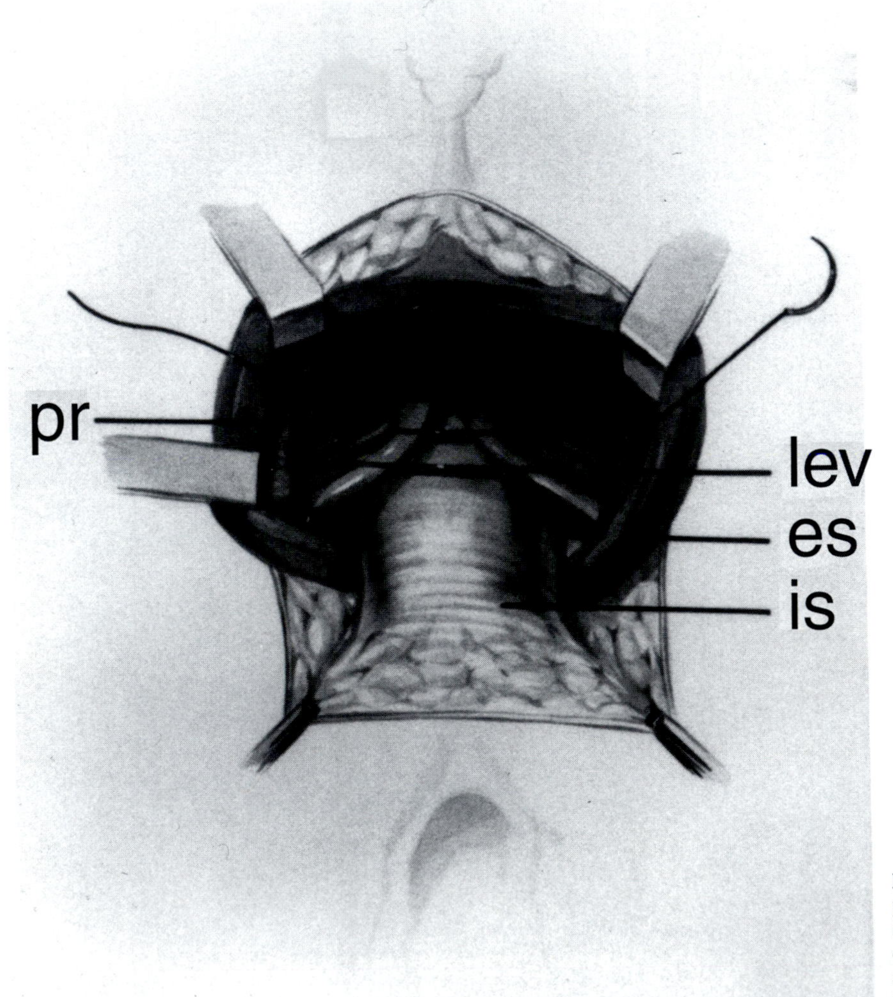

FIGURE 27–6. Postanal repair. Sutures are placed between halves of the levator muscles (*lev*) and the halves of the puborectalis (*pr*). *es* = external anal sphincter; *is* = internal anal sphincter. (Reprinted with permission from Cherry and Greenwald[29], p. 118, with permission.)

and external sphincter muscle are plicated posteriorly and the skin is closed in a V–Y fashion. A suction drain may be left in place for 2 to 3 days. The importance of constructing a posterior lattice has been challenged by some, who have omitted this from the procedure.[8]

Results

Some studies refuted the initial reports and raised doubt regarding the importance of restoring normal anatomy as the sole means of treating incontinence. Scheuer, Kuijpers, and Jacobs reported 39 patients who underwent postanal repair for neurogenic fecal incontinence.[8] Preoperative and postoperative manometry was performed and compared with functional results. They noted a statistically significant increase in squeeze pressure as a result of surgery, but no significant increase in resting pressure occurred. Furthermore, clinical results did not correlate with improvements in external sphincter function; 18% improved despite worsening external sphincter contractility, and 23% remained incontinent despite elevations in squeeze pressures. Overall, excellent results were obtained in only 15% of patients and good results in another 28%. They concluded that postanal repair may have restored anatomy, but that it did not improve function.

Orrom and colleagues prospectively studied 33 patients with idiopathic fecal incontinence.[11] Overlapping sphincteroplasty with anterior levatorplasty was performed in 16 patients; 17 underwent postanal repair. Satisfactory results were obtained in 64% of patients who underwent anterior sphincteroplasty and in 59% of those who underwent postanal repair. After surgery, the anorectal angle was measured radiographically. As expected, the anorectal angles were more obtuse in the anterior sphincteroplasty group than in the postanal group, yet functional results were not adversely affected. Furthermore, no significant change in the angle was demonstrated in the postanal repair group, although function did improve in some patients. In both treatment groups, patients with good results had signficant increases in squeeze pressures with improved sensation in the upper anal canal. The modest success of the postanal repair therefore has not been consistently attributed to restoration of the angle or to improvements in sphincter function; instead, improved fecal sensation and lengthening of the anal canal are probably the responsible factors.

OTHER PROCEDURES

In an attempt to improve the results of procedures for idiopathic fecal incontinence, Deen and associates performed a prospective randomized trial to compare postanal repair, anterior levatorplasty (plication of the puborectalis and external anal sphincter), and total pelvic floor reconstruction (postanal repair combined with anterior levatorplasty).[12] A total of 36 women were evaluated, 12 in each group. The women in the total pelvic floor reconstruction group were significantly younger than the women in the other groups. The three groups had similar severity of incontinence. Follow-up at 3 months revealed continence for solid and liquid stool in 3 patients (25%) after anterior levatorplasty, in 1 patient (8%) after postanal repair, and in 9 patients (69%) after total pelvic floor repair. At 2-years follow-up, no deterioration of function was noted. The authors concluded that total pelvic floor reconstruction was a viable option in the management of idiopathic fecal incontinence. A major criticism of this study, however, was the lack of preoperative and postoperative electrophysiologic studies; no pudendal latency measurements were reported. Thus despite randomization of the patients, equivalent stratification may not have occurred. Specifically, the number of patients in each group with true neurogenic incontinence versus those with idiopathic incontinence may not have been equivalent. Thus, although the concept of total pelvic floor reconstruction for neuropathic fecal incontinence is attractive, further clinical evaluation with objective physiologic data is needed.

NEOSPHINCTER PROCEDURES

Investigation is ongoing concerning neosphincters. Initial reports in the 1950s described the technique of graciloplasty for incontinence in children.[13,14] Pickrell and co-workers[13] transposed a nonstimulated gracilis muscle in 12 patients, ages 4 to 12 years, whose incontinence was due to congenital malformations in 11 instances and to trauma in 1. The results were excellent; all 12 patients gained voluntary control of feces and flatus. In 1983, Wee and Wong used a modification of this procedure to provide continence for patients who had undergone abdominoperineal resections for cancer.[15] Mercati and associates described a technique for electrically stimulated graciloplasty in 7 patients whose rectal cancer was also treated by abdominoperineal resection.[16] At a mean follow-up of 27 months, they reported slight-to-moderate fecal incontinence. All patients used a pad to control mucous discharge, and control was impaired in the presence of liquid stool. Manometric studies revealed a mean resting pressure of 12 mmHg and a mean squeeze pressure of 70 mmHg. All patients were satisfied with the procedure and could delay defecation at least 3 to 5 minutes.

The gracilis is a rapid-twitch, type-II-fiber muscle, whereas the internal anal sphincter is a fatigue-resistant type-I muscle. As such, appropriate voluntary contraction of the gracilis may be possible for only short periods of time (i.e., simulating the action of the external anal sphincter), but sustained activity is not possible. Thus, despite changes in the design of the transposition, suboptimal results continued. In 1990, Williams and associates[17] reported their experience with stimulated graciloplasty and noted that the electrical stimulation caused histopathologically confirmed electrophysiologic conversion of the gracilis from predominantly type II fibers to type I. Since the pioneering efforts by Williams, other authors have also reported success with the procedure and confirmed the histologic conversion.[17,19]

In addition to incontinence secondary to birth defects and radical operations for cancer; graciloplasty has also been used for neurogenic, idiopathic, and iatrogenic incontinence.[18,19] In such cases, prior operations usually were attempted and failed and graciloplasty is performed in an attempt to avoid colostomy. In these instances, complete continence has been seen in 46% to 65% of patients, whereas 15% to 34% were unchanged. Using manometry, increased squeeze pressures have been noted in those patients reporting improved sphincter function.

Current indications for stimulated graciloplasty include neurogenic and idiopathic incontinence, anorectal agenesis, and prior abdominoperineal resection for rectal cancer without evidence of local or distant recurrence.[20] Additionally, patients with obstetric or iatrogenic injuries who have failed one and perhaps two attempts at sphincteroplasty are candidates for this operation. Contraindications include patients whose gracilis muscle or its innervation have been damaged, and patients with spina bifida or generalized neurologic diseases such as multiple sclerosis. Patients with disseminated or locally recurrent cancer, Crohn's disease, cardiac pacemakers, and those who are unable to use the stimulator, are also not candidates for graciloplasty. The procedure is currently being performed in major centers throughout the United States and Great Britain.

Transposition of the gluteus maximus muscle has also been performed to attempt to restore fecal continence. Pearl and co-workers reported 7 patients, ages 26 to 65 years, who underwent bilateral gluteus muscle transposition.[21] Incontinence was due to iatrogenic causes in 4 patients, bilateral pudendal nerve damage in 2, and high imperforate anus in 1. No diverting colostomies were performed. After a 3-month follow-up, 3 patients were continent of solid stool, 2 were continent of liquid and solid stool, and 1 was continent of both stool and flatus. Although preoperative and postoperative manometry did not reveal changes in resting pressure, a markedly increased squeeze pressure was noted. Three patients (43%) developed surgical wound infections requiring prolonged hospitalization.

Another option for restoring fecal continence is the artificial anal sphincter. The device currently in use is a modification of the artificial urinary sphincter, which incorporates a balloon when inflated, occludes the anal canal.[22,23] Christiansen[24] reported 12 patients, 9 women and 3 men, median age 49 years, who underwent the procedure. Incontinence was secondary to neurologic causes in 9 patients, to trauma in 3. All 3 patients with traumatic causes had undergone previous unsuccessful attempts at reconstruction. Since instituting the current system, no revisions for malfunction have been required. A total of 10 patients have had functioning systems for more than 6 months; of these, 5 were completely continent with only occasional leakage of flatus. Slight leakage of flatus and liquid stool was reported in 3 patients. In addition, 2 patients with irritable bowel syndrome and frequent episodes of constipation developed outlet obstruction requiring the use of laxatives and enemas. Anal canal pressures were reported to be 5 to 38 cm H_2O with the sphincter cuff deflated, and 40 to 82 cm H_2O with it inflated.

COLOSTOMY

In certain cases of persistent incontinence following operative or nonoperative therapy, an end colostomy is preferable to a life of restricted social activities. It may even be of use in patients who are not candidates for an initial attempt at the various continence-restoring procedures discussed previously, although this decision must be made on an individual basis. The advent of the laparoscopy has facilitated a "relatively simple" method of fecal diversion without the need for a laparotomy.[35]

SUMMARY

With careful evaluation and selection, patients with fecal incontinence can be successfully treated surgically. A thorough preoperative evaluation should include a history of previous anorectal procedures, injury to the anal sphincters, or neurologic conditions. The evaluation may continue with anorectal manometry, electromyography, anal ultrasonography, and measurement of pudendal nerve terminal motor latencies. Physiologic studies have become widely available[36,37] and permit assignment of therapy and objective quantitation of treatment results. Moreover, these studies have challenged some tenets of the mechanisms of continence and the impact of current therapies upon those mechanisms.

Treatment of fecal incontinence is evolving; new techniques have become available to avoid the disability caused by either an incompetent sphincter or a colostomy. Treatment should be individualized depending on etiology of the incontinence and results of preoperative testing. An algorithm is presented in Figure 27–7.

Although early reports included only subjective functional results of surgery, more recent studies include both objective physiologic results and continence scores.[37] Continued preoperative and postoperative physiologic testing may allow us to achieve optimal results for all patients by comprehending both the patient's needs and the likelihood of a beneficial result from surgery.

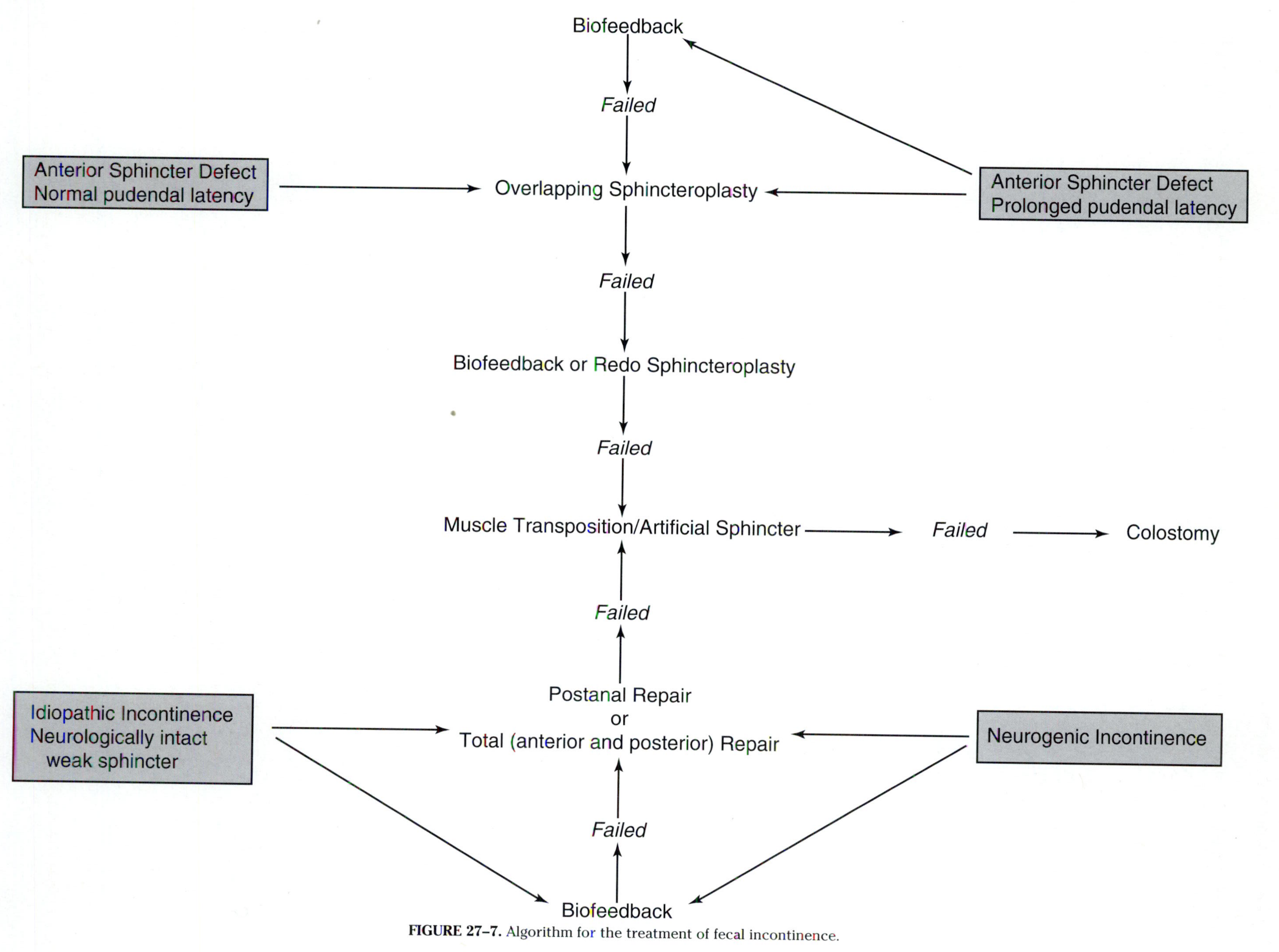

FIGURE 27–7. Algorithm for the treatment of fecal incontinence.

REFERENCES

1. Parks, AG, Porter, NH and Hardcastle, J: Syndrome of the descending perineum. Proc R Soc Med 59:477,1966.
2. Bannister, JJ, Gibbons C and Read, NW: Preservation of faecal continence during rises in intra-abdominal pressure: Is there a role for the flap-valve? Gut 28:1242,1987.
3. Bartolo, DCC, Roe, AM, Locke-Edwards, JC, et al: Flap-valve theory of anorectal incontinence. Br J Surg 73:1012,1986.
4. Fang, DT, Nivatongs, S, Vermeulen, ED, et al: Overlapping sphincteroplasty for acquired anal incontinence. Dis Colon Rectum 27:720,1984.
5. Arnaud, A, Sarles, JC, Sielezneff, I, et al: Sphincter repair without overlapping for fecal incontinence. Dis Colon Rectum 34:744,1991.
6. Parks, AG: Anorectal incontinence. Proc R Soc Med 68:681,1975.
7. Browning, GGP and Parks, AG: Postanal repair for neurogenic faecal incontinence: Correlation of clinical results and anal canal pressures. Br J Surg 70:101,1983.
8. Scheuer, M, Kuijpers, HC and Jacobs, PP: Postanal repair restores anatomy rather than function. Dis Colon Rectum 32:960,1989.
9. Pezim, ME, Spencer, RJ, Stanhope, CR, et al: Sphincter repair for fecal incontinence after obstetric or iatrogenic injury. Dis Colon Rectum 30:521,1987.
10. Labow, S, Miller, R, Cornes, H, et al: Perianal repair of rectal procidentia with an elastic sling. Dis Colon Rectum 23:467,1980.
11. Orrom, WJ, et al: Comparison of anterior sphincteroplasty and postanal repair on the treatment of idiopathic faecal incontinence. Dis Colon Rectum 34:305,1991.
12. Deen, KI, Oya, M, Ortiz, J, et al: Randomized trial comparing three forms of pelvic floor repair for neuropathic fecal incontinence. Update. Br J Surg 80:794,1993.
13. Pickrell, K, Masters, F, Georgiade, N, et al: Rectal sphincter reconstruction using gracilis muscle transplant. Plast Reconstr Surg 13:46,1954.
14. Pickrell, K, Georgiade, N, Maguire, C, et al: Transplantation of gracilis muscle to construct a rectal sphincter. Am J Surg 90:721,1955.
15. Wee, TK and Wong, SK: Functional anal sphincter reconstruction with the gracilis muscles after abdominoperineal resection. Lancet 2:1245,1984.
16. Mercati, U, Trancanelli, MD, Castaguoli, GP, et al: Use of the gracilis muscles for sphincteric construction after abdominoperineal resection. Dis Colon Rectum 34:1085,1991.
17. Williams, NS, et al: Restoration of gastrointestinal continuity and continence after abdominoperineal excision of the rectum using an electrically stimulated neoanal sphincter. Dis Colon Rectum 33:561,1990.
18. Christiansen, J, Sorensen, M and Rasmussen, OO: Gracilis muscle transposition for faecal incontinence. Br J Surg 77:1039,1990.
19. Konsten, J and Baeten, CGMI: Morphology of dynamic graciloplasty compared with the anal sphincter. Dis Colon Rectum 36:559,1993.
20. Wexner, SD: The gracilis neosphincter procedure for fecal incontinence. NICE Technologies, Ft. Lauderdale, FL, 1993.
21. Pearl, RK, Prasad, L, Nelson, RL, et al: Bilateral gluteus maximus transposition for anal incontinence. Dis Colon Rectum 34:478,1991.
22. Christiansen, J and Lorentzen, M: Implantation of artificial sphincter for anal incontinence. Lancet 1:244,1987.
23. Christiansen, J and Lorentzen, M: Implantation of artificial sphincter for anal incontinence. Report of five cases. Dis Colon Rectum 32:432,1989.
24. Christiansen, J: The artificial anal sphincter. Semin Colon Rectal Surg 3:98,1992.
25. Jorge, JMN and Wexner, SD: Etiology and management of fecal incontinence. Dis Colon Rectum 36:77,1993.
26. Laurberg, S, Swash, M and Henry, MM: Delayed external sphincter repair for obstetric tear. Br J Surg 75:786,1988.
27. Wexner, SD, Marchetti, F and Jagelman, DG: The role of sphincteroplasty for fecal incontinence re-evaluated: A prospective physiologic and functional review. Dis Colon Rectum 34:22–30,1991.
28. Blaisdell, PC: Repair of the incontinent sphincter ani. Surg Gynecol Obstet 70:692,1940.
29. Cherry, DA and Greenwald, ML: Anal incontinence. In Beck DE, Wexner SD (eds.): Fundamentals of Anorectal Surgery. McGraw-Hill, New York, 1992, pp 104–140.
30. Fleshman, JW, Peters, WR, Shemesh, EI, et al: Anal sphincter reconstruction: Anterior overlapping muscle repair. Dis Colon Rectum 34:793,1991.
31. Ctercteko, GC, Fazio, VW, Jagelman, DG, et al: Anal sphincter repair: A report of 60 cases and a review of the literature. Aust N Z J Surg 58:703,1988.
32. Jacobs, PPM, Scheuer, M, Kuijpers, JAC, et al: Obstetric fecal incontinence: Role of pelvic floor denervation and results of delayed sphincter repair. Dis Colon Rectum 33:494,1990.
33. Vaccaro, CA, Cheong, DMO, Wexner, SD, et al: The incidence and significance of pudendal neuropathy in patients with fecal incontinence. Presentation at the 13th Congress of the Association of Latin American Coloproctology, Margarita Island, Venezuela, September 19–23,1993.
34. Wexner, SD, Marchetti, F, Salanga, VD, et al: Neurophysiologic assessment of the anal sphincters. Dis Colon Rectum 34:606,1991.
35. Wexner, SD, Cohen, SM, Johansen, OB, et al: Laparoscopic colorectal surgery: A prospective assessment and current perspective. Br J Surg 80:1602,1993.
36. Karulf, RE, Coller, JA, Bartolo, DCE, et al: Anorectal physiology testing. A survey of availability and use. Dis Colon Rectum 34:464,1991.
37. Johansen, OB, Wexner, SD, Daniel, N, et al: Perineal rectosigmoidectomy in the elderly. Dis Colon Rectum 36:767,1993.

CHAPTER **28**

Rectovaginal Fistula

Anthony Senagore

A rectovaginal fistula (RVF) may cause significant discomfort and social embarrassment due to the passage of flatus or stool through the vagina. The degree of social exclusion that may result from such a condition is exemplified by an Ethiopian woman with surgically correctable blindness and an RVF. Given the option of which lesion to correct first, she chose closure of the RVF so that people would at least allow her to rejoin the community.[1]

CLASSIFICATION

Fistulas may occur anywhere along the length of the rectovaginal septum.[2,3] If the anorectal opening of the fistula tract is located at the dentate line of the anal canal, and the tract courses subcutaneously to the perineum or caudal-most vagina, such fistulas are considered anovaginal. Treatment consists of simple fistulotomy. This technique allows healing with minimal, if any, disruption of the sphincter. If an anovaginal fistula involves a significant amount of muscle, placement of a Seton suture may be necessary in order to avoid incontinence resulting from a one-stage fistulotomy.

A variety of classification schemes have been proposed based on the location of the fistula.[4,5] In actuality, these schemes are not helpful, because they do not take into consideration the etiology of the fistula and the integrity of the sphincter, factors that have an impact on the choice and success of repair.

ETIOLOGY

Although the relative frequency of causative factors varies institutionally, the most common cause overall is obstetric injury. Other causes are local malignancy, prior pelvic radiotherapy, inflammatory bowel disease, trauma, and perianal suppurative disease.[6–8]

Fistulas following vaginal delivery usually occur as a complication of a third-degree or fourth-degree perineal laceration,[9] the majority of which (90% or more) heal after prompt repair.[6,10,11] Venkatesh and colleagues reported 20,500 vaginal deliveries, of which 1,040 had third-degree or fourth-degree tears.[10] Only 101 (9.7%) of patients with third-degree or fourth-degree tears did not heal or developed complications. Of these, 67 (6.4% of the total) required surgical therapy, including 29 (2.8%) patients who underwent sphincter repair, and 25 (2.4%) who required repair of an RVF. Others have also reported a favorably low incidence of RVFs following complicated vaginal deliveries.[9,12–14] Risk factors include prolonged labor, high forceps delivery, shoulder dystocia, and midline episiotomy.[9,10]

CLINICAL EVALUATION

The severity of functional impairment is determined by both the size and cause of the fistula. The predominant symptom is the passage of flatus with or without liquid and solid stool through the vagina, which in turn may cause chronic vaginal irritation. In addition, patients may have varying degrees of sphincter impairment. These symptoms can be severely aggravated by diarrhea, which, if it occurs frequently, may herald an underlying inflammatory bowel disease.[15]

Underlying etiology determines the choice of operation as well as the prognosis following repair. For example, a patient who has had multiple vaginal deliveries or episiotomies may be incontinent because of sphincter tears or pudendal neuropathy, or both may exist simultaneously. In such a patient, RVF repair combined with sphincteroplasty may successfully eradicate the fistula, but incontinence may persist in the presence of neuropathy. Conditions such as inflammatory bowel disease or earlier radiotherapy for cancer can adversely affect attempts at local repairs. In these instances, the clinician may choose proctectomy or fecal diversion instead of local repair if the rectovaginal tissues are severely diseased.

Physical examination must include careful observation of the perineum, both at rest and with contraction of the pelvic floor. Stigmata of Crohn's disease (fleshy anal tags, multiple fissures, or fistulas) or radiotherapy changes (telangiectasias) are important findings. Equally important is the presence of a perineal body defect (foreshortening of the anovaginal distance), a finding frequently seen in obstetric injuries.

Digital rectal examination assesses the resting sphincter tone, strength and symmetry of the sphincter contraction, and the presence of any masses. Assessment of the thickness of the rectovaginal septum can be performed by simultaneous insertion of gloved digits transanally and transvaginally.

If a fistula is suspected but cannot be confirmed by physical examination, a variety of tactics may be employed. Most of these maneuvers involve placing easily identifiable substances into the rectum and then inspecting the vagina for their presence; included are methylene blue,[6] hydrogen peroxide,[16] barium followed by radiography of a vaginal tampon,[17] and soapy water.[18] Contrast studies of the gastrointestinal and genitourinary tract may not show a fistula although they may identify coexisting pathology; they should be obtained if symptoms warrant.[19] Computerized tomography of the pelvis may either locate the fistula or show anatomic changes suggestive of one.[20]

Essential steps taken prior to surgical intervention include determining the health of the rectovaginal tissue and adequacy of sphincter function. Proctosigmoidoscopy should be done to exclude inflammatory bowel disease, cancer, or radiation damage. If the patient reports fecal incontinence, verification of sphincter damage can be obtained by endoanal ultrasonography,[21,22] manometry,[23,24] and electrophysiologic testing.[25]

SURGICAL MANAGEMENT

Over twenty operative procedures have been described for repair of RVFs through transanal, transvaginal, transperineal, or transabdominal approaches. Surgical options are best discussed in terms of the type of injury, underlying disease processes, and those structures which require repair, rather than solely by the access route. This allows consideration of both physiologic and etiologic factors in the proper selection of the most suitable surgical repair. These fistulas can be divided into four injury groups: (1) simple rectovaginal fistula with or without anal sphincter disruption; (2) inflammatory bowel disease; (3) radiation injury; and (4) postoperative fistulas.

The overall physical condition of the patient must be considered. A debilitated patient with a severe perianal injury and loss of tissue, whether caused by trauma, radiation injury, or inflammatory bowel disease, may be better served by a well-constructed colostomy than by futile attempts at fistula repair. Conversely, the healthy patient with an isolated small rectovaginal fistula and no disruption of the anal sphincter mechanism can be treated appropriately with minimal anatomic disruption by closure of the fistula with an endoanal flap or transvaginal inversion.

RECTOVAGINAL FISTULA WITH OR WITHOUT ANAL SPHINCTER INJURY

"Simple" rectovaginal fistulas typically occur after an unsuccessful primary repair of a third-degree or fourth-degree perineal obstetric laceration.[10,11] They may also result from the progression or treatment of anal suppurative disease.[25,26] These fistulas occur low along the rectovaginal septum or may even arise from the anal canal.[7,25,27–29] Proper timing of fistula repair is important; if due to obstetric trauma, most become symptomatic within 7 days after delivery, but after 6 to 8 weeks, over 50% of these small RVFs close spontaneously.[10,30] Therefore, although successful repairs have been performed soon after onset,[29] it would seem more prudent to wait, allowing not only spontaneous healing, but also resolution of infection and inflammation, factors that can impair postoperative healing.

Preoperative preparation of patients should include a full mechanical bowel preparation consisting of a polyethylene glycol electrolyte lavage, or cathartics. Tap water enemas administered immediately before surgery may eliminate stool from the distal rectum. The patient should receive broad-spectrum intravenous antibiotics perioperatively, and although a variety of regimens have been recommended, therapy with a second-generation cephalosporin is adequate.[31] Nonabsorbable oral antibiotics may be administered as well.

Patients are positioned in either the prone jackknife or lithotomy position. Operative exposure is obtained by a bivalve retractor or by a Hill-Ferguson retractor inserted either transanally or transvaginally. Occasionally, it is helpful to use 4″ adhesive tape to retract the buttocks away from the operative field.

Transanal Endorectal Flaps

Originally proposed by Laird,[30] transanal approaches have gained in popularity for repairing fistulas involving the lower portions of the rectovaginal septum without coexisting sphincter disruption. Before using this approach, an anal ultrasound test should be done to detect occult sphincter injuries that should be repaired concomitantly if symptoms warrant. Rothenberger and colleagues reported a technique that uses a rectangular endorectal flap consisting of mucosa, submucosa, and circular muscle fibers. The flap is constructed from healthy proximal bowel wall; the flap base is twice as wide as its apex in order to preserve the blood supply[25] (Fig. 28–1). After the fistula tract has been excised, the flap is caudally advanced to cover the defect and is sutured in place with long-lasting absorbable material. In Rothenberger's series, successful healing was achieved in 32 of 35 patients.[25] Hoexter, Labow, and Moseson reported a similar high success rate and emphasized several points for optimum repair with an endorectal flap:

- The flap base should be located at least 4 cm proximal to the fistula.
- The fistula tract must be excised.
- The vaginal wound should be left open for drainage.
- A curvilinear incision should be made for the flap apex in order to avoid devascularization, which might occur with a straight transverse incision.[31]

Several others have had excellent results using this technique[17,29,32–34] (Table 28–1). Success diminishes with each succeeding attempt at repair, however; alternative approaches or even a colostomy should be considered if earlier operative attempts have failed.[8]

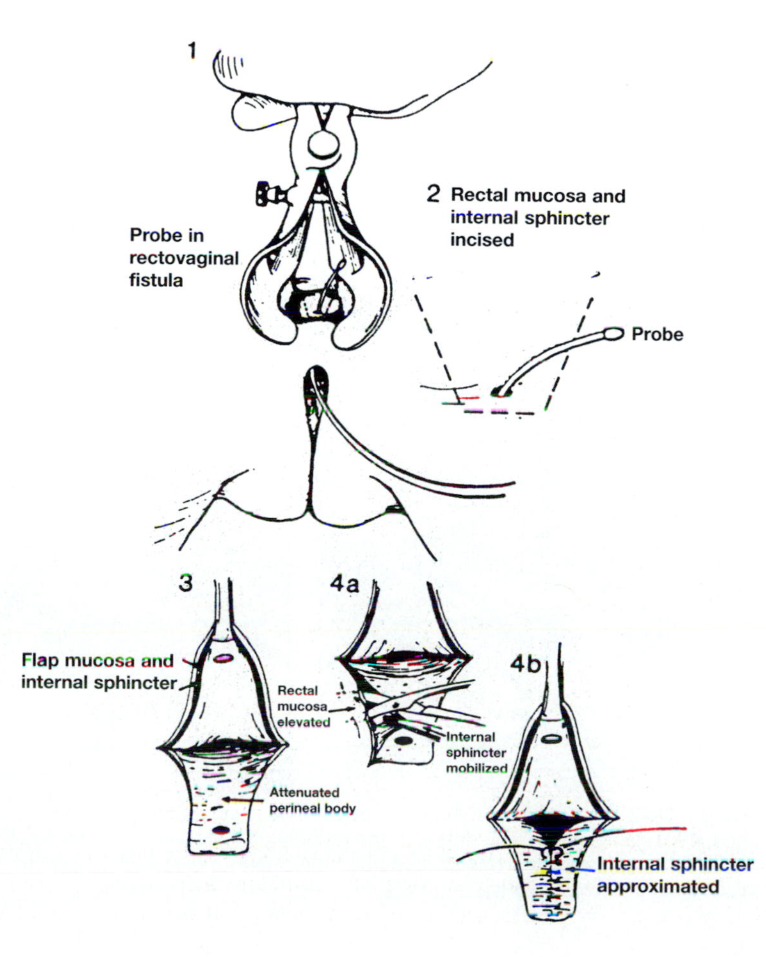

FIGURE 28–1. Fistula repair using a transanal approach. Steps 1 and 2 demonstrate identification of the rectovaginal fistula by placement of a probe from internal to external opening. Step 3 shows the elevation of the mucosal and muscular flap from just distal to the rectal opening of the fistula proximally. Steps 4a and 4b demonstrate mobilization of the internal sphincter and reconstitution of the internal sphincter continuity, if necessary. The flap is then lowered over the repair and the excess tissue, including the portion with the rectal fistula opening, is then excised. (Source: Adapted from Rothenberger, DA, et al: Endorectal advancement flap for treatment of simple rectovaginal fistula. Dis Colon Rectum 25:298, 1982, with permission.)

TABLE 28–1. Results Using Transanal Endorectal Flaps for Rectovaginal Fistulas

Author	Etiology	(%)	Concomitant Surgery	Successful	Effect of Prior Surgery	Successful	Complication
Lowry, et al.[8] (n = 81)	Obstetric Infection	74% 10%	Flap alone 69% Sphincteroplasty 31%	78% 88%	0 prior 1 prior 2 prior	88% 85% 55%	12%
Jones, et al.[34] (n = 23)	Obstetric Crohn's	26% 43%		76.9% 60.0%			
Wise, et al.[32] (n = 40)	Obstetric Infection	63% 20%	Flap alone 48% Sphincteroplasty 38% Rectocele 15%	Overall 95%	—	—	35%
Hoexter, et al.[31] (n = 35)	Crohn's disease excluded			Overall 100%			0%
Rothenberger[25] (n = 35)	Obstetric Infection	69% 3%	Flap alone 71% Sphincteroplasty 29%	Overall 86%	—	—	9%
Stern, et al.[17] (n = 10)	Obstetric Surgical trauma	60% 20%	Flap alone 50% Colostomy 30% Sphincteroplasty 20%	60% 100% 100%	—	—	—

Transvaginal Repair

Transvaginal repairs have also been described, but they are generally best performed for RVFs without anal sphincter disruption.[6,35,37] A simple transvaginal technique involves first making a circular incision around the fistula opening and excising the tract down into the rectal wall (Fig. 28–2). After the vaginal mucosa has been circumferentially elevated, a series of purse-string sutures are placed, which invaginate the rectovaginal septum into the rectum. The vaginal mucosa is then closed with simple sutures.

For larger fistula tracts, the vaginal mucosa must be sufficiently mobilized to obtain an adequate amount of tissue for closure without tension. With such larger defects, a series of mattress sutures should be employed.[37] Results are good (Table 28–2); there does not appear to be any clearcut advantage or disadvantage with a transvaginal approach in comparison to the transanal method. Experience and fa-

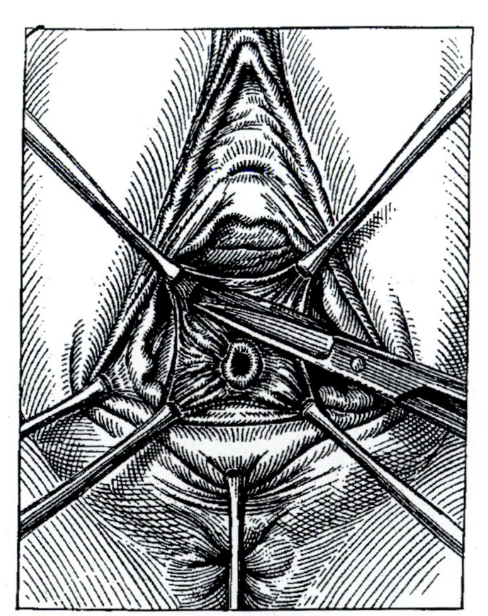

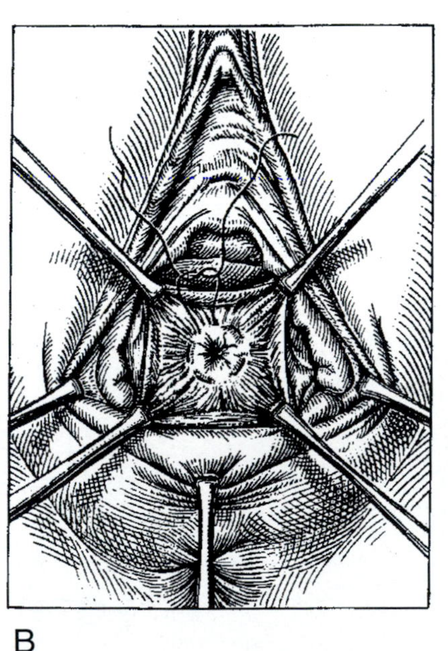

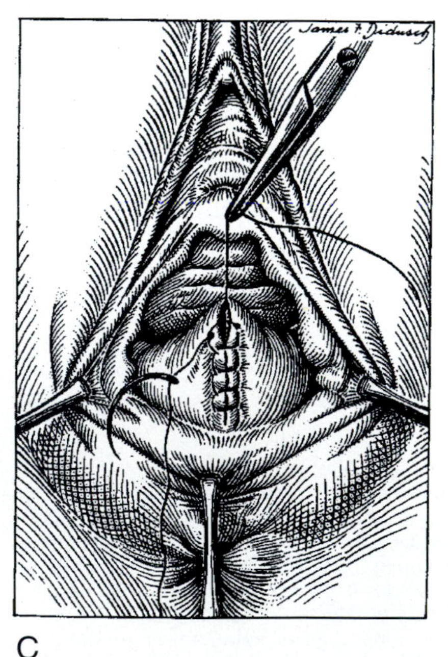

FIGURE 28–2. Transvaginal fistula repair. (A) The vaginal musoca is elevated circumferentially around the vaginal opening of the rectovaginal fistula tract. (B) The defect in the rectovaginal septum is closed by placement of a purse string suture. (C) The vaginal mucosa is then advanced over the defect to complete the repair. (Source: Mattingly, RF and Thompson, JD (eds.): TeLinde's Operative Gynecology, ed 7. JB Lippincott, Philadelphia, 1992, pp. 970–971, with permission.)

TABLE 28–2. Results Using Transvaginal Repair of Rectovaginal Fistulas

Author	Technique	—	Success
Given[35] (n = 26)	Conversion to complete laceration	—	100%
	Inversion into rectum	—	73%
Lescher[6] (n = 22)	Rectal inversion, layered	—	82%

miliarity with the anatomy dictate which method to choose.

Transperineal Approaches

For more extensive RVFs, particularly those associated with sphincter disruption, defects of the perineal body, or both, conversion of the fistula to a fourth-degree laceration (episioproctotomy) and reconstruction in layers can be performed.[35,36] With this technique, a probe or suture is placed through the fistula tract and a vertical perineal incision is made through the rectovaginal septum down to and including the fistula tract (Fig. 28–3). Rectal and vaginal mucosal flaps are then raised proximal to the fistula. Lateral dissection is needed to mobilize an adequate length of healthy tissue, especially sphincter muscle, which may have retracted away from the midline. After this has been completed, the rectovaginal septum and anal sphincter mechanism are reconstructed in layers using long-lasting, absorbable suture material.

An alternative to actually dividing the septum and whatever remnants of the sphincter still remain is a transperineal approach in which rectal and vaginal mucosal flaps are elevated after making a transverse incision midway between the anus and introitus[38,39] (Fig. 28–4). After the incision has been made, dissection may be undertaken either underneath the exter-

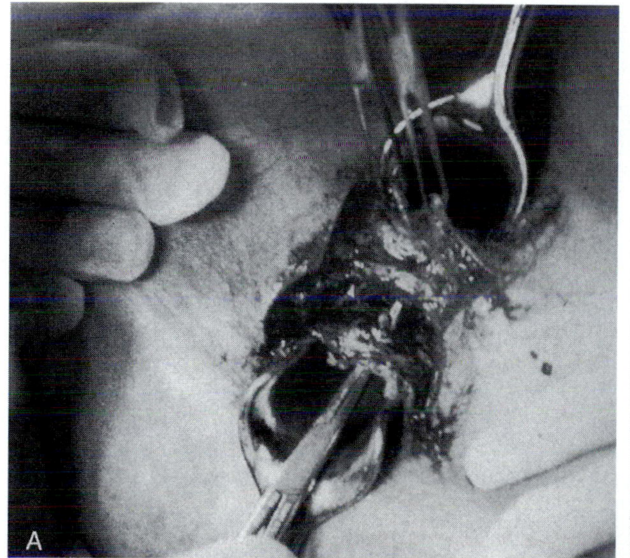

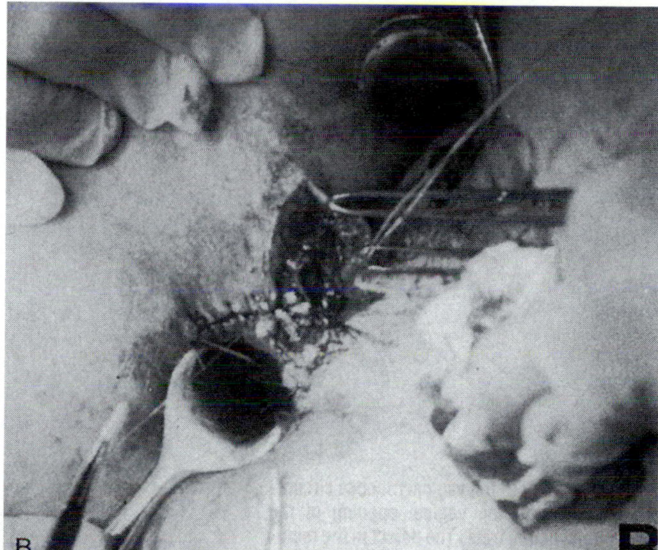

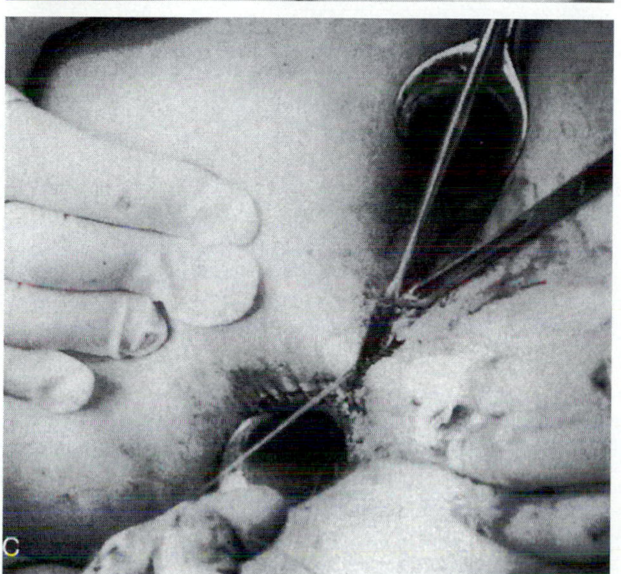

FIGURE 28–3. Mobilization of the skin, anoderm, and vaginal mucosa to a point proximal to the rectovaginal fistula tract. (*A*) The fistula tract and the rectovaginal septum have been divided to form a fourth-degree tear in the septum. (*B*) The rectovaginal septum is rebuilt with 2 to 3 layers of 2-0 polyglycolic acid suture. (*C*) The skin is closed over the repair, demonstrating a fully repaired rectovaginal septum. (Source: Mazier, WP, Levien, DH, Luchtefeld, MA and Senagore, AJ: Surgery of the Colon, Rectum, and Anus. WB Saunders, Philadelphia, 1995, p. 284, with permission.)

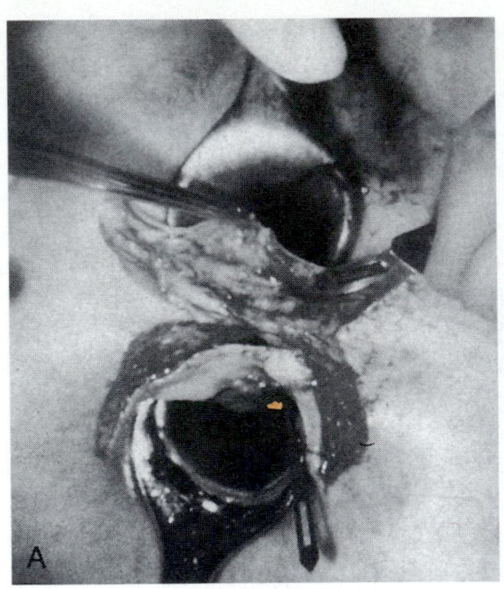

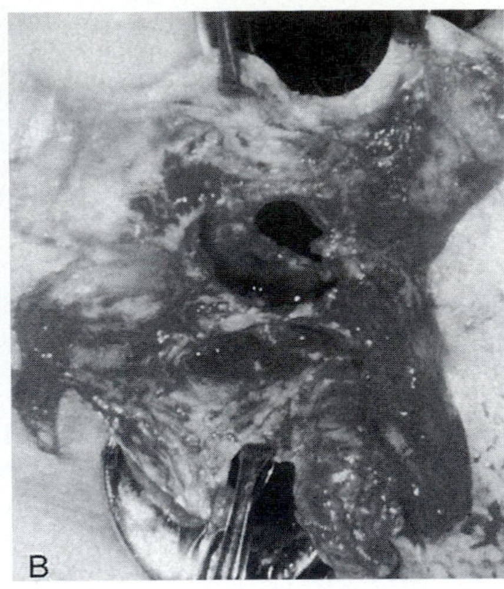

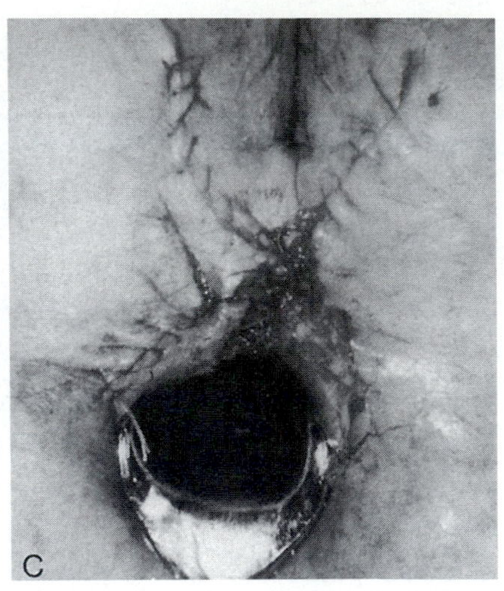

FIGURE 28–4. (*A*) Rectovaginal fistula with the probe going from rectum to vagina. An intersecting curvilinear incision is then made posterior to the vagina and anterior to the rectum to expose the rectovaginal septum. (*B*) The flap elevation is completed on either side of the rectovaginal septum without actual division of the rectovaginal fistula tract. The rectovaginal septum is then imbricated with 2 to 3 layers of 2-0 polyglycolic acid suture. (*C*) After the septum repair is completed, the skin is approximated. This completion picture demonstrates reconstitution of the perineal body with separation of the anal and vaginal orifices. (Source: Mazier, WP, Levien, DH, Luchtefeld, MA and Senagore, AJ: Surgery of the Colon, Rectum, and Anus. WB Saunders, Philadelphia, 1995, p. 285, with permission.)

nal sphincter within the intersphincteric plane, or extrasphincteric beneath the vaginal mucosa. In either case, the fistula is identified and excised; the rectal and vaginal mucosa are closed separately. The entire septum with or without sphincter are then imbricated in multiple layers, which adds bulk to the repair and discourages refistulization. The anovaginal distance is also increased if the skin edges are advanced during wound closure.[39–40]

RECTOVAGINAL FISTULA SECONDARY TO INFLAMMATORY BOWEL DISEASE

As has been alluded to previously, Crohn's disease frequently involves the anorectum and may cause complex fistulas. Management is initially nonsurgical, in the hopes that symptoms referable to the fistulas will respond to medical therapy for the enteric disease. After remission of the underlying disease has been produced, persistent symptomatic RVFs, if present, can be successfully managed surgically, and healing achieved.[34,41–44]

Bandy, Addison, and Parker reported 15 patients with RVFs secondary to Crohn's,[42] of whom 10 underwent primary repair through conversion to a fourth-degree laceration (episioproctotomy) and repair in layers as already described. Healing occurred in 9 of 10 patients during an average of 13 to 53 months follow-up. The remaining 5 patients in this series were treated using fecal diversion alone, which may be entirely appropriate for patients with significant anorectal disease and loss of reservoir function. Cohen and colleagues reported 14 patients with symptomatic RVFs, of whom 7 underwent proctocolectomy without attempting repair.[43] Of the remaining 7, 4 underwent episioproctotomy and reconstruction in layers, and 3 endoanal flap repair. Of the patients, 4 had good results; the 3 remaining subsequently required a diverting stoma. Sher reported 14 patients who underwent a transvaginal inversion of the fistula tract into the rectum.[41] All patients underwent a temporary loop ileostomy. The repairs healed in 13 of 14 patients, but the remaining patient was unable to have her ileostomy closed. Fry and associates reported on the use of the endorectal advancement flap without proximal diversion, which achieved healing in 5 of 6 patients with Crohn's disease.[44]

Thus, it appears that in selected cases of RVF secondary to Crohn's disease, successful surgical management can be anticipated in the face of quiescent rectal disease. These reports, however, represent small groups of highly selected patients, and repair of RVFs should be performed *only* for patients who have acceptable reservoir function, a compliant rectum, medically controlled disease, and adequate sphincter contractility. The vast majority of patients with severe perianal Crohn's disease ultimately need proctectomy.[45]

RADIATION-INDUCED RECTOVAGINAL FISTULA

Radiation-induced RVFs occur in 1% to 3% of patients treated for cervical carcinoma.[46–51] Corrective surgery is hampered by local radiation damage, which hinders dissection and identification of anatomic structures. In addition, the chronic microvascular injury associated with radiation results in a relative tissue hypoxemia, which contributes to poor healing after surgical intervention.[52] Recently, the use of hyperbaric oxygen has been advocated to promote healing and may be considered in severe cases prior to surgery.[53]

Important preoperative considerations include re-

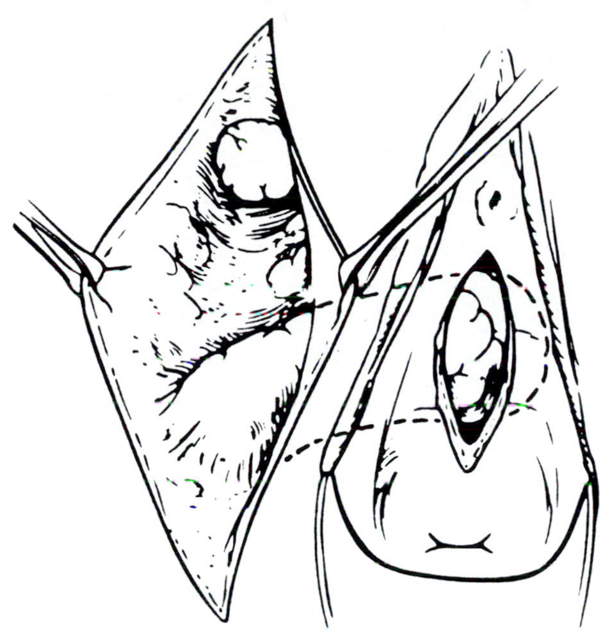

FIGURE 28–5. Repair of a rectovaginal fistula using an island flap developed by mobilization of one of the bulbocavernosus muscles. This muscle is then tunneled subcutaneously into the vagina so that it can be used to cover the rectovaginal fistula defect. The perineal incision is closed with an absorbable suture. (Source: Reprinted with permission from the American College of Obstetricians and Gynecologists (Obstet Gynecol 1990, 75:728).

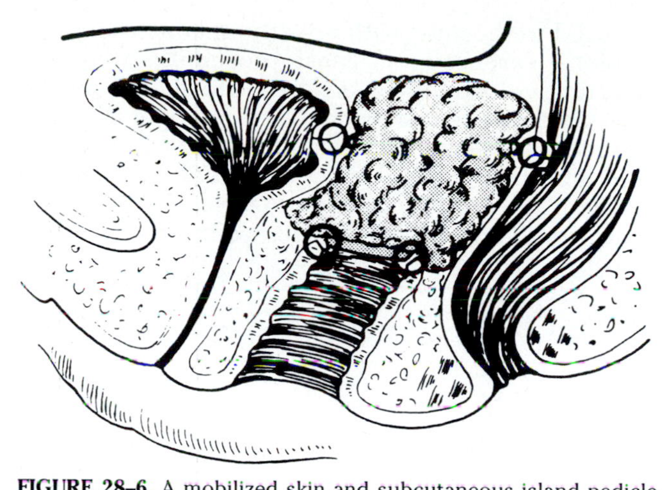

FIGURE 28–6. A mobilized skin and subcutaneous island pedicle flap is mobilized from the perineum and brought up to close the rectovaginal defect. The flap is positioned so that the skin faces into the vaginal lumen and the fatty tissue is used to separate the vaginal lumen from the rectum. (Source: Kelemen, Z and Lehoczky, G: Closure of severe vesico-vagino-rectal fistulas using Lehoczky's island flap. Br J Urol 59:155, 1987, with permission.)

viewing the method with which radiation was administered and excluding recurrent cancer as the cause of the fistula. Radium implants tend to injure less tissue than high-dose external beam radiotherapy, so that a fistula that results from implants may be amenable to simple transvaginal inversion of the tract.[35,36] A more complex procedure is required for RVFs occurring within a severely radiated rectum. Before attempting surgical correction of the fistula, a careful examination under anesthesia and biopsy of the fistula should be performed to exclude recurrent cancer. If cancer is present, local repair will fail; fecal diversion, alone or in conjunction with exenteration if the tumor is resectable, is preferable.

If larger defects or more severe radiation damage are present, nonirradiated well-vascularized tissue may be interposed between the rectum and vagina during take-down or repair of the fistula. A proximal diverting colostomy is often required in these cases to optimize healing. Local perineal tissue flaps such as bulbocavernosus muscle,[51,54–58] or skin and adipose tissue,[59] may be transferred into the rectovaginal septum during repair of the fistula. The graft is well vascularized and not only augments healing but also buttresses the septum and separates the rectum and vagina (Figs. 28–5 and 28–6).

Rectovaginal fistulas occurring within severely damaged tissues, which may be associated with diminished rectal compliance and reservoir capability may require radical approaches. The Bricker-Johnston colonic patch enlarges the capacity of the rectal reservoir with healthy nonirradiated proximal colon; results have been encouraging.[60–62] Three different techniques may be used, depending on the condition of the patient's tissues and her previous surgeries (Figs. 28–7, 28–8, and 28–9). Alternatively, the rectum may be resected, and proximal healthy colon anas-

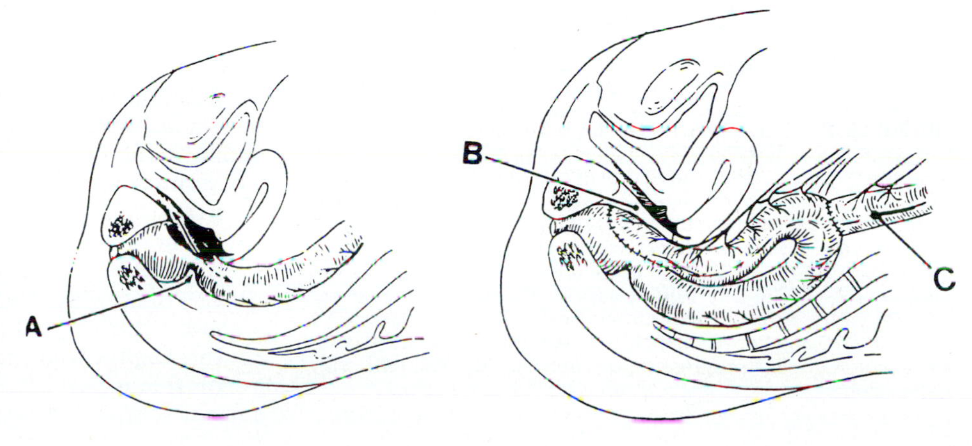

FIGURE 28–7. A Bricker-Johnston colonic onlay patch (Type I) in a patient who has a long segment of normal bypassed colon available for repair. (*A*) Web stricture at the level of the fistula. (*B*) If the posterior vaginal wall is unusable, a pedicle graft of labium majus with fat pad is used to substitute for the vagina to cover the suture line of the reconstruction. (*C*) A more proximal colocolostomy is then fashioned to reconstitute GI continuity. (Source: Bricker, EM, Johnston, WD and Patwardhan, RV: Repair of postirradiation damage to colorectum: A progress report. Ann Surg 193:556, 1981, with permission.)

tomosed to the anus with or without construction of a colonic reservoir.[63,64] These procedures require a diverting colostomy to ensure healing; the results have generally been good.[55,64–69] These operations do carry the potential for significant morbidity, however, and the physician must be sure that the risk is justified. Amelioration of symptoms and avoidance of major complications can be achieved with a diverting colostomy alone.

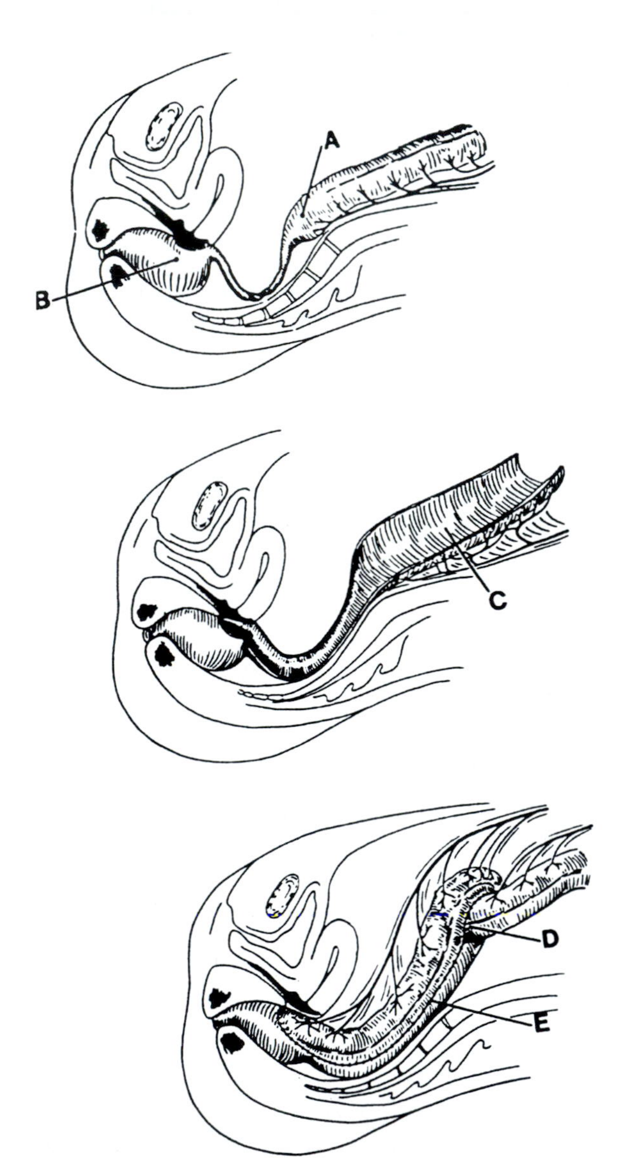

FIGURE 28–8. When a linear stricture exists and the patient has had a previous colostomy, the colonic onlay patch (Type II) may be applied using a "fillet-and-fold over" technique. Joining points (*A*) and (*B*) by a direct anastomosis may be difficult in these patients, but the fillet-and-fold over technique (*C*) provides a very adequate lumen; the entire stricture is openly divided and then the entire proximal bowel is folded down upon itself. (*D*) Proximal colon is attached using interrupted sutures. The long suture line (*E*) is made with a running stitch in one layer. (Source: Bricker, EM, Johnston, WD and Patwardhan, RV: Repair of postirradiation damage to colorectum: A progress report. Ann Surg 193:556, 1981, with permission.)

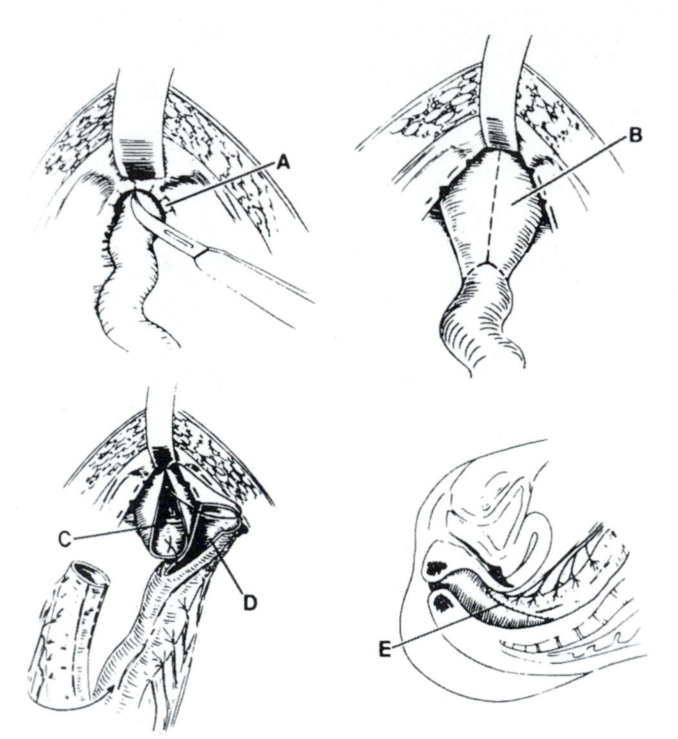

FIGURE 28–9. When the bypassed colon is not usable (because of irradiation damage, for instance), or when the patient has not had a colostomy, a Type III repair may be made. This is essentially a lower anterior resection, which removes all the irradiated bowel. (*A*) The shortened and constricted uterosacral arch is mobilized by multiple shallow incisions. (*B*) The ampulla of the rectum is exposed and incised longitudinally. The scarred rectosigmoid is then amputated, leaving a wide-open lumen for anastomosis (*C*). (*D*) Proximal colon is brought down and slit to fit the open ampulla. Placing all the sutures before bringing the structures into apposition may result in a wide-open anastomosis with less chance of a suture-line stricture (*E*). (Source: Bricker, EM, Johnston, WD and Patwardhan, RV: Repair of postirradiation damage to colorectum: A progress report. Ann Surg 193:557, 1981, with permission.)

POSTOPERATIVE RECTOVAGINAL FISTULAS

Any operative procedure involving dissection around the rectovaginal septum may cause fistulas. Rex and Khubchandani surveyed the membership of the American Society of Colon and Rectal Surgeons and identified 57 cases of RVF following low anterior resection for rectal cancer.[70] This procedure has been facilitated by the use of bowel-stapling devices which, although they permit the performance of deep pelvic anastomoses, may predispose to RVFs if not used properly. Most of the RVFs (53) occurred after a circular stapled anastomosis. Important points in avoiding this complication are:

- Mobilization and separation of the vagina away from the rectum
- Assurance that the vaginal cuff is not included in the staple lines prior to firing the instrument
- Use of autologous tissue such as omentum to separate the vaginal wound and rectal staple line if the vagina was inadvertently entered during the dissection

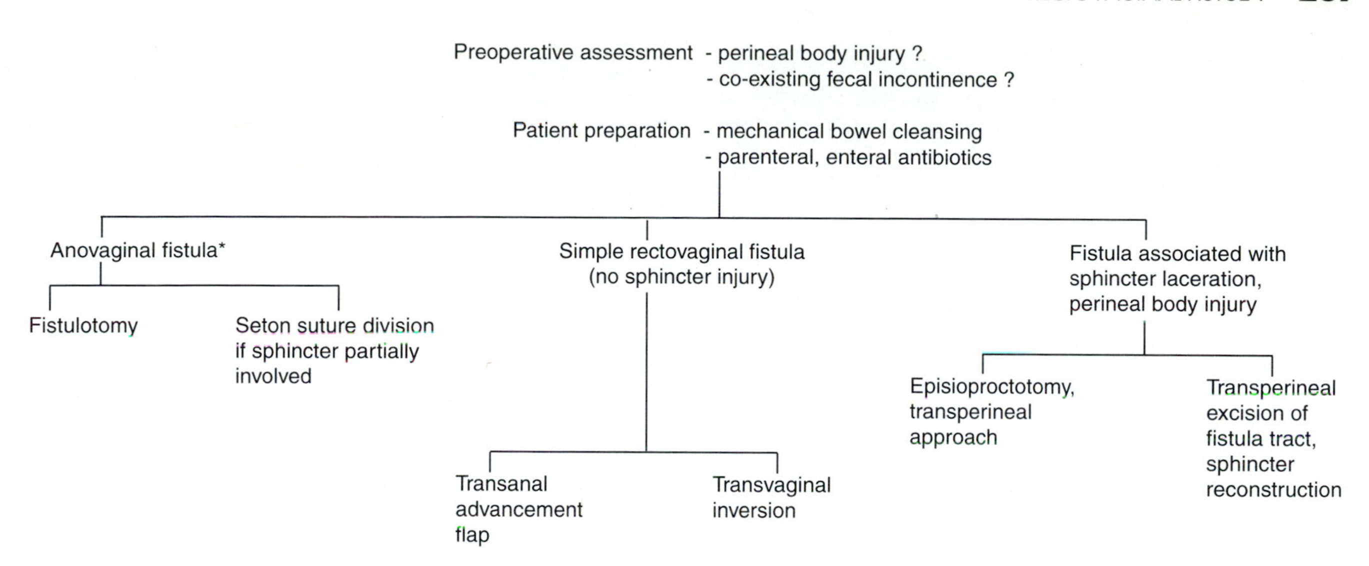

FIGURE 28–10. Options for obstetric rectovaginal fistulas.

If a fistula occurs, management usually requires temporary fecal diversion, followed by a repeated low anterior anastomosis, although transanal or transvaginal repairs have been used.[70]

Development of an RVF has also been described after ileoanal pouch surgery for ulcerative colitis or familial polyposis. This generally occurs as a complication of anastomotic healing or inadvertent entry into the vagina during the dissection, but the presence of unsuspected Crohn's disease should also be considered.[71] If significant pelvic sepsis is not present, transanal pouch advancement with coverage of the internal fistula opening has been highly successful.[71–73]

SUMMARY

Obstetric trauma causes most rectovaginal fistulas. If there is no associated sphincter dysfunction or alteration of the perineal anatomy, transrectal advancement flaps are usually successful in eradicating the fistulas. A transvaginal approach can be used as well. When sphincter or perineal injuries coexist with loss of tissue, a more extensive reconstruction is needed. This could be accomplished with transperineal conversion of the fistula to a complete laceration (episioproctotomy) with reconstruction in anatomic layers. A colostomy is rarely indicated at the initial repair, but because the likelihood of success diminishes with each attempt at repair, a colostomy may be indicated in reoperative cases. Surgical options are summarized in Figure 28–10.

Inflammatory bowel disease, prior irradiation, and iatrogenic nonobstetric injuries cause rectovaginal fistulas less frequently, but may be more difficult to treat. The same methods used to treat obstetric fistulas can be used in selected instances, but other considerations such as rectal compliance, reservoir capability, active inflammatory disease, and recurrent cancer determine which therapy to choose.

REFERENCES

1. Kelly, J: Fistulae of obstetric origin. Midwifery 7:71, 1991.
2. Block, IR, Rodriguez, S and Olivares, AL: The Warren operation for anal incontinence caused by disruption of the anterior segment of the anal sphincter, perineal body and rectovaginal septum: Report of five cases. Dis Colon Rectum 18:28, 1975.
3. Lawson, J: Rectovaginal fistulae following difficult labour. Proc R Soc Med 65:283, 1972.
4. Daniels, BT: Rectovaginal fistula: A clinical study. Thesis, University of Minnesota Graduate School, 1949.
5. Rosenshein, NB, Genadry, RR and Woodruff, JD: An anatomic classification of rectovaginal septal defects. Am J Obstet Gynecol 137:439, 1980.
6. Lescher, TC and Pratt, JH: Vaginal repair of the simple rectovaginal fistula. Surg Gynecol Obstet 124:1317, 1967.
7. Bandy, LC, Addison, A and Parker, RT: Surgical management of rectovaginal fistulas in Crohn's disease. Am J Obstet Gyencol 147:359, 1983.
8. Lowry, AC, Thorson, AG, Rothenberger, DA: et al: Repair of simple rectovaginal fistulas: influence of previous repairs. Dis Colon Rectum 31:676, 1988.
9. Goldaber, KG, Wendel, PJ, McIntyre, DD, et al: Postpartum perineal morbidity after fourth-degree perineal repair. Am J Obstet Gynecol 168:489–493, 1993.
10. Venkatesh, KS, Ramanujam, PS, Larson, DM, et al: Anorectal complications of vaginal delivery. Dis Colon Rectum 32:1039, 1989.
11. Goldberg, SM, Gordon, PH and Nivatvongs, S: Essentials of Anorectal Surgery. JB Lippincott, Philadelphia, 1980, pp. 319–327.
12. Brantley, JT, Burwell, JC: A study of fourth degree perineal lacerations and their sequelae. Am J Obstet Gynecol 80:711, 1960.
13. Legino, LJ, Woods, MP, Rayburn, WF, et al: Third and fourth degree perineal tears. 50 years' experience at a university hospital. J Reprod Med 33:423, 1988.

14. Harris, RE: An evaluation of the median episiotomy. Am J Obstet Gynecol 106:660, 1970.
15. Faulconer, HT and Muldoon, JP: Rectovaginal fistula in patient with colitis: Review and report of a case. Dis Colon Rectum 18:413, 1975.
16. Shieh, CJ and Gennaro, AR: Rectovaginal fistula: A review of 11 years experience. Int Surg 69:69, 1984.
17. Stern, H, Gamliel, Z, Ross, T, et al: Rectovaginal fistula: Initial experience. Can J Surg 31:359, 1988.
18. Carey, JC: A new method of diagnosing rectovaginal fistula: A case report. J Reprod Med 33:789, 1988.
19. Hudson, CH and Chir, M: Acquired fistulae between the intestine and the vagina. Ann R Coll Surg Engl 46:20, 1970.
20. Kuhlman, JE and Fishman, EK: CT evaluation of enterovaginal and vesicovaginal fistulas. J Comput Assist Tomogr 14:390, 1990.
21. Law, PJ, Kamm, MA and Bartram, CI: Anal endosonography in the investigation of faecal incontinence. Br J Surg 78:312, 1991.
22. Felt-Bersma, RJF, Klinkenberg-Knol, EC and Meuwissen, SG: Anorectal function investigations in incontinent and continent patients: Differences and discriminatory value. Dis Colon Rectum 33:479, 1990.
23. Felt-Bersma, RJF, Cuesta, MA, Koorevaar, M, et al: Anal endosonography: Relationship with anal manometry and neurophysiologic tests. Dis Colon Rectum 35:944, 1992.
24. Jacobs PP, et al: Obstetric fecal incontinence: Role of pelvic floor denervation and results of delayed sphincter repair. Dis Colon Rectum 33:494, 1990.
25. Rothenberger, DA, et al: Endorectal advancement flap for treatment of simple rectovaginal fistula. Dis Colon Rectum 25:297, 1982.
26. Belt, RL and Belt, RL, Jr: Repair of anorectal vaginal fistula utilizing segmental advancement of the internal sphincter muscle. Dis Colon Rectum 12:99, 1969.
27. Tancer, ML, Lasser, D and Rosenblum, N: Rectovaginal fistula or perineal and anal sphincter disruption, or both, after vaginal delivery. Surg Gynecol Obstet 171:43, 1990.
28. Pepe, F, Panella, M, Arikian, S, et al: Low rectovaginal fistulas. Aust N Z J Obstet Gynaecol 27:61, 1987.
29. Hankins, GD, et al: Early repair of episiotomy dehiscence. Obstet Gynecol 75:48, 1990.
30. Laird, DR: Procedures used in treatment of complicated fistulas. Am J Surg 76:701, 1948.
31. Hoexter, B, Labow, SB and Moseson, MD: Transanal rectovaginal fistula repair. Dis Colon Rectum 28:572, 1985.
32. Wise, WE, Jr, Aguilar, PS, Padmanabhan, A, et al: Surgical treatment of low rectovaginal fistulas. Dis Colon Rectum 34:271, 1991.
33. Senagore, A: Treatment of acquired anovaginal and rectovaginal fistulas. Seminars in Colon and Rectal Surgery 1:219, 1990.
34. Jones, IT, Fazio, VW and Jagelman, DG: The use of transanal rectal advancement flaps in the management of fistulas involving the anorectum. Dis Colon Rectum 30:919, 1987.
35. Given, FT, Jr: Rectovaginal fistula: A review of 20 years' experience in a community hospital. Am J Obstet Gynecol 108:41, 1970.
36. Hibbard, LT: Surgical management of rectovaginal fistulas and complete perineal tears. Am J Obstet Gynecol 130:139, 1978.
37. Mattingley, RF and Thompson JD (eds.): TeLinde's Operative Gynecology, ed 5. JB Lippincott, Philadelphia, 1977.
38. Wiskind, AK and Thompson, JD: Transverse transperineal repair of rectovaginal fistulas in the lower vagina. Am J Obstet Gynecol 167:694, 1992.
39. Corman, ML: Anorectal abscess and anal fistula: Rectovaginal fistula. In Corman, ML: Colon and Rectal Surgery, ed 3. JB Lippincott, Philadelphia, 1993, pp 171–180.
40. Hilsabeck, JR: Transanal advancement of the anterior rectal wall for vaginal fistulas involving the lower rectum. Dis Colon Rectum 23:236, 1980.
41. Sher, ME, Bauer, JJ and Gelernt, I: Surgical repair of rectovaginal fistulas in patients with Crohn's disease: Transvaginal approach. Dis Colon Rectum 34:641, 1991.
42. Bandy, LC, Addison, A and Parker, RT: Surgical management of rectovaginal fistulas in Crohn's disease. Amer J Obstet Gynecol 147:359, 1983.
43. Cohen, JL, Stricker, JW, Schoetz, DJ, Jr, et al: Rectovaginal fistula in Crohn's disease. Dis Colon Rectum 32:825, 1989.
44. Fry, RD, Schemesh, EI, Kodner, IJ, et al: Techniques and results in the management of anal and perianal Crohn's disease. Surg Gynecol Obstet 168:42, 1989.
45. Scott, NA, Nair, A and Hughes, LE: Anovaginal and rectovaginal fistula in patients with Crohn's disease. Br J Surg 79:1379, 1992.
46. Buchler, DA, Kline, JC, Peckham, BM, et al: Radiation reactions in cervical cancer therapy. Am J Obstet Gynecol 111:745, 1971.
47. Calame, RJ and Wallach, RC: An analysis of the complications of the radiologic treatment of carcinoma of the cervix. Surg Gynecol Obstet 125:39, 1967.
48. Joelsson, I: Radiotherapy of carcinoma of the uterine cervix with special regard to external irradiation. Acta Radiol 302(Suppl):1, 1970.
49. Muirhead, W and Green, LS: Carcinoma of the cervix. Am J Obstet Gynecol 101:744, 1968.
50. Stockbine, MF, Hancock, JE and Fletcher, GH: Complications in 831 patients with squamous cell carcinoma of the intact uterine cervix treated with 3000 rads or more whole pelvic irradiation. Am J Obstet Gynecol 108:293, 1970.
51. Villasanta, U: Complications of radiotherapy for carcinoma of the uterine cervix. Am J Obstet Gynecol 114:717, 1972.
52. Boronow, RC: Repair of the radiation-induced vaginal fistula utilizing the Martius technique. World J Surg 10:237, 1986.
53. Williams, JA, Jr, Clarke, D, Dennis, WA, et al: The treatment of pelvic soft tissue radiation necrosis with hyperbaric oxygen. Am J Obstet Gynecol 167:412, 1992.
54. Martius, H: Martius' Gynecological Operations: With Emphasis on Topographic Anatomy. Translated and edited by McCall, ML and Bolten, KA. Little, Brown & Company, Boston, 1957, p. 322.
55. Symmonds, RE: Loss of the urethral floor with total urinary incontinence. A technique for urethral reconstruction. Am J Obstet Gynecol 103:665, 1969.
56. White, AJ, Buchsbaum, HJ, Blythe, JG, et al: Use of the bulbocavernosus muscle (Martius procedure) for repair of radiation-induced rectovaginal fistulas. Obstet Gynecol 60:114, 1982.
57. Aartsen, EJ and Sindram, IS: Repair of the radiation induced rectovaginal fistulas without or with interposition of the bulbocavernosus muscle (Martius procedure). Eur J Surg Oncology 14:171, 1988.
58. Elkins, TE, DeLancey, JO and McGuire, EJ: The use of modified Martius graft as an adjunctive technique in vesicovaginal and rectovaginal fistula repair. Obstet Gynecol 75:727, 1990.
59. Kelemen, Z and Lehoczky, G: Closure of severe vesico-vaginorectal fistulas using Lehoczky's island flap. Br J Urol 59:153, 1987.
60. Bricker, EM and Johnston, WD: Repair of postirradiation rectovaginal fistula and stricture. Surg Gynecol Obstet 148:499, 1979.
61. Bricker, EM, Johnston, WD and Patwardhan, RV: Repair of postirradiation damage to colorectum: a progress report. Ann Surg 193:555, 1981.
62. Steichen, FM, Barber, HKR, Loubeau, JM, et al: Bricker-Johnston sigmoid colon graft for repair of postradiation rectovaginal fistula and stricture performed with mechanical sutures. Dis Colon Rectum 35:599, 1992.
63. Parks, AG, Allen, CL, Frank, JD, et al: A method of treating postirradiation rectovaginal fistulas. Br J Surg 65:417, 1978.
64. Lucarotti, ME, Mountford, RA and Bartolo, DCC: Surgical management of intestinal radiation injury. Dis Colon Rectum 34:865, 1991.
65. Nowacki, MP: Ten years of experience with Parks' coloanal sleeve anastomosis for the treatment of post-irradiation rectovaginal fistula. Eur J Surg Oncol 17:563, 1991.
66. Cooke, SAR and Wellsted, MD: The radiation-damaged rectum: Resection with coloanal anastomosis using the endoanal technique. World J Surg 10:220, 1986.
67. Nowacki, MP, Szawlowski, AW and Borkowski, A: Parks' coloanal sleeve anastomosis for treatment of postirradiation rectovaginal fistula. Dis Colon Rectum 29:817, 1986.
68. Cuthbertson, AM: Resection and pull-through for rectovaginal fistula. World J Surg 10:228, 1986.
69. Allen-Mersh, TG, Wilson, EJ, Hope-Stone, HF, et al: The man-

agement of late radiation-induced rectal injury after treatment of carcinoma of the uterus. Surg Gynecol Obstet 164:521, 1987.
70. Rex, JC and Khubchandani, IT: Rectovaginal fistula: Complication of low anterior resection. Dis Colon Rectum 35:354, 1992.
71. Fleshman, JW, McLeod, RS, Cohen, Z, et al: Improved results following use of an advancement technique in the treatemnt of ileoanal anastomotic complications. Int J Colorect Dis 3:161, 1988.
72. Fazio, VW and Tjandra, JJ: Pouch advancement and neo-ileoanal anastomosis for anastomotic stricture and anovaginal fistula complicating restorative proctocolectomy. Br J Surg 79:694, 1992.
73. Wexner, SD, Rothenberger, DA, Jensen, L, et al: Ileal pouch vaginal fistulas: Incidence, etiology and mangement. Dis Colon Rectum 32:460, 1989.

CHAPTER 29

Role of Physical Therapy

Rhonda Kotarinos • Linda T. Brubaker

For decades, physicians have prescribed Kegel's exercises to incontinent women. This type of exercise is most valuable when properly taught to an appropriately chosen patient. Although no normative values have been established for pelvic floor strength in women, it is clinically apparent that women vary greatly in their ability to perform pelvic floor exercises. Some women have such profound weakness that no contraction is palpable. These women will have difficulty exercising the pelvic floor appropriately and often will benefit from specialized attention to pelvic floor training by a dedicated physical therapist. The key to teaching pelvic floor exercise and a successful strengthening program is the ability of the patient to isolate and contract pelvic floor muscles. Biofeedback allows the patient to increase perception and then re-establish voluntary control.

When evaluating a patient with incontinence, the physical therapist should address the musculoskeletal system as a whole and the pelvic floor in isolation. As part of the general musculoskeletal examination, the therapist assesses posture, abdominal wall integrity, and strength of the hip girdle musculature. An individualized treatment plan is established for any muscle group contributing to dysfunction in the pelvic floor.

CORRECTION OF POSTURE

Posture plays an undeniable role in the treatment of incontinence. In 1909 Joel Goldthwait described the human form as a "delicately balanced machine made up of many parts each related to the others, and that which we call perfect health is simply the proper correlation of all these many parts."[1]

Goldthwait goes on to describe the importance of posture, not only to the structural aspects of the human but also to the functioning of the viscera as well.[1] He felt that when physicians present solutions to medical conditions, they should be offered to the patient only after great consideration as to the interactions not only locally but also to the whole system and all its functions. "It means that in the treatment of disturbances or displacements of organs, it is only half doing the work if the condition is treated locally, while an imperfect posture which may have been largely responsible for the trouble is allowed to go uncorrected."[1]

Therapists develop individual postural corrective exercise programs only after a thorough evaluation. Obvious areas of concerns with posture are kyphosis (with or without osteoporosis), scoliosis, and unequal leg length. Other concerns include muscle imbalances of the pelvis and hip.

The pelvic floor likely functions best when it is in the correct anatomic position. Logically, it follows that any musculoskeletal component that alters the positioning of the pelvis should be corrected. Tight muscle groups that tilt the pelvis anteriorly or posteriorly need to be stretched. As a muscle group is stretched, its antagonist must be strengthened to maintain a balance of length and strength about the joint. In a kyphotic posture, the abdominal wall is slack, allowing the pelvis to rotate anteriorly. Therapists use postural exercises to reduce the kyphosis and abdominal strengthening to assist in realigning the position of the pelvis.

The abdominal wall plays an important role in posture and in the maintenance and distribution of intraabdominal pressure. Penrose stated in his text of 1908 that the retentive power of the abdomen depends on the strength or rigidity of the abdominal wall.[2] Should a medically significant diastasis recti be discovered in the evaluation, the therapist should address it in the treatment plan. A diastasis is considered medically significant if a separation of more than two finger widths exists at or above the umbilicus and more than a finger width below the umbilicus.

Diastasis correction exercises may be performed with the patient in the supine position with knees bent. A folded sheet or towel is placed around the waist with the ends of the sheet crossed as if ready to be tied in a knot. The sheet should be firmly brought together to approximate the recti bellies, realigning them into a neutral position. After this realignment by supportive measures, the patient is instructed to raise her head from the treatment table without shoulder motion. Neck flexion will isolate the rectus abdominis. Each head lift should be held for 5 to 10 seconds and repeated 10 to 30 times.

The therapist should continue this exercise program until the size of the diastasis is no longer considered medically significant. After the diastasis is reduced, the therapist should initiate an individualized progressive program to strengthen the upper and lower abdominal areas.

RESTORATION OF THE PELVIC FLOOR

Restoration of the pelvic floor frequently requires muscle rehabilitation. The physical therapist plays an important role in selecting and supervising pelvic floor muscle training. Clinicians can improve the care of women with incontinence, prolapse, or both by applying these simple techniques.

The therapist should initially determine whether or not the patient can isolate and contract her pelvic floor muscles. If the patient has this capability, appropriate exercises can be used to strengthen the pelvic floor and surrounding musculature. When the patient is *not* able to isolate and contract the pelvic floor, however, the treatment plan must help the patient achieve this *initial* level of strength in her pelvic floor.

Women who cannot isolate and contract the pelvic floor cannot perform Kegel's exercises. Thus, the therapist may elect to use proprioceptive neuromuscular facilitation (PNF) techniques, cross transfer of training, or functional electrical stimulation, alone or in combination. The physical therapist may also try other facilitation techniques which do not require the expense of a stimulating device. The therapist may consider neuromuscular facilitation techniques such as quick stretch (stretch reflex) or tapping (stretch stimulus), because muscles are known to respond with greater force after the muscle has been stretched.

PROPRIOCEPTIVE NEUROMUSCULAR FACILITATION

The PNF exercise technique developed by Dr. Herman Kabat in the early 1940s can be used to facilitate an active contraction of the pelvic floor. In the PNF exercise approach, stronger muscle groups of the body are used to facilitate and strengthen weaker groups. Two diagonals of motion exist for each major body area. Each of these diagonals is further made up of two patterns that are antagonistic to each other.

Each pattern has three components: (1) flexion or extension, (2) abduction or adduction, and (3) internal or external rotation. The pattern most closely associated with facilitation of the pelvic floor is **extension, adduction,** and **external rotation** of the hip joint.

Sherrington demonstrated that when patterns of facilitation were performed against resistance, they promoted selective isolation.[3] Resisting hip extension, adduction, and external rotation has been shown to stimulate and facilitate the muscles of the pelvic floor. Resisting hip flexion, abduction, and internal rotation inhibits the muscles of the pelvic floor.[4]

This phenomenon may be demonstrated when evaluating a patient using surface electromyography (EMG) or pressure biofeedback. After initial baseline pelvic floor measurements are taken, the therapist can manually resist extension, adduction, and external rotation approximately 10 times to each hip. Immediate re-evaluation usually indicates increased EMG activity or increased pressure generation with a pelvic floor contraction.

CROSS TRANSFER OF TRAINING

Pelvic floor strength can also be enhanced using "cross transfer of training." This was originally described by Hellebrandt over 40 years ago. Hellebrandt did extensive studies to document that strengthening exercises to a limb will increase strength in the unexercised contralateral limb.[5] Until recently, only the transfer of strength had been described, but in 1992 Kannus and his co-workers reported a transfer of power and endurance.[6] Clinically, the physical therapist can establish a heavy-resistance, low-repetition strengthening exercise program for the hip girdle musculature. This facilitates the strengthening process of the pelvic floor muscles when the patient is unable to elicit an active pelvic floor contraction. Initiating the strengthening process in this manner allows a minimal isolated active contraction to develop without excessive inappropriate recruitment. After a minimal isolated contraction is present, the therapist can use biofeedback to continue the strengthening process while monitoring the patient's ability to isolate the contraction.

ELECTRICAL STIMULATION

Mechanisms of Action

For patients with marked pelvic floor weakness, electrical stimulation may be used as an important component of muscle re-education. Electrical stimulation for the treatment of urinary incontinence was introduced in 1963.[7] However, electrical stimulation for urinary incontinence was a component of the educational curriculum of physical therapy as early as 1950, approximately the time of Kegel's landmark work. Extensive physical therapy literature supporting the use of electrical stimulation for *muscle re-education*.

Electrical stimulation has traditionally been used to assist patients who have difficulty in voluntarily contracting a muscle secondary to disuse or trauma. Assuming the patient has at least partial innervation, an alternating current produces a muscular contraction by stimulating the afferent limb of the pudendal reflex.[8]

When electrical stimulation is necessary, the stimulation parameters must be specified. Few of these electrical parameters have been proven in randomized clinical trials. DeLitto and colleagues[9] found that following anterior cruciate ligament reconstructive surgery, electrical stimulation produced greater individual thigh strength gains than a standard manual exercise regimen did. Laughman and co-workers[10] demonstrated that electrical stimulation can strengthen normal quadriceps femoris muscles without voluntary effort. A review of the literature[11] found greater strength gains with electrical stimulation than with voluntary exercise in patients with certain disorders.

Electrical stimulation of the pelvic floor causes a reflex contraction of the paraurethral and periurethral muscles, as well as reflex inhibition of the detrusor muscle.[12] It is through this mechanism that electrical stimulation may affect both stress and urge incontinence. This is discussed in more detail in Chapter 18.

Electrical stimulation of the pelvic floor not only induces a reflex contraction of the striated muscle

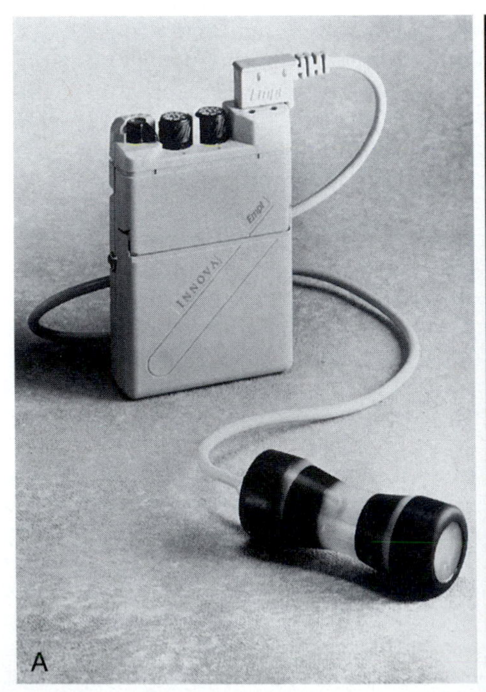

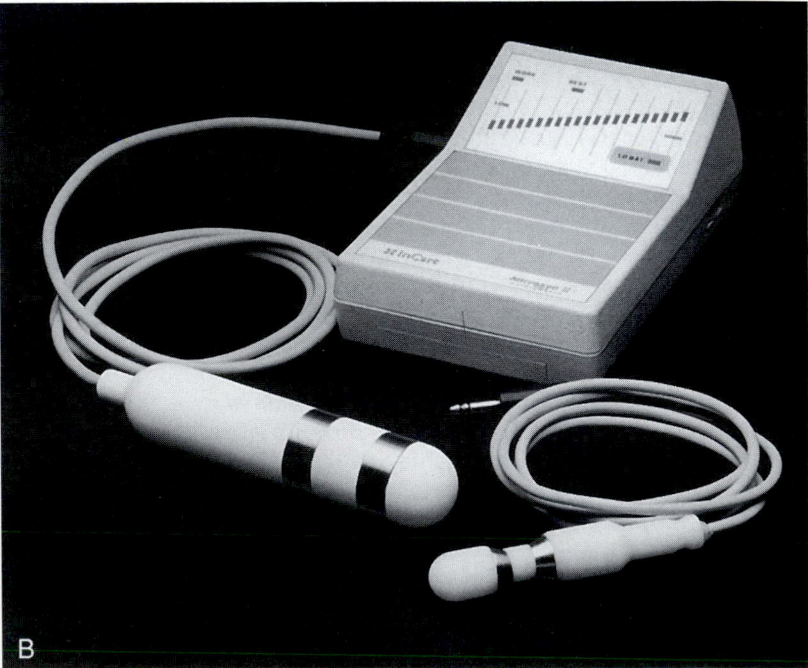

FIGURE 29–1. Home electrical stimulation units: (A) Innova (Empi, Inc., Minneapolis, MN) and (B) Microgyn II (InCare Medical Products).

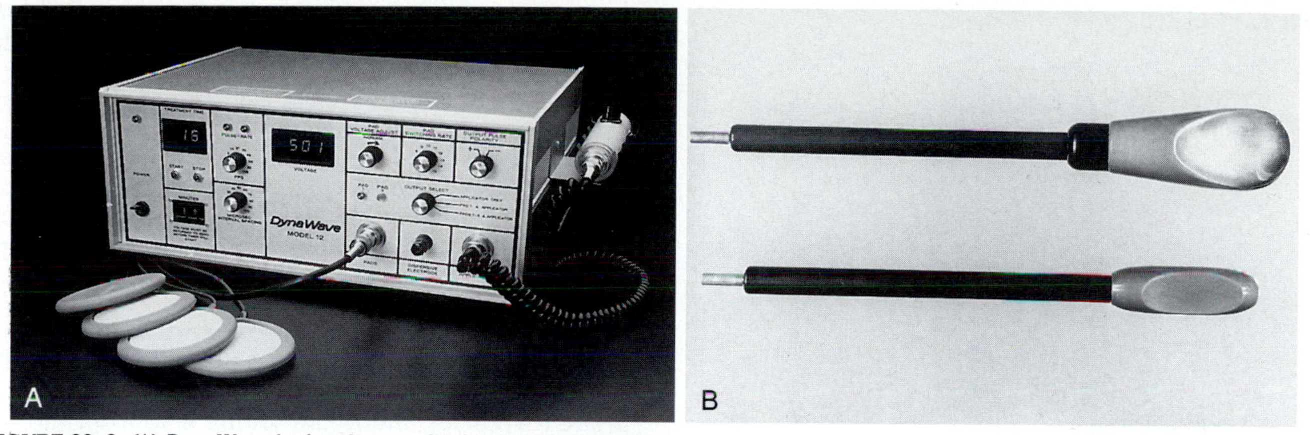

FIGURE 29–2. (A) DynaWave high-voltage pulsed galvanic stimulator with (B) vaginal and rectal probes (Dynawave Corporation).

but also produces a simultaneous inhibition of the detrusor muscle.[13] This is the proposed mechanism by which electrical stimulation is used to manage detrusor overactivity. Ideally, during the progression of treatment, strength of the pelvic floor contraction increases and the patient's own active contraction eventually becomes sufficient to provide the normal inhibition of the detrusor.

Types of Electrical Stimulators

Clinically, several types of electrical stimulators are available for transvaginal or transrectal stimulation. Some of these units were developed specifically for treatment of pelvic floor disorders (Fig. 29–1). As such, they have limited ability for alteration of electrical parameters. Typically, physical therapists have many other types of electrical stimulators at their disposal. These multipurpose clinical models afford the therapist greater variability in selecting parameters of treatment. Examples of vaginal and rectal electrodes for these multipurpose units are shown in Figure 29–2.

When using electrical stimulators that allow the therapist to select parameters, the settings used for stress incontinence are often based on alternating current at a frequency of 100 Hz, which is surged 6 to 10 times per minute.[14] The primary electrode is vaginal or rectal with a dispersive secondary electrode placed suprapubically on the anterior abdomen.

When a high-voltage pulsed galvanic unit is used, only one of the two active leads is required. The active lead is connected to the vaginal electrode and the dispersive electrode is placed suprapubically. Negative polarity is preferred for the vaginal electrode. Current parameters are often set at 80 pulses per second (PPS) to 100 PPS for 5 minutes in a continuous mode, followed by 20 minutes in an alternating or surged mode.[15]

If interferential equipment is used for management of stress incontinence or detrusor overactivity, a vaginal electrode is not required. The four plate or suction electrodes are typically placed in a crossed pattern over the lower abdominal and perineal area so that the intersection of the two interferential circuits is in the midline vaginal area (Fig. 29–3). Typical parameters for stress incontinence are 40 to 80 Hz fast sweep surged to produce a comfortable contraction approximating 2 seconds on and 6 seconds off. For detrusor overactivity, the parameters selected change to 0.5 to 15 Hz with a slow rhythmic sweep.[15]

BIOFEEDBACK THERAPY

Biofeedback therapy is also useful clinically, particularly for patients with weakened pelvic floor contractions.

During attempts to contract a weak pelvic floor voluntarily, it is common for accessory muscle groups, such as abdominals, gluteals, and adductors, to be recruited. In pelvic floor rehabilitation, biofeedback can be used to increase recruitment of the pelvic floor musculature while monitoring other muscles for inappropriate recruitment with surface EMG electrodes. Using this EMG biofeedback (Fig. 29–4), the patient can become aware of such inappropriate muscle recruitment, which enables the patient to

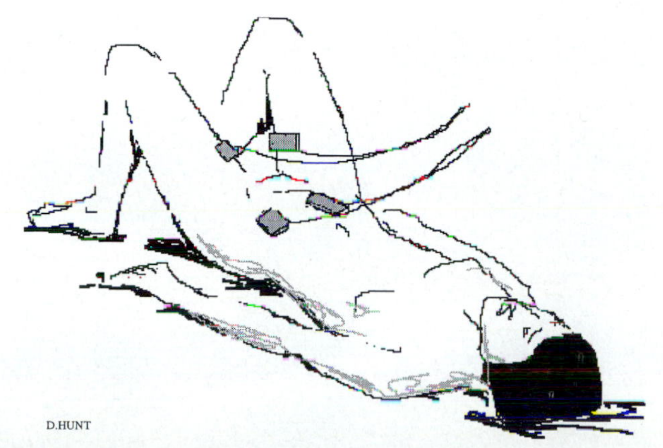

FIGURE 29–3. Typical electrode placement with interferential equipment for the management of incontinence.

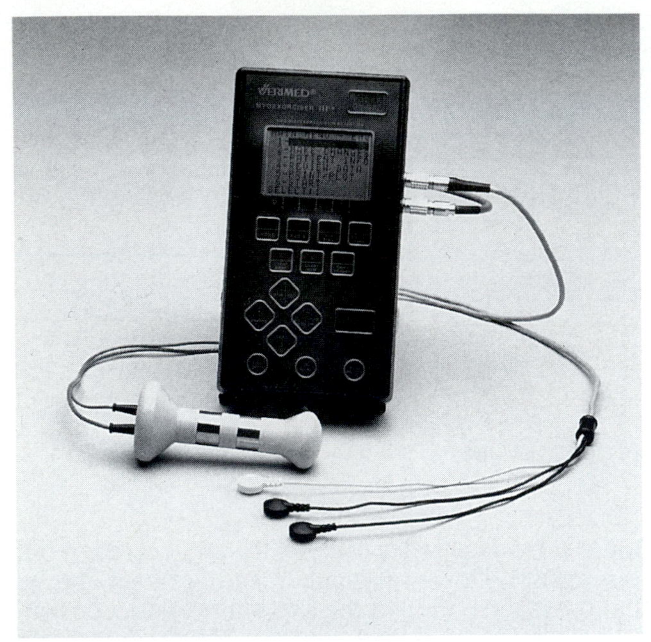

FIGURE 29–4. Myoexorciser II vaginal perineometer EMG biofeedback system (Verimed).

maintain relaxation of these inappropriate muscle groups, yet isolate and contract the pelvic floor muscles.

Biofeedback therapy specificially to augment levator ani strength can be accomplished with either a surface EMG device or an inflatable pressure-sensitive probe (Fig. 29–5). Surface electrode electromyographic (SEEMG) biofeedback measures muscle activity in microvolts. Pressure perineometers measure the force exerted on the probe in centimeters of water pressure. Biofeedback computer systems are available that use both methods, display the information on a video monitor, and produce an audible response (Fig. 29–6).

Biofeedback-assisted exercise has been shown by Burgio, Robinson, and Engel[16] to result in an 82% reduction in episodes of incontinence. They argue that the advantages of biofeedback over verbal feedback are: (1) instrumental feedback is graded specific to the response; (2) physiologic feedback is more precise; (3) instrumental feedback is continuous; and (4) physiologic feedback is immediate. Biofeedback, whether using SEEMG or pressure monitoring, is an excellent method for isolating the pelvic floor and teaching pelvic floor exercises by reinforcing appropriate responses and by inhibiting inappropriate responses.

STRENGTHENING PROGRAMS

After an isolated active contraction without excessive substitution can be demonstrated, whether during initial evaluation or after therapeutic intervention as previously discussed, a progressive strengthening program can be initiated. The therapist should develop an individualized program based on a strength assessment of the involved muscles. If the muscles cannot contract against gravity (in standing or sitting positions), the exercise program *must* eliminate gravity from the exercise. This can be accomplished by placing the patient in a supine position with knees bent and two to three pillows under the hips. In this position, the pelvic floor is in a gravity-*assisted* position.

When the patient can demonstrate a full active contraction against gravity, the therapist should advance the treatment plan so that the pelvic floor is

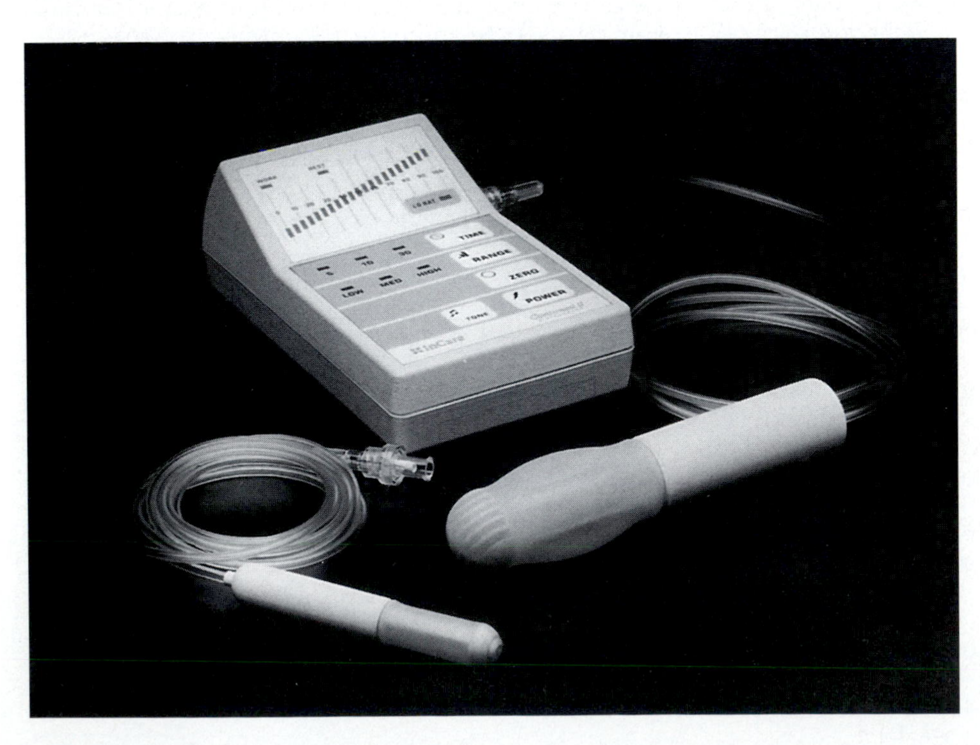

FIGURE 29–5. Contimed II pressure biofeedback system (InCare Medical Products).

exercised in a gravity-*resisted* position. The two gravity-resisted positions most often used are sitting or standing.

The individualized exercise protocol should also be varied as to the type of contractions, that is, quick or endurance. A typical protocol might be a sequence of 3 to 5 quick contractions, 5 seconds of rest, 5 seconds of contract and hold, 5 seconds of rest, repeating this sequence 10 to 30 times for 2 to 3 sessions a day. Although theories regarding exercise regimens for the pelvic floor are numerous, it is *essential* that *any* exercise program be personalized during its initial development and subsequent refinements.

Strength gains in any skeletal muscle are achieved only by subjecting the muscle to increasing loads. For the pelvic floor, therapists frequently use vaginal cones as a convenient system of progressive pelvic floor weights. A set of five weights ranging from 20 g to 70 g is currently available in the United States (Fig. 29–7). Cone therapy can be initiated during a regular office visit. The lightest cone is inserted into the standing patient's vagina. Muscular contraction should be noted for proper cone placement. If the cone can be held within the vagina for 1 minute, the patient is advanced to the next heaviest cone. This process is repeated until the cone cannot be held for 1 minute. This cone will be used to initiate the progressive strengthening program.

A typical program begins with the patient inserting the appropriate cone in the morning. The patient is instructed to be upright and go about her daily routine for 15 minutes, reinserting the weighted cone when she feels it is slipping out. The patient should have a conscious sensation of "holding" the cone. Cones which are placed too far posteriorly in the vagina do not effectively work the muscles. This routine is repeated later in the day. When the patient can hold this cone for the full 15 minutes without it slipping, she is instructed to progress to the next heaviest cone.

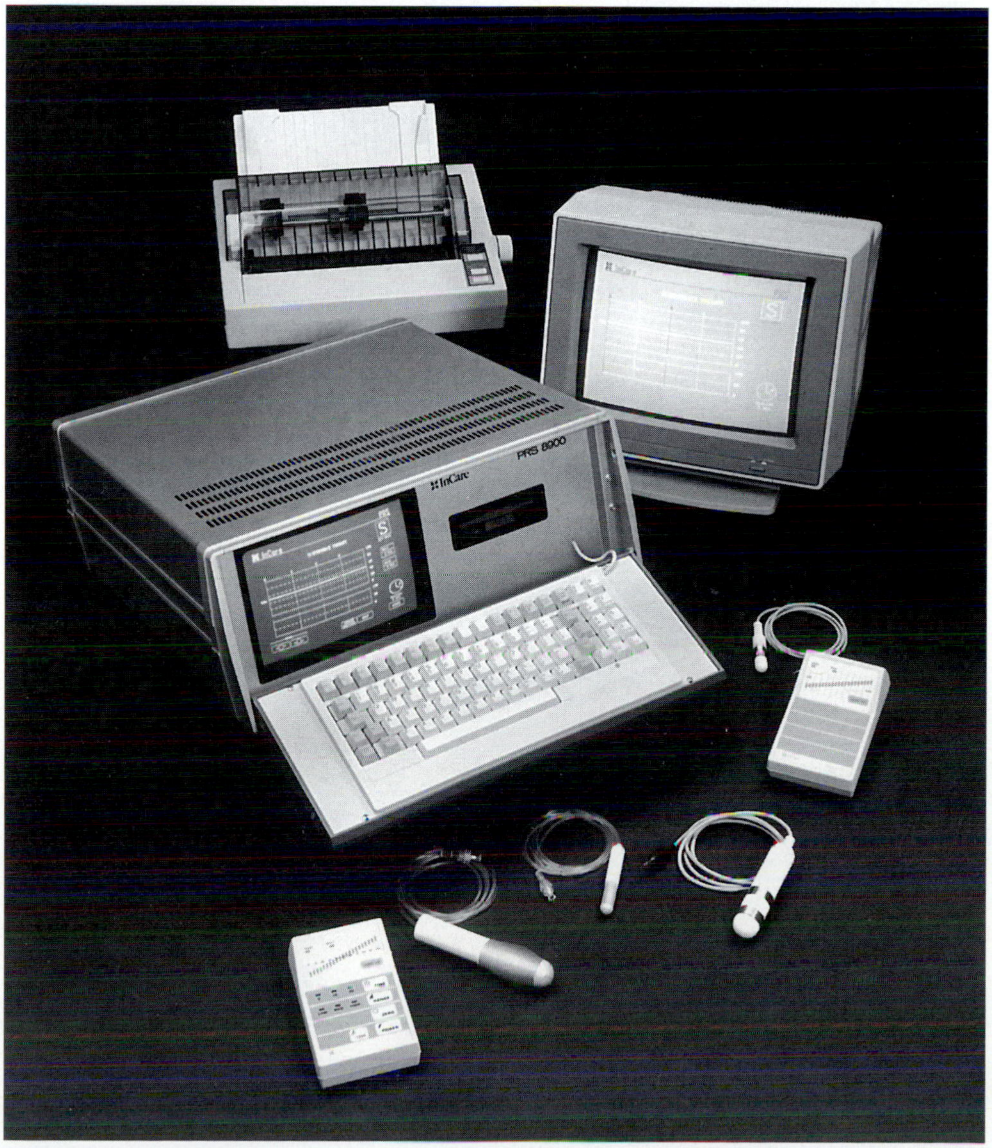

FIGURE 29–6. PRS8900 professional perineal re-education system (InCare Medical Products).

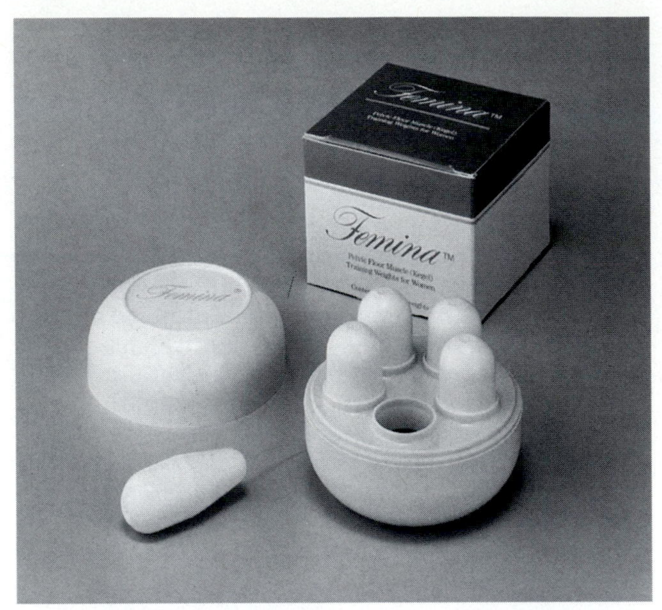

FIGURE 29–7. Femina pelvic floor muscle training weights (vaginal cones) for women (Dacomed).

After the patient can hold the heaviest cone for 15 minutes without its slipping, the patient is instructed to attempt more strenuous activities while holding the cone in place. This can include such functional activities as stair climbing, putting groceries away, or vaccuming. Ultimately, patients should strive to perform advanced daily life activities including exercise routines, walking, step classes, or low-impact aerobics.

SUMMARY

Pelvic floor rehabilitation can be accomplished with a wide variety of physical therapy techniques. Physicians providing care to women with pelvic floor dysfunction should consider these safe, commonsense techniques. Additionally, the outcome of surgical treatment of abnormalities in pelvic floor support or function may benefit from perioperative rehabilitative techniques.

REFERENCES

1. Goldthwait, JE: The relation of posture to human efficiency and the influence of poise upon the support and function of the viscera. Boston Medical and Surgical Journal 161:839,1909.
2. Penrose, CB: A Textbook of Diseases of Women. WB Saunders, Philadelphia, 1908, p 100.
3. Sherrington, LS: Selected Writings. Paul B. Hoever, New York, 1940.
4. Knott, M and Voss, DE: Proprioceptive Neuromuscular Facilitation: Patterns and Techniques. Harper & Row, New York, 1968.
5. Hellebrandt, FA: Cross education: Ipsilateral and contralateral effects of unimanual training. J Appl Physiology 4:136,1951.
6. Kannus, P, Alosa, D, Cook, L, et al: Effects of one-legged exercise on strength, power and endurance using isometric and concentric isokinetic training. Eur J Appl Physiol 64:117,1992.
7. Caldwell, KPS: The electrical control of sphincter incompetence. Lancet 1:174,1963.
8. Teague, CT and Merril, DC: Electric pelvic floor stimulation: mechanism of action. Investigative Urology 15:65,1977.
9. DeLitto, A, Rose, SJ, McKowen, JM, et al: Electrical stimulation versus voluntary exercise in strengthening thigh musculature after anterior cruciate ligament surgery. Physical Therapy 68:660,1988.
10. Laughman, RK, Youdos, JW, Garrett, TR, et al: Strength changes in the normal quadriceps femoris muscle as a result of electrical stimulation. Physical Therapy 63:494,1983.
11. Synder-Mackler, L and DeLitto, A: Two theories of muscle strength augmentation using percutaneous electrical stimulation. Physical Therapy 70:158,1990.
12. Kralj, B: The treatment of female urinary incontinence by functional electrical stimulation. In Ostegard, DR and Bent, AE (eds.): Urogynecology and Urodynamics, ed 3. Williams & Wilkins, Baltimore, 1991, p 508.
13. Godec, C, Cass, AS, and Ayala, GF, et al: Bladder inhibition with functional electrical stimulation. Urology 6:663,1975.
14. Kahn, J: Electrical modalities in obstetrics and gynecology. In Wilder E (ed.): Obstetric and Gynecologic Physical Therapy. Churchill Livingstone, New York, 1988, p 117.
15. Deller, AG: Physical principles of interferential therapy. In Savage B: Interferential Therapy. Faber & Faber, London 1988, p 96.
16. Burgio, KL, Robinson, JC and Engel, BT: The role of biofeedback in Kegel exercise training for stress urinary incontinence. Am J Obstet Gynecol 154:58,1986.

CHAPTER 30

Perineal Skin Care for the Bedridden Patient with Incontinence

Ruth C. McMyn

Incontinence is a challenging and distressing problem that can affect individuals of all ages. It may be transient, chronic, and vary significantly in degree and etiology. The International Continence Society[1] defines **urinary incontinence** (UI) as an objectively demonstrable condition in which involuntary loss of urine is a social or hygienic problem. **Fecal incontinence** (FI) is defined as the uncontrolled passage of stool through the rectum.[2]

COSTS OF INCONTINENCE

The economic impact of incontinence is contingent on (1) care setting; (2) degree of impairment; (3) patient functional status; and (4) management techniques.[3] Lacking specific data on the direct costs of FI, conclusions are based on the experience with UI. Hu[3] estimates direct health-care costs of UI to be greater than $10 billion, of which $7 billion are spent in community settings whereas $3.26 billion are spent in nursing homes. Skin irritation resulting from incontinence accounts for $112 million spent in the community and $70.6 million in nursing homes. These costs are generally not reimbursed by private insurance policies or federal Medicare/Medicaid programs.[3,4] Medicare will reimburse for *medically necessary* items (e.g., indwelling catheters) but not for *convenience* items (e.g., absorbent products).[5]

Labor resources must also be considered. The average time spent caring for a patient with an episode of incontinence in a nursing home is 8.68 minutes.[6] It has been estimated that in the United States more than 320,000 hours per day (12 million hours per year) are spent providing care to Medicaid-funded nursing home residents who are incontinent.[7]

Incontinence exacts many psychosocial costs and

may result in loss of independence and self-esteem. Social interactions suffer due to embarrassment, isolation, and depression. Family caregivers are also not exempt from these psychosocial costs; incontinence is frequently the deciding factor in admitting an individual to a nursing home.[8–12]

ETIOLOGY OF SKIN IRRITATION RELATED TO INCONTINENCE

Healthy, intact skin can be compromised by mechanical, chemical, and microbial forces. Although ammonia has been held as the responsible agent in the pathogenesis of diaper dermatitis, it is currently believed to play only a minor role in skin irritation associated with incontinence.[13,14] *Moisture* and the *interaction* between urine and feces are recognized as causes of diaper dermatitis.

Proglonged contact of the epidermis with moisture results in increased hydration of the stratum corneum, which raises the coefficient of friction of the affected skin and makes it more susceptible to damage from abrasion and erosion.[15] Furthermore, increased epidermal hydration results in greater transepidermal permeability and microbial growth.[15] These factors leave the skin vulnerable to penetration by irritating environmental substances and increased proliferation of micro-organisms.

Healthy skin is normally acidic. As urine and feces come in contact with each other, fecal urease facilitates degradation of urinary urea, releasing ammonia that elevates skin pH.[14] The resultant alkaline pH is not only a skin irritant in itself, but also a promoter of fecal enzyme activity.[14] Such enzymes include proteases and lipases, which are major skin irritants.[16] Additionally, fecal bile salts potentiate lipase activity and intensify existing skin damage.[16] These caustic effects are all heightened by an alkaline pH.

MANAGEMENT TECHNIQUES

Skin-care management accompanying intractable incontinence must be tailored to the severity of the problem and to the individual patient. The goals are to keep skin clean, dry, supple, and odor-free. Many skin-care options are available.

INVASIVE DEVICES

The decision to use an indwelling urethral catheter for long-term management of UI should be made judiciously. The associated morbidity is well known and includes nearly universal bacteriuria.[17,18] Indications for chronic indwelling catheter use may include

- Overflow incontinence recalcitrant to other therapies
- Prevention of wound or pressure-ulcer contamination by urine
- Painful and sometimes terminal illnesses.[18]

The smallest catheter adequate to allow drainage should be used; a 5 to 10 mL balloon is generally sufficient.[19,20] Optimal catheter material (e.g., silicon, latex, Teflon) has yet to be determined.[18] A closed system should be maintained, with a drainage bag containing an antireflux inlet valve. Bedridden patients should use at least a 2-liter–capacity drainage bag that can be affixed to the side of the bed or attached to a floor stand. Catheters should be secured to prevent unnecessary irritation and trauma and change schedules should be tailored to individual patient needs.[19,21,22] Routine catheter-care protocols should be followed at all times (e.g., aseptic technique, adequate fluid intake).

Clean intermittent catheterization (CIC) may be an appropriate management option for overflow incontinence.[18] Its lower morbidity makes it preferable to long-term indwelling catheters.[23–25] Caution must be exercised with immunosuppressed individuals. Advanced age and immobility, including bedridden status, are not contraindications to instituting CIC. Depending on the patient's functional status, assistive devices or caregiver training may be necessary. CIC may, however, be impractical in certain nursing home and residential settings.

Rectal tubes are an extremely controversial management option for liquid diarrhea. These tubes—with or without balloon tips—are typically large-diameter catheters connected to hanging bedside drainage bags. Currently no data support the clinical safety of these devices, so they should not be considered the treatment of choice. If used, rectal tubes should be a *short-term* intervention and are contraindicated in the presence of rectal pathology, neutropenia, or hypocoagulable states. Strict protocols for the use of these devices should include measures to minimize the risk of mechanical or ischemic damage to the anal canal and bowel wall. The perineum should be inspected regularly for leakage around the tube, which can lead to skin irritation and breakdown.

EXTERNAL DEVICES

Although seldom seen, portable female urinals are available in the United States. They are generally constructed of plastic with a bottle-shaped body and openings of varied widths and contours. Urinal neck angles should be steep enough to prevent spillage while in use and handles large enough to accommodate patients with dexterity problems. Female urinals cannot be left in place for extended periods without risking skin irritation and pressure necrosis on skin surfaces in direct contact with the device. This factor limits their usefulness in the management of intractable UI.

Bedpans are manufactured in various materials and multiple designs. Whenever possible, a sitting position should be replicated by elevating the head of the bed. An overbed trapeze can facilitate positioning. A fracture pan may be most appropriate for patients with limited hip flexion. As with female uri-

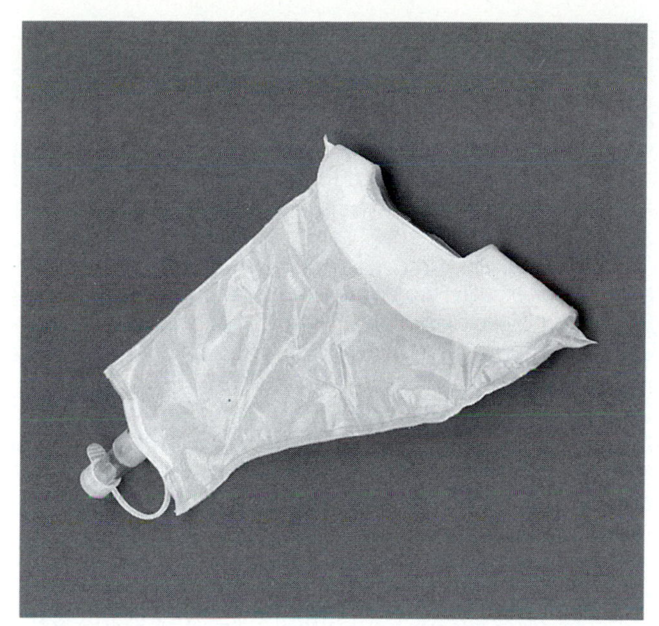

FIGURE 30–1. Female external urine collection device (Hollister Female Urinary Pouch, Hollister Incorporated, Libertyville, IL).

nals, ischemic skin damage can occur if patient contact with bedpans is prolonged. Generally, the usefulness of bedpans is limited in bedridden patients with incontinence.

The adult female external urine collection device (analogous to the male condom catheter) is a one-piece pouch-like appliance made of flexible, odor-proof plastic with a synthetic adhesive skin barrier (Fig. 30–1). It encompasses the vulva and can be attached to a hanging bedside drainage bag. Studies of this device reveal a median time of patient's wearing them of 43 hours.[26] Local reactions are minimal and confined to transient periurethral erythema[26,27]; the incidence of bacteriuria was reportedly lower than that for indwelling urethral catheters.[26] These devices are contraindicated in patients with urinary retention and in those individuals unable to assume the lithotomy application position safely.[26] Patients should be monitored regularly for leakage while wearing this device.

Adult external fecal collection devices are available as flexible, odor-proof rectal pouches. These devices adhere to the perianal area with synthetic skin barriers (Fig. 30–2), and can be attached to hanging bedside drainage bags or closed with clamps, depending on fecal consistency. Wear-time for these devices is 24 hours or longer.[28–30] Rectal pouches are most effective when applied *before* skin irritation and breakdown have developed. Patients should be checked regularly for leakage and skin soilage.

ABSORBENT PRODUCTS

Absorbent products are not only the most widely used method of treating intractable incontinence but also are the most widely sold health-care product in the United States.[31] Diapers, because of their roll-on application, are among the absorbent products most workable with bedridden patients. They are available in both reusable and disposable forms.

Although **reusable diapers** vary in design and composition, they are most often rectangular cotton cloth with a multi-ply center strip. Cloth diapers may or may not have a waterproof outer layer. Plastic pants are frequently added to those diapers without a backing to protect the patient's immediate surroundings, but an early study of diaper dermatitis[32] warns that an occlusive diaper cover (i.e., plastic pants) can affect skin hydration and increase the coefficient of friction, thus placing skin integrity at risk.

Most **disposable diapers** are of similar construction. A soft, quick-dry inner surface covers an absorbent cellulose core. Many disposable diapers also contain a superabsorbent polymer in their core, designed to bind fluids in a gel matrix. The composition, volume, and distribution of such polymers within the diaper core varies by manufacturer. The outermost layer of disposable diapers is generally waterproof polyethylene or polypropylene material.[33,34] Specialty features available on disposable diapers include elasticized waist and leg bands, contour fitting, external wetness indicator strips, and reusable adhesive closure tabs.

Studies with infants comparing a conventional disposable with a superabsorbent disposable and in another study of conventional disposable, superabsorbent disposable, and reusable cloth diapers revealed reduced skin wetness,[35,36] closer to normal skin pH values,[35,36] and less skin irritation[33,35,36] associated with the use of superabsorbent disposable diapers. These improvements are attributed to the ability of the gel matrix to keep moisture away from the patient's skin as well as to diminish the likelihood of urine-fecal mixing, thereby reducing the potential for an ammonia-related increase in skin pH.

Protective underpads are also common in the management of bedridden patients who are incontinent.

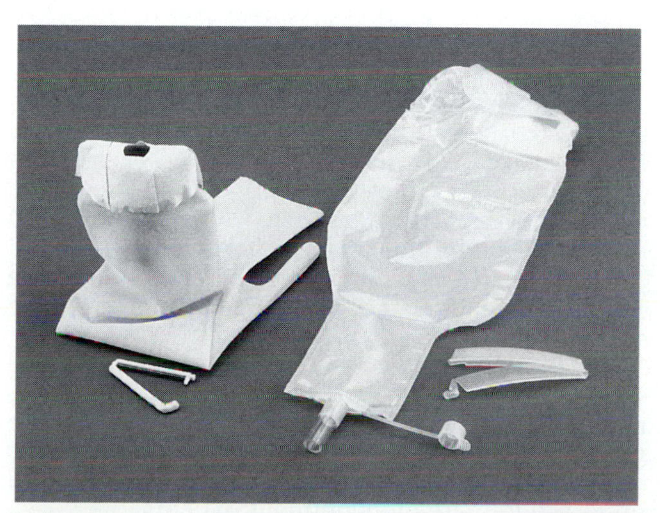

FIGURE 30–2. External fecal collection devices. *Left,* Bard FCD Self-Adhesive Fecal Containment Device (Bard Patient Care Division: C.R. Bard, Inc., Murray Hill, NJ). *Right,* Hollister Drainable Fecal Incontinence Collector (Hollister Incorporated, Libertyville, IL).

TABLE 30–1. Selection Criteria for Absorbent Products

- Type and severity of incontinence
- Patient functional status
- Care setting
- Patient comfort and response
- Product cost and availability
- Tensile strength
- Absorbency/saturation capacity/dispersion pattern
- Anti-bunch/anti-shift construction
- Odor control properties
- Maintenance requirements (storage, laundry vs. disposal)
- Environmental impact (fuel and air/water pollution vs. solid waste disposal)

Underpads are constructed in layers similar to diapers. They are available in a variety of sizes and come in both reusable and disposable forms.

Although absorbent products are also available in the form of pads with inserts, padded pant and pad-and-strap systems, these are generally impractical for bedridden individuals. Such systems tend to risk leakage with the patient in a recumbent position.

Many factors must be considered before selecting any absorbent product for long-term management (Table 30–1). The use of all absorbent products must be accompanied by meticulous local skin care so as to avoid skin irritation and breakdown.

TOPICAL AGENTS

Topical agents for routine skin care of incontinent patients include a skin cleanser, moisturizer, and barrier product. Commercial cleansers for patients with incontinence are available in spray and foam formulations. They are generally pH-balanced and contain emulsifiers, which precludes the need for vigorous scrubbing and potential friction-related skin damage. Some commercial cleansers do not need to be rinsed off, others contain deodorizers.

Soap and water are also acceptable cleansers. Soap should be of a mild, pH-balanced variety. The water should be tepid. Minimal force should be applied to the skin during the cleansing process.[37]

Supple skin is less likely to break. Poorly hydrated stratum corneum becomes inflexible and inelastic and is associated with cracking and fissuring.[38] Application of topical moisturizing agents appears to be clinically beneficial to dry skin.[38–40] Most moisturizing creams and lotions have a petrolatum base and contain other agents such as mineral oil, vegetable oil, lanolin, or paraffin. They should be applied to the skin after cleansing.

Finally, skin repeatedly exposed to moisture should be protected with a moisture-barrier ointment or skin sealant. Moisture-barrier ointments are generally petrolatum-based, whereas skin sealants are copolymer films. Waterproof skin sealants are preferred for care of incontinent patients.

Routine skin care of incontinent patients should be provided after every instance to prevent skin irritation and breakdown. Once skin is denuded, however, occlusive skin pastes become the topical agent of choice. These pastes are generally manufactured with a zinc-oxide–petrolatum base and are designed to adhere to broken skin. They should be reapplied as often as necessary to prevent contamination of skin by feces and urine.

Fungal rashes (e.g., *Candida albicans*) are not uncommon in patients with incontinence as a result of the moisture present in the perineal and buttock areas. Antifungal preparations are readily available in powder, cream, and ointment forms. Several manufacturers of the aforementioned incontinence ointments and pastes have incorporated antifungal agents into their products. If skin infections do not respond to these measures, consultation with a dermatologist should be obtained.

When choosing a specific topical agent for long-term use, efficacy, cost, and availability should be considered. Agents containing fragrances and dyes may act as allergens, and products with a high alcohol content should be avoided because of their drying effects on skin.

ODOR CONTROL

Multiple options are available for the management of incontinence-related odor. Adequate hydration and diet manipulation are helpful, whereas nonprescription oral chlorophyllin copper-complex tablets may be appropriate in certain circumstances.

Commercial appliance deodorizers, deodorizing skin cleansers, and room sprays are common. An *odor eliminator* may be preferable to a product that simply masks odors. Reusable equipment and devices should be cleaned thoroughly according to the

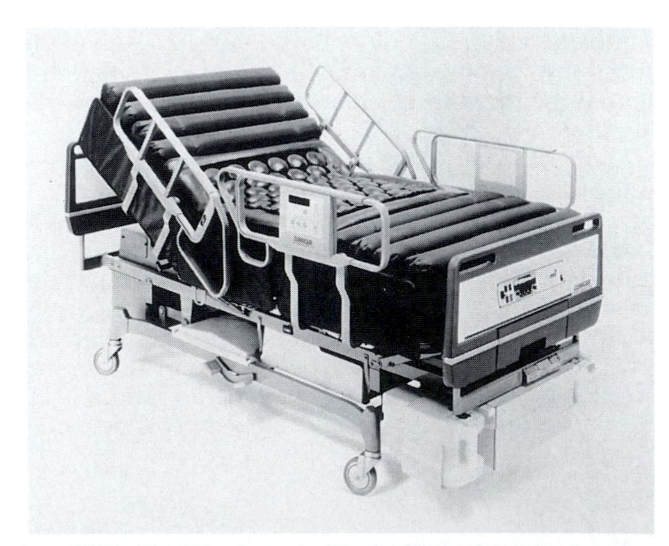

FIGURE 30–3. Clensicair Incontinence Management System (Support Systems International, Inc., Charleston, SC).

manufacturer's instructions. Single-use products should be promptly and properly discarded.

NEW TECHNOLOGY

Recently, a new incontinence-management bed system has been introduced combining pressure relief and incontinence skin cleansing (Fig. 30–3). This system addresses (1) immobility associated with incontinence; (2) the role of moisture in predisposing skin to irritation and breakdown; and (3) FI in association with pressure ulcers in hospitalized, bedridden patients.[41] Patients are supported on pressure-relieving, low–air-loss therapy cells covered by a quick-drying filter sheet. A moisture detector is triggered after every incontinence, aspirating effluent away from the patient's skin to a collection reservoir. Cleansing is accomplished with a low-pressure spray wand delivering a warmed solution of the caregiver's choice. Intake and output measurements are easily retrieved.

SURGICAL INTERVENTION

It may be necessary to consider surgery as a management (vs. corrective) option in cases of severe, intractable incontinence and skin breakdown refractory to conservative treatment. Diversionary surgery can be used in patients with urinary and fecal incontinence.

COMMUNITY RESOURCES

Patients and caregivers may benefit from contact with an incontinence support group (Table 30–2). Help for Incontinent People (HIP), Inc. is a nonprofit patient advocacy and educational organization. Its publications include a comprehensive resource guide to incontinence products. The Simon Foundation is another, similar, resource.

SUMMARY

Incontinence is pervasive and costly. It affects large numbers of women, many of whom have accompanying functional impairments. Skin-care management techniques must be used in conjunction with efforts to identify the source of incontinence. Treatment and management must be tailored to the cause and overall patient-care goals to ensure optimal clinical outcomes.

TABLE 30–2. Community Resources

HIP, Inc.	Simon Foundation
P.O. Box 544	P.O. Box 815
Union, S.C. 29379	Wilmette, IL 60091
1-800-BLADDER	1-800-23-SIMON
1-800-579-7900	1-708-864-3913

REFERENCES

1. Bates, P, Bradley, WE, Glen, E, et al: The standardization of terminology of lower urinary tract function. J Urol 121:551,1979.
2. Kiff, ES: Faecal incontinence. BMJ 305:702,1992.
3. Hu, TW: Impact of urinary incontinence on health-care costs. J Am Geriatr Soc 38:292,1990.
4. Krazner, D: Skin care products for the incontinent: How to select products. Continuing Care 8:15,1989.
5. Mitteness, LS: Social aspects of urinary incontinence in the elderly. AORN J 56:731,1992.
6. Creason, NS: Costing urinary incontinence in nursing homes. Contemporary Long Term Care 10:84,1987.
7. Cella, M: The nursing costs of urinary incontinence in a nursing home population. Nurs Clin North Am 23:159,1988.
8. Mohide, EA: The prevalence and scope of urinary incontinence. Clin Geriatr Med 2:639,1986.
9. Hu, TW: The economic impact of urinary incontinence. Clin Geriatr Med 2:673,1986.
10. Szurszewski, JH, Holt, PR and Schuster, M: Proceedings of a workshop entitled "Neuromuscular function and dysfunction of the gastrointestinal tract in aging." Dig Dis Sci 34:1135,1989.
11. Resnick, NM: Older women's health: Contemporary and emerging health issues. Urinary Incontinence. Public Health Rep 102(suppl):67,1987.
12. Ouslander, JG, Kane, RL and Abrass IB: Urinary incontinence in elderly nursing home patients. JAMA 248:1194,1982.
13. Leyden, JJ, Katz, S, Stewart, R, et al: Urinary ammonia and ammonia-producing microorganisms in infants with and without diaper dermatitis. Arch Dermatol 113:1678,1977.
14. Berg, RW, Buckingham, KW and Stewart, RL: Etiologic factors in diaper dermatitis: The role of urine. Pediatr Dermatol 3:102,1986.
15. Zimmerer, RE, Lawson, KD and Calvert, CJ: The effects of wearing diapers on skin. Pediatr Dermatol 3:95,1986.
16. Buckingham, KW and Berg, RW: Etiologic factors in diaper dermatitis: The role of feces. Pediatr Dermatol 3:107,1986.
17. Warren, JW, Tenney, JH, Hoopes, JM, et al: A prospective microbiology study of bacteriuria in patients with chronic indwelling urethral catheters. J Infect Dis 146:719,1982.
18. Urinary Incontinence Guideline Panel: Urinary Incontinence in Adults. Clinical Practice Guideline, Number 2. Agency for Health Care Policy and Research, Public Health Service, U.S. Department of Health and Human Services, Rockville, MD, 1992.
19. Constantino, G: Catheterization. In Jeter, K, Faller, N and Norton, C (eds.): Nursing for Continence. WB Saunders, Philadelphia, 1990, p 241.
20. Gray, M, Siegel, SW, Troy, R, et al: Management of urinary incontinence. Doughty, DB (ed): Urinary and Fecal Incontinence: Nursing Management. Mosby-Yearbook, St. Louis, 1991, p 95.
21. Kunin, CM, Chin, QF and Chambers, S: Indwelling urinary catheters in the elderly. Relationship of "catheter life" to formation of encrustations in patients with and without blocked catheters. Am J Med 82:405,1987.
22. Wong, ES: Guidelines for prevention of catheter-associated urinary tract infections. Am J Infect Control 11:28,1983.
23. Webb, RJ, Lawson, AL and Neal, DE: Clean intermittent self-catheterization in 172 adults. Brit J Urol 65:20,1990.
24. Maynard, KM and Diokno, AC: Urinary infection and complications during clean intermittent catheterization after spinal cord injury. J Urol 132:943,1984.
25. Bennett, CJ and Diokno, AC: Clean intermittent self catheterization in the elderly. Urology 24:43,1984.
26. Johnson, DE, Muncie, HL, O'Reilly, JL, et al: An external urine collection device for incontinent women. Evaluation of long-term use. J Am Geriatr Soc 38:1016,1990.

27. Johnson, DE, O'Reilly, JL and Warren, JW: Clinical evaluation of an external urine collection device for nonambulatory incontinent women. J Urol 141:535,1989.
28. Basch, A and Jensen, L: Management of fecal incontinence. In Doughty, DB (ed.): Urinary and Fecal Incontinence. Nursing Management. Mosby-Yearbook, St. Louis, 1991, p 235.
29. Duso, S: Product notebook: A new fecal containment device. A cast study describing one use of the Bard FCD fecal containment device. Ostomy Wound Management 38:38,1992.
30. Freedman, P: The rectal pouch: A safer alternative to rectal tubes. Am J Nurs 91:105,1991.
31. Newman, DK: The treatment of urinary incontinence in adults. Nurse Pract 14:21,1989.
32. Boisits, EK and McCormack, JJ: Diaper dermatitis and the role of predisposition. In Maibach, HI and Boisits, EK (eds.): Neonatal Skin Structure and Function. Marcel Dekker, New York, 1982, p 191.
33. Lane, AT, Rehder, PA and Helm, K: Evaluations of diapers containing absorbent gelling material with conventional disposable diapers in newborn infants. Am J Dis Child 144:315,1990.
34. Wong, DL, Brantly, D, Clutter, LB, et al: Diapering choices: A critical review of the issues. Pediatric Nursing 18:41,1992.
35. Campbell, RL, Seymour, JL, Stone, LC, et al: Clinical studies with disposable diapers containing absorbent gelling materials: Evaluation of effects on infant skin condition. J Am Acad Dermatol 17:978,1987.
36. Davis, JA, Leyden, JJ, Grove, SL, et al: Comparison of disposable diapers with fluff absorbent and fluff plus absorbent polymers: Effects on skin hydration, skin pH, and diaper dermatitis. Pediatr Dermatol 6:102,1989.
37. Panel for the Prediction and Prevention of Pressure Ulcers in Adults: Pressure Ulcers in Adults: Prediction and Prevention. Clinical Practice Guideline, Number 3. Agency for Health Care Policy and Research, Public Health Service, U.S. Department of Health and Human Services, Rockville, MD, 1992.
38. Kligman, AM: Regression method for assessing the efficacy of moisturizers. Cosmetics and Toiletries 93:27,1978.
39. Kantor, I, Ballinger, WG and Savin, RC: Severely dry skin: Clinical evaluation of a highly effective therapeutic lotion. Cutis 30:410,1982.
40. Wehr, R, Krochmal, L, Whitmore, C, et al: Efficacy of alpha keri after showering for treatment of xerosis. Cutis 37/38:384,1986.
41. Allman, RM, Laprade, CA, Noel, LB, et al: Pressure sores among hospitalized patients. Ann Intern Med 105:337,1986.

SECTION SIX

DISORDERS OF SUPPORT

CHAPTER 31

Posterior Vaginal Support Defects

Linda T. Brubaker • Dee E. Fenner
Theodore J. Saclarides

Support defects in the posterior vaginal wall are commonly associated with enterocele alone or with rectocele formation. This chapter reviews the etiology, diagnosis, and treatment of these support entities. Although these disorders have been documented in men, this chapter focuses on rectoceles and enteroceles in women.

RECTOCELE

A **rectocele** may be defined as an outpouching of the rectum beyond its normal contours. Although rectoceles are frequently diagnosed, it is increasingly clear that they can vary widely in appearance and the degree to which they are responsible for the patient's symptoms. Furthermore, severity of symptoms does not always correlate with the extent of anatomic distortion. One must be certain, therefore, that what is a common physical or radiographic finding is pathologic. To this end, the evaluation of a rectocele must include determining the patient's need for assisted defecation, such as support of the posterior vaginal wall or perineal body. Difficult defecation may also be indicated by a feeling of incomplete emptying.

ETIOLOGY

It is generally believed that rectocele formation is related to vaginal delivery.[1] Although no epidemiologic studies substantiate this concept, the vast majority of clinicians consider that rectocele formation is a delayed result of rectovaginal septum thinning or separation.

In the absence of vaginal delivery, chronic straining or unusually forceful increases in abdominal pressure may be clinically associated with rectocele formation.

PREVALENCE

The incidence and prevalence of rectoceles in asymptomatic women is unknown. Moreover, the lack of a standardized definition limits comparison of clinical studies. Although it is clinically apparent that there are changes in vaginal support caused by vaginal childbirth and aging, the range of anatomic variation has not been studied. Bartram, Turnbull, and Lennard-Jones reported a series of 20 asymptomatic patients (10 female, 10 male) referred for barium enema who consented to proctography.[2] They defined rectocele as any ballooning of the anterior or posterior rectal wall beyond the normal rectal contours. Using this definition, anterior rectocele was found in 8 of 10 female patients. Freimanis and co-workers reported a series of 21 asymptomatic patients (14 women) with normal physical examination. She found that 77% of the women had rectoceles that were subjectively graded as small, moderate, or large.[3] Shorvon and colleagues studied 23 asymptomatic women and 25 asymptomatic men under age 35. Using a definition similar to Bartram, 48% of women had a rectocele more than 1 cm in depth; a single subject had a rectocele more than 2 cm in depth.[4] It is certain that some anterior rectal wall movement is normal during straining, but the point at which this movement should be considered abnormal has not been established.

EXAMINATION AND EVALUATION

Physical examination is the mainstay of diagnosis, and virtually all major gynecology textbooks outline how the physical examination should be performed. In the United States, most gynecologists strongly prefer the dorsal lithotomy position for supine examination because it allows a complete view of vaginal supports. As discussed in Chapter 4, however, prolapse is a gravity-dependent disorder. Therefore, examination of the patient in the upright position is mandatory, in order to fully reproduce maximum anatomic distortion. In fact, the position of the examination may be an important variable. Delemarre and associates reported a series of 51 patients who were examined in both the supine and left lateral decubitus positions.[5] In 15 patients, the rectocele grade was higher in the decubitus position, whereas in 5 patients, the grade was lower.

Transrectal assessment of septal thickness, strength, and bulging is also commonly used in the diagnosis of rectocele. Experienced examiners indicate an ability to determine the integrity of this tissue. This skill has yet to be tested, however, for sensitivity, specificity, and reproducibility. An alternative examination technique uses a combined rectovaginal examination. The examiner places two fingers on the posterior wall of the vagina and the index finger of the opposite hand in the rectum. The vaginal fingers are pressed against the rectal finger while the patient forcibly strains. In small increments, the vaginal fingers are moved toward the hymen until the rectocele is seen to bulge into the vagina. This is an ancillary examination technique that may be useful in localizing a discrete rectovaginal septum defect.

During physical examination, it is also helpful to ask the patient to demonstrate any assistive maneuvers that she uses to complete defecation. Women who apply pressure to the perineal body may have a different anatomic defect compared with women who support the posterior vaginal wall.

Usually a rectocele is diagnosed when physical examination indicates a weakening or separation of the rectovaginal septum that allows protrusion of the rectum into the vaginal canal. Although this is a common definition, it is also highly subjective. Imaging studies, especially fluoroscopic ones, have been used to study rectoceles. As with physical examination, no standardized radiographic definition or staging system exists. Most rectoceles are anterior, that is, oriented toward the vagina. Posterior rectoceles are distinctly less common than anterior rectoceles.

The vast majority of rectoceles are "low," that is, at the perineal body (Fig. 31–1). The literature commonly refers to "mid" and "high" rectoceles, but we have only seen such defects in patients with unsuccessful prior posterior colporrhaphy. In these instances, the initial repair was not extended cephalad to the upper limit of the defect, as suggested by Nichols[6] (Fig. 31–2).

During defecography, the excursion of the anterior wall is quite variable throughout the dynamic study, depending on the phase of defecation. The measurement of the anterior rectal wall should be specified in relationship to the progress of defecation—for

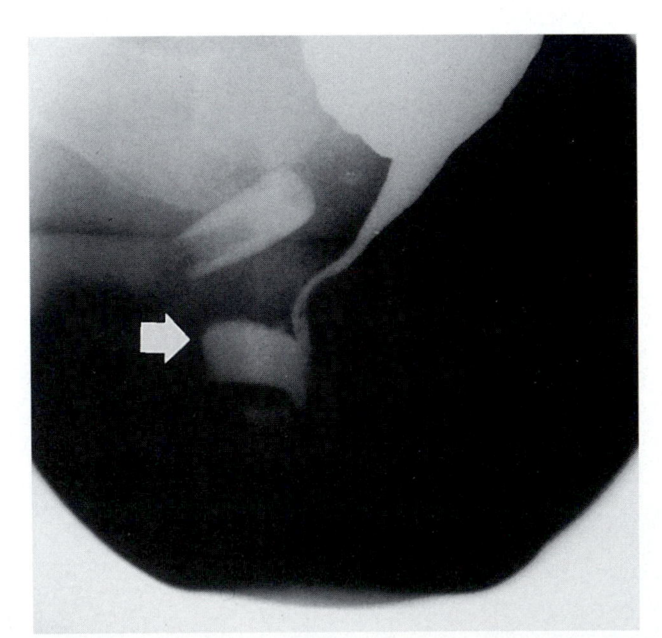

FIGURE 31–1. Classic anterior, low rectocele (arrow), located distally, just above the perineal body.

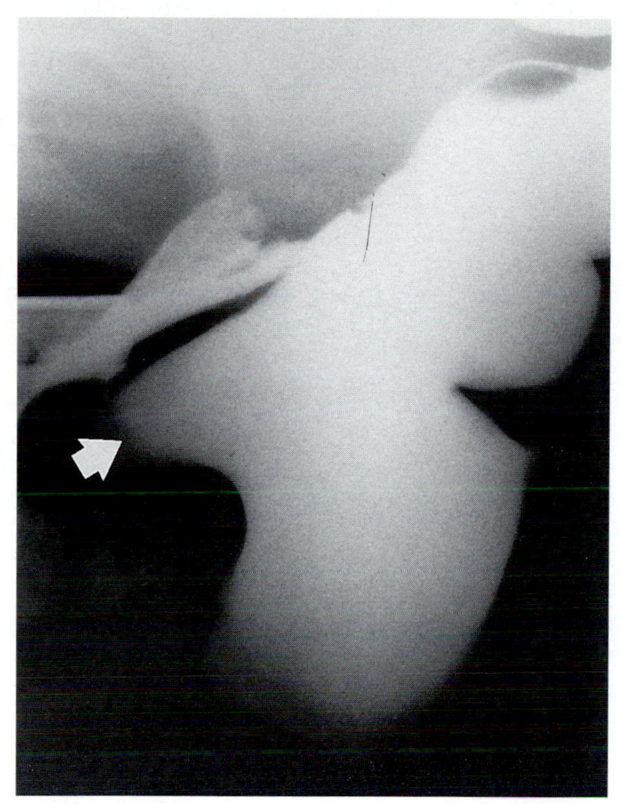

FIGURE 31–2. High rectocele (arrow) seen only in patients with prior posterior wall surgery. (Courtesy of J. Thomas Benson.)

example, early defecation, during defecation, end defecation, and after defecation. Delemarre and colleagues compared quantitative analysis with subjective grading of rectoceles on defecography. Rectoceles were measured at their maximum excursion as determined retrospectively by review of videotape. A maximum anatomic defect of 20 mm or more was always graded as severe. Of 25 patients with rectoceles smaller than 20 mm, 2 patients (left lateral decubitus) and 5 patients (lithotomy) were clinically graded as having only small or absent rectoceles on the basis of physical examination.

Delemarre also examined variation among investigators in the interpretation of defecographic findings. In 29% of the examinations, observers disagreed. These same observers also reviewed magnetic resonance images (MRI) of 14 of these patients, with even more interobserver differences in MRI interpretation. In addition, the anatomic deformities were generally graded less severely with MRI than with defecography.[5] This is likely related to the supine position during study.

In addition to the extent of anatomic distortion of the anterior rectal wall, rectoceles may be described by their functional characteristics. A common fluoroscopic finding is an anatomic pouching that retains contrast despite the patient's best efforts to evacuate completely (both on the radio-opaque commode and the private toilet). The significance of retained contrast has yet to be determined. Although retention of contrast does not correlate with the extent of anatomic distortion by the rectocele,[7] intuitively it may implicate the rectocele as the cause of dysfunctional defecation.

STAGING

Most physicians have been taught to examine the posterior vaginal wall while the patient is forcefully straining. The extent of the anatomic distortion is then graded by one of several proposed grading scales. These grading scales, orginally used for uterine prolapse, have significant limitations when applied to the posterior vaginal wall. For example, the prolapsing structure has no defined upper limit, unlike the uterus. In addition, it is not uncommon to see perineal skin that has been superficially closed in lieu of a properly reconstructed perineal body. Such perineal skin may artificially limit the excursion of prolapsing tissue.

Although no standardized quantitative nomenclature for the description of prolapse exists, anatomic support defects may be quantified. For example, the extent of the defect may be measured with reference to a relatively fixed point, such as the hymen. Such a system allows comparison of multiple examiners or allows a single examiner to quantify change in an individual patient over time.

ASSOCIATED DISORDERS

An isolated rectocele is an unusual finding. Generally, clinicians should rule out associated support defects in other areas before embarking on a surgical procedure designed to correct an isolated finding. When earlier surgery has failed, unusual forms of prolapse that were initially missed may be present, including enterocele (anterior and posterior) and sigmoidocele. Enteroceles usually cause posterior vaginal support defects; in such cases, there is thinning of the rectovaginal septum and the clinical diagnosis of isolated rectocele is mistakenly made (Fig. 31–3). Fluoroscopic evaluation is frequently needed to identify all support defects; this is especially important for posterior vaginal wall abnormalities, where rectocele, enterocele, and sigmoidocele may coexist.

Rectoceles (and other posterior vaginal support defects) may affect coital activity. Patients may relate discomfort from the large protrusions, fear of (or actual) loss of retained feces, and decreased libido due to a perceived loss of sexual desirability.

INDICATIONS AND TECHNIQUES FOR OPERATIVE REPAIR

An asymptomatic rectocele does not warrant surgical intervention despite what some gynecologic textbooks recommend. Clearly, surgery is justified when symptoms are attributable to the fascial defect,

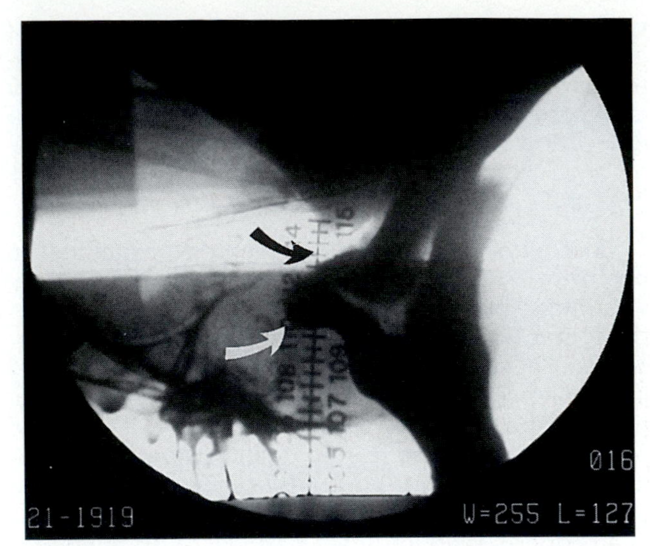

FIGURE 31–3. Coexisting rectocele (white arrow) and enterocele (black arrow).

such as the need to assist with defecation digitally. Typically patients describe needing to press on the perineal body or to press posteriorly on the vaginal wall to empty the trapped fecal material (Fig. 31–4). Additional symptoms worthy of surgical correction include bothersome protrusion of posterior vaginal skin overlying the rectocele defect.

Traditional rectocele repairs rely on plication of an extensive length of rectovaginal fascia. These repairs have been described and modified by Goff.[8] The traditional posterior colporrhaphy is shown in Fig. 31–5. The posterior vaginal mucosa is opened in the midline to expose the underlying rectovaginal fascia. This fascia can be identified by its avascular nature and by its course, which is a direct continuation of the uterosacral ligaments up to the sacrum when the superior portions of the fascia are intact. The upper fascia is plicated in the midline using long-lasting absorbable sutures that incorporate only fascia while

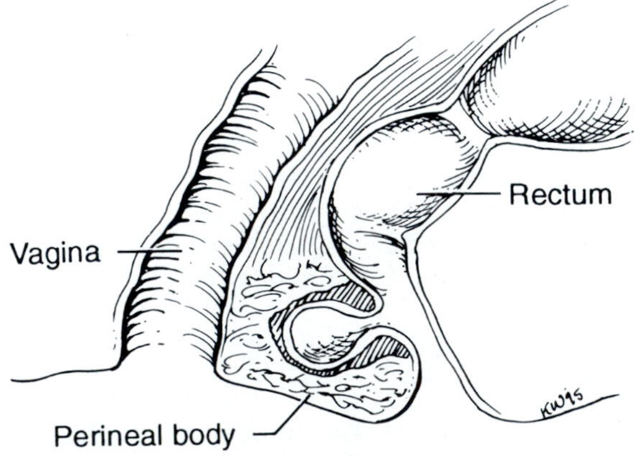

FIGURE 31–4. Classic picture of stool trapping above the perineal body. Patients who use manual evacuation press on either the posterior wall of the vagina or the perineal body.

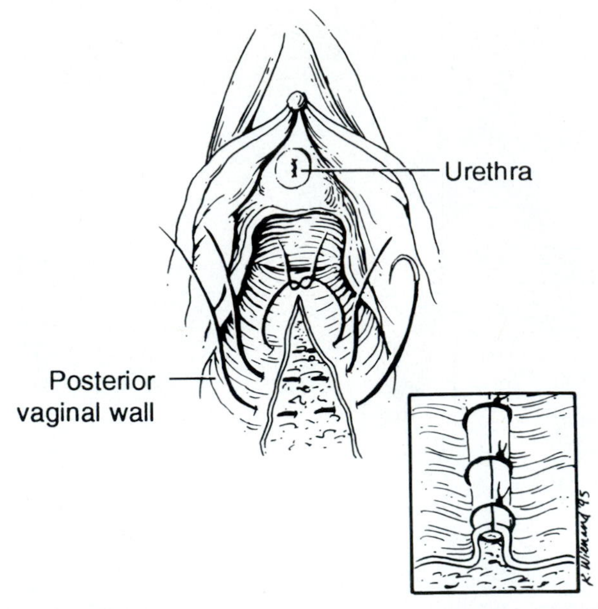

FIGURE 31–5. Rectocele repair, performed with traditional posterior colporrhaphy technique.

avoiding both only fascia while avoiding both skeletal muscle and vaginal wall. Sutures are placed at close intervals to avoid bunching or ridge formation in the posterior wall, because this may cause postoperative dyspareunia. It is important to maintain the normal anatomic relationship of these tissues, keeping the rectovaginal fascia intact as a free layer that is capable of sliding with reference to the vaginal tube. Excision of the vaginal mucosa should be done cautiously, resisting the common temptation to remove large amounts of tissue. The etiologic defect of the rectocele is not primarily in the vaginal mucosa, and this tissue should be removed only when redundancy is likely to be problematic.

An alternative approach to rectocele repair relies on identification and repair of a fascial separation that has permitted the rectum to come into direct contact with the vaginal tube. Such defects can be identified at the time of surgical dissection and can be mentally visualized during fluoroscopic images of posterior vaginal wall defects (Fig. 31–6). The rectovaginal fascia has often been pulled away from the perineal body or never reattached at the time of vaginal delivery. During rectocele repair, the posterior vaginal skin is opened in the midline, exposing the transverse edges of the rectovaginal fascial defect, complete exposure and visualization of which is necessary before repair is possible. The fascial edges are then reattached to the perineal body with delayed absorbable or fine permanent suture material. Frequently, antecedent perineal body reconstruction is necessary. The fascia should be firmly and widely attached to the perineal body (Fig. 31–7). The overlying vaginal skin is closed hemostatically.

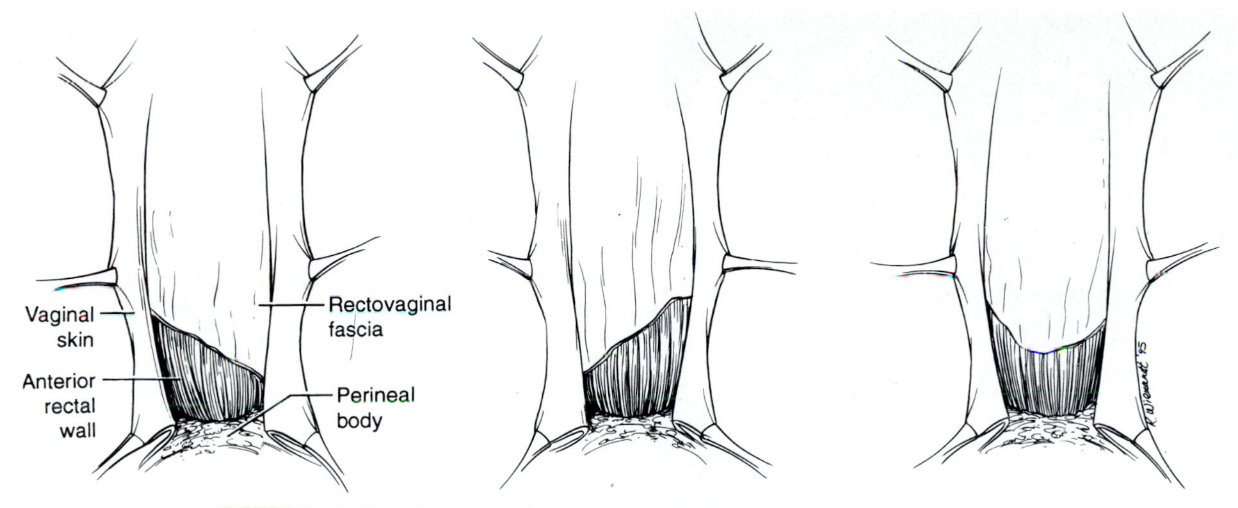

FIGURE 31–6. Line drawing of the rectocele fascial defect seen during fluoroscopy.

ENTEROCELE

Enterocele has been defined as a herniation of the pelvic peritoneum beyond the normal confines of the cul-de-sac.[9] Enteroceles most commonly form posterior to the vagina and dissect into the rectovaginal space, but an enterocele may be found anterior or lateral to the vagina.[10] As with a rectocele, it is rarely an isolated defect and more commonly occurs with other pelvic floor defects including uterine or vaginal vault prolapse, cystocele, and rectocele.

ETIOLOGY

Kuhn and Hollyock measured the adult cul-de-sac depth in 44 women undergoing diagnostic laparoscopy or tubal ligation;[11] the average depth was 5.3 cm ± 0.5 cm in nulliparous patients and 5.4 cm ± 0.4 cm in multiparous patients when the distance from the uterosacral ligament to the apex of the cul-de-sac was measured. In 5 of 17 multiparous women, there was a clinical diagnosis of enterocele, even though they were asymptomatic. Studies to date suggest that there is no direct relationship between cul-de-sac depth and enterocele formation. Zacharin demonstrated this lack of correlation in Chinese women whose deep cul-de-sac is associated with excessive vaginal and rectal mobility, but not associated with pulsion enterocele.[12]

The traditional classification of enteroceles was described by Nichols,[13] who suggested four etiologic subtypes: traction, pulsion, iatrogenic, and congenital. Iatrogenic enteroceles are unfortunately becoming more common. Changes in pelvic anatomy, particularly alteration of the normal vaginal axis, may result in formation of enteroceles. Burch first noted in his initial report of 53 cystourethropexies that 4 patients, or 7.5%, subsequently developed enteroceles.[14] The elevation of the anterior vaginal wall may change the axis of the vagina, opening the cul-de-sac to increased abdominal pressure. Such enteroceles clinically appear to be related to post-hysterectomy vaginal vault prolapse.

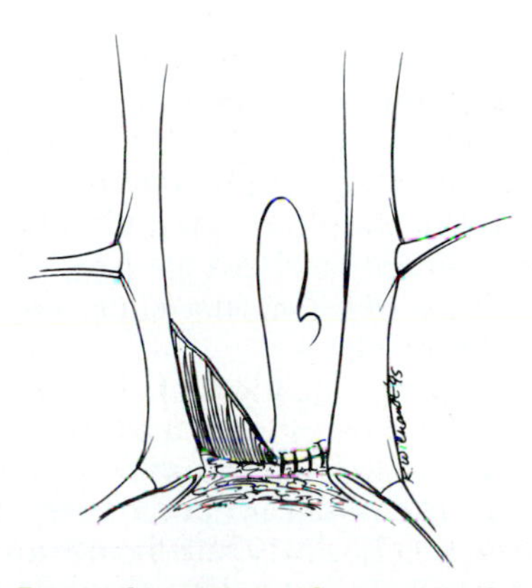

FIGURE 31–7. Rectocele repair involving reattachment of the rectovaginal septum to the perineal body.

EXAMINATION AND EVALUATION

The diagnosis of an enterocele should be suspected clinically when the patient reports a pressure or dragging sensation in the pelvis, especially when standing or bearing down. Stretching of the small-bowel mesentery during strain or the Valsalva maneuver may cause colicky lower abdominal pain or lower back pain. In addition, she may report noticing a bulge at the introitus while cleaning the perineum or during intercourse.

During physical examination, the patient should be asked to bear down in order to distend the hernia. Beneath a thin, postmenopausal vagina, peristalsis of small bowel may be seen. A bimanual examination with the index finger in the rectum is helpful but not infallible to differentiate a rectocele from an entero-

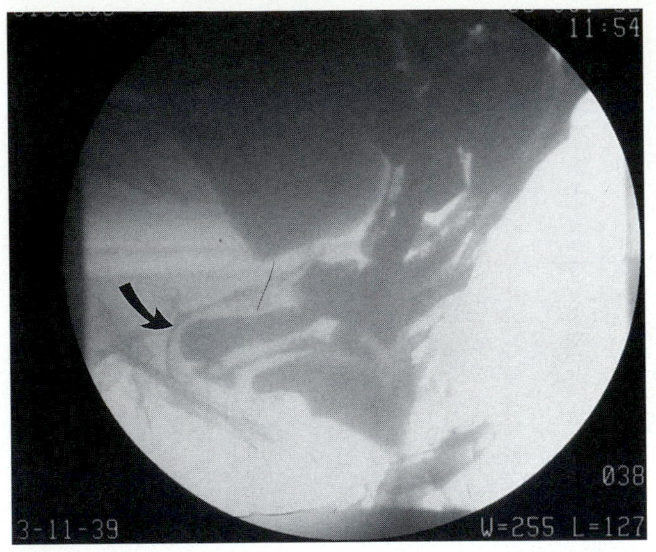

FIGURE 31–8. Postoperative enterocele (arrow) secondary to failed Moschowitz's obliteration of the cul-de-sac.

cele. The enterocele can frequently be palpated sliding down the rectovaginal septum between the index finger and thumb. Unless the defect is maximally demonstrated in the supine position, this maneuver should be repeated with the patient standing and straining to maximize prolapse and hernia formation.

Clinical examination alone is not always accurate in identifying all pelvic floor defects. Kelvin and colleagues[15] studied 74 consecutive patients with pelvic prolapse using defecography. Thirteen patients had enteroceles by defecography while physical examination detected only seven of these. Undoubtedly, missed enteroceles contribute to higher recurrence rates of "persistent" vault prolapse. This is especially true in patients who have undergone surgery earlier for pelvic-floor support defects. In these patients, defecography has proven most valuable in diagnosing enteroceles, as well as other pelvic floor defects.

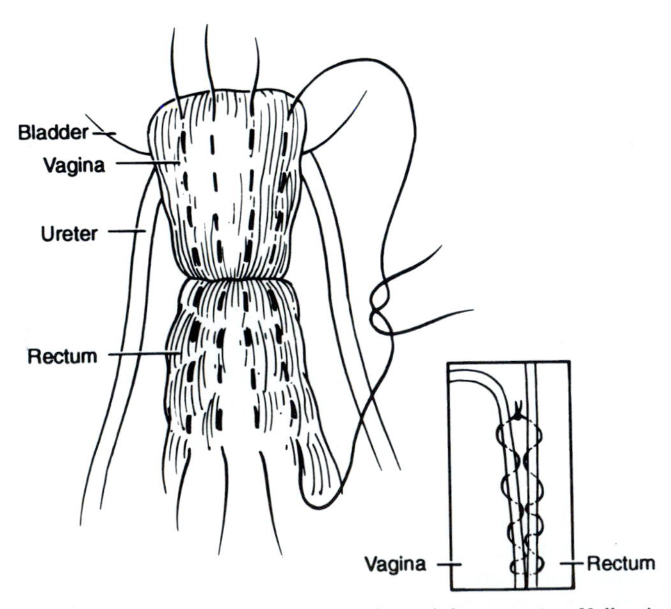

FIGURE 31–9. Vertical closure of the cul-de-sac using Halban's technique.

TABLE 31–1. Surgical Principles of Enterocele Repair

1. Identification of coexisting defects
2. Excision or obliteration of sac
3. High ligation of sac orifice
4. Support below

INDICATIONS AND TECHNIQUES FOR OPERATIVE REPAIR

The first step of enterocele repair is to recognize the enterocele, its probable cause, and coexisting defects.[13] The entire sac must then be exposed, dissected, and either excised or obliterated. The orifice of the sac should be occluded by high ligation.[13] This can be accomplished by placing a double pursestring circumferentially either abdominally or vaginally as described by Moschowitz,[16] who originally proposed this technique as a cure for rectal prolapse. Moschowitz postulated that rectal prolapse was a form of hernia and so set out to devise an operation in which the principles for the cure of a hernia could be carried out. Both on physical examination and at dissection, he noted the presence of an enterocele in conjunction with rectal prolapse. When performed for rectal prolapse, obliteration of the cul-de-sac is usually unsuccessful, but it has worked well as a prophylactic and primary repair of an enterocele.

A disadvantage of this method is suture slippage, which can leave a small hole through which small bowel can herniate, resulting in a persistent enterocele or strangulation. A postoperative enterocele secondary to suture slippage is shown in Figure 31–8. Alternatively, vertical closure of the cul-de-sac with Halban's stitches may be preferable (Fig. 31–9).[17] Unfortunately, no data support the efficacy or success of any type of enterocele repair.

Surgical technique must include grasping the peritoneum carefully before needle placement to prevent placing the sutures too deeply and through the rectal wall. Both ureters should be identified before and after suture placement to check for ligation or kinking. As in the closure of all hernia sacs, permanent sutures should be used.

In addition to high ligation of the sac, horizontal support along the levator plate and reconstruction of a normal upper vaginal axis must be provided.[13] This latter aspect of the repair is accomplished by pulling the vaginal apex superiorly and posteriorly. Ligation of the hernia sac alone is not adequate to support the upper vagina (Table 31–1).

SUMMARY

Posterior vaginal support defects present a diagnostic and therapeutic challenge that may be made even more difficult by previous unsuccessful operations. Differential diagnosis includes rectocele, enterocele, and sigmoidocele; physical examination alone is not infallible in distinguishing among these entities. Evaluation must include examination in a gravity-dependent position to maximize the abnormality and defecography to determine the exact nature of the defect and identify coexisting pathology. Failure to diagnose and treat these other defects may contribute to poor surgical results.

Deciding whether the repair should be performed by a gynecologist or by a general or colorectal surgeon is not as critical as choosing a clinician with experience and familiarity with the anatomy, both normal and abnormal. Transvaginal repairs of rectoceles provide better exposure than a transrectal approach and offer the distinct advantage of being able to address other support defects as well. Before embarking on surgery, however, one must be sure that the rectocele is likely to be responsible for whatever symptoms the patient is experiencing. We know that rectoceles can be found in asymptomatic patients, so their significance in patients with vague symptoms must be questioned.

REFERENCES

1. Yoshioka, K, Matsui, Y, Yamada, O, et al: Physiologic and anatomic assessment of patients with rectocele. Dis Colon Rectum 34:704–708, 1991.
2. Bartram, CI, Turnbull, GK and Lennard-Jones JE: Evacuation proctography: An investigation of rectal expulsion in 20 subjects without defecatory disturbance. Gastrointest Radiol 13:72–80, 1988.
3. Freimanis, MG, Wald, A, Caruana, B and Bauman, DH: Evacuation proctography in normal volunteers. Invest Radiol 26:581–585, 1991.
4. Shorvon, PJ, McHugh, S, Diamant, NE, et al: Defecography in normal volunteers: Results and implications. Gut 30:1737–1749, 1989.
5. Delemarre, JBVM, Kruyt, RH, Doornbos, J, et al: Anterior rectocele: Assessment with radiographic defecography, dynamic magnetic resonance imaging, and physical examination. Dis Colon Rectum 37:249–259, 1994.
6. Nichols, DH: Rectocele and perineal defect. In Nichols DH (ed.): Gynecologic and Obstetric Surgery. Mosby-Year Book, St. Louis, 1993, pp 363–385.
7. Ting, KH, Mangel, E, Eibl-Eibesfeldt, B and Muller-Lissner, SA: Is the volume retained after defecation a valuable parameter at defecography? Dis Colon Rectum 35:762–767, 1992.
8. Goff, BH: A practical consideration of the damaged pelvic floor with a technique for its secondary reconstruction. Surg Gynecol Obstet 46:866, 1968.
9. Nichols, H and Randall, CL: Vaginal Surgery. Williams & Wilkins, Baltimore, 1976, pp. 62–63.
10. Wilensky, AV and Kaufman, PA: Vaginal hernia. Am J Surg 49:31–41, 1940.
11. Kuhn, RJP and Hollyock, VE: Observations on the anatomy of the rectovaginal pouch and septum. Obstet Gynecol 59:445, 1982.
12. Zacharin, RF: Pulsion enterocele: Review of functional anatomy of the pelvic floor. Obstet Gynecol 55:135, 1980.
13. Nichols, DH: Types of enterocele and principles underlying choice of operation for repair. Obstet Gynecol 40:257–263, 1972.
14. Burch, JC: Urethrovaginal fixation to Cooper's ligament for correction of stress incontinence, cystocele, and prolapse. Am J Obstet Gynecol 81:281–290, 1961.
15. Kelvin, FM, Maglinte, DD, Hornback, JA, et al. Pelvic prolapse: Assessment with evacuation proctography (defecography). Radiology 184:547–551, 1992.
16. Moschowitz, AV: The pathogenesis, anatomy, and cure of prolapse of the rectum. Surg Gynecol Obstet 15:7–21, 1912.
17. Halban, J: Gynäkoligische Operationslehre. Urban & Schwarzenberg, Berlin-Vienna, 1932, p. 172.

CHAPTER **32**

Vaginal Vault Prolapse

M. Chrystie Timmons • W. Allen Addison

The vaginal vault constitutes the cephalad extreme of the vaginal canal. This part of the vagina can prolapse toward, through, and beyond the introitus, regardless of whether a hysterectomy has been previously performed. Significant vaginal vault prolapse is a complex condition which confronts the clinician with a difficult challenge to manage. The multitude of treatment options, historical and current, surgical and nonsurgical, attests to the magnitude of this problem.

Effective management of vaginal vault prolapse requires knowledge of anatomy (normal and abnormal), expertise in accurate physical diagnosis, and skill in assessment of the clinical applicability of diagnostic tests. The surgeon dedicated to treating vaginal vault prolapse must be able to tailor the surgery to meet each patient's needs optimally. This mandates proficiency in the performance of a number of surgical approaches and precludes adherence to a single approach.

ETIOLOGY

Inasmuch as the vast majority of instances of urogenital prolapse occur in parous women, it has long been accepted that the major cause of support defects is vaginal delivery.[1] This probably results from detachment and attenuation of supporting tissues, but recent research suggests that partial denervation of pelvic floor muscles during delivery may play a role.[2] This mechanism in no way negates the predisposing effects of vaginal delivery in causing disorders of support, including those that progress to vaginal vault prolapse. Additional factors that may predispose to prolapse include those that generate chronic increases in intra-abdominal pressure with resulting stress on the pelvic floor. These include chronic pulmonary disease, repetitive occupational or recreational straining, constipation, and attempts to look thinner by wearing tight foundation garments.

Pelvic relaxation can accelerate rapidly after menopause or may exhibit worrisome progression with aging in general. Estrogen deprivation is known to decrease collagen content in tissues.[3] Pelvic support structures possess sex–steroid hormone receptors, the presence of which has not been demonstrated in nonpelvic supporting tissues.[4] Even with exogenous estrogen support, continued progression of pelvic relaxation can be observed with aging; the extent to which this may be related to earlier nerve damage caused by vaginal delivery, or to other neuropathy, is unknown.

Another important cause of vaginal vault prolapse is prior gynecologic surgery. DeLancey[5] has attributed the development of posthysterectomy vaginal eversion to disruption of the three levels of vaginal support. In this study on cadavers, different levels of disruption clearly correlated with different clinical presentations (enteroceles, cystoceles and rectoceles, and complete vaginal eversion). The concept of maintaining or re-establishing vaginal support during hysterectomy is not new.[6] General acceptance of this concept is evidenced by ongoing attempts to develop techniques that, during hysterectomy, may prevent subsequent enterocele formation and vaginal prolapse. Admonitions for attention to the cul-de-sac during hysterectomy continue to appear in the reports of experienced surgeons.[7–9]

Alteration of the axis of the upper vagina from its normal horizontal to a more anteriorly displaced position may also predispose to vaginal vault prolapse.[10] This alteration can occur after operations involving fixation of the vagina to anterior structures such as Cooper's ligament in Burch's colposuspensions[11] or to the pubic symphysis, as done in the Marshall-Marchetti-Krantz procedure.

In summary, although multiple causes of vaginal vault prolapse exist, increased understanding and recognition of risk factors should lead to a lower incidence of this problem. Decreasing pelvic floor and perineal stress at the time of delivery has been shown to decrease urogenital prolapse later in life.[2,12] Timely institution of estrogen-replacement therapy should enhance the maintenance of collagen and muscle of pelvic supporting structures in older women. Patients at increased risk because of their habits, occupation, or recreational stresses can be counseled regarding possible lifestyle changes intended to avoid repetitive increases in intra-abdominal pressure. Finally, and possibly most importantly, all surgeons performing procedures that can have negative effects on vaginal support mechanisms must be attuned to preserving and re-establishing support to the vagina in the course of surgery. Put simply, uterosacral–cardinal ligament plication and attention to Douglas's cul-de-sac must not be neglected.

DIAGNOSIS

Accurate diagnosis of vaginal vault prolapse and identification of other discrete support defects that are invariably present are essential for successful management and treatment. A precise medical history and a meticulous pelvic examination constitute the most important elements for diagnosis. The predominant symptoms reported by patients with vaginal eversion result from the vaginal prolapse itself (protrusion, pressure, difficulty in walking or sitting, coital impairment) and from concomitant prolapse of adjacent organs (urinary incontinence, frequency and urgency of urination, difficulty in initiating the urinary stream, fecal soiling, or difficulty defecating). The goal of the pelvic examination is to assess the degree of vaginal vault prolapse and to identify those support defects allowing the prolapse. A comprehensive pelvic examination should include a systematic grading of support defects of the six sites of potential prolapse along the vaginal canal (i.e., bladder, urethra, uterus, cul-de-sac, rectum, and perineum) while the patient is straining in the lithotomy position as described by Baden and Walker.[13] The patient should also be examined in the standing position, without straining, if any discrepancy between symptomatology and lithotomy examination seems to be present. Obviously, complete vaginal vault prolapse and eversion represent the maximum loss of support at all sites with accompanying paravaginal defects of the lateral vaginal walls (Fig. 32–1).

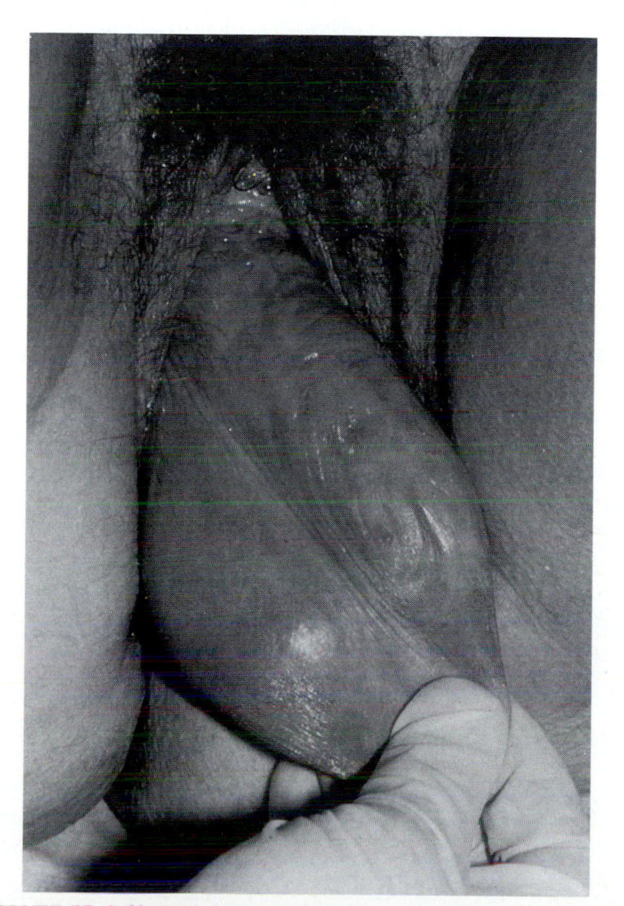

FIGURE 32–1. Vaginal vault prolapse with loss of all site-specific support.

Imaging techniques that have recently evolved are also potentially useful for diagnosis of specific defects of pelvic support. Evacuation proctography is more accurate than physical examination in the diagnosis of enterocele in patients with significant posterior compartment defects.[14] Fast magnetic resonance imaging (MRI) has been used to dynamically display support defects of all three compartments simultaneously.[15] A system of radiographic grading showed good correlation of radiographic findings with physical examination. Goodrich and associates[16] used conventional and snapshot MRI in five normal multiparous women and five women with pelvic prolapse both before and after surgical correction. The images showed a slightly higher degree of prolapse in patients diagnosed with mild prolapse on physical examination, excellent correlation with the physical diagnosis of moderate and severe prolapse, and excellent postoperative correction of all defects of support.

Magnetic resonance studies have the major disadvantage of studying prolapse with the patient in the supine position. A more promising technique has been described using dynamic fluoroscopy for total pelvic floor evaluation with the patient sitting at rest, when performing Kegel's exercises, and when defecating. All pelvic viscera, including the bladder, vagina, rectum, and small bowel, are opacified with contrast material before fluoroscopy. This technique was used in a study by Brubaker and colleagues[17] of 30 women with prolapse beyond the introitus. With this technique, they demonstrated improved diagnostic accuracy of the specific components of the vaginal prolapse. This technique may be useful for patients with confusing physical findings, unusual symptomatology, or recurrent prolapse. It would also be an excellent way to document restoration of normal anatomy after surgery. The ultimate role of imaging techniques in investigating and managing vaginal prolapse remains to be established.

Regardless of which technique is used to enhance accuracy of preoperative diagnosis, the surgeon must carefully assess the physical findings at the time of surgery. Satisfactory surgical correction of vaginal vault prolapse must entail confirmation of defects in anterior and posterior vaginal wall support, as well as correction of these persistent defects after suspension of the vagina. Indeed, an accurate final assessment of defects of the anterior or posterior vaginal wall can only be made after vaginal vault suspension.

MANAGEMENT

There are several important considerations in determining the management of vaginal vault prolapse, including patient age, lifestyle, general health, symptomatology, and degree of prolapse. In general, younger or more active patients benefit from the strongest support provided by the most durable operation. The frail, elderly, or sedentary patient may be managed nonsurgically initially or by surgical techniques that may be less extensive but still afford strength and durability. If the vaginal vault bulges beyond the introitus, however, surgical correction is indicated, except in the rare patient who cannot tolerate surgery and can successfully use a pessary.

Another consideration in managing uterovaginal prolapse is the patient's desire for preservation of fertility or retention of the uterus. If the prolapse descends beyond the introital opening, uterine suspension is usually indicated. With lesser degrees of uterovaginal prolapse, nonsurgical management can be attempted.

Preservation of fertility is an important concern but is infrequently expressed by most patients; instead, restoration and preservation of vaginal coital function is the usual goal. Many patients with posthysterectomy vaginal prolapse have had prior operations for prolapse and incontinence and may present with already compromised vaginal caliber, depth, and coital dysfunction. Obviously, any procedure that further compromises and foreshortens the vagina is contraindicated. Conversely, an elderly woman with no desire for retention of vaginal coital function may not object to a procedure that results in vaginal obliteration or compromise.

The general categories of nonsurgical and surgical management of vaginal vault prolapse are listed in Table 32–1. The categories of surgical management are by necessity broad. Many different operations have been developed some of which are of historical interest only. The diversity of surgical techniques in the literature attests to the clinical challenge of managing vaginal vault prolapse while understanding no "perfect" operative approach with consistent efficacy, durability, and universal applicability exists. The surgical options discussed in this chapter are limited to currently used operations.

NONSURGICAL MANAGEMENT

Nonsurgical management of vaginal vault prolapse consists of pelvic floor–muscle exercises and pessaries. Exercises originated with the universally known

TABLE 32–1. Management of Vaginal Vault Prolapse

Nonsurgical
- Pelvic floor muscle exercises
  - Kegel's exercises
  - Biofeedback
  - Vaginal cones
- Pessaries

Surgical
- Vaginal
  - Suspensions
  - Obliterative procedures
- Abdominal
  - Vaginopexies
  - Abdominal sacral colpopexy

Kegel maneuvers. Although regular performance of contractions of the pubococcygeal muscle may improve pelvic floor–muscle tone and stress urinary incontinence, no evidence exists that these exercises successfully manage significant vaginal vault prolapse. Likewise, biofeedback with sensors and computer display programs has refined the instruction and performance of pelvic floor exercises. Weighted vaginal cones have been used to promote steady contraction of the pelvic floor muscles around the cone to prevent its extrusion. A search of the literature provides no evidence in terms of prospective, blinded, randomized studies demonstrating that enhanced pelvic floor–muscle tone leads to control or regression of vaginal vault prolapse.

Since antiquity, management of uterovaginal prolapse has been attempted using an almost endless variety of types of pessary. Indications for pessary use in the current management of uterovaginal prolapse are limited. Examples include pregnant patients, patients wishing to retain reproductive capacity without resorting to surgery, and patients with vaginal prolapse in whom surgery is prohibitively dangerous. Additionally, the patient who refuses, or who must delay, surgery may derive some relief from pessary use. Pessary retention may not be possible for the patient with total vaginal eversion and complete loss of support. Details of pessary selection and use, including recent designs, are presented in Chapter 34.

SURGICAL MANAGEMENT

The principles of surgery for vaginal vault prolapse include correction of support defects and restoration of normal anatomy and function. Whether a vaginal or abdominal approach is chosen, surgery must include excision of the enterocele sac or obliteration of the cul-de-sac, resuspension of the vaginal vault to adequate supporting tissues, using either natural or synthetic material, and repair of all concomitant defects of pelvic support.

Vaginal Approaches

Vaginal approaches can be divided into two categories: suspensions and obliterative procedures. In either approach, it is our belief that culdoplasty is essential. Most patients with vaginal vault prolapse require colpoplastic repair of the anterior and/or posterior vaginal walls, the rare exception being the patient whose prolapse results from a central enterocele in the presence of sustained anterior and posterior wall support. Given[18] reported excellent results with recurrent prolapse in only 2 of 68 patients with vaginal vault prolapse who underwent only culdoplasty with colpoplastic repairs.

The most common transvaginal suspension in current use is the sacrospinous ligament suspension. After culdoplasty has been performed and anterior defects have been addressed, the vaginal vault is suspended, generally unilaterally, to the sacrospinous ligament by means of sutures placed in the ligament and then secured to the vaginal vault as described by Nichols.[19] Excellent results have been reported by Morley and DeLancey.[20] Likewise, Shull and colleagues[21] reported excellent results in correcting vault prolapse but did note the propensity for recurrence of anterior vaginal wall relaxation after sacrospinous ligament suspension. Alternative suspension sites include obturator internus fascia and iliococcygeus fascia.[22] Attachment to the obturator internus fascia is analogous to abdominal paravaginal defect repairs done transvaginally. In our opinion, the iliococcygeus fascial attachment provides effective cuff suspension with less risk of nerve or vascular damage than does sacrospinous ligament suspension.

The second category of vaginal approaches for vault prolapse involves obliterative procedures. The Neugebauer-LeFort operation is an obliterative procedure, which maintains the uterus in situ while one performs anterior-posterior closure of the vaginal walls. This can also be performed if the patient had an earlier hysterectomy. It is best suited for the elderly patient, because it is less extensive. Large studies with long-term follow-up have documented durable reduction of the prolapse,[23,24] but urinary incontinence is a worrisome sequela. Our preference for a vaginal obliterative procedure is meticulous culdoplasty (generally, modified Miller's procedure) with extensive colpoplastic repairs and extensive partial colpectomy with colpocleisis. This leaves a markedly shortened vagina of narrow caliber, but the vesical neck is not placed on downward traction, which might predispose to incontinence. This procedure is well tolerated by even the frail and elderly patient and is durable. With all the vaginal obliterative procedures, the patient and her sexual partner must understand preoperatively that vaginal coital function will not be possible after the surgical procedure.

Abdominal Approaches

The underlying principle of abdominal approaches for treatment of vaginal vault prolapse is to attach the vaginal vault to a supporting structure with natural or synthetic material. The vaginal vault has been attached to the anterior rectus fascia by strips or ox fascia[25] or fascia lata,[26] to Cooper's ligaments that had been detached and tunneled beneath the round ligaments,[27] and to external oblique muscle fascia in like fashion.[28] These operations are rarely used today. Baden and Walker[29] described excellent results by placing sutures bilaterally at the vaginal cuff angles and presacral uterosacral ligaments, performing a culdoplasty, and then tying the cuff suture to the corresponding suture on each side.

Abdominal sacral colpopexy with attachment of the prolapsed vaginal vault to the sacral periosteum with a suspensory sling of synthetic material has

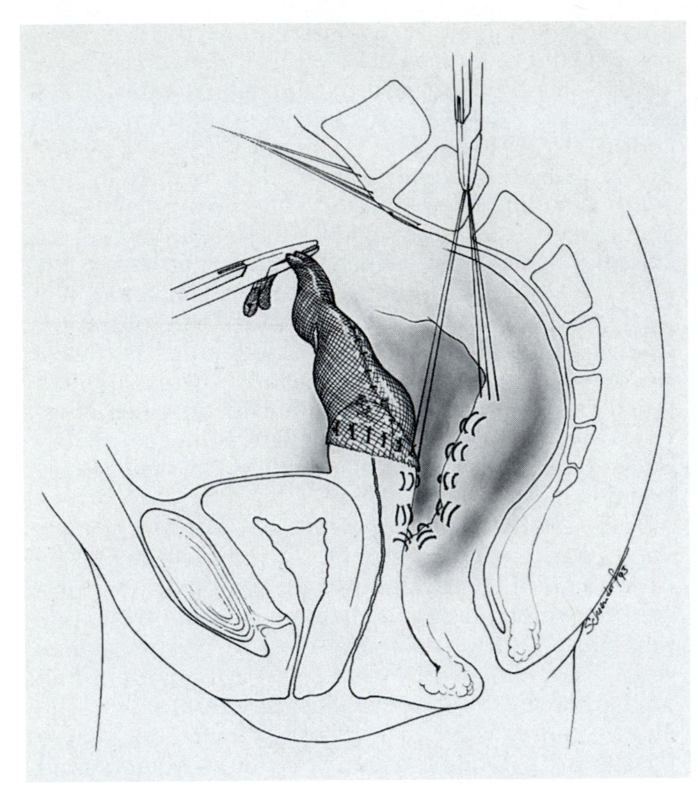

FIGURE 32–2. Abdominal sacral colpopexy technique. Attachment of suspensory mesh around the entire vaginal vault and placement of Halban's culdoplasty sutures.

been shown to be effective with little risk of recurrent prolapse in two large series with long-term follow-up.[30,31] The basic appearance of the techniques performed are shown in Figure 32–2. A full description of the technique we currently employ has been reported.[31] Culdoplasty is always performed. The tension on the mesh between the vaginal vault and the sacrum should be sufficient to provide support but not so tight as to straighten the anterior vaginal wall excessively, thus predisposing the patient to postoperative urinary incontinence.

In total uterovaginal prolapse, abdominal sacral colpopexy can be performed in conjunction with abdominal hysterectomy. Because the risk of infection from mesh may be higher, care should be taken to avoid placing synthetic material or attaching sutures near the cuff. In addition, the cuff should be closed with additional imbricating layers over the suture line (Fig. 32–3).

Preservation of Fertility and Surgical Management

Surgical management of total uterovaginal prolapse does not preclude uterine preservation. Nichols[33] has described an abdominal approach with construction of a sacrocervical ligament of fascia lata or a sacrospinous cervicopexy where the cervix is sewn on one side to the sacrospinous ligament and coccygeus muscle complex. Richardson, Scotti, and Ostergard[34] also described success in treating uterovaginal prolapse with sacrospinous ligament suspension in five women, but no ensuing pregnancies occurred. Nesbitt[35] performed a combination bladder neck and lower uterine suspension to Cooper's ligament. Again, only one of his 16 patients underwent the procedure for fertility preservation and she developed tubal occlusion from pelvic inflammatory disease soon after the procedure and was thereafter unable to become pregnant. In India, uterovaginal prolapse is apparently common in young women; Allahbadia[36,37] described two series with good subsequent fertility and delivery outcomes, comparing several different uterine conservative approaches. Finally, the prolapsed uterus may be resuspended and attached to the sacral periosteum with synthetic material or to the anterior abdominal wall in patients with bladder exstrophy.[32]

SURGICAL FAILURE

Any patient who has had recurrent urogenital prolapse remains at risk for recurrent prolapse after a surgical procedure. Any surgeon would be foolish to guarantee permanent correction postoperatively in patients with vaginal vault prolapse. Understanding potential, and often avoidable, causes for surgical failure, however, can help the surgeon reduce the chances of surgical failure in any given patient. If surgical failure does occur, careful evaluation must be performed to attempt to determine the cause of failure in order to provide appropriate management of the recurrent prolapse.

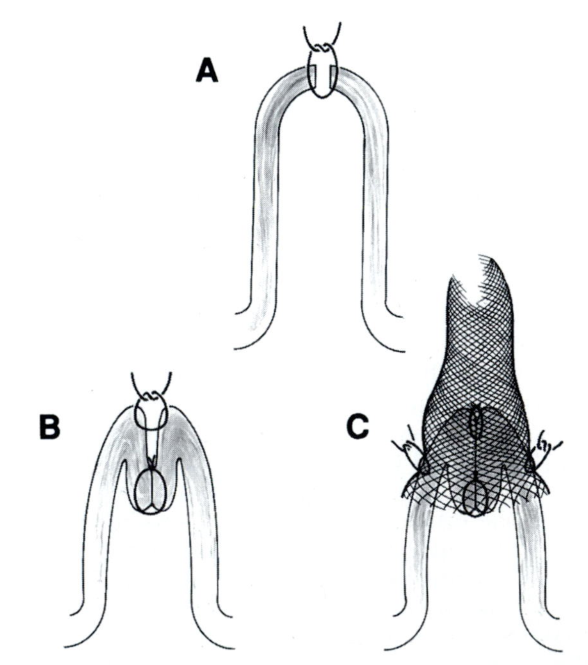

FIGURE 32–3. Recommended cuff closure and attachment of suspensory mesh when sacral colpopexy is performed with hysterectomy.

Causes

Many potential causes for recurrent vaginal vault prolapse after corrective surgery exist. Some are related to patient factors, such as poor tissues and impaired healing potential (chronic diabetes, malnutrition, collagen dysfunction), chronic pathologic increases in intra-abdominal pressure or patient failure to comply with recommendations to avoid activities that generate severe increases in intra-abdominal pressure.

Most causes for failure, however, are probably related to surgical technique. First, the diagnosis may have been incomplete. In vaginal vault prolapse, it is essential to recognize accurately all support defects and to treat them. For example, if an anterior wall defect is not diagnosed, and a patient undergoes vaginal suspension alone, she is likely to have persistence or progression of the untreated anterior compartment. If the diagnosis is correct, an incorrect operation may have been chosen; for example, a young, active woman who undergoes only a culdoplasty may well experience recurrent prolapse. Even if the diagnosis and operative plan are correct, performance of the surgery can be suboptimal. Use of too few sutures, sutures that are too weak, or sutures that are placed too superficially can certainly predispose to failure.[38]

Evaluation

When surgical failure or recurrent prolapse ensues, the surgeon must then proceed with a meticulous, site-specific evaluation of the prolapse. The careful, detailed history must focus not only on the symptoms of vaginal prolapse but also on the chronology and associated activities that may have led to recurrence. Again, the pelvic examination must be careful and comprehensive, as if there was no history of earlier failures of repair. In our experience, the diagnosis most frequently missed by a referring physician is a middle compartment defect with enterocele leading to vaginal vault descent.

Because previous surgery may distort anatomy, imaging techniques may be a useful adjunct to evaluate recurrent vaginal vault prolapse accurately. This might be especially helpful to determine the extent of residual support from the previous procedures.

Management

Management of recurrent vaginal vault prolapse deserves an especially thoughtful approach. One may choose to repeat the original operation, if evidence indicates the failure results from suboptimal technique. For example, in a failed sacral colpopexy, the top of the vagina may have been poorly secured to a narrow suspensory material.[38] Alternatively, the clinician may elect to perform a different operation for repeat surgical correction. For example, a patient who has earlier vaginal procedures that failed might do well with an abdominal procedure. If earlier vaginal suspension was performed using natural material, synthetic material could be considered for a repeat procedure. Finally, any patient with recurrent vaginal vault prolapse must be approached surgically using those techniques that are specified in the literature to afford the greatest durability.

SUMMARY

Vaginal vault prolapse, both before and after hysterectomy, continues to constitute a formidable management challenge. Physicians treating patients with this problem must be capable of individualizing management to the best advantage of each patient. The ability to individualize management appropriately requires familiarity with a spectrum of surgical and nonsurgical approaches and demands ongoing awareness and inclusion of new developments in this field.

REFERENCES

1. Gainey, HL: Postpartum observation of pelvic tissue damage: Further studies. Am J Obstet Gynecol 70:800, 1955.
2. Smith, ARB, Hosker, GL and Warrell, DW: The role of partial denervation of the pelvic floor in the aetiology of genitourinary prolapse and stress incontinence of urine. A neurophysiological study. Br J Obstet Gynaecol 96:24, 1989.
3. Brincat, M, Kabalan, S, Studd, JW, et al: A study of the decrease of skin collagen content, skin thickness, and bone mass in the postmenopausal woman. Obstet Gynecol 70:840, 1987.
4. Smith, P, Heimer, G and Norgren, A: Steroid hormone receptors in pelvic muscles and ligaments in women. Gynecol Obstet Invest 30:27, 1990.
5. DeLancey, JOL: Anatomic aspects of vaginal eversion after hysterectomy. Am J Obstet Gynecol 166:1717, 1992.
6. Symmonds, RE and Pratt, JH: Vaginal prolapse following hysterectomy. Am J Obstet Gynecol 79:899, 1960.
7. Symmonds, RE and Sheldon, RS: Vaginal prolapse after hysterectomy. Obstet Gynecol 25:61, 1965.
8. Cruikshank, SH: Preventing posthysterectomy vaginal vault prolapse and enterocele during vaginal hysterectomy. Am J Obstet Gynecol 156:1433, 1987.
9. Borenstein, R, Elchalal, U, Goldschmit, R, et al: The importance of the endopelvic fascia repair during vaginal hysterectomy. Surg Gynecol Obstet 175:551, 1992.
10. Nichols, DH, Milley, PS and Randall, CL: Significance of restoration of normal vaginal depth and axis. Obstet Gynecol 36:251, 1970.
11. Wiskind, AK, Creighton, SM and Stanton, SL: The incidence of genital prolapse after the Burch colposuspension. Am J Obstet Gynecol 167:406, 1992.
12. Ranney, B: Decreasing numbers of patients for vaginal hysterectomy and plasty. S D J Med 43:7, 1990.
13. Baden, WF and Walker, T: Fundamentals, symptoms, and classification. In Baden, WF and Walker, T (eds.): Surgical Repair of Vaginal Defects. JB Lippincott, Philadelphia, 1992, p 9.
14. Kelvin, FM, Maglinte, DD, Hornback, JA, et al: Pelvic prolapse: Assessment with evacuation proctography (defecography). Radiology 184:547, 1992.
15. Yang, A, Mostwin, JL, Rosenshein, NB, et al: Pelvic floor descent in women: dynamic evaluation with fast MR imaging and cinematic display. Radiology 179:25, 1991.

16. Goodrich, MA, Webb, MJ, King, BF, et al: Magnetic resonance imaging of pelvic floor relaxation: Dynamic analysis and evaluation of patients before and after surgical repair. Obstet Gynecol 82:883, 1993.
17. Brubaker, L and Given, FT, Jr: Pelvic floor evaluation with dynamic fluoroscopy. Obstet Gynecol 82:863, 1993.
18. Given, FT: "Posterior culdeplasty": Revisited. Am J Obstet Gynecol 153:135, 1985.
19. Nichols, DH: Sacrospinous fixation for massive eversion of the vagina. Am J Obstet Gynecol 142:901, 1982.
20. Morley, G and DeLancey, JOL: Sacrospinous ligament fixation for eversion of the vagina. Am J Obstet Gynecol 158:872, 1988.
21. Shull, BL, Capen, CV, Riggs, MW, et al: Preoperative and postoperative analysis of site-specific pelvic support defects in 81 women treated with sacrospinous ligament suspension and pelvic reconstruction. Am J Obstet Gynecol 166:1764, 1992.
22. Shull, BL, Capen, CV, Riggs, MW, et al: Bilateral attachment of the vaginal cuff to iliococcygeus fascia: An effective method of cuff suspension. Am J Obstet Gynecol 168:1669, 1993.
23. Hanson, GE and Keettel, WC: The Neugebauer-le Fort operation: A review of 288 colpocleises. Obstet Gynecol 34:352, 1969.
24. Ubachs, JMH, Van Sante, J and Schellekens, LA: Partial colpocleisis by a modification of LeFort's operation. Obstet Gynecol 42:415, 1973.
25. Ward, GE: Ox fascia lata for reconstruction of round ligaments and correcting prolapse of the vagina. Arch Surg 36:163, 1938.
26. Beecham, CT and Beecham, JB: Correction of prolapsed vagina or enterocele with fascia lata. Obstet Gynecol 42:542, 1973.
27. Langmade, CF: Cooper ligament repair of vaginal vault prolapse. Am J Obstet Gynecol 92:601, 1964.
28. Richardson, AC and Williams, GA: Treatment of prolapse of the vagina following hysterectomy. Am J Obstet Gynecol 105:90, 1969.
29. Baden, WF and Walker, T: Abdominal approach to superior vaginal defects. In Baden, WF and Walker, T. (eds.): Surgical Repair of Vaginal Defects. JB Lippincott, Philadelphia, 1992, p 119.
30. Synder, TE and Krantz, KE: Abdominal-retroperitoneal sacral colpopexy for the correction of vaginal prolapse. Obstet Gynecol 77:944, 1991.
31. Timmons, MC, Addison, WA, Addison, SB, et al: Abdominal sacral colpopexy in 163 women with posthysterectomy vaginal vault prolapse and enterocele: Evolution of operative techniques. J Reprod Med 37:323, 1992.
32. Addison, WA and Timmons, MC: Abdominal approach to vaginal eversion. Clin Obstet Gynecol 36:995, 1993.
33. Nichols, DH: Fertility retention in the patient with genital prolapse. Am J Obstet Gynecol 164:1155, 1991.
34. Richardson, DA, Scotti, RJ and Ostergard DR: Surgical management of uterine prolapse in young women. J Reprod Med 34:388, 1989.
35. Nesbitt, REL: Uterine preservation in the surgical management of genuine stress urinary incontinence associated with uterovaginal prolapse. Surg Gynecol Obstet 168:143, 1989.
36. Allahbadia, GN: Reproductive performance following sleeve excision anastomosis operation for genital prolapse. Aust N J Obstet Gynaecol 32:149, 1992.
37. Allahbadia, GN: Obstetric performance following conservative surgery for pelvic relaxation. Int J Gynecol Obstet 38:293, 1992.
38. Addison, WA, Timmons, MC, Wall, LL, et al: Failed abdominal sacral colpopexy: observations and recommendations. Obstet Gynecol 74:480, 1989.

CHAPTER 33

Cystocele

Anita Pillai-Allen • J. Thomas Benson

Cystoceles, although a common clinical diagnosis, present a significant challenge for those treating pelvic floor disorders. They may be considered the nemesis of the pelvic surgeon. Controversy exists in their definition, diagnosis, and treatment; this chapter attempts to review current understanding of this problem.

DEFINITION

Any abnormal descent of the anterior vaginal wall and bladder base at rest or with strain is considered a cystocele. Although classification systems exist, the opinions of two well-known authors are summarized below. A.C. Richardson[1–2] has described cystoceles based on four anatomic defects noted in the pubocervical fascia and its attachments (Fig. 33–1). He theorizes that cystoceles occur secondary to "breaks in the continuity of bladder support."

Lateral or *paravaginal defects* occur when pubocervical fascia detaches from the fascia overlying the obturator internus and levator muscles, at the arcus tendineus fascia pelvis (white line). This results in descent of the lateral vaginal sulci. This type of defect is most commonly seen, and may be unilateral or bilateral.[3] Often, it is unilateral with predominance on the right side for unknown reasons. Frequently, urethrovesical junction hypermobility and stress urinary incontinence are present.

Transverse defects occur when pubocervical fascia detaches from its central attachment at the pericervical ring of fibromuscular tissue. This is also where the cardinal and uterosacral ligaments attach. When this type of defect occurs alone, it can produce a large cystocele with anterior vaginal fornix obliteration but with normal lateral and vesical neck support. Frequently, a voiding dysfunction may result, with increased residual urine volumes.

Central defects occur when the pubocervical fascia breaks in the midline underneath the bladder base. It can result in urethrovesical junction hypermobility and stress urinary incontinence, if the break extends

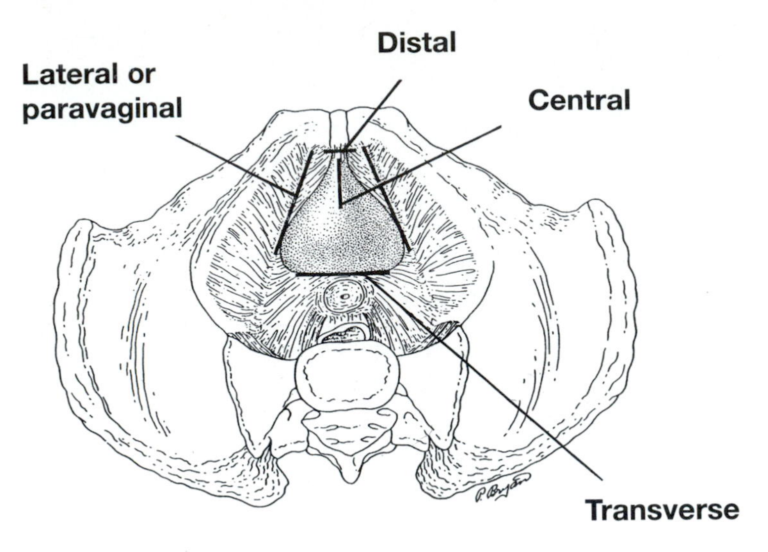

FIGURE 33–1. A. C. Richardson has described four anatomic defects in the pubocervical fascia and its attachments that may result in cystocele formation. (Source: Richardson, AC, Lyons, JB and Williams, NL: A new look at pelvic relaxation. Am J Obstet Gynecol 126:568, 1976, with permission.)

to the vesical neck. If this defect occurs alone, lateral sulci and the anterior vaginal fornix will be intact.

The rarest defect described is a *distal defect.* It represents detachment of the pubocervical fascia distally from the urogenital diaphragm.

D.H. Nichols[4–9] describes cystoceles as *anterior* or *posterior*, based on their position relative to the interureteric ridge. An *anterior cystocele* represents varying degrees of rotational descent of the urethra and vesical neck during strain.[10]

A *posterior cystocele* represents a descent of the bladder base posterior to the interureteric ridge with an intact urethrovesical junction. The posterior cystocele may be further distinguished as either a distention-type or displacement-type cystocele.

A *distention cystocele* (Fig. 33–2) is attributed to the overstretching and thinning of the anterior vaginal wall associated with parturition. It can worsen with atrophy of the intrinsic structural components of the vaginal wall caused by aging, estrogen deprivation, or both. Clinically, anterior vaginal wall rugae are diminished or absent.

A *displacement cystocele* (Fig. 33–3) is attributed to

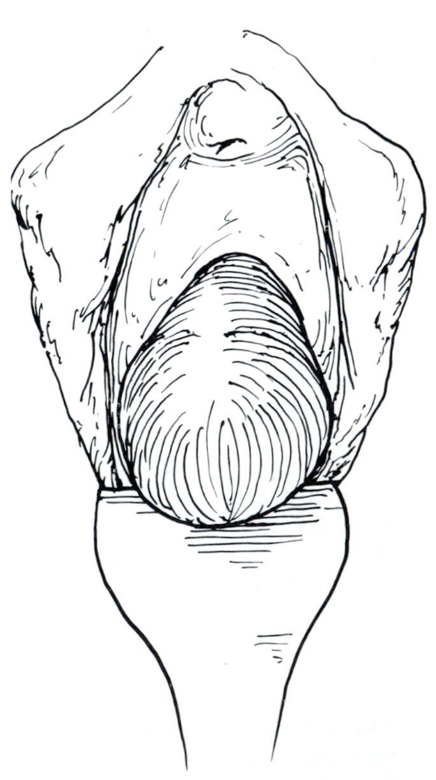

FIGURE 33–2. A distention cystocele.

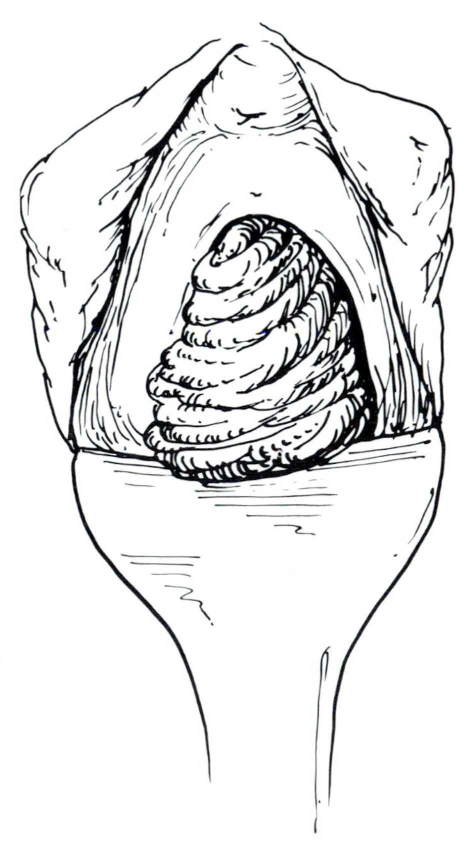

FIGURE 33–3. A displacement cystocele.

elongation or loss of lateral vaginal support from the arcus tendineus fascia pelvis. Clinically, rugae are well preserved but loss of lateral sulci is noted. Combinations of anterior and posterior cystoceles are common.

Although these classifications differ, points of similarities exist in these two paradigms of cystocele. Regardless of the terminology, emphasis should be placed on thorough evaluation of each patient's anatomic abnormality. Until a standardized terminology is formulated, narrative descriptions may be more helpful in communications between examiners. An opportunity to communicate is lost when descriptive terms are replaced by single digit grades (i.e., 1–4).

DIAGNOSIS AND GRADING

The history and physical examination have been the cornerstones of diagnosis of prolapse. Women may report "heaviness," "pressure," "a feeling of something falling," or a "protrusion" or "bulge" at the introitus. There may be associated vaginal irritation, low back pain, or difficulty during sexual intercourse. Most symptoms are exacerbated by standing for a long time or by physical exertion. Occasionally, large cystoceles may cause voiding difficulties requiring digital maneuvers to initiate or complete urination.[4–6] If incomplete emptying occurs, increased residual urine and urinary stasis[4–6] may result in recurrent urinary tract infections. Urinary frequency, urgency, nocturia, or incontinence may be associated complaints.

Although this chapter primarily discusses cystoceles, it is important to remember the dynamic relationship between all compartments of the pelvic floor; a wholistic approach is crucial.[11,12]

Diagnostic tests are not required for evaluation of a cystocele itself, but are essential to assess the patient for lower urinary tract dysfunction. This is particularly important if the patient is symptomatic or if surgical therapy is planned.

NONSURGICAL MANAGEMENT

Management of pelvic support abnormalities includes both nonsurgical and surgical options. Asymptomatic patients do not require intervention. Patients who have minimal symptoms, or only mild to moderate degrees of prolpase may opt for treatment with a pessary.[13] The pessary has a dual function as a diagnostic tool and a supportive treatment (see Chapter 34).

SURGICAL MANAGEMENT

Surgical management remains the primary mode of therapy for cystoceles. Traditionally, anterior colporrhaphy with vesical neck plication has been the procedure of choice. Several authors[5,6,14–16] have described their techniques of anterior colporrhaphy based on modifications of the original Kelly plication stitch,[17] introduced in 1913 for relief of urinary incontinence. The mere presence of so many variations of anterior colporrhaphy implies that imperfect results are obtained clinically. Although few studies have directly addressed long-term follow-up, failure rates as high as 40% to 45% have been noted.[18,19] As a result, we have abandoned the use of standard anterior colporrhaphy for cystocele correction. The paravaginal repair, discussed subsequently, is most commonly performed when surgery is undertaken. In the following discussion, techniques for both abdominal and vaginal paravaginal repair are described.

Before surgical therapy, the patient's preoperative status should be optimized. All pre-existing medical illnesses are evaluated and treated appropriately, with particular attention to cardiovascular disease, pulmonary disease, diabetes, and genitourinary infections. Estrogen deficiency is treated if no contraindications to it exist to improve vaginal tissue. Weight reduction is encouraged for obese patients. Smokers are advised to quit to reduce surgical morbidity and to improve long-term results. Pelvic floor exercises are taught and written instructions reviewed.[20,21] Physical therapy is frequently used when pelvic floor weakness is noted. Potential risks and complications of the procedures are explained, and postoperative instructions and expectations are outlined.

ABDOMINAL PARAVAGINAL REPAIR

Abdominal paravaginal repair[1,2,22,23] is indicated for pure lateral or displacement-type cystoceles. It is performed to reattach the vagina and overlying pubocervical fascia to its correct anatomic position at the arcus tendineus fascia pelvis. The arcus, or the white line, extends from the inferior pubic symphysis along the pelvic side wall to the ischial spine (Fig. 33–4).

The patient is placed in a modified dorsal lithotomy position using Allen's universal stirrups. A 20-Fr Foley catheter is placed for drainage of the bladder and identification of the urethrovesical junction. A Pfannenstiel incision is taken through the rectus fascia. The retropubic space is exposed by retraction of the rectus muscles. The peritoneum is dissected from the underside of the muscle and the transversalis fascia is sharply incised over the posterior surface of the pubic bone. Gentle, blunt dissection is performed laterally along the superior pubic ramus until the obturator canal is palpated. Dissection is now directed inferiorly to the ischial spine, often using the blunt tip of a suction apparatus. The Vital Vue (Vital Vue Metric, San Diego, CA) provides both illumination and irrigation, which can be extraordinarily helpful when performing this procedure. The bladder is

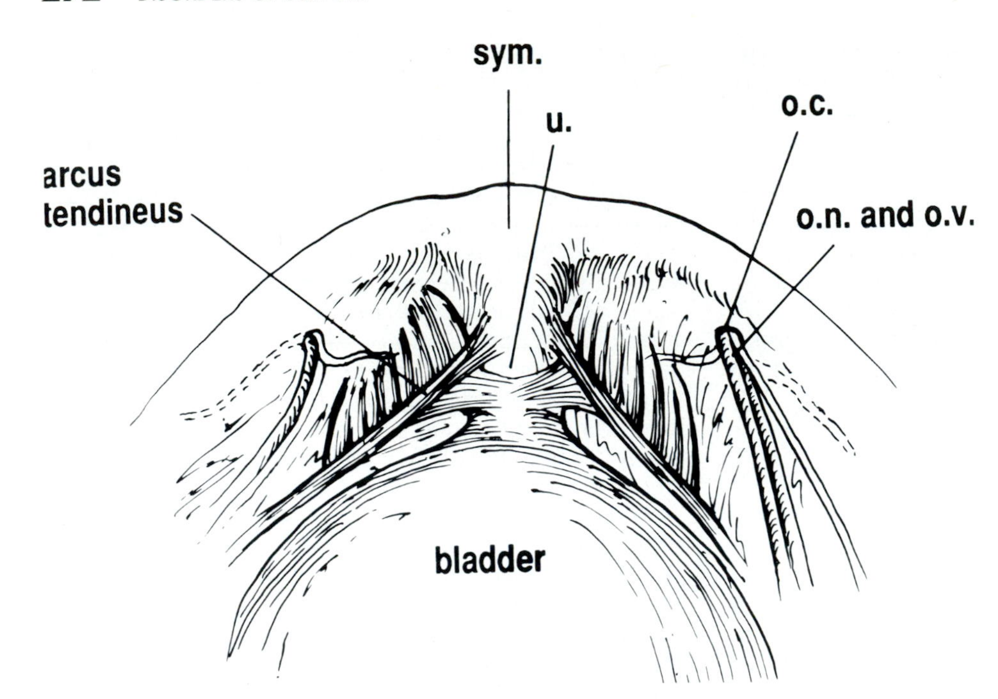

FIGURE 33–4. The arcus, or white line, extends from the inferior pubic symphysis (sym.) along the pelvic side wall to the ischial spine. u = urethra; o.c. = obturator canal; o.n. = obturator nerve; o.v. = obturator vein.

then retracted medially and the prominent veins along the lateral vaginal sulcus are exposed (Fig. 33–5). The operator's nondominant hand is placed into the vagina to elevate the lateral vaginal sulcus (Fig. 33–6). An assistant continues to retract the bladder medially during suture placement. The first stitch incorporates the entire vaginal muscularis for approximately 1 cm anterior to the ischial spine; one must also encircle the prominent lateral sulcus veins (Fig. 33–7). The lateral suture is then taken through the obturator fascia at the level of detachment of the fascial arcus. Additional stitches are placed anteriorly at 1-cm increments, along the vaginal sulcus toward the pubic ramus (Fig. 33–8). Sutures are tied after all the stitches have been placed. Permanent suture material is strongly recommended. The procedure is then performed on the opposite side. If anatomic stress incontinence was diagnosed preoperatively, a Burch-type[24,25] retropubic urethropexy may be performed. Suprapubic teloscopy or cystoscopy is then performed to verify ureteral patency and absence of intraluminal permanent suture. The bladder is filled with 10% dextrose through the Foley catheter, while 5 mL of indigo carmine are given intravenously. Rarely, a cystotomy is required for adequate assessment.

VAGINAL PARAVAGINAL REPAIR

Vaginal paravaginal repair was originally described in 1909 by White.[26,27] Theoretically, this technique may be used when a lateral or displacement cysto-

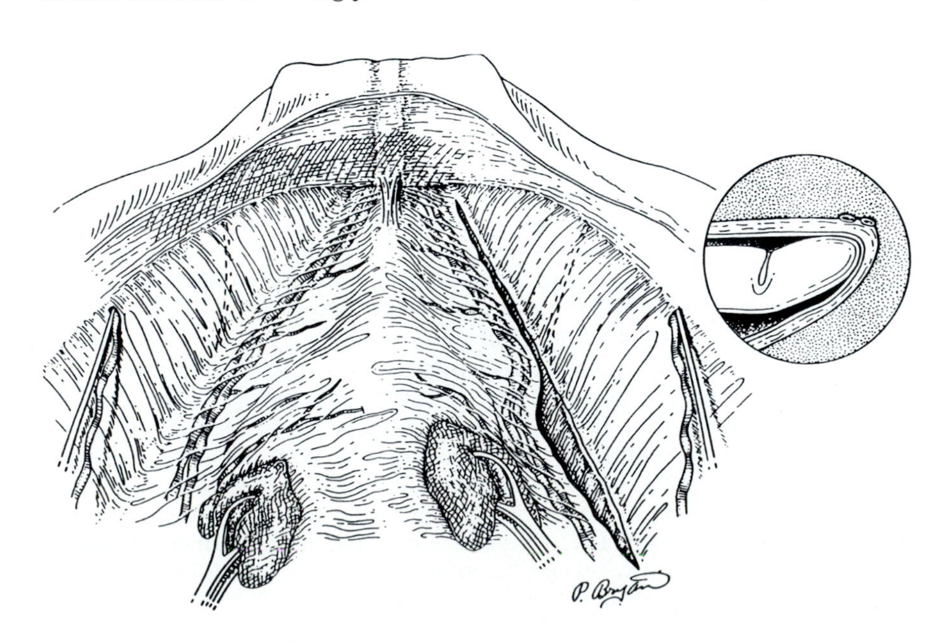

FIGURE 33–5. During an abdominal paravaginal repair, the bladder is retracted medially and the prominent veins along the lateral vaginal sulcus are exposed. (Source: Richardson, AC, Lyons, JB and Williams, NL: A new look at pelvic relaxation. Am J Obstet Gynecol 126:568, 1976, with permission.)

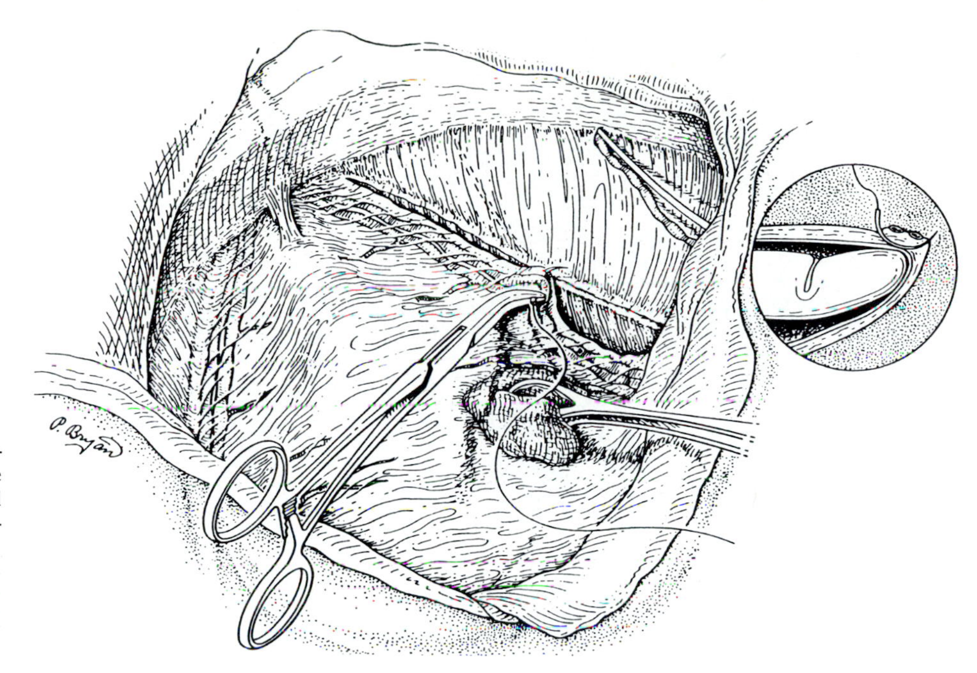

FIGURE 33–6. The operator's nondominant hand is then placed into the vagina to elevate the lateral vaginal sulcus. The bladder is retracted medially during suture placement. (Source: Richardson, AC, Lyons, JB and Williams, NL: A new look at pelvic relaxation. Am J Obstet Gynecol 126:568, 1976, with permission.)

cele requires correction but the clinician wishes to avoid a laparotomy because of the patient's obesity or coexisting medical illnesses. This repair permits simultaneous correction of vaginal, perineal, or rectal disorders with a local approach. Restoring normal anatomy by reattaching the vagina to the arcus tendineus fasciae pelvis is achieved by the vaginal repair, just as with the abdominal paravaginal cystocele repair. If a midline vaginal incision is used, central or transverse apical defects may be corrected simultaneously by standard plication techniques. Benson and colleagues observed 60 patients treated with the vaginal paravaginal cystocele repair (with or without midline plication) over a 14-month period. Protrusion of the anterior vaginal wall through the introitus during the Valsalva maneuver with the patient in the upright position was noted after a 2-year follow-up in 50% of the patients, with the majority of these being central or distention-type cystoceles. This led to the modification of the vaginal paravaginal cystocele repair to incorporate mesh[28,29] (as described subsequently) when significant central or distention components coexisted with lateral defects on preoperative cystocele diagnosis (Fig. 33–9).

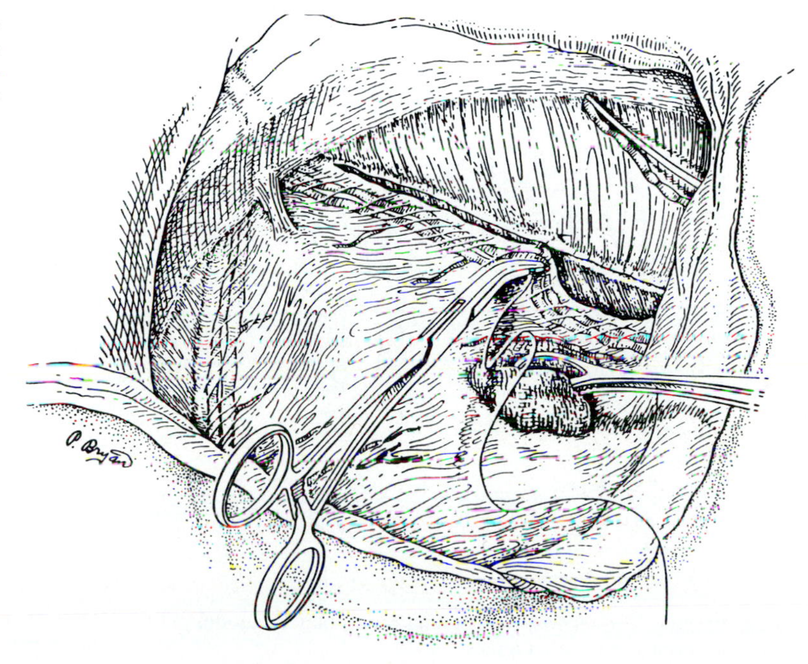

FIGURE 33–7. The vaginal stitch incorporates the entire vaginal muscularis, approximately 1 cm anterior to the ischial spine, encircling the prominent lateral sulcus veins. The lateral suture is placed through the obturator fascia at the level of fascial detachment. (Source: Richardson, AC, Lyons, JB and Williams, NL: A new look at pelvic relaxation. Am J Obstet Gynecol 126:568, 1976, with permission.)

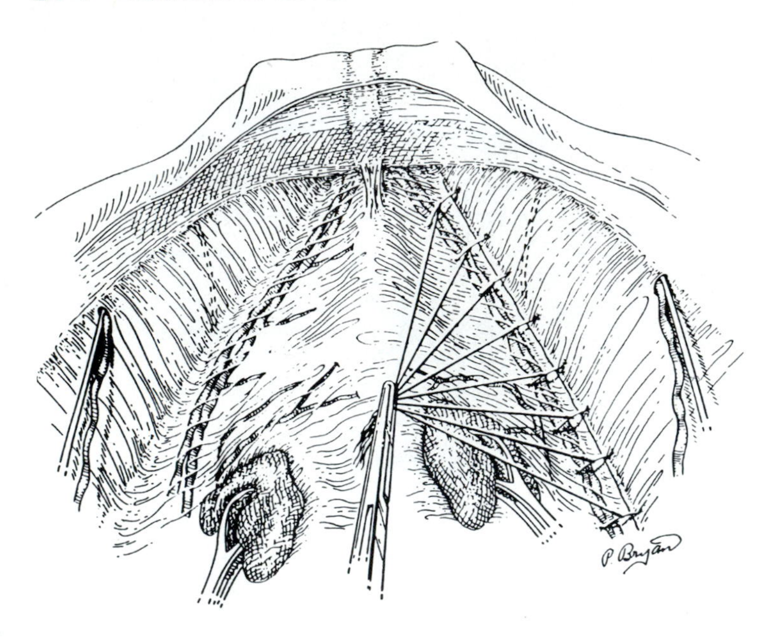

FIGURE 33–8. Additional stitches are placed anteriorly at 1-cm increments, along the vaginal sulcus toward the pubic ramus. (Source: Richardson, AC, Lyons, JB and Williams, NL: A new look at pelvic relaxation. Am J Obstet Gynecol 126:568, 1976, with permission.)

Vaginal Paravaginal Cystocele Repair with Prolene Mesh

The patient is placed in the dorsal lithotomy position and a 20-Fr Foley catheter is placed to drain the bladder. It is then clamped and used throughout the procedure to aid in identification of the urethrovesical junction. A midline vaginal incision is made (Fig. 33–10) and marking sutures are placed laterally on the anterior vaginal wall at the level of the urethrovesical junction and ischial spine. These markers guide the surgeon in placing the sutures properly along the anterior vaginal wall for elevation to the arcus tendineus fasciae pelvis. A piece of prolene mesh is cut in a trapezoidal shape using the marking sutures as a guide; it is then soaked in antibiotic solution of gentamicin and bacitracin. The mesh will later be incorporated into the vaginal paravaginal cystocele repair to lie like a hammock between the pelvic side walls, giving support to the entire bladder base. It may also provide a framework for scarification and collagen deposition.

Allis's clamps are placed in the midline from the urethrovesical junction to the vaginal apex. Saline solution is injected into the proper avascular surgical

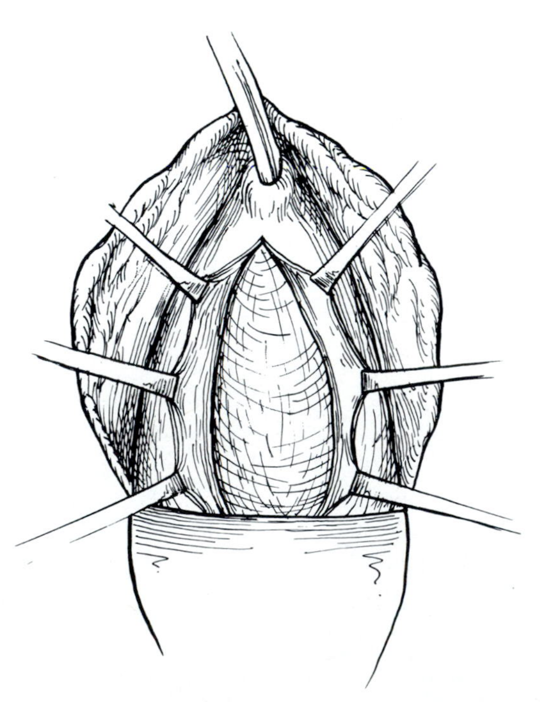

FIGURE 33–9. The vaginal paravaginal repair may be modified to augment poor fascia using a mesh.

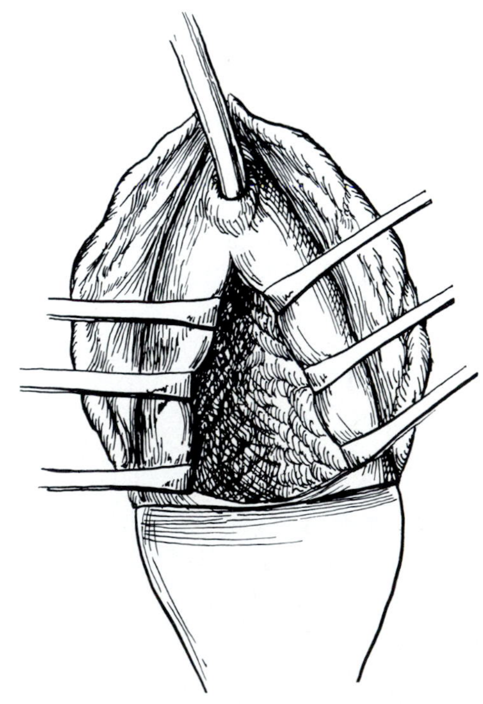

FIGURE 33–10. The vaginal paravaginal repair begins with a midline vaginal incision.

plane. The midline incision is made and the vaginal mucosa sharply dissected to completely delineate the cystocele (Fig. 33–11). Dissection is then carried lateral to the urethrovesical junction so the operator's finger can bluntly puncture through the urogenital diaphragm to enter the space of Retzius. Occasionally, sharp puncture is required. The posterior surface of the superior pubic ramus is palpated and blunt dissection is performed laterally until the obturator canal is reached (Fig. 33–12). The operator's finger is now swept inferiorly toward the ischial spine. Caution must be taken to avoid injury to the obturator nerve and vessels by always remaining posterior and inferior to the obturator canal. The Breisky-Navratil retractor is used gently to retract the bladder medially. Under direct visualization, a Deschamps ligature carrier is used to place permanent sutures in the obturator internus fascia at 1-cm increments beginning near the ischial spine and extending along the arcus tendineus to the pubis symphysis. Structures in danger of injury include the internal pudendal nerves and vessels by the ischial spine, obturator nerves and vessels by the obturator canal, and the inferior hypogastric nerve plexus overlying the iliococcygeal muscle.)[30] These sutures are tagged and then incorporated into the prolene mesh with the base of the trapezoid aligned at the level of the ischial spine and the apex at the urethrovesical junction (Fig. 33–13). After being placed through the prolene mesh proportionally, the sutures are now sewn into the vaginal wall using the markers as a guide. The same procedure is performed on the opposite side. The mesh is secured in a hammock-like fashion, underneath the bladder base with lateral attachments to the obturator internus fascia at the pelvic side walls (Fig. 33–14). It should not be overly

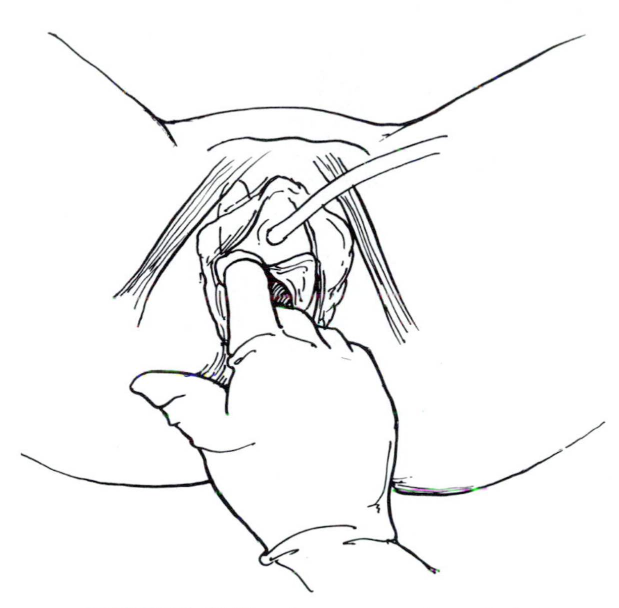

FIGURE 33–12. The obturator canal is palpated.

taut, because postoperative bladder dysfunction or erosion may result. On the other hand, if placed too loosely, the mesh does not provide the supportive function for which it is intended. Copious irrigation with the antibiotic solution (using the "Vital Vue" device) is performed throughout the procedure. Routinely a Pereyra-type[31,32] or Nichols-type[33] urethropexy is performed prophylactically for elevation of the urethrovesical junction, secondary to occurrence

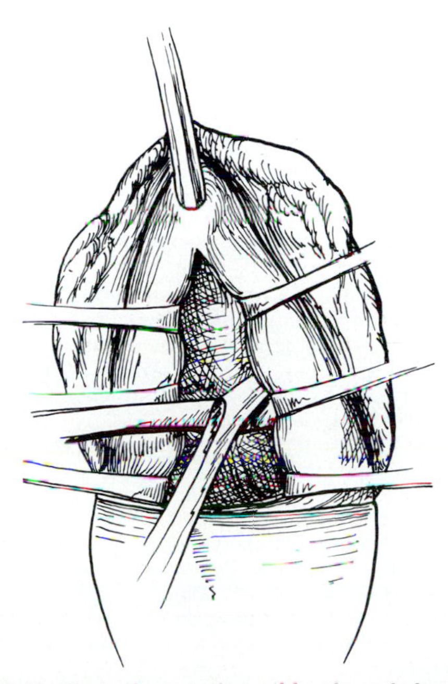

FIGURE 33–11. Dissection continues bluntly and sharply into the space of Retzius.

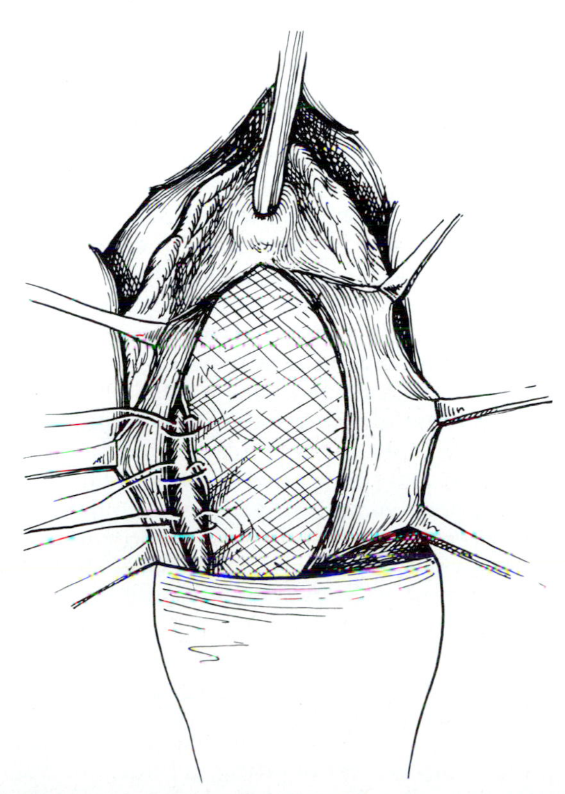

FIGURE 33–13. Previously placed marking sutures are used to attach a permanent mesh to the arcus tendineus.

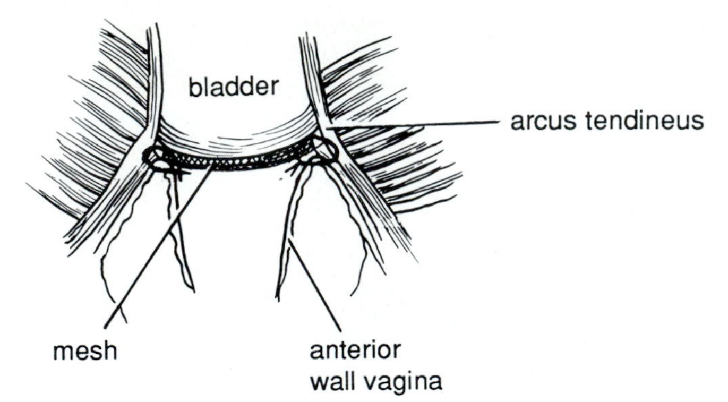

FIGURE 33–14. A trapezoid of mesh is used to elevate the bladder.

of genuine stress urinary incontinence postoperatively in patients without evidence of stress incontinence on preoperative testing. We theorize that this incontinence most likely results from disruption of urethral supports or neuropathy created during the vaginal dissection.[34] The vaginal mucosa is trimmed and then closed in a two-layer fashion with 2-0 polyglactin sutures. The bladder is then drained, filled with 300 mL of 10% dextrose solution. Indigo carmine is given intravenously. Urethrocystoscopy is performed to document bilateral ureteral patency and absence of suture within the bladder. A suprapubic tube is placed using direct cystoscopic guidance. The patient is given prophylactic intravenous antibiotics for the first 24 hours and then changed to an oral regimen such as doxycycline and metronidazole for 10 days. Routine management of bladder drainage and voiding trials are instituted.

Preliminary assessment of 24 women who underwent this mesh procedure has shown promising results.[35] In comparison with 50 women who had a standard vaginal paravaginal cystocele repair, overall failure rates were significantly reduced.[35]

The use of the abdominal wedge resection[36] of the anterior vaginal wall in patients with significant central cystocele is not recommended due to unacceptable recurrence rates. If a patient has a significant central cystocele in addition to a paravaginal defect, the vaginal paravaginal cystocele repair with mesh placement may be considered.

There may be a role for absorbable mesh in this procedure. No data support this approach, however, and clinical trials will be needed. Because the vaginal route produces neuropathy, the abdominal route may be preferred. Although these procedures are more extensive and more costly in the short term, they may be more economically beneficial if recurrence rates are reduced.

RECURRENCES

Recurrent cystoceles are approached cautiously. If the patient desires reoperation, all anterior vaginal wall defects must be carefully delineated. Surgical therapy should be individualized for the patient's specific anatomic defects; the same procedure should not be performed for every anterior-wall prolapse. Attention is given to meticulous technique in order to restore normal anatomy. Most importantly, all other pelvic support abnormalities must be repaired concurrently.

FOLLOW-UP

Follow-up observation of patients is essential in determining the subjective and objective success of surgical therapy. Postoperative evaluations at 2 weeks, 6 weeks, 6 months, and 1 year are recommended. Thereafter, yearly visits are sufficient so long as patients remain asymptomatic.

At each visit, patients are interviewed for symptoms of prolapse and urinary, sexual, and anorectal dysfunction. A pelvic examination is performed, with emphasis on the anterior vaginal wall. Pelvic floor muscle strength is reassessed, and daily performance of Kegel's exercises is emphasized. Physical therapy is used on an individual basis.

Support of the anterior vaginal wall remains a challenge to the pelvic surgeon. We hope the information summarized in this chapter is thought-provoking and will inspire readers to seek nuances in diagnosis and therapy with each patient they treat.

REFERENCES

1. Richardson, AC, Lyons, JB and Williams, NL: A new look at pelvic relaxation. Am J Obstet Gynecol 126:568, 1976.
2. Richardson, AC, Edmonds, PB and Williams, NL: Treatment of stress urinary incontinence due to paravaginal fascial defect. Obstet Gynecol 57:357, 1981.
3. Benson, JT: Female pelvic floor disorders: Investigation and management. WW Norton & Company, New York, 1992, p. 280.
4. Nichols, DH: Vaginal prolapse affecting bladder function. Urol Clin North Am 12:329, 1985.
5. Nichols, DH and Randall, CL: Vaginal Surgery, ed 3., Williams & Wilkins, Baltimore, 1989, p. 239.
6. Nichols, DH: Gynecologic and Obstetric Surgery. Mosby-Year Book, St. Louis, 1993, p. 334.
7. Nichols, DH: Effects of pelvic relaxation on gynecologic urologic problems. Clin Obstet Gynecol 21:759, 1978.
8. Nichols, DH: Surgery for pelvic floor disorders. Surg Clin North Am 71:927, 1991.
9. Ball, TL: Anterior and posterior cystocele. Clin Obstet Gynecol 9:1062, 1966.
10. Enhorning, G, Miller, ER and Hinman, F: Urethral closure studied with cineroentgenography and simultaneous bladder–urethra pressure recording. Surg Gynecol Obstet 108:507, 1964.
11. Wall, LL and DeLancey, JOL: The politics of prolapse: A revisionist approach to disorders of the pelvic floor in women. Perspect Biol Med 34:486, 1991.
12. Benson, JT: The compartmentalization of the female pelvic floor. Int Urogynecol J 2:195, 1991.
13. Brubaker, LT: The vaginal pessary. American Urogynecologic Society Quarterly Report 9(3):1991.
14. Schram, M: Cystocele etiology. N Y State J Med 76:370, 1976.
15. Schram, M and Schram, D: Cystocele repair: A modified technique. Obstet Gynecol 29:447, 1967.
16. Kennedy, E: Urinary incontinence relieved by restoration and maintenance of normal position of the urethra. Am J Obstet 41:116, 1941.
17. Kelly, HA: Incontinence of urine in women. Urol Cutan Rev 17:291, 1913.

18. Baden, WF and Walker, T: Urinary stress incontinence: Evaluation of paravaginal repair. Fem Patient 2:89, 1987.
19. Stanton, SL and Tenagho, EA: Preface. In Stanton SL, Tenagho EA (eds.): Surgery of Female Incontinence. Springer-Verlag, New York, 1980.
20. Ferguson, KL, McKey, PL, Bishop, KR, et al: Stress urinary incontinence: Effect of pelvic muscle exercise. Obstet Gynecol 75:671, 1990.
21. Kegel, A: Progressive resistance exercise in the functional restoration of the perineal muscles. Am J Obstet Gynecol 56:238, 1948.
22. Shull, BL and Baden, WF: A six year experience with paravaginal defect repair for stress urinary incontinence. Am J Obstet Gynecol 160:1432, 1989.
23. Youngblood, JP: Paravaginal repair. Contem OB/GYN 35:28, 1990.
24. Burch, JC: Urethrovaginal fixation to Cooper's ligament for correction of stress incontinence, cystocele and prolapse. Am J Obstet Gynecol 81:281, 1961.
25. Tenagho, EA: Colpocystourethropexy: The way to do it. J Urol 116:751, 1976.
26. White, GR: An anatomic operation for the cure of cystocele. Am J Obstet Dis Wom Child 65:286, 1912.
27. White, GR: Cystocele, a radical cure by suturing lateral sulci of vagina to white line of pelvic fascia. JAMA 53:1701, 1909.
28. Friedman, EA and Meltzer, RM: Collagen mesh prosthesis for repair of endopelvic fascial defects. Am J Obstet Gynecol 106:430, 1970.
29. Moore J, Armstrong, JT and Willis, SH: The use of Tantalum mesh in cystocele with critical report of ten cases. Am J Obstet Gynecol 69:1127, 1955.
30. Benson, JT: Female Pelvic Floor Disorders: Investigation and Management. WW Norton & Company, New York, 1992, p. 289.
31. Pereyra, AJ, Lebherz, TB, Growden, WA, et al: Pubourethral supports in perspective: Modified Pereyra procedure for urinary incontinence. Obstet Gynecol 59:643, 1982.
32. Karram, MM and Bhatia, NN: Transvaginal needle bladder neck suspension procedures for stress urinary incontinence: A comprehensive review. Obstet Gynecol 73:906, 1989.
33. Nichols, DH and Milley, PS: Identification of pubourethral ligaments and their role in transvaginal surgical correction of stress incontinence. Am J Obstet Gynecol, 115:123, 1973.
34. Benson, JT and McClellan, E: The effect of vaginal dissection on the pudendal nerve. Obstet Gynecol 82:387, 1993.
35. Caputo, RM and Benson, JT: Vaginal paravaginal repair with mesh placement for cystocele. American Urogynecologic Society Annual Meeting, November 1993, San Antonio, TX.
36. Macer, GA: Transabdominal repair of cystocele, a 20 year experience, compared with the traditional vaginal approach. Am J Obstet Gynecol 131:203, 1978.

CHAPTER 34

Use and Care of the Pessary

Linda T. Brubaker • Michael Heit

The pessary is a classic gynecologic instrument, which has been used for several generations; many variations of it have been introduced over the past 200 years by both patients and physicians. Current indications for pessary use are limited to support of prolapsing pelvic organs and temporary repositioning of an incarcerated pregnant uterus. Other indications had been considered but have fallen into disfavor because of a lack of scientific support (e.g., infertility secondary to uterine malposition, cervical incompetence, and treatment of pelvic pain).

Although a rare indication, the strongly retroverted or anteverted uterus may become incarcerated at the pelvic brim at the end of the first trimester of pregnancy. Such patients may present with pelvic pain or acute urinary retention. Treatment includes manual repositioning of the uterus, which can be augmented, if indicated, with pessary placement to prevent recurrence until the uterus is large enough to stay above the symphysis.

A pessary offers a nonsurgical option for patients with prolapse of the pelvic organs.[1,2] Although this disorder is generally managed surgically, certain patients can be treated with nonoperative means if social or medical reasons delay planned definitive surgery, or if the patient's strong preference or poor medical condition rule out surgery.[3] Alternatively, the pessary may appeal to women who have undergone unsuccessful surgical correction for prolapse. This nonsurgical option provides a psychologic, physiologic, and financial respite before another surgical attempt at definitive repair is made.

PREREQUISITES FOR PESSARY PLACEMENT

There are several prerequisites for pessary placement. Most important is that the patient must be available for active follow-up, by either the physician placing the appliance or a willing alternative caregiver, such as a nurse or physician's assistant.[4] Pessaries should not be placed in cognitively impaired patients unless the caretaker can promise proper follow-up visits. The other main consideration is the thickness of the vaginal tissues. Unestrogenized vaginal tissues are generally prone to erosions by any vaginal foreign body. Consequently, a pessary is rarely placed in a markedly hypoestrogenic vagina. Vaginal or oral estrogen should be given according to the prevailing clinical guidelines. Perineal sensory deficits are a contraindication to pessary placement, because such patients with this disorder may not be able to report dangerous erosions or abnormalities in bowel or bladder emptying.

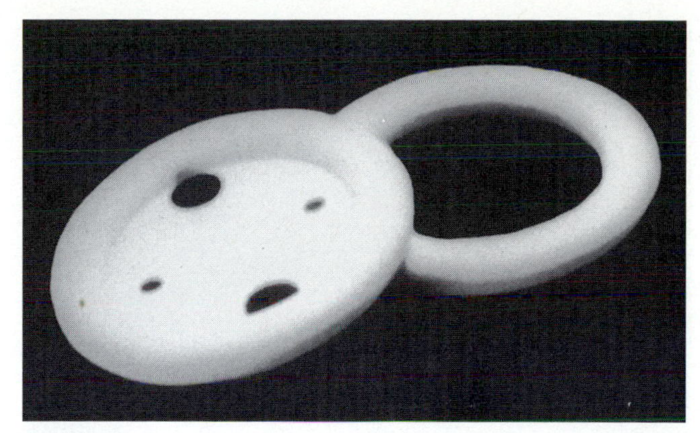

FIGURE 34–1. A ring pessary and a ring with support. (Courtesy of Milex Products, Chicago, IL.)

FITTING

Pessary fitting should begin following a discussion with the patient about the diagnosis and the treatment options. If the patient wishes to proceed with pessary placement, the physician should have at hand a variety of sizes and types of pessaries. With the patient in the lithotomy position, a confirmatory pelvic examination estimates the size of the pessary to be inserted. This pessary is then gently inserted, striving to keep pressure off the urethra. After the pessary has been placed in the vagina, it is prudent to ask the patient to bear down forcefully. If the pessary is immediately expelled in the supine position, it is unsuitable and must be resized. After the proper size and type have been selected and successfully inserted, the patient is asked to return to the sitting position. At this point, it is helpful to allow the patient some time to privately "test" her pessary with various maneuvers including standing, squatting, and the Valsalva maneuver, among others. Generally, this test is best accomplished in the privacy of a washroom or examination room. After approximately 5 minutes, the physician should return and assess the patient's comfort and the position of the pessary. If the pessary is causing discomfort (e.g., uncomfortable rectal pressure) it is not properly fitted and will not be a successful intervention for this patient, in whom a different design or size should be tried.

PESSARY OPTIONS: TYPES OF PESSARIES

Although a wide variety of pessaries is available, most practitioners find that using two or three familiar types is sufficient for patients' requirements and most patients can be managed by selecting a pessary from a relatively small office inventory.

RING AND RING WITH SUPPORT

This type of pessary (Fig. 34–1) is one of the simplest to fit, insert, and explain to patients. The form and placement mimics that of a contraceptive diaphragm. These pessaries are made of plastic or rubber and are available in sizes 0 to 13. In our practice, approximately 75% of patients use this model. It is particularly useful for prolapse that is predominantly anterior or anteroapical.

These pessaries should be inserted into the vagina by bending the device into a half-moon at it flexion point. Using an oblique orientation, the pessary is then pushed into the vagina and allowed to open to its full diameter. The pessary should be placed snugly behind the pubic symphysis. Posteriorly, the rim should be placed posterior to the cervix (if present). With proper fitting, a single finger-width should remain between the pessary and the pubic symphysis. Once properly fitted, the flexion point should be rotated off the midline to reduce the risk of spontaneous pessary explusion.

DOUGHNUT

The doughnut pessary is preferred by many gynecologists. This pessary (Fig. 34–2) is somewhat thicker than the ring type. It is made of rubber and is supplied in sizes 0 to 6 (2″–3½″ in diameter). Although this type of pessary is relatively easy to fit, it tends to be more difficult than the ring for patients

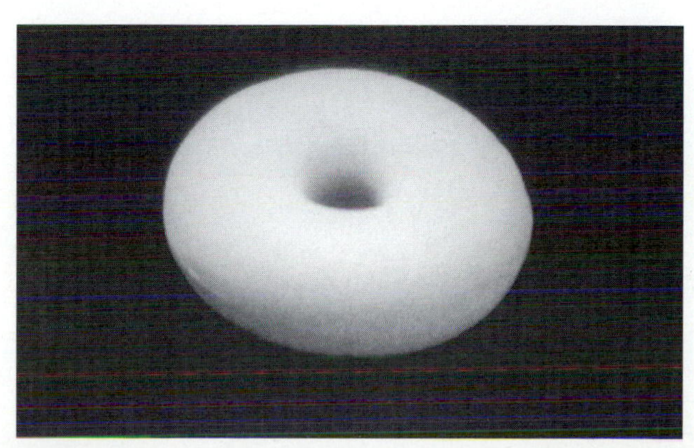

FIGURE 34–2. A doughnut pessary. (Courtesy of Milex Products, Chicago, IL.)

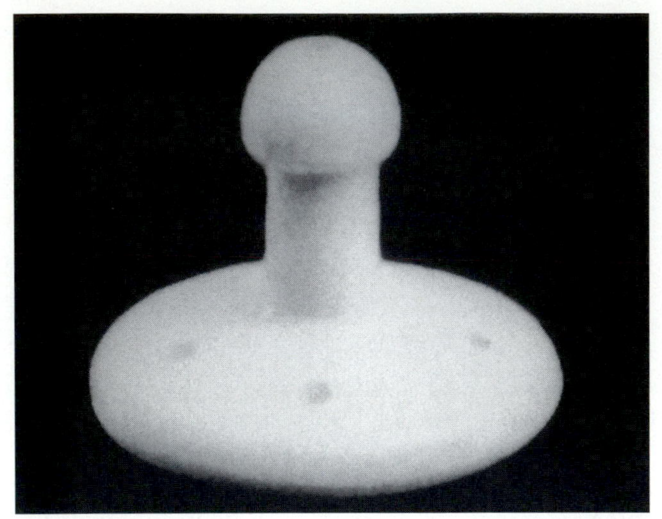

FIGURE 34–3. A Gellhorn pessary. (Courtesy of Milex Products, Chicago, IL.)

to manage on their own. In comparison to the ring or ring with support, the doughnut provides sufficient support for more severe forms of prolapse. Adequate integrity of the introital opening is essential for retention of this pessary.

Insertion of the doughnut pessary mimics insertion of the ring pessaries, with only minor differences. The doughnut pessary does not have a flexion point. Therefore, the physican should compress the pessary as much as possible and insert the device into the vaginal canal fully, only then releasing the compression. The doughnut should fit comfortably when opened in the vagina.

THE GELLHORN PESSARY

The Gellhorn pessary (Fig. 34–3) is used for patients with moderate to severe prolapse. This pessary relies on the integrity of the perineal body for its retention. It is placed with the stem portion positioned posteriorly, inside the introitus. This pessary is available in diameters from 1½″ to 3½″. This pessary is favored by Sulak, Kuehl, and Shull.[5]

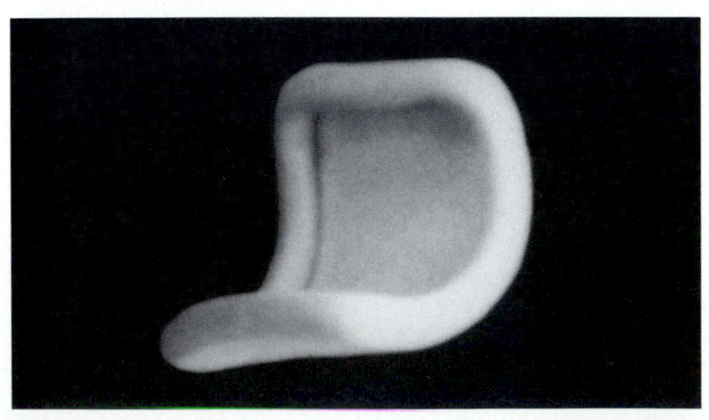

FIGURE 34–4. A Gehrung pessary. (Courtesy of Milex Products, Chicago, IL.)

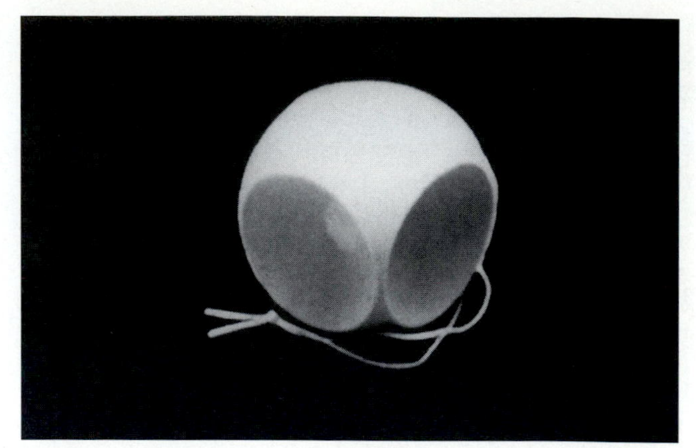

FIGURE 34–5. A cube pessary. (Courtesy of Milex Products, Chicago, IL.)

The Gellhorn pessary is placed with the wide, flat surface toward the anterior vaginal wall. The knob handle rests on the posterior vaginal wall, gaining support from the perineal body. It is best introduced into the vagina in an oblique manner, taking unnecessary pressure off the urethra.

THE GEHRUNG PESSARY

The Gehrung pessary (Fig. 34–4) is designed to provide differential support to the anterior vaginal wall. Bladder support and the effect on continence have not been studied scientifically.

This pessary is folded onto itself and placed obliquely into the vagina. After it is in the vaginal canal, it is allowed to open into its full arch form. The base of the arch rests on the posterior walls and the curve supports the anterior wall.

CUBE AND INFLATO-BALL

The cube pessary (Fig. 34–5) provides support in the absence of introital or perineal integrity. The vast majority of gynecologists rarely use this pessary, however, because it frequently causes a vaginal discharge with an unmistakably strong odor, reminiscent of a forgotten tampon. In general, this pessary should be used as a temporary measure for only a few days, such as when support is needed just before definitive surgical repair.

The Inflato-ball (Fig. 34–6) provides general support for the prolapsing vaginal structures. This pessary is made of rubber and has a filling port, which allows inflation and deflation of the supportive structure. The advantages include less risk of erosion and greater ease of insertion and removal. Patients decline or accept this device simply based on a description of the design.

The cube and Inflato-ball are fitted simply by approximating the capacity of the vagina, visually selecting the pessary that best approximates this volume, and inserting it to confirm proper size selection.

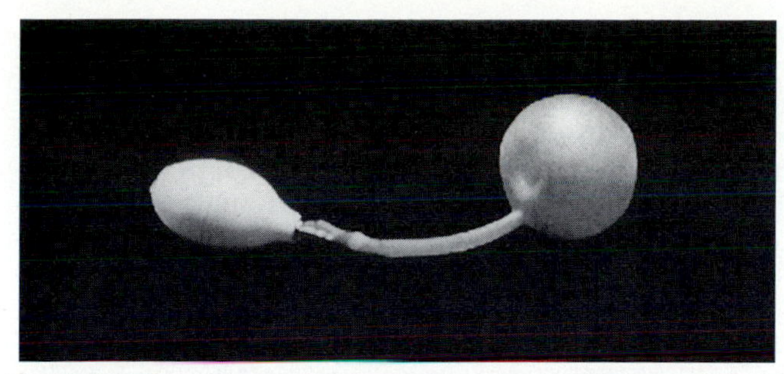

FIGURE 34–6. Inflato-ball pessary. (Courtesy of Milex Products, Chicago, IL.)

THE HODGE, SMITH-HODGE, AND RISSER PESSARIES

These pessaries are used primarily for repositioning of the uterus (Fig. 34–7). Although these designs may provide support to certain patients with prolapse, they are less commonly used than those listed above.

DISCUSSIONS AFTER FITTING

After the pessary is properly fitted and is providing adequate support of the prolapsing pelvic organs, the physician should discuss bowel and bladder control. Patients with prolapse frequently have coexisting dysfunction of bowel and bladder control. Urinary incontinence is particularly common, occurring in an estimated 30% to 60% of women with prolapse.

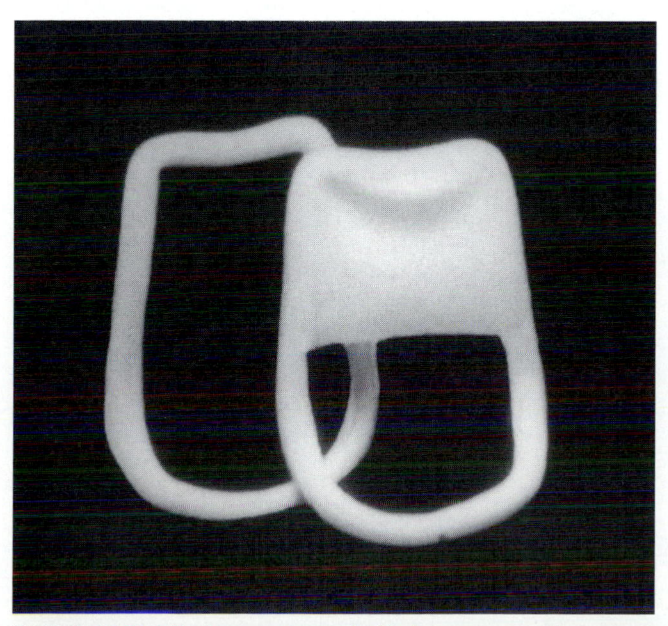

FIGURE 34–7. A Hodge pessary and a Hodge pessary with support. (Courtesy of Milex Products, Chicago, IL.)

These women may notice worsening of incontinence and should be forewarned. Paradoxically, some may notice decreased incontinence, presumably due to some level of urethral obstruction caused by the pessary. Women who have not experienced urinary incontinence should be specifically warned that they have a risk of "potential" incontinence which has previously been masked by the prolapse. These patients may exhibit incontinence after the prolapse has been reduced. Such patients must understand that the incontinence is not caused by the pessary, but simply by the unmasking of an underlying disorder.

Despite efforts to fit a pessary carefully, the only way to know if the pessary is effective for an individual patient is to have her wear the device for 2 to 3 days. If the pessary has been well chosen and properly fitted, the patient will report excellent symptom relief, no new symptoms, and no awareness that the pessary is in situ. Alternatively, patients may report no relief symptoms, *new* symptoms (such as urinary incontinence), or dislodgement or loss of the pessary. These patients may wish to try another pessary or may wish to proceed to presurgical counseling.

FOLLOW-UP

After proper fitting and discussion of bladder control, the physician should see the patient within 2 or 3 days to be sure the pessary is comfortable and has been retained, and that the patient has no new symptoms, such as urinary incontinence or difficulties with defecation. At the first follow-up visit, the pessary should be removed and the vagina inspected for erosions. If all is well, the physician can discuss options for management. Many women are quite capable of pessary management and can be easily taught to remove, clean, and reinsert their pessaries. Such self-reliance gives them a great deal of freedom, allowing fewer visits to the physician. Many patients prefer to remove the pessary at night, in anticipation of sexual activity. This nightly removal offers additional protection against erosions. Other patients may prefer to wear their pessary continuously, day and night, with removal on only a weekly basis. Although no scientific data direct such recommendations, it seems prudent to suggest that pessary care should occur at a minimum of every 6 to 8 weeks.

The physician may elect to continue to provide pessary care. Patients should present at approximately 6- to 8-week intervals. Shorter intervals are appropriate for patients with low estrogen levels and thin vaginal walls. Longer intervals may be used in patients with more normal levels of estrogen who are reliable in symptom reporting. Patients with pessaries should be actively observed. The neglected pessary, although rare, may be a source of serious morbidity. There is no shortage of case reports of neglected pessaries which have eroded into a variety of pelvic viscera.[3,6,7]

PESSARY CLEANING AND REPLACEMENT

Modern pessaries may be cleaned with simple soap and water. Although some discoloration of the plastic or rubber may occur, this is not harmful. The pessary should be replaced when there is cracking or a loss of supportive characteristics such as spring-like flexion. For patients who live long distances from their physician, and for women who travel or spend certain seasons of the year elsewhere, it is wise to provide a *spare* pessary in case the pessary regularly used becomes lost or damaged.

MANAGEMENT OF EROSIONS

Vaginal erosion occurs in a minority of patients. Assuming adequate estrogenization of the tissues, erosions can generally be managed by "pessary rest." The general principle is simply to decrease the time that the pessary is in the vagina. Occasionally, a smaller or different type of pessary may be indicated. For patients who are managing their own pessaries, nightly removal is often successful in managing erosions. Patients who rely on their physician for management may require removal of the pessary for 2 to 4 weeks until the erosion has healed. When the pessary is then reinserted, evaluations should resume at more frequent intervals. Recurrent erosions are an indication for discontinuation of pessary use. Erosions that are refractory to periods when the pessary is not used are suspicious for malignant or premalignant disease and should be biopsied.

DISCONTINUATION OF PESSARY USE

The pessary may be discontinued for a number of reasons. The most common is a desire for definitive surgical correction. Others include new onset or worsening of bowel or bladder symptoms. Recurrent erosions or the inability to comply with management requirements are also indications for discontinuation of pessary use.

DIAGNOSTIC USE OF THE PESSARY

The pessary has two main diagnostic uses. The first is to determine symptom relief with prolapse replacement. The second is to uncover urinary incontinence that is masked by obstruction of the urinary outflow tract.[9,10] Bergman, Koonings, and Ballard[11] studied 67 continent women with cystocele protruding at least beyond the vaginal orifice. Each woman underwent a comprehensive urogynecologic examination and multichannel urodynamic study. Of these women, 17 had leakage of urine and 7 others had poor abdominal pressure transmission when the cystocele was reduced with a pessary. Poor abdominal pressure transmission is considered to be an abnormal condition associated with urinary incontinence. These patients underwent successful anti-incontinence operations as part of the repairs of their prolapse. Those women with preserved abdominal pressure transmission underwent prolapse repair alone, without development of urinary incontinence. A similar use of the pessary was reported by Fianu, Kjaelgaard, and Larsen[12] who uncovered latent stress incontinence in 6 of 41 women undergoing preoperative evaluation for cystocele repair.

SUMMARY

The use and care of the vaginal pessary is valuable knowledge for physicians caring for women with prolapse. Familiarity with available pessary designs, their proper fitting, and appropriate management completes the full spectrum of patient care for women with prolapse.

REFERENCES

1. Brubaker, L: Conservative treatment of prolapse: Use and care of the vaginal pessary. In: Hajj, SN and Evans, WJ (eds.): Clinical Postreproductive Gynecology. Appleton & Lange, Norwalk, CT, 1993, pp 119–27.
2. Colmer, WM: Use of the pessary. Am J Obstet Gynecol 65:170, 1953.
3. Wood, NJ: The use of vaginal pessaries for uterine prolapse. Nurse Pract 17:31–38, 1992.
4. Miller, DS: Contemporary use of the pessary. In Sciarra J (ed): Clinical Gynecology, vol 1. Harper & Row, New York, 1991, pp 1–12.
5. Sulak, PJ, Kuehl, TJ and Shull, BL: Vaginal pessaries and their use in pelvic relaxation. J Reprod Med 38:919–923, 1993.
6. Goldstein, I, Wise, GJ and Tancer, ML: A vesicovaginal fistula and intravesical foreign body: A rare case of the neglected pessary. Am J Obstet Gynecol 163:589–591, 1990.
7. Meinhardt, W: Bilateral hydronephrosis with urosepsis due to neglected pessary. Case report. Scand J Urol Nephrol 27:419–420, 1993.
8. Ott, R, Richter, H, Behr, J and Scheele, J: Small bowel prolapse and incarceration caused by a vaginal ring pessary. Br J Surg 80:1157, 1993.
9. Bhatia, NN and Bergman, A: Pessary test in women with urinary incontinence. Obstet Gynecol 65:220, 1985.
10. Bhatia, NN, Bergman, A and Gunning, JE: Urodynamic effects of a vaginal pessary in women with stress urinary incontinence. Am J Obstet Gynecol 147:876–884, 1983.
11. Bergman, A, Koonings, PP and Ballard, CA: Predicting postoperative urinary incontinence development in women undergoing operation for genitourinary prolapse. J Obstet Gynecol 158:1171–1175, 1988.
12. Fianu, S, Kjaeldgaard, A, and Larsson, B: Preoperative screening for latent stress incontinence in women with cystocele. Neurourol Urodynam 4:5–7, 1985.

CHAPTER 35

Preprolapse Syndromes

José M. Dominguez • Theodore J. Saclarides

This chapter discusses three conditions that are considered precursors of rectal prolapse: solitary rectal ulcer syndrome (SRUS), colitis cystica profunda (CCP), and descending perineum syndrome (DPS). These conditions may be seen in both men and women and may also be seen without a prolapse component. The etiology, clinical presentation, diagnosis, and treatment of each condition is addressed.

SOLITARY RECTAL ULCER SYNDROME

SRUS is a benign condition of the rectum whose etiology is not known, but as with many disorders that are incompletely understood, many theories about its pathogenesis have been proposed.[1–6] The first description of SRUS was provided by Cruveilhier in the 1830s,[7] but not until 1969 were the classic presentation and pathology set forth by Madigan and Morson.[1] Treatment of this condition may be problematic and frustrating for both patient and physician, because a standardized, successful therapeutic regimen has yet to be established.

ETIOLOGY

Multiple theories have been proposed, yet none adequately explain all aspects of this condition and so it is difficult to separate associated conditions from cause.[4] Most authors believe that SRUS is caused by varying degrees of rectal prolapse in conjunction with muscular dysfunction of the pelvic floor.[3,8]

Abnormal Puborectalis Activity

Inappropriate contraction (rather than relaxation) of the puborectalis muscle during defecation has been implicated as a cause of SRUS.[9] Supporting this theory is that increased electromyographic (EMG) activity of the puborectalis during straining has been noted in patients with SRUS.[10,11] This observation, however, has also been witnessed in some patients with constipation unassociated with SRUS, as well as in patients with idiopathic perineal pain without any coexisting defecation disorders.[12] Furthermore, inappropriate puborectalis contraction is not seen in all patients with SRUS and clearly fails to explain the chronic straining many of these patients experience. These findings, taken in conjunction with the doubt raised about the value of an obtuse anorectal angle in facilitating defecation, have diverted research and investigation into areas other than the puborectalis.

Abnormal Activity of the External Sphincter

Inappropriate activity (increased EMG activity) of the external sphincter muscle has been noted in some patients with SRUS. This finding has been seen more frequently in the ulcerating than in the nonulcerating forms of SRUS, yet is not consistently found in all patients with SRUS.[13]

Rectal Prolapse

SRUS has been considered a manifestation or precursor of rectal prolapse. This is supported by the frequent observation of internal intussusception of the rectum during defecography in patients with SRUS.[13–17] Furthermore, external prolapse subsequently occurs in 40% of these patients.[10] In comparing the manometric findings of patients with SRUS with those with prolapse, patients with SRUS demonstrated higher rectal voiding pressures during the Valsalva maneuver as well as higher resting anal-canal pressures. This high transmural pressure gradient seems to promote ulceration of the rectal wall and, because the anal sphincter is also under high pressure, external prolapse and decompression of the intraluminal pressure does not occur.[13] As people age and perineal descent and neuropathy commence, the sphincter weakens, allowing external prolapse of the rectum, lowering of the intraluminal pressure, and healing of the ulcer.[13] This evolution over time may explain why patients with SRUS are much younger than those with external prolapse.

CLINICAL PRESENTATION

Although cases of SRUS have been reported in the pediatric literature, the average age at presentation is in the third decade; only rarely are patients older than 70.[1,13,14,18,19] There is a slight female predominance.[13,18,19] Presenting symptoms are vague and nonspecific and include rectal bleeding, tenesmus, pelvic pain, mucus discharge, and constipation. There is usually a history of prolonged straining with defecation and a sensation of incomplete evacuation. Patients may resort to enemas, suppositories, and self-digitation to evacuate stool; as a result, many spend excessive time daily to initiate and complete bowel movements.

PATIENT EVALUATION

Evaluation of the patient should begin with a digital examination followed by proctoscopy. Digital rectal examination may reveal induration, usually of the anterior rectal wall. Endoscopically, most ulcers will be seen 5 to 12 centimeters from the anal verge and may be either solitary or multiple.[1,9,20–23] Although most lesions are ulcerating, occasionally they may be exophytic and grossly mimic a neoplasm.[18,20,24] It is possible, therefore, for these lesions to be neither solitary nor ulcerating; the correct diagnosis is made using results of a biopsy. The lesion may vary in size from a few millimeters to several centimeters, may be circumferential, and may have a white or gray fibrinous exudate covering its base. Bleeding may occur because of the friable nature of the lesion, so that biopsy is essential to exclude an ulcerating malignancy.

After a malignancy has been excluded, defecography is performed to define the defecation disorder more clearly. A spectrum of defecographic findings has been seen in SRUS (Table 35–1).[13–17] Included are anterior mucosal prolapse, internal rectal prolapse, and complete procidentia (full thickness, external prolapse). Other abnormalities seen include rectoceles, failed relaxation of the puborectalis muscle, and abnormal anorectal angles.

Abnormal EMG activity of the puborectalis and sphincter muscles has been described in SRUS.[13] During defecography, paradoxic contraction of the puborectalis during defecation is seen as persistence of an abnormally acute anorectal angle as well as extrinsic impingement of the posterior rectal wall.[14–17] Failure of the puborectalis to relax can also be demonstrated with EMG in some patients with SRUS. The reliability of this finding is debatable, because it is also seen in a multitude of defecatory problems and in patients who are completely asymptomatic.

TABLE 35–1. Solitary Rectal Ulcer Syndrome: Findings on Defecography

Reference	N	Complete Procidentia %	Internal Intussusception* %	Rectocele %	Failed Puborectal Relaxation %
Kuijpers[14]	19	0 (0%)	13 (68%)	0 (0%)	5 (26%)
Mahieu[15]	43	19 (44%)	15 (35%)	2 (5%)	4 (9%)
Womack[13]	18	5 (28%)	10 (56%)	0 (0%)	NR
Goei[16]	16	1 (6%)	8 (50%)	1 (6%)	4 (25%)
Mackle[17]	22	0 (0%)	9 (41%)	6 (27%)	5 (23%)

NR = Not reported; * = Including anterior rectal wall prolapse

PATHOLOGY

Histologic examination of the ulcer biopsies show characteristic obliteration of the lamina propria with fibroblasts that are arranged at right angles to a hypertrophied muscularis mucosa.[1,20,21,25,26] Regenerative changes are usually seen in the crypt epithelium. Other findings include erosion or ulceration of the mucosa, dilated or cystic mucosal glands, goblet-cell depletion, and infiltration with acute and chronic inflammatory cells.[27] Localized CCP may be found.[2,21]

TREATMENT

SRUS is difficult to treat successfully; a wide variety of both conservative and surgical treatments have been proposed. Initial measures should include dietary fiber supplements to facilitate defecation and strict avoidance of prolonged straining. Glycerine suppositories may ease defecation.[28] Numerous topical agents such as epinephrine, antihistamines, steroids, arsenic, bismuth, decicaine, ichthammol, mercury, witch hazel, silver nitrate, heavy metals, snake venom, and tannic acid have been tried and usually failed.[1] Sucralfate enemas have been used with success in a small number of patients.[29] Physiotherapy with biofeedback and retraining may be beneficial in patients with elevated external anal sphincter pressures.[5]

When conservative treatment fails to provide adequate results, surgical treatment may be considered. Local excision has been reported but has low success rates; at least 70% of patients have recurrence of their SRUS.[30] Clearly, patients with external rectal prolapse and SRUS should be considered for surgery; options include transabdominal rectopexy, anterior resection, or perineal proctectomy if one wishes to avoid a laparotomy because of advanced patient age or coexisting medical problems. These surgical approaches usually yield less favorable success rates in patients with internal or occult prolapse; it is thus controversial whether they should be performed for internal prolapse. Nicholls and Simson,[19] however, combined posterior rectopexy with anterior rectopexy in patients with internal prolapse and achieved favorable results in 12 of 14 patients.

In rare situations in which conservative and standard surgical treatment have failed, patients may be considered for more aggressive treatment. This could include proctectomy with coloanal anastomosis or abdominoperineal resection, but before embarking on such a radical approach, the patient's symptoms must be sufficiently severe to justify this choice of therapy.

SUMMARY

SRUS is a benign disorder of the rectum whose etiology is not clearly understood. It may be secondary to prolapse, straining, elevated voiding pressure, and abnormal pressure gradients between the rectal vault and anal canal. In this respect, SRUS may be an early manifestation of rectal procidentia, occurring when anal outlet pressures are too high to permit external intussusception. Defecography, endoscopy with biopsy, and anal manometry are helpful in establishing diagnosis and guiding treatment. Conservative measures such as use of fiber supplements and avoidance of straining are the first line of treatment. Physiotherapy and biofeedback may be helpful. Surgical treatment is indicated primarily if external rectal prolapse occurs in conjunction with SRUS. The standard prolapse operations, however, have not yielded acceptable results when used for internal prolapse. Early results of anteroposterior rectopexy are encouraging.

COLITIS CYSTICA PROFUNDA

CCP is another obscure, benign condition of the colon and rectum; it may exist in either a diffuse or a localized form.[31–35] When localized to the rectosigmoid, CCP is associated with rectal prolapse. As a result of similar morphology and gross appearance, one must perform a biopsy on these lesions in order to differentiate CCP from a well-differentiated mucinous adenocarcinoma.

HISTORICAL PERSPECTIVE

This condition was first described in 1766 by Stark[36] who reported two cases associated with chronic dysentery.[36] Because submucosal cysts may appear grossly polypoid, Virchow[37] in 1863 coined the term **colitis cystica polyposa**. Goodall and Sinclair in 1957 termed the condition **colitis cystica profunda**, in order to differentiate it from **colitis cystica superficialis**, which can be seen in pellagra.[38] The first large series was reported in 1967 by Wayte and Helwig,[33] who reported 24 cases from the files of the Armed Forces Institute of Pathology.

ETIOLOGY

Many theories regarding the etiology of CCP have been proposed. They fall into two categories: congenital and acquired. Most authors do not support the congenital theory, because very few of these lesions have been reported in large pediatric autopsy series.[39]

An acquired etiology is supported by the fact that most cases are found in association with diseases that produce chronic irritation and inflammation, including ulcerative colitis, Crohn's disease, dysentery, previous surgery, irradiation, rectal prolapse, rectal intussusception, trauma, polyposis syndromes, and solitary rectal ulcer syndrome.[31,40–44] Epstein and associates[39] theorized in 1966 that weakness in the muscularis mucosa caused by inflammation allowed herniation of mucosa into the submucosa, causing cyst formation. Most authors agree that CCP is the end result of a chronic cycle of inflammation and healing.

TABLE 35–2. Colitis Cystica Profunda: Localized versus Diffuse Forms

	Localized (Rectosigmoid)	Diffuse
Percentage of Cases	85%	15%
Location	Rectum (5–12 cm from anal verge)	Reported throughout colon
Associated condition	Internal rectal prolapse Complete rectal prolapse Self-digitation Suppositories	Ulcerative colitis Crohn's disease Radiation damage Dysentery Anastomosis Colostomy
Treatment	Steroid enemas High-fiber diet Treat prolapse if present	Directed toward cause of colonic irritation Resection

The localized form is typically found 5 to 12 centimeters from the anal verge, usually on the anterior rectal wall.[31] This is also the site where solitary rectal ulcers occur, perhaps owing to trauma secondary to internal rectal intussusception. This injury may then lead to CCP or SRUS. The diffuse variety of CCP may be seen in cases of inflammatory bowel disease and dysentery[31] (Table 35–2).

CLINICAL PRESENTATION

All ages may be affected, but most patients are in their third decade. There does not seem to be a gender preference.[31,45] In order of decreasing frequency, common presenting symptoms are bleeding, mucus discharge, diarrhea, tenesmus, abdominal discomfort, and rectal pain.[31]

A careful history may yield complaints of frequent straining, constipation, or rectal prolapse. Patients may experience a feeling of incomplete evacuation and may require suppositories or even need to perform self-digitation to produce a bowel movement.[2,38,41]

Physical findings vary depending on location and extent of disease. If confined to the rectosigmoid, digital rectal examination may reveal a mass or nodularity of the rectal mucosa; rectal prolapse may be seen during straining. The stools may be hemoccult positive.

Endoscopic examination may show submucosal bulging, erythema of the overlying mucosa, and ulceration. Biopsy of the lesion is important to rule out malignancy, but superficial biopsies may fail to yield a diagnosis of CCP because of the intramural location of the cysts.[31,42,46–49]

PATIENT EVALUATION

Before initiating treatment, the correct diagnosis must be obtained. The entire colon must be examined endoscopically to rule out associated pathology that may be causing these changes. Results of multiple biopsies must be obtained and evaluated by an experienced gastrointestinal pathologist. In cases localized to the rectosigmoid, defecography may identify abnormalities in defecation and pelvic floor function, such as internal prolapse. If this is identified and symptoms warrant, treatment, whether medical or surgical, must be instituted when CCP is confined to this region. Transrectal ultrasound also has been used in the diagnosis of CCP.[50]

PATHOLOGY

Mucinous cysts are found below the muscularis mucosa; most are found in the submucosa, but they have been seen in the muscularis propria and serosa as well.[46,47] The lining of the cysts varies from a columnar to a squamous epithelium. The overlying mucosa frequently shows a chronic inflammatory infiltrate and superficial ulceration.

TREATMENT

Initial treatment consists of nonsurgical methods to facilitate bowel movements and reduce inflammation. Corticosteroid enemas should be the first line of treatment. A diet high in fiber is also used in cases of constipation and straining.[31]

Patients who do not improve with conservative medical therapy may be considered for surgical treatment.[51–54] Options include local excision with and without repair of prolapse, colon resection, anterior resection with either colorectal or coloanal anastomosis, diverting colostomy, and fulguration. Only if all measures have been exhausted and the patient remains profoundly symptomatic should abdominoperineal resection be considered.[31]

SUMMARY

CCP is a benign disease generally seen in association with disorders causing colitis or proctitis. Differentiating CCP from well-differentiated mucinous adenocarcinoma is critical. If the patient has rectal prolapse, it should be addressed if the symptoms are to be successfully treated.

DESCENDING PERINEUM SYNDROME

DPS was first described by Parks, Porter, and Hardcastle in 1966.[55] This condition is the result of chronic straining, which causes pudendal neuropathy and pelvic floor muscular weakness.[56] Progressive injury may lead to fecal incontinence.[57] Nonsurgical and surgical treatments have been employed with variable success.

ETIOLOGY

Straining at stool causes repeated and prolonged pelvic floor descent. As a result, the pudendal nerve is progressively stretched, and this, in turn, causes denervation of the pelvic floor musculature and further descent.[56,58] This descent allows continued and greater injury to the pudendal nerve.

DPS has been reported in paratroopers wearing harnesses that lacked perineal support. The shock of the parachute's opening and the subsequent impact when hitting the ground cause rapid unsupported descent of the perineum, which may lead to pudendal nerve injury.[59]

CLINICAL PRESENTATION

Most cases reported in the literature occur in females.[56,57,60] who may report a feeling of incomplete evacuation and obstructed defecation. A history of chronic constipation, laxative abuse, and excessive straining during defecation may be present. Associated complaints include tenesmus, dull perineal pain, and urgency. Occasionally, patients with anterior rectal mucosal prolapse may complain of skin irritation and itching caused by mucus or bloody discharge. Incontinence may also be the initial reason for presentation.

PATIENT EVALUATION

DPS should be suspected in patients with a history of excessive straining with defecation. Parks originally defined DPS as an anal margin below a line from the pubis to the coccyx (pubococcygeal line) at rest and a descent of greater than 3 to 4 centimeters with straining.[55] Findings on physical examination may be confirmed radiographically using defecography or by taking measurements with a perineometer.[56,61,62] Physical examination reveals bulging of the anus, which is best seen during straining. Prolapse of anterior rectal mucosa may be present and should not be confused with prolapse of hemorrhoids.[57]

The diagnosis of DPS is supported by the results of other physiologic tests, in addition to defecography and physical examination. Anal manometry may show anal sphincter weakness; pudendal-nerve motor latency testing may show neuropathy.[57,60] Defecography permits radiographic determination of the anorectal angle in relationship to the pubococcygeal line. If the angle is greater than 2 centimeters below the pubococcygeal line at rest or greater than 3 centimeters below during straining, the diagnosis of DPS is confirmed.[62]

The use of a perineometer has also been reported. The anal verge is measured to the ischial tuberosities bilaterally. Oettle and associates[62] reported that the perineometer measurement of descent underestimated the corresponding defecography value by 60%.

TREATMENT

Once diagnosed, DPS warrants treatment in order to prevent further pudendal nerve damage and possible incontinence. Initial treatment involves conservative measures to decrease the amount of straining. Patients who pass hard stool should be given a regimen of stool softeners such as dietary fiber supplements. The use of daily suppositories to regulate bowel movements is frequently required. A program of pelvic-floor–muscle strengthening exercises should be considered, especially in patients with weakness apparent on manometry. Biofeedback techniques can be helpful in this regard.

Lesaffer and Milo[63] described a **perineum device** used in the treatment of DPS.[63] This board-like instrument has an anal and urogenital gap for defecation and voiding. Between these apertures is a "saddle-like elevation," which supports the perineum. This prevents abnormal descent, which may worsen pre-existing pudendal-nerve damage.

Surgical management is reserved for patients who have failed conservative measures and who have disabling symptoms of tenesmus, pelvic discomfort, and obstructed defecation. Transabdominal procedures that suspend the rectum by direct suture rectopexy or by using mesh may be considered. Patients with colonic motility disorders documented on transit studies may benefit from colon resection. Nicholls[59] described transperineal retrorectal levatorplasty; key steps in this procedure include suspension of the posterior rectal wall to the presacral fascia and reapproximation of the levator muscles posteriorly.[59] Various surgical approaches may ultimately correct the anatomic abnormalities, but normal function is much more difficult to obtain.

SUMMARY

DPS is a condition seen in patients with long histories of constipation and excessive straining. Early diagnosis and treatment are important to prevent progressive pudendal nerve injury that may lead to incontinence. Conservative measures, the mainstay of treatment, are measures to facilitate defecation without straining.

REFERENCES

1. Madigan, MR and Morson, BC: Solitary ulcer of the rectum. Gut 10:871, 1969.
2. Levine, DS: "Solitary" rectal ulcer syndrome. Are "solitary" rectal ulcer syndrome and "localized" colitis cystica profunda analogous syndromes caused by rectal prolapse? Gastroenterology 92:243, 1987.
3. Pescatori, M, Maria, G, Mattana, C, et al: Clinical picture and pelvic floor physiology in the solitary rectal ulcer syndrome. Dis Colon Rectum 28:862, 1985.
4. Eckardt, VF, Kanzler, G and Remmele, W: Anorectal ergotism: Another cause of solitary rectal ulcers. Gastroenterology 91:1123, 1986.
5. Mackle, EJ and Parks, TG: Solitary rectal ulcer syndrome: Aetiology, investigation and management. Dig Dis 8:294, 1990.
6. Thomson, H and Hill, D: Solitary rectal ulcer: Always a self-induced condition? Br J Surg 67:784, 1980.
7. Cruveilhier, J: Ulcère chronique du rectum. In: Anatomie pathologique du corps humain, Maladies du Rectum 2:4, 1830.
8. Sun, WM, Read, NW, Donnelly, TC, et al: A common pathophysiology for full thickness rectal prolapse, anterior mucosal prolapse and solitary rectal ulcer syndrome. Br J Surg 76:290, 1989.
9. Keighley, MRB and Shouler, P: Clinical and manometric fea-

tures of the solitary rectal ulcer syndrome. Dis Colon Rectum 27:507, 1984.
10. Rutter, KRP and Riddell, RH: The solitary ulcer syndrome of the rectum. Clin Gastroenterology 4:505, 1975.
11. Snooks, SJ, Nicholls, RJ, Henry, MM, et al: Electrophysiological and manometric assessment of the pelvic floor in the solitary rectal ulcer syndrome. Br J Surg 72:131, 1985.
12. Jones, PN, Lubowski, DZ, Swash, M, et al: Is paradoxical contraction of puborectalis muscle of functional importance? Dis Colon Rectum 30:667, 1987.
13. Womack, NR, Williams, NS, Holmfield, JH, et al: Pressure and prolapse: The cause of solitary rectal ulceration. Gut 28:1228, 1987.
14. Kuijpers, HC, Schreve, RH and Hoedemakers, HTC: Diagnosis of functional disorders of defecation causing the solitary rectal ulcer syndrome. Dis Colon Rectum 29:126, 1986.
15. Mahiev, PHG: Barium enema and defaecography in the diagnosis and evaluation of the solitary rectal ulcer syndrome. Int J Colorectal Dis 1:85, 1986.
16. Goei, R, Baeten, C and Arends, JW: Solitary rectal ulcer syndrome: Findings at barium enema study and defecography. Radiology 168: 303, 1988.
17. Mackle, EJ, Mills, JOM and Parks, TG: The investigation of anorectal dysfunction in the solitary rectal ulcer syndrome. Int J Colorectal Dis 5:21, 1990.
18. Martin, CJ, Parks, TG and Biggart, JD: Solitary rectal ulcer syndrome in Northern Ireland, 1971–1980. Br J Surg 68:744, 1981.
19. Nicholls, RJ and Simson, JNL: Anteroposterior rectopexy in the treatment of solitary rectal ulcer syndrome without overt rectal prolapse. Br J Surg 73:222, 1986.
20. Britto, E, Borges, AM, Swaroop, VS, et al: Solitary rectal ulcer syndrome: Twenty cases seen at an oncology center. Dis Colon Rectum 30:381, 1987.
21. Niv, Y and Bat, L: Solitary rectal ulcer syndrome: Clinical, endoscopic, and histological spectrum. Am J Gastroenterol 81: 486, 1986.
22. Saul, SH and Sollenberger, LC: Solitary rectal ulcer syndrome: Its clinical and pathological underdiagnosis. Am J Surg Pathol 9:411, 1985.
23. Thomson, G, Clark, A, Handyside, J, et al: Solitary ulcer of the rectum—or is it? A report of 6 cases. Br J Surg 68:21, 1981.
24. Yamagina, H: Protruded variants in solitary ulcer syndrome of the rectum. Acta Pathol Jpn 38:471, 1988.
25. Chanvitan, A and Nopanitaya, W: Solitary rectal ulcer: Electron microscopy study of two cases. Dis Colon Rectum 29:421, 1986.
26. Franzin, G, Dina, R, Scarpa, A, et al: "The evolution of the solitary ulcer of the rectum": An endoscopic and histopathologic study. Endoscopy 14:131, 1982.
27. Levine, DS, Surawicz, CM, Ajer, TN, et al: Diffuse excess mucosal collagen in rectal biopsies facilitates differential diagnosis of solitary rectal ulcer syndrome from other inflammatory bowel disease. Dig Dis Sci 33:1345, 1988.
28. Lam, TCF, Lubowski, DZ and King, DW: Solitary rectal ulcer syndrome. Baillieres Clin Gastroenterol 6:129, 1992.
29. Spiliadis, C, Skandalis, N and Emmanouildis, A: Treatment of solitary rectal ulcer syndrome with sucralfate enema. Gastrointest Endosc 35:131, 1989.
30. Jalan, KN, Brunt, PW and Maclean, N: Benign solitary rectal ulcer of the rectum: A report of 5 cases. Scand J Gastroenterol 5:143, 1970.
31. Guest, CB and Reznick, RK: Colitis cystica profunda: Review of the literature. Dis Colon Rectum 32:983, 1989.
32. Tedesco, FJ, Sumner, HW and Kassens, WD: Colitis cystica profunda. Am J Gastroenterol 65:339, 1976.
33. Wayte, DM and Helwig, EB: Colitis cystica profunda. Am J Clin Pathol 48:159, 1967.
34. Rosen, Y, Vaillant, JG and Yermakov, V: Submucosal mucous cysts at a colostomy site: Relationship to colitis cystica profunda and report of a case. Dis Colon Rectum 19:453, 1976.
35. Dippolito, AD, Aburano, A, Bezouska, CA, et al: Enteritis cystica profunda in Peutz-Jeghers syndrome: Report of a case and review of the literature. Dis Colon Rectum 30:192, 1987.
36. Stark, W: Specimen septem histories et dissectiones dysentericorum exhibens. Leiden, The Netherlands: Leiden University, 1766. Thesis.
37. Virchow, R: Die Krankhaften Geschwulste, vol 1. Auguste Hirschwald, Berlin; 1863; p 243.
38. Goodall, HB and Sinclair, ISR: Colitis cystica profunda. J Path Bacteriol 73:33, 1957.
39. Epstein, SE, Ascari, WQ, Ablow, RC, et al: Colitis cystica profunda. Am J Clin Pathol 45:186, 1966.
40. Valiulis, AP, Gardiner, GW and Mahoney, LJ: Adenocarcinoma and colitis cystica profunda in a radiation-induced colonic stricture. Dis Colon Rectum 28:128, 1985.
41. Peterkin, GA, Moroz, K and Kondi, ES: Proctitis cystica profunda in paraplegics: Report of three cases. Dis Colon Rectum 35:1174, 1992.
42. Black, HC, Gardner, WA and Weidner, MG: Localized colitis cystica profunda: A benign lesion simulating malignancy. Am Surg 38:237, 1972.
43. Bentley, E, Chandrasoma, P, Cohen, H, et al: Colitis cystica profunda: Presenting with complete intestinal obstruction and recurrence. Gastroenterology 89:1157, 1985.
44. Black, WC, Gomez, LS, Yuhas, JM, et al: Quantitation of the late effects of x-radiation on the large intestine. Cancer 45:444, 1980.
45. Martin, JK, Culp, CE and Weiland, LH: Colitis cystica profunda. Dis Colon Rectum 23:488, 1980.
46. Silver, H and Stolar, J: Distinguishing features of well-differentiated mucinous adenocarcinoma of the rectum and colitis cystica profunda. Am J Clin Pathol 51:493, 1969.
47. Stolar, J and Silver, H: Differentiation of pseudoinflammatory colloid carcinoma from colitis cystica profunda. Dis Colon Rectum 12:63, 1969.
48. Schein, M, Veller, M and Decker, GAG: Colitis cystica profunda simulating rectal carcinoma: A case report. S Afr Med J 72:289, 1987.
49. Yashiro, K, Murakami, Y, Iizuka, B, et al: Localized colitis cystica profunda of the sigmoid colon. Endoscopy 17:198, 1985.
50. Hulsmans, FJ, Tio, TL, Reeders, JW, et al: Transrectal US in the diagnosis of localized colitis cystica profunda. Radiology 181:201, 1991.
51. Walker, JP, Wiener, I and Rowe, EB: Colitis cystica profunda: Diagnosis and management. South Med J 79:1167, 1986.
52. Guy, PJ and Hall, M: Colitis cystica profunda of the rectum treated by mucosal sleeve resection and colo-anal pullthrough. Br J Surg 75:289, 1988.
53. Barcia, PJ and Washburn, ME: Colitis cystica profunda: An unusual surgical problem. Am Surg 45:61, 1979.
54. Herman, AH and Nabseth, DC: Colitis cystica profunda: Localized, segmental and diffuse. Arch Surg 106:337, 1973.
55. Parks, AG, Porter, NH, and Hardcastle, J: The syndrome of the descending perineum. Proc R Soc Med 59:477, 1966.
56. Henry, MM, Parks, AG, and Swash, M: The pelvic floor musculature in descending perineum syndrome. Br J Surg 69:470, 1982.
57. Read, NW, Bartolo, DC, Read, MG, et al: Differences in anorectal manometry between patients with hemorrhoids and patients with descending perineum syndrome: implications for management. Br J Surg 70:656, 1983.
58. Bartolo, DC, Read, NW, Read, MG, et al: Differences in anal sphincter function and clinical presentation in patients with pelvic floor descent. Gastroenterology 85:68, 1983.
59. Nicholls, DH: Retrorectal levatorplasty for anal and perineal prolapse. Surg Gynecol Obs 154:251, 1982.
60. Bartolo, DCC, Read, MG, and Read, NW: The saline contingence test: Dynamic studies in faecal incontinence, haemorrhoids and the descending perineum syndrome. Acta Gastroenterol Belg 48:39, 1985.
61. Ambrose, S, and Keighley, MRB: Outpatient measurement of perineal descent. Ann R Col Surg Engl 67:306, 1985.
62. Oettle, GJ, Roe, AM, Bartolo, DC, et al: What is the best way of measuring perineal descent? A comparison of radiographic and clinical methods. Br J Surg 72:999, 1985.
63. Lesaffer, L and Milo, R: Descending perineum syndrome: Control defecogram with a "perineum device," perspective in prevention and conservative therapy. J Belge Radiol 71:709, 1988.

CHAPTER **36**

Rectal Prolapse

Steven J. Stryker

Rectal prolapse, or procidentia, refers to the protrusion of full-thickness rectal wall through the anal canal to the anal verge or beyond. Despite the recognition of this uncommon condition for millennia, agreement about its etiology and optimal treatment is lacking.

ETIOLOGY

Several theories have been proposed regarding the causes of rectal prolapse, but two mechanisms, herniation and intussusception, that explain this condition in anatomic terms are worthy of further discussion. Moschcowitz[1] compared rectal prolapse to other sliding hernias involving abdominal viscera and suggested that the protruding rectum represented the end result of herniation of the anterior rectal wall, which began at the level of Douglas's pouch. More recently, Broden and Snellman[2] conducted a series of elegant cineradiographic studies that clearly demonstrated a circumferential intussusception 6 to 8 cm above the anal verge as the initiating event in the progression of the rectum out of the anal orifice. This intussusception theory was subsequently confirmed by Theuerkauf, Beahrs, and Hill.[3] As Gordon[4] points out, these theories of herniation and intussusception complement one another and most likely describe different aspects of the same process.

Anatomic abnormalities associated with rectal prolapse are remarkably consistent (Fig. 36–1). These include: (1) a diastasis of the levator ani musculature; (2) an abnormally deep Douglas's pouch, essentially in contact with the levator ani; (3) attenuated mesorectal attachments between the rectum and the endopelvic fascia laterally and posteriorly; and (4) an elongated rectosigmoid colon.[5] Despite the fact that most surgical techniques developed for the treatment of rectal prolapse seek to correct one or more of these anatomic defects, these findings are felt to be secondary rather than the cause of chronic prolapse.

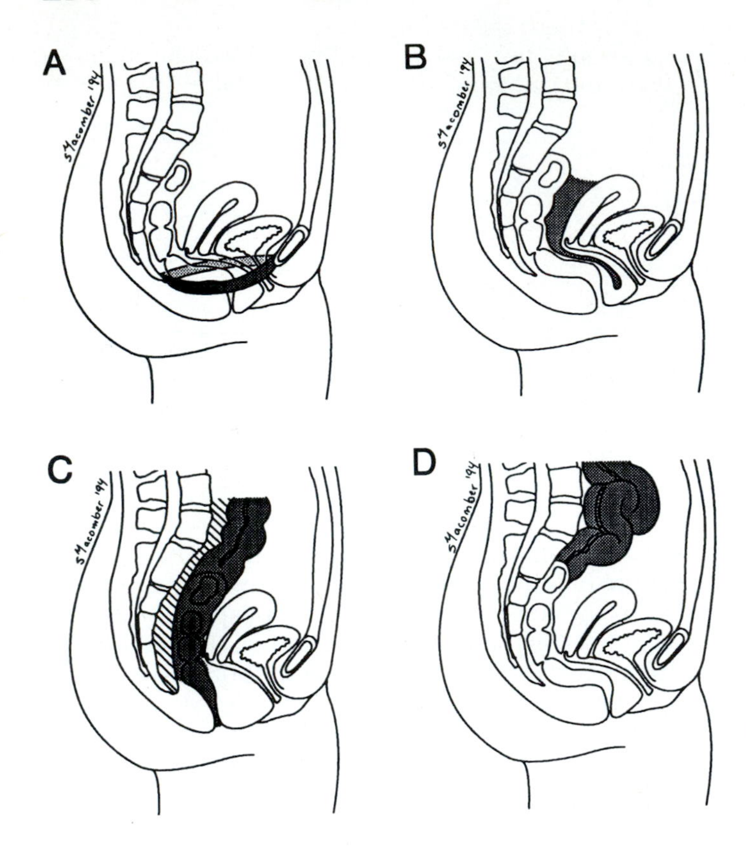

FIGURE 36–1. Anatomic abnormalities associated with rectal prolapse. (*A*) Diastasis of levator musculature. (*B*) Deep recto-vaginal Douglas's pouch. (*C*) Elongated mesorectum with lax sacral attachment. (*D*) Redundant sigmoid colon.

In adults, rectal prolapse occurs predominantly in women, by a 6-fold to 10-fold difference than in men. Although the incidence seems evenly distributed by age for men, the incidence of rectal prolapse in women increases with age, with a peak occurring during the seventh decade of life.[6]

Several predisposing factors or associated conditions have been linked to rectal prolapse. A history of chronic straining to defecate is reported by most patients, with 52% having intractable constipation and 15% chronic diarrhea.[7] Congenital or acquired neurologic disorders that result in denervation of the pelvic floor, such as spina bifida, multiple sclerosis, or tabes dorsalis, are known to predispose to rectal prolapse. Surprisingly, multiparity and the risk of birth injury to the pelvic floor musculature have *not* been conclusively proven to produce rectal prolapse,[8] although many patients may have associated uterine or bladder prolapse.[6,9] The frequent association of these latter two conditions with rectal prolapse suggests a common underlying cause. Conversely, nulliparity is frequently identified as a predisposing factor to prolapse. What is unclear, however, is whether nulliparity is an independent variable or whether it is related to other accepted predisposing factors (e.g., constipation).

Finally, a disproportionately large percentage of patients with rectal prolapse have a background of psychiatric illness or other conditions requiring institutionalization.[10] The exact role of mental illness in the development of prolapse is unclear. One might hypothesize that inappropriate and prolonged straining to defecate in the face of an empty rectal ampulla might be one cause. Another might be the constipating effects of many of the medications used in the treatment of psychiatric disorders.

CLINICAL FEATURES AND EVALUATION

Evaluation of patients with rectal prolapse begins with taking a detailed, symptom-specific history. Patients may or may not be aware of their specific diagnosis; many complain of varying degrees of protrusion, alteration of fecal continence, or both. The duration of symptoms should be determined, along with the level of activity required to elicit the protrusion. Early in the development of rectal prolapse, the protrusion may be only infrequently noted, usually during straining. As the condition progresses over several years, the prolapse occurs with ever-decreasing effort; ultimately the rectum promptly everts with assumption of upright posture and ambulation. As increased frequency and ease of prolapse are noted by the patient, fecal incontinence may ensue. The examining physician should attempt to quantitate the degree of incontinence by asking questions regarding the ability to control flatus and stool of varying consistency, ranging from liquid to solid. The level of social disability caused by less-than-perfect continence should be determined as well.

During the initial physical examination, the prolapse is usually reduced and may be difficult or impossible to detect, especially in the prone or left-lateral decubitus position. Suspected rectal prolapse is best demonstrated by having the patient sit on the toilet and strain. Observation in this position will frequently define the nature and extent of the patient's complaint of protrusion; in fact, this may be the only way to differentiate a true full-thickness rectal prolapse from large, prolapsing internal hemorrhoids. The concentric folds of rectal prolapse are usually easily distinguishable from the quadrant radial orientation of internal hemorrhoids (Fig. 36–2). Digital examination helps to exclude a rectal mass but is mainly useful in estimating the degree of sphincter laxity. Flexible sigmoidoscopy performed at the time of the initial office visit may show erythema, granularity, or superficial ulceration of the distal 8 to 10 cm of mucosa. It also excludes coexisting pathology (e.g., neoplasia, diverticular disease) that may influence the operative approach to the correction of the prolapse. A finding of squamous metaplasia of the mucosa suggests chronic prolapse.

Some authors suggest additional diagnostic studies, including colonoscopy, cineradiography, anorectal manometry, anorectal EMG, and colonic transit-time studies.[11,12] Colonoscopy (or barium enema) occasionally reveals unsuspected proximal neoplasms in the elderly patient presenting with rectal prolapse. Although the neoplasm does not cause the prolapse, its definitive management usually takes precedence over treatment of the prolapse. Cineradiography (dynamic proctography) is most useful when the diagnosis of rectal prolapse is suspected but not confirmed by physical examination. In addition to demonstrating varying degrees of prolapse, cineradiography may identify unsuspected fecal incontinence, a rectocele, or an enterocele. Anal manometry and anal EMG quantify the extent of sphincter impairment associated with rectal prolapse but have not, as yet, proven useful in treatment planning. Finally, colonic transit studies to identify a subset of patients with "slow-transit constipation" may be used preoperatively in individuals with unusually severe constipation associated with prolapse. Although abnormalities are often discovered when these studies are pursued, the results seldom alter the initial management of the prolapse. Therefore, these studies should be used *selectively* to evaluate signs or symptoms not immediately attributable to the prolapse.

TREATMENT

Whether or not the underlying cause of rectal prolapse can be identified or treated, the anatomic derangements that allow the rectum to evert must be dealt with for a satisfactory surgical outcome. The multitude of repairs described reflects the various attempts to correct these anatomic abnormalities. This section focuses on the most widely used prolapse repairs. All have acceptable morbidity and mortality rates, but differences become apparent with respect to recurrence rates and functional outcomes.

TRANSPERINEAL REPAIRS

A transperineal approach to correct rectal prolapse appears to be a straightforward attempt to directly deal with the protruding gut segment. Indeed, due to acceptably low operative morbidity and mortality rates, various perineal procedures have been used in the management of rectal prolapse for more than 100 years. In addition to low complication rates, perineal approaches cause less pain, have shorter hospital stays, and allow a faster return to normal activity. Furthermore, they can be performed under a local or regional anesthetic without a laparotomy.

The Thiersch Procedure

Encirclement of the anal outlet (anal cerclage) was first described by Thiersch in 1891. Nonabsorbable material is inserted circumanally through a series of two or more small counterincisions; thus anal canal expansion is limited and protrusion of the rectum is prevented (Fig. 36–3). The material, usually a monofilament suture, is tightened while the surgeon's finger or a #18 Hegar dilator traverses the anal canal to gauge diameter properly. Other materials, such as sil-

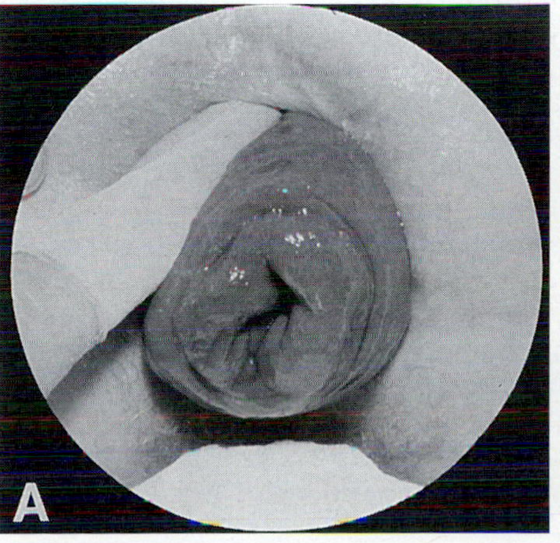

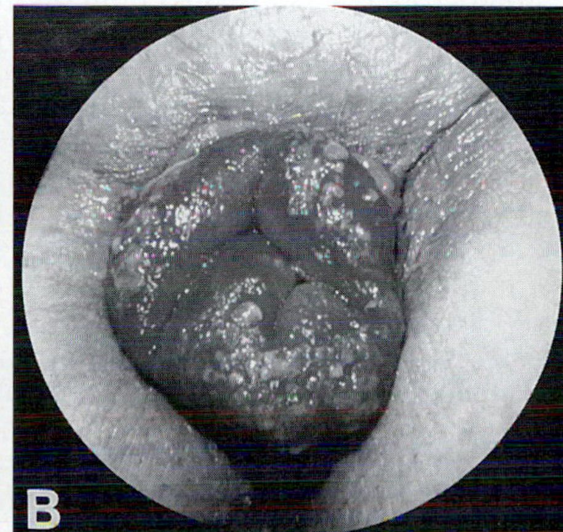

FIGURE 36–2. (*A*) Full thickness rectal prolapse. (*B*) Prolapsing internal hemorrhoids.

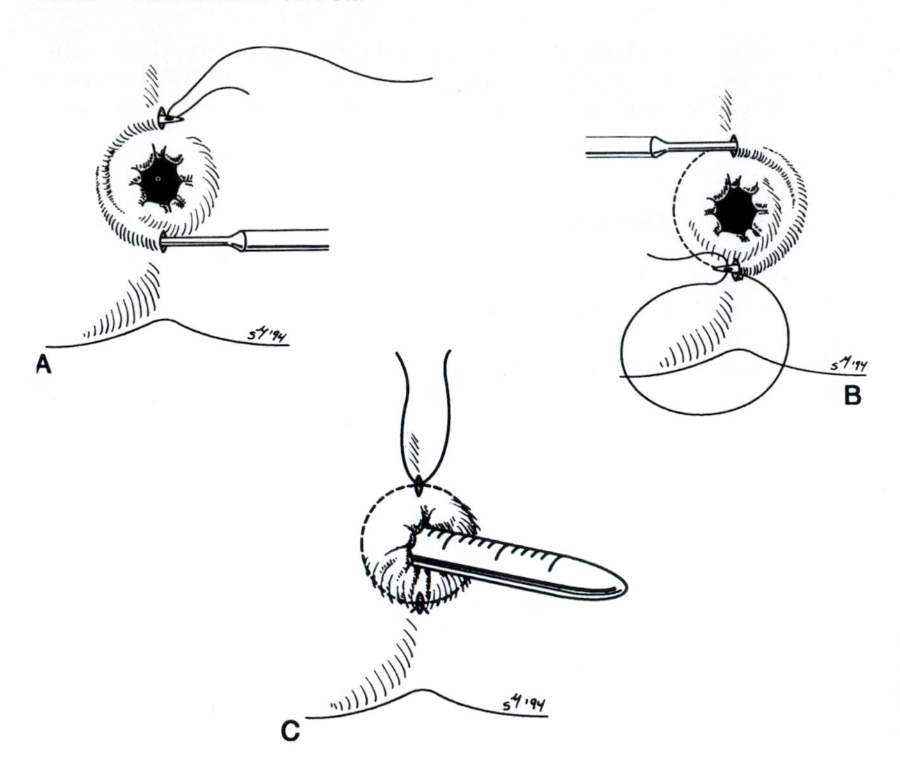

FIGURE 36–3. Thiersch's procedure. (*A*) Using a curved needle, the thread has been placed around the right 180 degrees of the anus. (*B*) The anus has been completely encircled. (*C*) The suture is tightened around the dilator.

icone rubber tubing and strips, polypropylene mesh, and stainless steel wire, have also been employed. One major advantage of this procedure is the ability to perform it using local anesthesia.

Postoperative bowel management is problematic because fecal impaction commonly follows the Thiersch procedure. Complications encountered less frequently include suture breakage, erosion, infection, and rectovaginal fistula. Because a satisfactory outcome is achieved in only half the patients so treated, this procedure is only rarely used. It does remain an option, however, for "high-risk" surgical patients and nonambulatory residents of nursing homes and psychiatric facilities who have troublesome prolapse.[13]

Transperineal Resection

Transperineal resection (e.g., perineal rectosigmoidectomy) has been a common method for treating full-thickness prolapse since early in this century and it remains a useful option in select individuals. Prolapse that readily occurs in the standing position or prolapse that is irreducible can be easily managed using this approach. The procedure is performed in either the lithotomy or prone jackknife position. Eversion of the rectum through the anal canal is accomplished by gentle traction, and a circumferential, full-thickness incision is made 1 to 2 cm proximal to the dentate line (Fig. 36–4). Dissection is undertaken in the intramural space, the redundant segment is straightened and exteriorized and the mesentery serially divided. An anterior and/or posterior levatoroplasty is performed, as suggested by Altemeier and colleagues.[10] Following levatoroplasty, the anterior peritoneum is reapproximated and the mobilized segment amputated. Anastomosis between the proximal colon and the distal rectal mucosa is then accomplished by suture or staple technique and the anastomosis allowed to retract upward into the anal canal. Anastomotic dehiscence, bleeding, or stricture occur infrequently; operative mortality is less than 1%.

The Delorme Procedure

A third perineal operation for rectal prolapse, the Delorme procedure, differs from the Altemeier procedure in that a full-thickness resection and anastomosis are not performed. Following eversion of the prolapsing segment, mucosal stripping is begun approximately 1 cm above the dentate line and continued in a sleeve-like fashion proximally for 10 cm or more. Blood loss during this dissection is minimized by a submucosal injection of a 1:200,000 epinephrine solution. After the mucosal dissection has been completed, the mucosal segment is divided proximally and the denuded muscular tube is plicated by a series of longitudinally placed sutures. This "bunches up" the redundant rectum just above the levator ani muscle and brings the proximal mucosal incision down to the anal canal, where it can be readily anastomosed to the distal mucosal edge.[14]

Like other perineal operations for rectal prolapse, the Delorme procedure is ideally suited for frail, elderly patients who might not tolerate general anesthesia or a laparotomy. Morbidity is similar to that of perineal rectosigmoidectomy. One clear-cut dis-

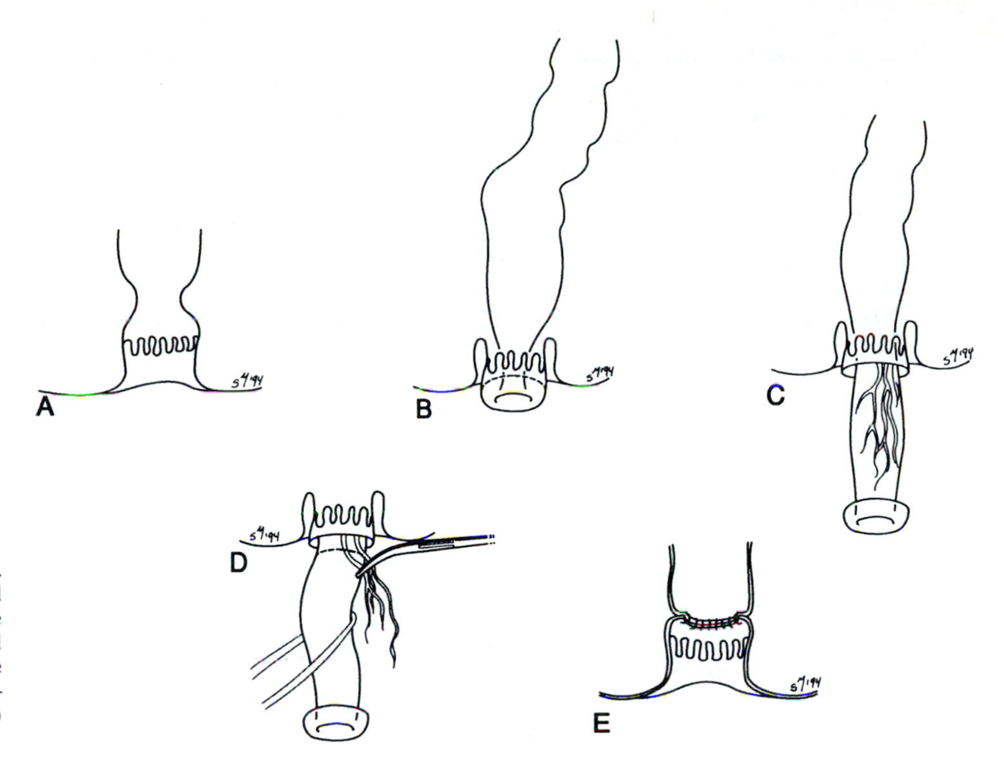

FIGURE 36–4. Rectosigmoidectomy. (*A*) Normal anatomy of the anorectal region. (*B*) Prolapsed segment. The incision is made along the dotted line. (*C*) Complete eversion of the prolapsed segment. (*D*) Serial ligation of the rectal mesentery. (*E*) Completed coloanal anastomosis.

advantage is the technically cumbersome submucosal dissection, which discourages more frequent use of this approach.

Recurrence Rates Following Perineal Repair

The single most useful parameter in comparing the various surgical approaches is the recurrence rate. After the period of postoperative morbidity and mortality has passed, recurrence rate becomes the simplest means of assessing the success of a given procedure. Recurrence rates were originally thought to reach a plateau after the second or third year following repair.[15] More recently, however, it has become clear that late recurrences do indeed occur, rendering greater credibility and importance to studies with *long-term* follow-up.[16,17]

Perineal procedures have been historically regarded as having higher recurrence rates. This was felt to be an acceptable compromise when used in high-risk patients undergoing procedures associated with lower perioperative morbidity. Recurrence rates for Thiersch's repairs are difficult to derive from the literature due to a paucity of follow-up information; most recurrences follow removal of the implant for complications such as infection, erosion, breakage, or fecal impaction. These complications occur in 25% to 50% of patients treated by Thiersch-type repairs.[13,18] Perineal rectosigmoidectomy has shown a wide range of recurrence rates over the years, ranging from no recurrence to 58%.[10,19] Improvements in technique as suggested originally by Altemeier and colleagues[10] and more recently by Prasad[20] (levator plication, posterior rectopexy) have decreased the recurrence rates to less than 5%. The Delorme operation is associated with recurrence rates in the 6% to 17% range.[14,21]

TRANSABDOMINAL REPAIRS

Transabdominal approaches are the most frequently used, chiefly because of their lower recurrence rates and the opportunity they provide for addressing associated intraabdominal pathology. Most transabdominal procedures involve either sacral suspension-fixation (to the anterior or posterior rectal wall) or resection of the sigmoid (anterior resection with or without suture rectopexy). In either case, the rectal vault is preserved, thus enhancing postoperative function, in contrast to perineal rectosigmoidectomy, which causes the sigmoid colon to assume reservoir function. In the latter case, compliance and storage may be diminished.

Suspension and Fixation

Anterior Rectopexy (Ripstein's Repair). Anterior rectopexy with mesh was originally described by Ripstein and Lanter in 1963.[22] This classic suspension-fixation technique sought to correct the lack of both sacral fixation and normal curvature of the rectum found in patients with prolapse. In the Ripstein repair, the attenuated posterior mesorectal attachment to the presacral fascia is divided down to the levator ani musculature. The proximal lateral stalks are similarly divided to facilitate placement of a nonabsorbable mesh transversely across the anterior midrectal wall. Teflon, Marlex, and more recently, Gore-Tex have been used as the mesh (sling) material, which is wrapped circumferentially. The mesh is then sutured to the presacral fascia after the rectum is firmly pulled in a cephalad and posterior position along the sacral curvature (Fig. 36–5). Additional sutures may be placed between the mesh and the rectum to prevent slippage in the early postoperative period, but care must be taken to leave sufficient room between the mesh and the bowel wall (one or two fingerbreadths) or between the mesh and the sacrum to prevent narrowing or angulation.

Complications following the Ripstein repair include fecal impaction, pelvic abscess, hemorrhage, mesh erosion, or mechanical small-bowel obstruction. A survey conducted by Gordon and Hoexter[23] reported a 17% complication rate and a 4% reoperation rate for these problems. Notably, fecal impaction, rectal stricture, or both occurred in 8% of patients. As mentioned in the preceding paragraph, considerable care should be exercised to prevent wrapping the mesh too tightly across the surface of the rectum. This complication has led many surgeons, including Ripstein himself, to abandon anterior rectopexy in favor of posterior rectopexy.

Posterior Rectopexy. Posterior rectopexy is similar to the Ripstein repair in that it involves the same suspension-fixation principles to restore the rectosacral attachments. It differs in that the mesh surrounds the rectum posteriorly, leaving an anterior gap (Fig. 36–6). This approach was originally described by Wells in 1959,[24] who used an Ivalon sponge (polyvinyl alcohol sponge) to encircle the rectum. This sponge is subsequently slowly absorbed. The anterior gap seems to prevent compression and stricture of the rectum and minimizes the potential for fecal impaction; furthermore, the extraperitoneal location of the mesh may decrease the incidence of postoperative bowel obstruction. The remainder of the technique is very similar to the Ripstein anterior rectopexy. Because Ivalon sponge has never been approved for prolapse surgery in the United States, Teflon, Marlex, and Gore-Tex have been used instead, with satisfactory results. Another alternative is to use an absorbable polyglycolic mesh (Vicryl), as originally described by Arndt and Pircher.[25]

Complications following posterior rectopexy are similar to those that may occur after the Ripstein repair, including presacral hemorrhage, pelvic abscess, and small-bowel obstruction. As already mentioned, a major advantage of posterior rectopexy is the avoidance of stricture and fecal impaction. One additional advantage of a posterior wrap is that most of the mesh lies in contact with thick mesorectal tissues posteriorly and laterally, allowing little contact with the bare anterior rectal wall. Theoretically, this should result in a lower incidence of erosion of prosthetic mesh into the rectum.

Resection

The alternative to suspension-fixation procedures in the treatment of rectal prolapse has been resection of varying lengths of the sigmoid colon or rectum. This practice is based on the theory that prolapse cannot occur if the intussusceptum is suspended and the mobile colon at risk for prolapse is resected. The first report of anterior resection for

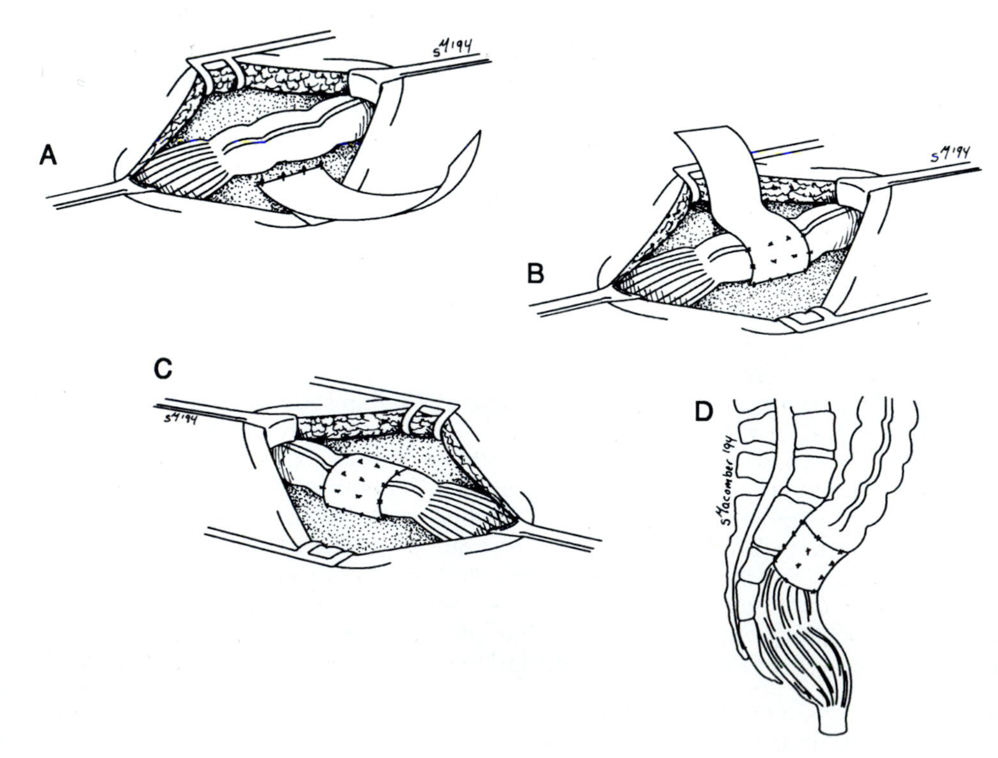

FIGURE 36–5. Anterior rectopexy (Ripstein's procedure). (*A*) Rectum mobilized, pulled cephalad. Mesh being sutured to one side of presacral fascia. (*B*) Anterior wrap across the rectum. (*C*) and (*D*) Completed wrap and suture to sacral fascia.

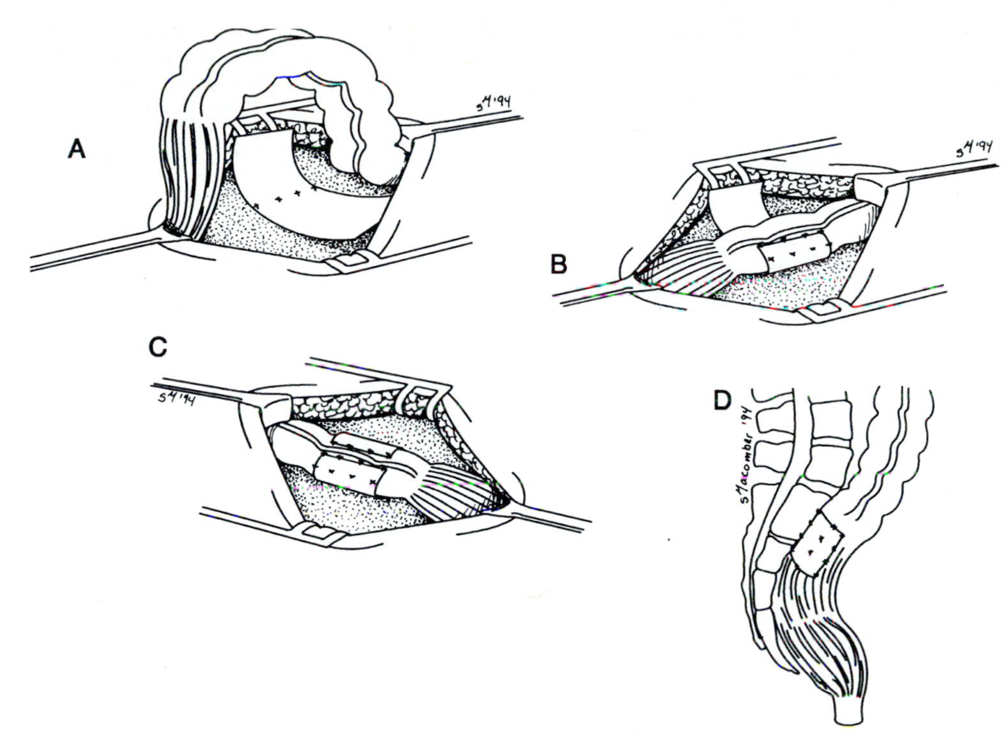

FIGURE 36–6. Posterior rectopexy. (*A*) Rectum mobilized, lifted upward. (*B*) Posterior wrap around the rectum. (*C*) Anterior gap seen. (*D*) Wrap completed.

prolapse was made by Muir[26] in 1962. Subsequently, Frykman and Goldberg[27] advanced the principle of combining sigmoid resection with suture rectopexy in the treatment of prolapse.

The procedure requires mobilization of the sigmoid colon in preparation for resection. The lateral peritoneal reflections of the rectosigmoid and upper rectum are divided bilaterally, but the middle and distal portions of the lateral stalks are preserved. The mesorectum is separated from the sacrum distally to the pelvic floor. The rectum is then retracted superiorly and posteriorly and a sutured rectopexy is performed bilaterally to the upper sacral segments. The sigmoid colon is then resected and an anastomosis without tension is performed between the descending colon and the upper rectum, just proximal to the rectopexy.[27]

Complications following anterior or sigmoid resection for prolapse are no different than when performed for other indications. Major complication rates range from 12% to 39%[17] and include large- or small-bowel obstruction, pelvic sepsis, hemorrhage, wound dehiscence, and anastomotic leak. Anastomotic leak is less likely if the anastomosis is performed between two peritonealized portions of bowel (i.e., using the upper rectum rather than the lower rectum for the distal anastomotic segment).

Resectional procedures have potential advantages over the suspension-fixation procedures in two areas. First, they may decrease the troublesome constipation that frequently persists or even worsens after other types of prolapse repair.[28] The extent of resection can vary according to the anatomy and the severity of the preoperative functional abnormality. Secondly, anterior resection is an operation *commonly* performed by surgeons for other pathologic conditions. This familiarity allows surgeons not trained in suspension-fixation techniques to carry out an effective prolapse repair with expectations for acceptable morbidity and low recurrence.

Recurrence Rates Following Abdominal Repair

The abdominal approaches to rectal prolapse are felt by many to be associated with the lowest recurrence rates. Several series reporting on the Ripstein repair give recurrence rates of nothing to 10%, with the largest single report showing a 2.3% rate.[23] Posterior rectopexy series likewise show a range of recurrences from no recurrence to 20%, with a collective average of 4.5%.[3,6,8,16] Anterior resection with or without rectopexy is associated with a 2% to 9% recurrence rate in the few large series reported.[17,29]

FUNCTIONAL ABNORMALITIES PERSISTING AFTER PROLAPSE REPAIR

Approximately 50% of patients with rectal prolapse have chronic constipation that may persist in many patients following surgical repair and may, in fact, worsen after the Ripstein repair.[30] Postoperative straining has been implicated in the development of recurrent prolapse.[16] Regardless of the operative approach used, successful postoperative management should include instruction about bowel routine and avoidance of both constipation and straining. Rarely, severe or worsening constipation following prolapse repair may require subtotal colectomy for relief.[28] The role of preoperative screening for colonic transit abnormalities in patients with rectal prolapse is currently being investigated.[28]

Fecal incontinence is present in approximately 50% of patients presenting with rectal prolapse.[3,21] Electrophysiologic studies have shown deficiencies in internal anal sphincter[31] and external anal sphincter[32] function. In such patients, continence improves following abdominal repairs in 60%;[12] improvement in continence is less frequently seen following perineal prolapse repairs. Patients with persistent fecal incontinence should be managed with measures initially used in any incontinent patient (i.e., perineal strengthening exercises, dietary modification, thick suspensions of bulk-forming laxatives, and bowel "retraining" techniques). Despite these measures, noticeable improvement in continence may take up to 12 months. If *disabling* incontinence persists more than 6 to 12 months postoperatively, consideration may be given to anal cerclage, sphincteroplasty, postanal repair or, in extreme instances, diverting colostomy.

SUMMARY AND RECOMMENDATIONS

This chapter attempts to present a variety of operative procedures commonly employed in the treatment of rectal prolapse. Each has its own advantages and disadvantages. Esoteric procedures of limited availability or practicality have been omitted.

Clearly, the major factor dictating the operative approach to rectal prolapse is the patient's overall medical condition. If the clinician seeks low recurrence rates for an otherwise healthy individual, an abdominal approach is favored. Posterior rectopexy with mesh is an excellent option. Sigmoid colon resection with or without suture rectopexy is also appropriate, especially if there is associated sigmoid pathology or constipation.

For poor-risk individuals with prolapse, a perineal approach is preferable. Rectosigmoidectomy with levator ani plication is appropriate for most of these patients. Thiersch-type procedures should be reserved for nonambulatory patients and those with limited life expectancy. Finally, both laparoscopic resection and laparoscopic rectopexy have been described for the treatment of prolapse and may someday be applicable to poor-risk patients who are not candidates for laparotomy and transabdominal repair.[33,34]

REFERENCES

1. Moschcowitz, AV: The pathogenesis, anatomy, and cure of prolapse of the rectum. Surg Gynecol Obstet 15:7, 1912.
2. Broden, B and Snellman, B: Procidentia of the rectum studied with cineradiography: A contribution to the discussion of causative mechanism. Dis Colon Rectum 11:330, 1968.
3. Theuerkauf, FJ, Jr, Beahrs, OH and Hill, JR: Rectal prolapse: Causation and surgical treatment. Ann Surg 171:819, 1970.
4. Gordan, PH: Rectal procidentia. In Gordon, PH, and Nivatvongs, S (eds.): Principles and Practice of Surgery for the Colon, Rectum, and Anus. Quality Medical Publishing, St. Louis, 1992, p 450.
5. Ibid, p 452.
6. Küpfer, CA and Goligher, JC: One hundred consecutive cases of complete prolapse of the rectum treated by operation. Br J Surg 57:481, 1970.
7. Mann CV: Rectal prolapse. In Morson, BC and Heinemann, W (eds.): Diseases of the Colon, Rectum, Anus. Medical Books, London, 1969, p 238.
8. Boutsis, C and Ellis, H: The Ivalon-sponge-wrap operation for rectal prolapse: An experience with 26 patients. Dis Colon Rectum 17:21, 1974.
9. Corman, ML, Veidenheimer, MC and Coller, JA: Managing rectal prolapse. Geriatrics 29:87, 1974.
10. Altemeier, WA, Culbertson, WR, Schowengerdt, C, et al: Nineteen years' experience with the one-stage perineal repair of rectal prolapse. Ann Surg 173:993, 1971.
11. Metcalf, AM and Loening-Baucke, V: Anorectal function and defecation dynamics in patients with rectal prolapse. Am J Surg 55:206, 1988.
12. Williams, JG, Wong, WD, Jensen, L, et al: Incontinence and rectal prolapse: A prospective manometric study. Dis Colon Rectum 34:209, 1991.
13. Vongsangnak, V, Varma, JS and Smith, AN: Reappraisal of Thiersch's operation for complete rectal prolapse. J R Coll Surg Edinb. 30:185, 1985.
14. Uhlig, BE and Sullivan, ES: The modified Delorme operation: Its place in surgical treatment for massive rectal prolapse. Dis Colon Rectum 22:513, 1979.
15. Mann, CV and Hoffman, C: Complete rectal prolapse: The anatomical and functional results of treatment by an extended abdominal rectopexy. Br J Surg 75:34, 1988.
16. Boulos, PB, Stryker, SJ and Nicholls, RJ: The long-term results of polyvinyl alcohol (Ivalon) sponge for rectal prolapse in young patients. Br J Surg 71:213, 1984.
17. Schlinkert, RT, Beart, RW, Jr, Wolff, BG, et al: Anterior resection for complete rectal prolapse. Dis Colon Rectum 28:409, 1985.
18. Hurt, TM, Fraser, IA and Maybury, NK: Treatment of rectal prolapse by sphincteric support using silastic rods. Br J Surg 72:491, 1985.
19. Porter, N: Surgery for rectal prolapse. Br Med J 3:113, 1971.
20. Prasad, ML, Pearl, RK, Abcarian, H, et al: Perineal proctectomy, posterior rectopexy, and postanal levator repair for the treatment of rectal prolapse. Dis Colon Rectum 29:547, 1986.
21. Christiansen, J and Kirkegaard, P: Delorme's operation for complete rectal prolapse. Br J Surg 68:537, 1981.
22. Ripstein, CB and Lanter, B: Etiology and surgical therapy of massive prolapse of the rectum. Ann Surg 157:259, 1963.
23. Gordon, PH and Hoexter, B: Complications of the Ripstein procedure. Dis Colon Rectum 21:277, 1978.
24. Wells, C: New operation for rectal prolapse. Proc R Soc Med 52:602, 1959.
25. Arndt, M and Pircher, W: Absorbable mesh in the treatment of rectal prolapse. Int J Colorectal Dis 3:141, 1988.
26. Muir, EG: Treatment of complete rectal prolapse in the adult. Proc R Soc Med 55:1086, 1962.
27. Frykman, HM and Goldberg, SM: The surgical treatment of rectal procidentia. Surg Gynecol Obstet 129:1225, 1969.
28. Madoff, RD, Williams, JG, Wong, WD, et al: Long-term functional results of colon resection and rectopexy for overt rectal prolapse. Am J Gastroenterol 87:101, 1992.
29. Watts, JD, Rothenberger, DA, Buls, JG, et al: The management of procidentia: 30 years experience. Dis Colon Rectum 28:96, 1985.
30. Sayfan, J, Pinho, M, Alexander-Williams, J, et al: Sutured posterior rectopexy with sigmoidectomy compared to Marlex rectopexy for rectal prolapse. Br J Surg 77:143, 1990.
31. Broden, G, Dolk, A and Holmstrom, B: Recovery of the internal anal sphincter following rectopexy: A possible explanation for continence improvement. Int J Colorectal Dis 3:23, 1988.
32. Neill, ME, Parks, AG and Swash, M: Physiologic studies of the anal musculature in faecal incontinence and rectal prolapse. Br J Surg 68:531, 1981.
33. Munro, W, Avramovic, J and Roney, W: Laparoscopic rectopexy. J Laparoendosc Surg 3:55, 1993.
34. Senagore, AJ, Luchtefeld, MA and MacKeigan, JM: Rectopexy. J Laparoendosc Surg 3:339, 1993.

SECTION SEVEN

FUTURE CONSIDERATIONS, RESEARCH

CHAPTER 37

The Frontiers of Female Pelvic Floor Disorders

Linda T. Brubaker • Theodore J. Saclarides

Various authors in this book have emphasized the critical interactions of anatomy and function of the female pelvic floor—it is truly an amazing ecosystem! Disorders of incontinence, pelvic organ prolapse, disordered defecation, and pelvic pain are frequently interrelated. Yet these physiologic interactions are far from completely understood. In fact, given the wide gaps in our knowledge, it is amazing that we are able to achieve our current degree of clinical success. An understanding of the etiology, natural history, and pathophysiology of pelvic floor disorders is essential for rational evaluation and treatment. It is with hope and anticipation that we look forward to exploring the new frontiers for female pelvic floor disorders.

Several opportunities may allow us to maximize our approach in these new frontiers. First, there is a pressing financial component which mandates efficient and effective treatment of pelvic floor disorders. These disorders are costly when left untreated, and with a larger aging population, these health-care costs are no longer viewed as avoidable. These financial concerns, combined with inconsistencies in treatment, have prompted the U.S. government to publish guidelines for the evaluation and treatment of urinary incontinence.

Beyond the direct financial costs lie the disruption to the individual's quality of life, measurement of which is elusive and difficult to quantify, yet which commands a growing interest. Certainly the majority of pelvic floor disorders are not life-threatening but rather threaten the quality of life. At present, we have an incomplete understanding of the effects of simple maladies and common interventions on an individual's quality of life. As scientific understanding of these domains increases, physicians and allied providers should be able to refine treatment strategies.

It is gratifying that a growing number of physicians and ancillary health providers are recognizing pelvic floor disorders as having primary clinical and research interest. Historically in gynecology, the treatment of urinary incontinence and pelvic organ prolapse was a pursuit occurring late in a physician's career. This observation gave rise to the saying, "The obstetrician-gynecologist spends the first half of his career by supporting the perineum (at delivery) and the second half of his career *being supported by* the perineum." More recently, a cadre of younger gynecologists has been able to concentrate on the evaluation and care of patients with pelvic floor disorders, as have physicians in other disciplines, such as urology, general surgery, and colon and rectal surgery. These surgeons have an obligation to observe, record, and communicate information keenly. An important frontier will be conquered when pelvic floor surgical reports contain comprehensive information on both anatomic support and physiologic functions of the pelvic viscera. Failure to report suboptimal surgical outcomes must stop; clinical outcomes, for better or worse, must be reported honestly. Those who would judge another's surgical prowess must do so in a scientific forum with comprehensive pelvic floor assessment, rather than in an isolated report of one's own surgical success, narrowly defined.

Finally, it is increasingly recognized that superior outcomes occur when a multidisciplinary approach to pelvic floor disorders is used. Given the complex inter-relationships of these disorders, it is simply not feasible for any single clinician to possess the fund of knowledge or the spectrum of clinical skills to address the full range of pelvic floor disorders optimally. Physicians, in particular, may feel financial constraints that cause them to fan the fires of "turf battles." Although possibly effective in the short term, this philosophy is likely to backfire in the long run, as patients experience incomplete resolution of their symptoms. Appropriate consultation and referral signify that a physician is secure, both personally and professionally. Such physicians will ultimately attract a broad-based patient population who will be trusting and confident in their physician's recommendations.

The challenges of the pelvic floor are many, but the dedication and scientific abilities of physicians and allied providers are phenomenal. Clinical care will improve dramatically as health-care providers embrace a multidisciplinary, scientifically critical approach to evaluation and treatment.

Index

Page numbers followed by an "f" indicate a figure; page numbers followed by a "t" indicate a table

ISBN 0-8036-0075-5
90000>
EAN
9 780803 600751